advances
in ulcer disease

advances in ulcer disease

Proceedings of a Symposium on the Pathogenesis and Therapy of Ulcer Disease

Munich,
March 13-14, 1980

editors:
K.-H. HOLTERMÜLLER
J.-R. MALAGELADA

EXCERPTA MEDICA 1980
AMSTERDAM-OXFORD-PRINCETON

International Congress Series No. 537
ISBN Excerpta Medica 90 219 9504 2
ISBN Elsevier North-Holland 0 444 90187 6

Library of Congress Cataloging in Publication Data

Symposium on the Pathogenesis and Therapy of Ulcer
    Disease, Munich, 1980.
    Advances in ulcer disease.

    (International congress series; no. 537)
    Includes indexes.
    1. Peptic ulcer--Congresses. 2. Peptic ulcer--
Surgery--Congresses. I. Holtermüller, K.-H.
II. Malagelada, J.-R. III. Title. IV. Series.
[DNLM: 1. Duodenal ulcer--Congresses. 2. Stomach
ulcer--Congresses. W3 EX89 no. 537 1980 / WI 360
S9895a 1980]
RC821.S92 1980   616.3'43   80-25800

Publisher:
Excerpta Medica
305 Keizersgracht
1000 BC Amsterdam
P.O. Box 1126

Sole Distributors for the USA and Canada:
Elsevier North-Holland Inc.
52 Vanderbilt Avenue
New York, NY 10017

Printed in The Netherlands by Casparie, Amsterdam

Preface

Writing a book about ulcer disease in 1980 is a challenging task, for ulcer disease is in the midst of an explosion of new knowledge. Significant advances have occurred in both basic and clinical aspects of the disease. Concepts are being constantly revised, as new data become available. A traditional textbook approach would have almost surely produced a volume already outdated by the time it reached its potential readers. Instead, we invited key scientists around the world whose active programs and leadership in specific areas of research allowed them to give a detailed analysis of the currently available knowledge about ulcer disease. All participants assembled for 2 days of scientific presentations and open debate in Munich. We are deeply grateful to these colleagues for their generous help which produced thoughtful papers in particularly controversial and exciting areas. In many instances, the work contains not only an update on the topic, but also important hints about future research directions.

To spare our readers tedious transcriptions, we have summarized these discussions with the help of Drs. S. Bonfils, W. Dölle, W.P. Fritsch, W. Lorenz, G. Strohmeyer, and K.G. Wormsley. The latter also summarized and gave his personal viewpoints on the issues discussed during the round table on 'Future research directions in the medical therapy of ulcer disease'.

We also felt compelled to ask some friends to assist us in the task of reviewing, criticizing, and complementing selected areas that reached beyond our editorial expertise. Drs. A.J. Cameron, T.P. Dousa, R.A. Levine, M.I. Samloff, W. Schreiber and V. Schumpelick, performed this important task. Some of them also contributed with critical overviews, printed at the end of each section. Dr. Grossman honored us by contributing his overview of the topic, that closed the meeting and the book. Mr. Aart Brouwer of Smith Kline Dauelsberg, Germany, provided encouragement and generous support to make all of this possible.

The result of all this effort is the volume we now present to our readers for them to judge. We hope they will not be disappointed. This volume should provide a solid base of information both of practical value and as a point of departure for further discoveries. If we manage to capture the interest and approval of our readers we, and the rest of the contributors, will feel that our work has been worthwhile.

Professor Dr. Karl-Hans Holtermüller
I. Medizinische Klinik und Poliklinik
Langenbeckstraße 1
6500 Mainz
Federal Republic of Germany

Dr. Juan-Ramon Malagelada
Mayo Clinic and Mayo Foundation
Gastroenterology Research Unit
Rochester, MN 55901
U.S.A.

Contents

Introductory remarks*

L. Demling
Medizinische Klinik mit Poliklinik, Universität Erlangen-Nürnberg, Federal Republic of Germany

Today, it is thought that peptic ulceration arises from an imbalance between aggressive and protective factors. In general terms this idea is certainly correct, for the healing of an ulcer can be accelerated both by reducing aggressive factors through the administration of antacids or H_2-blockers and by strengthening the protective action of the gastric mucus (for example, by administration of carbenoxolone).

The endoscopist never observes the development of a peptic ulcer, but merely its gradual healing. In this respect, the peptic lesion has something of the characteristics of a myocardial infarction. And, indeed, it is possible that a local disturbance in blood flow is involved in the genesis of an ulcer.
Thus, the aggressive gastric juice develops its corrosive effect rapidly and locally, leading to impaired blood flow. When gastritis causes a reduction in the resistance of the mucosal membrane, the back-diffusion of the hydrochloric acid in the gastric juice is seen as the pathogenic meeting point of peptic activity, inflammation and vascular process. It is feasible that the blood vessels of the gastric mucosa are damaged by the back-diffusing H-ions, so that spasms or thrombotic processes disturb the flow of blood within them; this process can be accelerated by the decrease of blood flow which accompanies an increase of H-ion output under certain circumstances (for example, stress). Our own investigations using autoradiography (HTO) and mass spectroscopy (D^{18} water) provided proof that hydrogen ions, but not whole water molecules, back-diffuse into an experimentally-damaged gastric mucosa, but not into the intact mucous membrane.

A quite different theoretical model is the idea that, in gastric ulceration, a certain amount of acid and pepsin does not leave the glandular channel to

---

* Excerpt from the Welcome Address given by Professor Dr. L. Demling at the opening of the symposium.

enter into the gastric lumen at all, but rather, as in the case of trypsin in the development of pancreatitis, moves off in the wrong direction by diffusing into the interstitial tissue. The experimental intramucosal injection of gastric juice has demonstrated what damage acid and pepsin can do there: the result is chronic ulceration.

It is possible that gastritis gives rise to changes in the tissue surrounding the glandular channels, thus causing them to leak. The development of ulcers at the line dividing gastritis from normal mucosa could be explained by the fact that, at this point, relatively abundant amounts of acid are produced near damaged tissue. Perhaps, however, gastritis merely promotes such leakage and has only a localizing effect, while other processes are responsible for breaking open the glandular channel.

This idea does not apply to duodenal ulcer, since no hydrochloric acid is produced in the duodenal mucosa. However, theoretical models differing from those so far considered might also be examined, such as the idea that ulceration in the duodenum is not produced by the acid 'breaking into' the mucosa, but that its absorption or transfer might lead to a pathogenic effect. If we assume that the absorption of acid in the duodenum is a physiological process, then it is possible that, as a result of changes in the interstitial tissue, this acid might also follow the wrong path. It is conceivable that an additional mechanism in the duodenum promotes the uncontrolled penetration of the normally harmless acid. Might not the amino precursor uptake and decarboxylation cells responsible for dealing with the biogenic amines provide the initial triggering mechanism, in the form of tissue damage which permits entry to the acid? Brunner's glands are found mainly between the pylorus and the papilla of Vater, and extend into the submucosa. Could it be possible that, under certain circumstances, they might provide the corrosive gastric juice with an access pathway?

Ladies and gentlemen, I should not wish to conclude this welcoming address without paying tribute to the man who is our guest of honor today and at whose suggestion this symposium came into being.

Our colleague, Professor Hans-Peter Wolff, exemplifies the fact that the field of internal medicine cannot be torn apart and robbed of its intrinsic coherence. An active investigator in the fields of nephrology and hypertension, he established the connection to gastroenterology with his work on the pathogenesis of ascites and the metabolism of aldosterone in liver diseases. Special thanks and recognition are due to him for the fact that, while delving deeply into particulars, he has retained a view of the whole and has also promoted international cooperation.

It is our hope that, during this symposium, an atmosphere may be created which will be conducive to the sowing of seeds of new and fertile ideas. The creative hypothesis is the requisite for the art of recognizing interrelationships in this world. When we are able to hypothesize, we free ourselves from slavery to unknown forces, and become their master.

Chapter I: Heterogeneity of ulcer disease*

* The review paper for this chapter appears on pages 545–550.

Genetic aspects of ulcer disease*

J.I. Rotter and M.I. Grossman
Division of Medical Genetics, Departments of Medicine and Pediatrics, Harbor-UCLA Medical Center, Torrance; and Center for Ulcer Research and Education, Wadsworth V.A. Hospital, UCLA School of Medicine, Los Angeles, California, U.S.A.

Introduction

The familial aggregation of peptic ulcer disease and its association with such clear-cut genetic factors as blood group O and nonsecretor status is well established. However, the genetics of this disorder or group of disorders has, until recently, been poorly delineated. Polygenic inheritance was the prevailing hypothesis proposed for peptic ulcer, based primarily on the finding of blood group associations and the exclusion of a simple mode of inheritance for all ulcer disease. We have proposed genetic heterogeneity as an alternative hypothesis, which could explain both the familial aggregation of peptic ulcer disease and the lack of a simple Mendelian pattern of inheritance [1]. This concept states that peptic ulcer is not one disease, but a group of disorders with different genetic and environmental causes. Initially based on indirect evidence, genetic heterogeneity has now received direct support from genetic studies using subclinical markers such as serum pepsinogen I [2, 3]. The unravelling of the genetic heterogeneity of peptic ulcer has important clinical and etiologic implications, for if what is termed a 'disease' is in reality a number of disorders that are grouped together because of some common clinical feature, these distinct disorders may differ markedly in genetics, pathophysiology, interaction with environmental agents, natural history and response to therapy.

J.I. Rotter holds a Clinical Investigator Award (AM 00523) and a March of Dimes Basil O'Connor Starter Grant (5-245). M.I. Grossman is a Veterans Administration Senior Medical Investigator. *This work was supported in part by grant AM 17328 to CURE (Center for Ulcer Research and Education).

Peptic ulcer is among the most common of chronic diseases. This results in a number of problems for genetic studies. Is a relative of a patient with peptic ulcer affected because he has the same genotype, shares the same environment, or simply has, by chance, a common disorder? The age of onset of peptic ulcer varies markedly. Therefore, it is impossible to say whether an individual who is clinically unaffected at any given time will become affected later in life. Like many common diseases, genetic studies of peptic ulcer have suffered from confusion engendered by the use of varying definitions of 'affected' by different investigators. Thus, 'affected' may in one case refer to any individual who has abdominal pain, yet in another case it may only apply to one with an endoscopically-demonstrated crater. However, the greatest obstacles to genetic studies have been our ignorance concerning the basic defect(s) in this disorder or group of disorders, and the unavailability of genetic markers to detect individuals with the mutant genotype prior to its clinical manifestation.

Despite these difficulties, we have known for many years that genetic factors play a role in the etiology of peptic ulcer, based on 3 lines of evidence: family studies, twin studies, and blood-group studies.

Genetic factors

The first approach in looking for genetic factors in a common disease is to determine whether familial aggregation is present, comparing the incidence of the disease in relatives of patients with its incidence in the general population. If increased, this is often the first indication that genetic factors are important in a disease. Family aggregation was noted in the late 1800's but, as with many diseases, the majority of initial reports presented one or few pedigrees with no control data. Subsequently, individuals with peptic ulcer were shown to have an 'increased family history' of the disease [4–6]. Most reports indicated a positive family history in 20–50% of individuals with peptic ulcer, compared to 5–15% in controls. While this information has been used to support the importance of genetic factors, it is of little value in testing genetic hypotheses since the prevalence of a positive family history will vary greatly with the type of interview, family size, number of relatives included, and with the criteria used for defining an affected individual. A more accurate assessment of familial aggregation is obtained by comparing the prevalence of the disorder among specific relatives of an affected individual to that found among similar relatives of a control group. This has been done in several excellent studies [5, 7–12], and the consistent observation was that the frequency of peptic ulcer was 2–3 times greater in first-degree relatives of peptic ulcer patients than in first-degree relatives of controls or the general population (Table I). Because these differences persisted across generations and social classes, genetic factors were presumed to explain these findings.

Familial aggregation can conceivably be due to common environmental as well as common genetic factors. Twin studies represent an approach to resolving the questions of the relative influence of genetics and environment. The frequency of concordance (both members of the twin pair affected) of monozygotic (identical) twins is compared with that of dizygotic (fraternal) twins. Monozygotic twins share all genes, and should be concordant for disorders with pure genetic etiology. Dizygotic twins share only half their genes and are no more alike genetically than any pair of siblings. If the characteristic being studied is genetically determined, with no environmental influence, then one would expect 100% concordance in monozygotic twins, and less in dizygotic twins. If the disorder is entirely environmental, one should see equal concordance between monozygotic and dizygotic twins. If an interaction between a genetic predisposition and an environmental agent is necessary for clinical expression, one would expect to find a higher concordance among monozygotic than dizygotic twins, but not 100%. In fact, the concordance for peptic ulcer in monozygotic twins was found to be less than 100% but consistently higher than that in dizygotic twins in a number of published studies (Table II). This difference persisted when dizygotic twins were restricted to pairs of like sex. We can conclude from these twin studies that a large part of the observed familial aggregation is due to genetic factors.

The third early line of evidence for genetic factors in ulcer came from studies of blood-group association. The goal of such disease association studies is to determine the prevalence of a disorder among individuals with well-defined genetic traits, such as blood groups or serum enzyme polymorphisms (also known as qualitative gene markers). If there is a positive association between a given disease and a particular allele of a well-defined genetic locus, then the genetically determined trait is usually considered to be of importance in the pathogenesis of the disorder under study [20, 21]. Soon after the original association between blood group A and gastric cancer was described, the same group of investigators demonstrated that peptic ulcer was associated with blood group O [22]. Individuals with blood group O have a 30–40% greater incidence of peptic ulcer than those with other blood groups [4, 23, 24]. One might question whether this relatively small increased risk is real. Yet this observation has been repeated by many investigators in many countries, and in different racial and ethnic groups throughout the world. The physiologic basis for the blood group O association remains unknown. Attempts have been made to relate it to the acid secretory capacity of the

Table I: Peptic ulcer in families.

Study	Proband's diagnosis	Relatives studied	Criteria	Frequency in relatives of ulcer proband (%)	Frequency in relatives of controls or in population controls (%)
Doll and Buch [8]	Peptic ulcer	Brothers	Hospital	11.5	4.6
		Sisters	Records (60%);	2.8	0.9
		Fathers	patient's	16.4	4.5
		Mothers	account (40%)	4.3	—
Wretmark [9]	Peptic ulcer	Brothers	History	15.0	6.6-8.1
		Fathers	from	14.8	3.6
		Mothers	propositus	7.4	1.2
Kuennsberg [10]	Duodenal ulcer	Sons	History	7.9	2.4
		Daughters	from propositus	5.1	0.7
Monson [11]	Peptic ulcer	Fathers	History	24.5	14.4
		Mothers	from	9.5	4.5
		Brothers	propositus	14.3	6.5
		Sisters		3.7	1.6
Jirasek [5]	Duodenal ulcer	Parents	History	14.7	
		Sibs	from	9.9	
	Duodenal-gastric ulcer	Parents	propositus	10.0	
		Sibs		8.0	1.5-4.8
	Pyloric ulcer	Parents		8.0	
		Sibs		7.1	
	Gastric ulcer	Parents		12.1	
		Sibs		6.8	
Kubickova and Vesely [12]	Duodenal ulcer	First degree	History	9.5	1.7
		Second degree	from	2.9	0.5
		Third degree	propositus	1.4	0.22

Table II: Peptic ulcer in twins.

Study	Criteria	Number of pairs	Concordance (%)	
			MZ	DZ
Camerer [13]	Often clinical	14	14	14
Huhn [14]	Questionnaire, then X-ray	13	80	0
Doig [15]	X-ray	10	50	12.5
Harvald and Hauge [16]	Hospitalized	112	18	7.2
Marshall et al. [17]	X-ray	58[1]	14.3	6.3
Eberhard [18]	X-ray	112	11.3	5.8
Pollin et al. [19]	Medical records	837[2]	11.3	5.8
Gotlieb–Jensen [6][3]	X-ray of all twins	181	52.6	35.7

[1]Very young population.
[2]Duodenal ulcer only. Based on follow-up of U.S. WW II veterans, whose care is still under the Veterans Administration.
[3]An excellent detailed study using the Danish twin registry. Should be compared with Harvald and Hauge [16], same twin source, to show what detailed investigation and an extra 10 years of follow-up reveals.

stomach as defined by serum pepsinogen or maximal acid output, but no consistent relationship has been delineated [4, 24–26].

The next polymorphic genetic marker found to be associated with peptic ulcer was nonsecretor status [27]. Nonsecretors are 40–50% more likely to have a duodenal ulcer than secretors [4, 23, 24].

The effect of the 2 genes, O and nonsecretor, on the risk for ulcer seem to be multiplicative [20, 24, 28]. The relative risk for duodenal ulcer in a blood group O individual is 1.3 (30% increase over a non-O individual), and the relative risk for duodenal ulcer in a nonsecretor is 1.5 (increased 50% over a secretor). Individuals who are both O and nonsecretor have a relative risk for duodenal ulcer of approximately 2.5 (hence the term multiplicative).

Many other gene marker associations have been reported with peptic ulcer [29]. As can be seen in Table III, some 8 different genetic systems have been implicated at one time or another as predisposing to peptic ulcer, making peptic ulcer the most 'associated' disorder in man. Some of these associations, notably blood group O and blood group nonsecretor, are so well established that they are undeniably real. Others, such as Rh positivity, are of such small effect (relative risk 1.1 for duodenal ulcer) that they must remain of questionable importance. The other associations listed in Table III have been examined only in a few or even single studies, and so must be considered tentative.

*Table III: Gene marker associations with peptic ulcer.**

Polymorphic allele with increased risk for ulcer	Genetic marker system	Number of reports	Relative risk	Comments
O	ABO	>200	1.3	Well-established
Nonsecretor	ABH secretor	~40	1.5	Well-established
Rh +	Rh	~30	1.1	Very small relative risk
Taster	PTC tasting	2	1.4-2.7	
Decreased alpha-1 antitrypsin activity	Alpha-1-antitrypsin	5	1.4-3.0	? a partial explanation of ulcer pulmonary disease association
Pg^A	Urinary pepsinogen phenotyping	1	2.4	? related to quantitative pepsinogen I
B5	HLA	2 (1 negative)	2.9	? an immunologic form of ulcer
G6PD deficiency	glucose-6-phosphate dehydrogenase	1	2.2	—

* Most associations are with duodenal ulcer. Nonsecretor and alpha-1-antitrypsin are associated with duodenal and gastric ulcer.

What can we conclude regarding the genetics of ulcer from this wealth of association data? There are 2 major possibilities. One is that each of these genes has a small effect in predisposing to peptic ulcer, a true polygenic system. The other is that each predisposes to a specific subgroup of peptic ulcer. If the latter hypothesis is true then, as subgroups are delineated, one would expect stronger associations in certain subgroups and no associations in others. In contrast, if these predispositions are truly polygenic in nature, then these associations should occur across ulcer groups.

Our understanding of the nature of these various associations to peptic ulcer would be greatly enhanced if we were able to delineate the physiologic basis of each of them. In the case of blood group O and nonsecretor status, the pathophysiologic relationships to ulcer remain unknown after more than 20 years of study. This is probably because the degree of the association is so small. It has been calculated that both O and nonsecretor combined contribute only 2.5–3% of the genetic variance to ulcer [30, 31]. In cases of alpha-1-antitrypsin deficiency, HLA antigens and urinary pepsinogen phenotype, there are clinical or theoretical clues for the association. Thus, even though the latter associations are still statistically tentative, the possibility of a pathophysiologic relationship makes them of interest.

Genetic interpretations

It has thus been clear for a number of years that genetic factors predispose to peptic ulcer, but the mode of inheritance of this genetic predisposition has not been resolved. For over a decade, the hypothesis of polygenic inheritance was used to explain the genetics of peptic ulcer [4, 30, 32]. Polygenic or multifactorial inheritance refers to the concept that the hereditary component of a given disorder is due to the contribution of many genes acting together (polygenic), resulting in a continuum of genetic predisposition toward the disorder [33]. Thus clinical disease would exist when the presence of a sufficient number of genes, perhaps in combination with environmental factors (i.e., multifactorial) exceeds a threshold level. The relatives of index patients share genes in common with the patients in direct proportion to the closeness of their relationship. The multifactorial model thus predicts that such relatives will share some of the disease-predisposing genes and hence will be shifted toward the threshold for disease and have a higher disease frequency than the general population.

However, polygenic inheritance has often been used as an excuse or last resort in explaining disease genetics. Thus, many disorders that did not show monogenic patterns of inheritance were labeled 'multifactorial' without demonstration that they satisfied the criteria for use of that model.

Peptic ulcer was placed in the polygenic category for 2 principal reasons. First, the inheritance of all ulcer disease could not be explained by any simple, single genetic defect − that is, the genetics of ulcer was not compatible with simple autosomal-dominant, autosomal-recessive or X-linked modes of inheritance. Secondly, the demonstrations of the 2 gene marker associations mentioned earlier, blood group O and blood group nonsecretor status, provided some direct support for the polygenic hypothesis since more than one gene seemed to contribute a small but measurable tendency toward peptic ulcer and the presence of both genes had a multiplicative effect. However, while there may be a polygenic contribution peptic ulcer, the alternative mechanism of genetic heterogeneity is probably much more important.

Genetic heterogeneity has been proposed as an alternative hypothesis which can explain both the familial aggregation of peptic ulcer disease and the lack of a simple Mendelian pattern of inheritance [1, 34]. Furthermore, genetic heterogeneity would better account for the varying physiologic disturbances and diverse clinical manifestations that have been described in peptic ulcer patients. The concept of genetic heterogeneity states that a particular clinical disorder is, in reality, a group of distinct diseases with different etiologies, both genetic and nongenetic, which by a variety of pathogenetic mechanisms result in a similar clinical picture. In the absence of subclinical markers to help separate the different diseases, a number of distinct disorders may be lumped together in a common genetic analysis, masking the existence of subsets of a variety of simply inherited disorders in such a way that the familial aggregation observed would appear to conform with the polygenic model. Indeed, in almost every clinical disease studied with this concept in mind, genetic heterogeneity has been found. This includes rare disorders such as the mucopolysaccharidoses [35] and the chondrodystrophies [36], and common disorders such as hyperlipidemia [37] and diabetes mellitus [38–40]. Thus it would not be surprising to find that peptic ulcer disease also consists of a heterogeneous group of disorders, due to a variety of genetic and environmental causes [1, 39, 41].

Heterogeneity of a common disease can be demonstrated by several methods, including: the existence of rare genetic syndromes with peptic ulcer, ethnic variability, clinical suggestions of heterogeneity, physiologic evidence for heterogeneity, heterogeneity of association with genetic polymorphisms, and genetic studies utilizing subclinical markers. Advances in all these areas have contributed to our knowledge of ulcer heterogeneity. Because of limitations of space we shall discuss each only briefly, except the last, on which we shall focus in some detail.

The existence of rare, distinct genetic syndromes associated with peptic ulcer is an immediate demonstration of genetic heterogeneity. The best known is multiple endocrine adenoma syndrome, type I (MEA-I, Werner syndrome), characterized by pituitary, parathyroid, and pancreatic adenomas [42–44]. The pancreatic adenomas may secrete gastrin, resulting in a severe ulcer diathesis (Zollinger-Ellison syndrome). Until the association of ulcer disease with the other endocrine tumors was recognized, the dominant pattern of inheritance elucidated and the biochemical marker of increased plasma gastrin levels characterized, this specific entity was lost among the mass of peptic ulcer patients. Gastrinoma of the pancreas and associated ulcer disease may also occur as a sporadic mutation without familial aggregation and without endocrine tumors in other organs [44]. Systemic mastocytosis is another multisystem syndrome complicated by peptic ulcer, in this case because of histamine excess [29]; both dominant and recessive pedigrees have been described. Another rare dominant syndrome was recently described which consists of a tetrad of abnormalities: essential tremor, congenital nystagmus, a narcolepsy-like sleep disturbance, and severe duodenal ulceration [45]. Other genetic syndromes in which an increased incidence of ulcer has been suggested include alpha-1-antitrypsin deficiency, hyperparathyroidism (this association may be solely through MEA-I), cystic fibrosis, carcinoid syndrome (sometimes associated with gastrinoma), and a recently described 'stiff-skin syndrome' [29]. The recognition of these disorders is important not just for the implications for genetic heterogeneity, but because they illustrate that different pathogenetic mechanisms (e.g., excess gastrin or excess histamine) can result in peptic ulcer.

Patients with these disorders should have specific genetic counseling and therapy. MEA-I is an excellent example of how the alert physician, by making an accurate diagnosis, can then screen asymptomatic family members for the presence of subclinical disease and, by detecting the endocrine tumors early, prevent or ameliorate many of their manifestations. The existence of these rare disorders also suggests that what we recognize as 'common' peptic ulcer may, in fact, comprise several disorders.

The marked ethnic variability in the prevalence and, especially, in the clinical features of peptic ulcer constitutes epidemiologic evidence for heterogeneity [29, 46]. While duodenal ulcer is usually more common than gastric ulcer, in a few cases, such as in Japan, gastric ulcer is more frequent. The absolute incidence also varies widely; e.g., the frequency of duodenal ulcer in Southwest American Indians is one-fourtieth that of United States whites. Male/female ratios varies widely as well, from over 30 to 1 in rural Africa and India to about 2–3 to 1 in the United States. Most significantly, there is extensive ethnic and geographic variation in clinical characteristics such as age of onset and complications. In rural India the complication of pyloric stenosis is the indication for surgery in 80% of cases, whereas in Western countries it is an infrequent indication [47].

The demonstration of clinical, physiologic, or genetic differences within a disorder that can be consistently related to other clinical features, such as ulcer location or age of onset, can also suggest genetic heterogeneity. Much of the evidence indicating that gastric and duodenal ulcer are separate and distinct disorders had been gathered in this fashion, using the ulcer location as the dividing criterion and then comparing other features (age of onset, complications, male/female ratio, acid secretion, etc.). Some of the earliest definitive evidence that gastric and duodenal ulcer were separate disorders was presented in the Doll and Kellock study, which demonstrated that the increased familial risk for ulcer was site specific, i.e., if the index patient had gastric ulcer then gastric and not duodenal ulcer was increased among his relatives, while if the index patient had duodenal ulcer then duodenal and not gastric ulcer was increased in his family [48]. This is also known as independent segregation. Twin studies supported this separation, as the ulcer location was usually concordant when both members of a twin pair were affected [6]. In an analogous fashion, Doll and Kellock's study also suggested that combined ulcer (gastric plus duodenal) may also segregate independently [48], and this was supported by the epidemiologic studies of Bonnevie, which demonstrated that the incidence of duodenal and gastric ulceration in the same patient is some 20 times that expected from the relative frequencies of these 2 disorders in the population [49].

Heterogeneity within duodenal ulcer has also been suggested by using age of onset as a dividing criterion. Childhood duodenal ulcer may well be genetically distinct from adult duodenal ulcer, analogous to the separation of juvenile- from maturity-onset diabetes [29]. Investigators have been impressed by the frequency of a 'positive family history' [32], and one study has reported that the first- and second-degree relatives of childhood duodenal ulcer patients are affected with a frequency twice that of relatives of adult probands [50]. In Hong Kong, Lam and Ong grouped their duodenal ulcer patients by age of onset and found that their early-onset group (onset below age 20 years) had a significantly stronger family history, had a frequency of blood group O similar to that of controls, more frequently presented with gastrointestinal bleeding as the first manifestation of the disease and rarely had complications such as perforation, obstruction, intractable pain or secondary gastric ulcer; in contrast, their late-onset group (onset after age 30 years) had an infrequent family history of ulcer disease, had an increased incidence of blood group O, presented less frequently with gastrointestinal bleeding and had an increased frequency of complications such as perforation, pyloroduodenal stenosis, severe pain, virulent ulcer and secondary gastric ulcer [51].

Another means of looking for heterogeneity clinically is to examine the association of ulcer with other diseases within families. Based on preliminary observations in certain families, we have proposed that the association of ulcer with certain chronic diseases may occur because of the inheritance of a common defect that predisposes to both diseases [41]. This may account for observations of the familial aggregation of ulcer disease and renal stones (without hyperparathyroidism), ulcer and coronary artery disease, and ulcer and chronic obstructive pulmonary diseases. In the latter case, it has often been assumed that the ulcer is secondary to the pulmonary disease, yet the association is both with chronic pulmonary disease and lung cancer [52], which have been shown to have a common familial component [53]. Although cigarette smoking is associated with both lung disease and ulcer, it does not fully account for the assocation of lung disease and ulcer. In addition, we have recently observed that in many, if not most, cases the ulcer disease precedes the pulmonary disease [54].

There is extensive evidence for physiologic heterogeneity in peptic ulcer. For example, mean levels of acid secretion and of serum pepsinogen I are decreased in gastric ulcer patients, whereas in duodenal ulcer patients these are increased [55, 56]. It has been suggested that combined ulcer patients have a different pathophysiology, exhibiting a positive correlation of gastric acid output and gastrin response [57]. Physiologic evidence for heterogeneity within duodenal ulcer includes: the occurrence of duodenal ulcer in both acid hypersecretors and normosecretors, the identification of hyperpepsinogenemic I and normopepsinogenemic I duodenal ulcer patients, marked variability in the gastrin response to a protein meal and the observation that the rate of gastric emptying differs among duodenal ulcer patients [1, 29]. The recent suggestion of an association of an HLA antigen with duodenal ulcer [58] and the report of antibodies to secretory IgA in certain duodenal ulcer patients [59] hint that there may be an immunological form of peptic ulcer. Yet each of these abnormalities is found in some but not all ulcer patients. Thus, rather than looking for a single defect in all ulcer patients, we should be emphasizing the differences between patients as clues to delineate different disorders.

Further evidence of heterogeneity is the observation that different forms of the disorder differ in their associations with genetic polymorphisms. Thus the blood group association helped to further separate gastric from duodenal ulcer, since blood group O was found to be associated with duodenal ulcer (with or without associated gastric ulcer), but not with primary gastric ulcer [3, 23].

Genetic studies utilizing subclinical markers

Possibly the most powerful method of demonstrating genetic heterogeneity is the use of family studies to test whether the reported physiologic abnormalities have a genetic basis and, if so, whether they serve as subclinical markers [21, 29, 39]. Subclinical markers (predictors) are abnormalities proposed to have a role in the pathogenesis of the disease under study. They thus detect more individuals with the abnormal genotype, in addition to detecting those with overt disease. They are useful in genetic studies, because in many disorders not all individuals with the mutant genotype may manifest the disorder (reduced penetrance), or, if they do, the clinical features may be too mild to be readily apparent (variable expressivity), or there may be a delayed age of onset of the disease, with the result that younger genetically-predisposed individuals would be clinically normal. Thus subclinical markers maximize the number of affected individuals that can be detected. Before the indentification of subclinical markers in peptic ulcer, individuals genetically predisposed to ulcer could not be detected until its clinical manifestations were full blown.

Subclinical markers can also be used to detect heterogeneity within a clinical syndrome. The simple fact that a given potential marker does not occur in all individuals with a clinically-similar disorder does not mean that it is unimportant in a given subgroup of these individuals, who may have a distinct but previously unrecognized disease. For example, sickling of the red cells is an excellent subclinical marker in some patients with anemia, whereas G6PD levels is a valid subclinical marker in other anemia patients. If anemia was considered a single disease, then both sickling and G6PD levels would be rejected as good subclinical markers, since neither occurs in all affected individuals. Similary, in peptic ulcer, many biochemical and physiologic abnormalities have been described in some but not all ulcer patients. The proposition that distinct ulcer syndromes can be defined by the stratification of patients into groups according to different markers is being borne out by appropriate genetic-physiologic studies. This has been done for several physiologic traits, including serum pepsinogen I, gastric emptying, and gastrin response to a protein meal.

The most extensive studies have utilized the radioimmunoassay of serum pepsinogen I (PG I), as developed by Samloff and co-workers [56, 60]. Human serum pepsinogens, the precursors of pepsin, have been separated into 2 immunochemically-distinct groups, one of fast electrophoretic mobility, which is confined to the acid secreting part of the stomach (pepsinogen I, PG I), and the other of slower mobility, which is found throughout the stomach and in the first part of the duodenum (pepsinogen II, PG II) [61–63].

Studies of some 120 duodenal ulcer sibships have shown that about half of duodenal ulcer patients have hyperpepsinogenemia I (hyper PG I) and the other half have normopepsinogenemia I (normo PG I), both on a familial basis [3]. That is, the hyper PG I duodenal ulcer and normo PG I duodenal ulcer for the most part segregate independently (within any one sibship, most patients with duodenal ulcer are either hyper PG I or normo PG I). Both forms of duodenal ulcer exhibit an increased risk to sibs for ulcer (some 20–25% of the sibs affected) compared to the population risk. Thus both forms demonstrate familial aggregation with a presumably genetic basis. Other risk factors did not distinguish between the 2 groups, such as blood groups or the male/female ratio, which was 3 to 1 in both groups. Results in a small series of twins also support this separation of hyper and normo PG I duodenal ulcer [64].

Sibling studies and studies of extended families have also demonstrated that the familial aggregation of elevated PG I is consistent with autosomal dominant inheritance [2, 3]. In the sibship studies, 36 of 83 clinically normal sibs of the hyper PG I sibships had elevated PG I [3]. Segregation analysis of the trait of elevated PG I yielded segregation ratios bracketing the value of 0.5, supporting autosomal dominant inheritance of this trait. In the extended families studied, the vertical transmission of elevated PG I was also characteristic of autosomal dominant inheritance. In each generation, approximately 50% of the offspring of members with elevated PG I had an elevated PG I, all offspring of normo PG I members had normal PG I, and there was male-to-male transmission of hyperpepsinogenemia. Thus, these studies have delineated a major genetic factor, elevated serum pepsinogen I, which can identify individuals at risk and which may account for the major genetic predisposition of some half of duodenal ulcer patients. This does not mean that an elevated serum pepsinogen I itself predisposes to ulcer. More likely, it identifies those individuals with an increased mass of chief and parietal cells who are genetically predisposed on the basis of producing excess pepsin and acid. In family and sibling studies of hyperpepsinogenemic I patients, some 40% of the relatives with elevated pepsinogen I have clinical duodenal ulcer. Other factors, environmental and/or genetic, must therefore also play a role in disease expression.

Thus these accumulated studies suggest that there are at least 2 genetic subtypes of duodenal ulcer. In the hyper PG I type, the genetic predisposition to duodenal ulcer in apparently normal sibs can be identified by an elevated serum PG I level. The second type is characterized by normopepsinogenemia I both in the ulcer proband and in the proband's sibs. This latter type of ulcer also appears to have a genetic basis, as demonstrated by its familial aggregation; we assume that there are other markers which identify individuals at risk, and we are seeking to discover them. One should not conclude from these studies that there are only 2 forms of duodenal ulcer. The use of other subclinical markers might further subdivide these broad groups. Additional studies utilizing other physiologic characteristics are just starting to further subdivide the hyperpepsinogenemic I and normopepsinogenemic I duodenal ulcer groups. There appears to be a subgroup of the normopepsinogenemic I class in which rapid gastric emptying seems to be the inherited physiological abnormality predisposing to ulcer [65]. Familial hyperpepsinogenemic I duodenal ulcer seems also to be separable into different groups. A group of patients with a markedly exaggerated gastrin response to a protein meal from an antral source (antral G cell hyperfunction) have also been shown to have hyperpepsinogenemia I [66, 67]. In addition, both the gastrin and pepsinogen I abnormalities were shown to have a familial basis. Both the rapid emptying and postprandial hypergastrinemia appeared to follow autosomal dominant inheritance patterns.

Thus pepsinogen I, gastric emptying, and gastrin response to a meal have been demonstrated to be useful markers in genetic studies. There are a variety of additional potential subclinical markers for genetic studies of peptic ulcer (Table IV). The only one of these examined in a family study has been maximum acid secretion: Fodor et al. measured maximum acid output in 160 duodenal ulcer patients, 113 non-ulcerated first-degree relatives, and 155 healthy controls without a family history of ulcer, and found that acid secretion in the family members was intermediate between the ulcer patients and controls, regardless of blood group or secretor status [68]. Since only mean values were reported, it is not known whether there was any segregation of an elevated acid secretion, but the considerable overlap between normals

Table IV: Subclinical markers of peptic ulcer [29].

Confirmed in genetic studies

   Maximum acid secretion
   Serum pepsinogen I (PG I)
   Gastric emptying
   Gastrin response to a meal

Potential markers

   Serum pepsinogen II (PG II)
   Abnormalities of acid secretion
     Increased acid response to a meal
     Increased sensitivity to gastrin
     Decreased inhibition of acid release (by acid, by distension)
   Abnormalities of gastrin
     Decreased inhibition of gastrin release by acid
   Alpha-1-antitrypsin levels
   Antibodies to secretory IgA
   Plasma noradrenaline
   Secretin-induced histamine release in skin
   Smooth muscle contracting factor
   Acetycholinesterase levels (serum, red cells)
   Salivary response to citric acid
   Gastritis, duodenitis
   Duodenogastric reflux and pyloric sphincter dysfunction

---

and ulcer patients would complicate such analysis. It would be worthwhile, however, to re-examine Fodor's data with modern genetic analytic techniques.

It should be noted that the genetic-family method of studying potential markers is not only useful for demonstrating heterogeneity. By showing cosegregation of the disease and the physiologic marker in certain families it can, equally importantly, help demonstrate that a particular abnormality does in fact have a clear pathophysiologic relationship to at least one type of peptic ulcer. Such studies can thus resolve any doubt about whether a given abnormality is a 'real' observation in peptic ulcer patients.

A genetic classification and implications

Thus, the accumulating evidence suggests that the genetic predisposition to peptic ulcer is not due principally to the cumulative effect of multiple, additive predisposing genes, each having a small effect (the polygenic hypothesis), but rather that there are multiple forms of peptic ulcer, each with a different genetic basis. A classification of peptic ulcer genetic heterogeneity is given in Table V. It should be noted that polygenic inheritance and genetic heterogeneity are not necessarily mutually exclusive. There may well be a polygenic background upon which major predisposing genes act. Alternatively, one of

Table V: Proposed classification of peptic ulcer genetic heterogeneity.

---

1. Peptic ulcer associated with rare genetic syndromes
    A. Multiple endocrine adenomatosis, Type I (gastrinoma)
    B. Systemic mastocytosis
    C. Tremor-nystagmus-ulcer syndrome
2. Gastric ulcer
3. Combined gastric and duodenal ulcer
4. Hyperpepsinogenemic-I duodenal ulcer
    A. Without postprandial hypergastrinemia
    B. With postprandial hypergastrinemia
5. Normopepsinogenemic-I duodenal ulcer
    A. Without rapid gastric emptying
    B. With rapid gastric emptying
6. Childhood duodenal ulcer
7. Immunologic form of duodenal ulcer*
8. Peptic ulcer associated with other chronic diseases*
    A. Peptic ulcer and chronic lung disease
    B. Duodenal ulcer and renal stones
    C. Duodenal ulcer and coronary artery disease

---

* Tentative subdivision.

the various heterogeneous forms may be polygenic in origin.

Can these new subclinical markers, such as pepsinogen I, gastric emptying and gastrin response, be used to define the risk for ulcer in order to counsel ulcer patients and their families? At this point it seems that such efforts are premature, and will remain premature until we gain more basic knowledge regarding the specific diagnosis, prognosis and therapy of each of these different disorders. The rare genetic syndromes that feature peptic ulceration should certainly be identified, as these require specific counseling and therapy [29]. However, even though it is clear at this time that the hyper PG I relative of a hyper PG I duodenal ulcer patient may be at high risk for ulcer (about 40%) [3], it is unclear what either physicians or individuals would do, or could do, with such information until we have learned more about what converts genetic predisposition into clinical disease.

Thus, further studies should proceed in several directions. All of the physiologic and biochemical abnormalities that have been identified in some members of the peptic ulcer population should be evaluated in appropriately designed genetic studies. These potential subclinical markers must be studied in concert, to determine which cosegregate and to delineate as completely as possible the phenotype of a specific disorder. When a specific disorder is delineated, intensive physiologic and biochemical study of affected family members should be performed, with the goal of identifying the biochemical-genetic abnormality. As markers are confirmed for individuals at risk for various types of ulcer disorders, they should be incorporated into clinical and epidemiologic studies, to identify the specific environmental influences which convert genetic predisposition into clinical disease and to delineate the natural history of each disorder. Clinical studies must incorporate traits which identify the different forms of ulcer, as these different diseases may well have specific modes of therapy and/or prevention. We can anticipate some future day when a physician who finds an ulcer crater in the stomach or duodenum would regard this as the beginning rather than the end of the diagnostic process, and would then proceed to specific therapy, counseling, and prevention for the particular form of the disease found in that patient.

Summary

Evidence that genetic factors are important in predisposing to peptic ulcer came from traditional family, twin, and disease association studies. However, the mode of inheritance of this predisposition remained unclear. Polygenic inheritance became the most commonly accepted explanation. In contrast, we proposed genetic heterogeneity as an alternative hypothesis that can explain both the familial aggregation and the lack of a simple Mendelian pattern of inheritance for all ulcer disease. Evidence for heterogeneity of peptic ulcer now includes clinical evidence, ethnic variability, physiologic differences, the existence of rare genetic syndromes, heterogeneity of association with genetic polymorphisms and genetic studies utilizing subclinical markers. The last 3 of these provide direct evidence of ulcer genetic heterogeneity, and genetic studies utilizing such physiologic characteristics as serum pepsinogen I have provided the most powerful support for the hypothesis of genetic heterogeneity of 'common' peptic ulcer. About 50% of patients with duodenal ulcer have increased serum pepsinogen I, which appears to be transmitted as an autosomal dominant trait. The full extent of the heterogeneity of the peptic ulcer diathesis remains to be determined.

Acknowledgments

We wish to especially acknowledge our collaborators, Drs. David L. Rimoin and I. Michael Samloff. We also thank Alycia Bittick and Ellen Bruce for their secretarial assistance.

References

1. Rotter, J.I. and Rimoin, D.L. (1977): Peptic ulcer disease − a heterogeneous group of disorders? *Gastroenterology 73*, 604.
2. Rotter, J.I., Sones, J.Q., Samloff, I.M. et al. (1979): Duodenal ulcer disease associated with elevated serum pepsinogen I, an inherited autosomal dominant disorder. *N. Engl. J. Med. 300*, 63.
3. Rotter, J.I., Petersen, G.M., Samloff, I.M. et al. (1979): Genetic heterogeneity of familial hyperpepsinogenemic I and normopepsinogenemic I duodenal ulcer disease. *Ann. Intern. Med. 91*, 372.
4. McConnel, R.B. (1966): Gastric and duodenal ulcer. In: *The Genetics of the Gastrointestinal Disorders*, p. 76. Oxford University Press, London.
5. Jirasek, V. (1971): Hereditary factors in the etiology of peptic ulcer. *Acta Univ. Carol. Med. 17*, 383.
6. Gotlieb-Jensen, K. (1972): *Peptic Ulcer: Genetic and Epidemiological Aspects Based on Twin Studies*. Munksgaard, Copenhagen.
7. Levin, A.E. and Kuchur, B.A. (1936): On the clinico-genetical differentiation of ulcerous diseases (Russian). *Proc. Maxim Gorky Med.-Genet. Res. Inst. 4*, 181.
8. Doll, R. and Buch, J. (1950): Hereditary factors in peptic ulcer. *Ann. Eugen. 15*, 135.
9. Wretmark, G. (1953): The peptic ulcer individual, a study in heredity, physique and personality. *Acta Psychiatr. Scand., Sup. 84*.
10. Kuenssberg, E.V. (1962): Are duodenal ulcer and chronic bronchitis family diseases? *Proc. R. Soc. Med. 55*, 299.
11. Monson, R.R. (1970): Familial factors in peptic ulcer, the occurrence of ulcer in relatives. *Am. J. Epidemiol. 91*, 453.

12. Kubickova, Z. and Vesely, K.T. (1972): The value of investigation of the incidence of peptic ulcer in families of patients with duodenal ulcer. *J. Med. Genet. 9,* 38.
13. Camerer, J.W. (1936): *Z. Menschl. Vererb-U. Konstit. Lehre 19,* 416 (Quoted in Gotlieb Jensen, 1972).
14. Huhn, G. (1939): *Magenerkrankungen bei Zwillingen.* Hamburg (Quoted in Gotlieb Jensen, 1972).
15. Doig, R.K. (1957): Illness in twins: duodenal ulcer. *Med. J. Aust. 2,* 617.
16. Harvald, B. and Hauge, M. (1958): A catamnestic investigation of Danish twins. *Acta Genet. 8,* 287.
17. Marshall, A.G., Hutchinson, E.O. and Honisett, J. (1962): Heredity in common diseases, a retrospective survey of twins in a hospital population. *Br. Med. J. I,* 1.
18. Eberhard, G. (1968): Peptic ulcer in twins. A study in personality, heredity and environment. *Acta Psychiatr. Scand., Sup. 205.*
19. Pollin, W., Allen, M.G., Hoffer, A. et al. (1969): Psychopathology in 15,909 pairs of veteran twins: evidence for a genetic factor in the pathogenesis of schizophrenia and its relative absence in psychoneurosis. *Am. J. Psychiatry 126,* 597.
20. McConnel, R.B. (1963): Associations and linkage in human genetics. *Am. J. Med. 34,* 692.
21. Rotter, J.I. and Rimoin, D.L. (1979): Diabetes mellitus: the search for genetic markers. *Diabetes Care 2,* 215.
22. Aird, I., Bentall, H.H., Mehigaro, J.A. and Roberts, J.A.F. (1954): The blood groups in relation to peptic ulceration and carcinoma of the colon, rectum, breast and bronchus. *Br. Med. J. 2,* 315.
23. Mourant, A.E., Kopec, A.C. and Domaniewska-Sobczak, K. (1978): *Blood Groups and Diseases: A Study of Associations of Diseases with Blood Groups and Other Polymorphisms.* Oxford University Press, Oxford.
24. Langman, M.J.S. (1973): Blood groups and alimentary disorders. *Clin. Gastroenterol. 2,* 497.
25. Lam, S.K. and Sircus, W. (1975): Studies in duodenal ulcer, the clinical evidence for the existence of two populations. *Q. J. Med. 44,* 369.
26. Prescott, R.J., Sircus, W., Lai, C.L. and Lam, S.K. (1976): Failure to confirm evidence for existence of two populations with duodenal ulcer. *Br. Med. J. 2,* 677.
27. Clarke, C.A., Edwards, J.W., Haddock, D.R.W. et al. (1956): ABO blood group and secretor character in duodenal ulcer. *Br. Med. J. 2,* 725.
28. Doll, R., Drane, H. and Newell, A.C. (1961): Secretion of blood group substances in duodenal, gastric and stomach ulcer, gastric carcinoma, and diabetes mellitus. *Gut 2,* 352.
29. Rotter, J.I. (1980): Peptic ulcer disease – more than one gene, more than one disease. In: *Progress in Medical Genetics,* New Series, Vol. IV, p. 1. Eds: A.G. Steinberg, A.G. Bearn, A.G. Motulsky and B. Childs. Saunders, Philadelphia.
30. Roberts, J.A.F. (1965): ABO blood groups, secretor status and susceptibility to chronic diseases: an example of genetic basis for family predispostions. In: *Genetics and the Epidemiology of Chronic Diseases,* p. 77. Eds: J.V. Neel, M.W. Shaw and W.J. Schull. U.S. Government Printing Office, Public Health Service. Publication No. 1163.
31. Edwards, J.H. (1965): The meaning of the associations between blood groups and disease. *Ann. Hum. Genet. 29,* 77.

32. Cowan, W.K. (1973): Genetics of duodenal and gastric ulcer. *Clin. Gastroenterol.* *2*, 539.
33. Carter, C.O. (1969): Genetics of common disorders. *Br. Med. Bull. 25*, 52.
34. Rotter, J.I., Gursky, J.M., Samloff, I.M. and Rimoin, D.L. (1976): Peptic ulcer disease – further evidence for genetic heterogeneity. (Abstract.) In: *Vth International Congress of Human Genetics*, p. 96. Eds: S. Armendares and R. Lisker. Excerpta Medica, Amsterdam-Oxford-Princeton.
35. McKusick, V.A. (1978): The William Allan Memorial award lecture. Genetic nosology: three approaches. *Am. J. Hum. Genet. 30*, 105.
36. Rimoin, D.L. (1975): The chondrodystrophies. In: *Advances in Human Genetics*, Vol. 5, p. 1. Eds: H. Harris and K. Hirschhorn. Plenum Publishing Corp., New York.
37. Motulsky, A.G. (1976): The genetic hyperlipidemias. *N. Engl. J. Med. 294*, 823.
38. Creutzfeldt, W., Kobberling, J. and Neel, J.V. (1976): *The Genetics of Diabetes Mellitus.* Springer-Verlag, Berlin.
39. Rotter, J.I., Rimoin, D.L. and Samloff, I.M. (1978): Genetic heterogeneity in diabetes mellitus and peptic ulcer. In: *Genetic Epidemiology*, p. 381. Eds: N.E. Morton and C.S. Chung. Academic Press, New York.
40. Rotter, J.I. (1979): Genetic heterogeneity within diabetes mellitus, a review. In: *Genetic Analysis of Common Diseases: Applications to Predictive Factors in Coronary Heart Disease*, p. 135. Eds: C.F. Sing and M.H. Skolnick. Alan R. Liss, New York.
41. Rotter, J.I. Rimoin, D.L. and Samloff, I.M. (1979): Genetic heterogeneity in peptic ulcer. *Lancet I*, 1088.
42. Ballard, H.S., Frame, B. and Hartsock, R.J. (1964): Familial multiple endocrine adenoma-peptic ulcer complex. *Medicine Baltimore 43*, 481.
43. Rimoin, D.L. and Schimke, R.N. (1971): Multiple endocrine adenomatosis. In: *Genetic Disorders of the Endocrine Glands*, p. 200. C.V. Mosby Co., St. Louis.
44. Lamers, C.B., Stadil, F. and Van Tongeren, J.H. (1978): Prevalence of endocrine abnormalities in patients with the Zollinger-Ellison syndrome and their families. *Am. J. Med. 64*, 607.
45. Neuhauser, G., Daly, R.F., Magnelli, N.C. et al. (1976): Essential tremor, nystagmus and duodenal ulceration. *Clin. Genet. 9*, 81.
46. Susser, M. (1967): Causes of peptic ulcer, a selective epidemiologic review. *J. Chronic Dis. 20*, 435.
47. Tovey, F.I. (1979): Progress report, Peptic ulcer in India and Bangladesh. *Gut 20*, 329.
48. Doll, R. and Kellock, T.D. (1951): The separate inheritance of gastric and duodenal ulcers. *Ann. Eugen. 16*, 231.
49 Bonnevie, O. (1975): The incidence in Copenhagen County of gastric and duodenal ulcers in the same patient. *Scand. J. Gastroenterol. 10*, 529.
50 Sedlachova, M. and Seemonova, E. (1973): Genealogical investigation in a group of children with duodenal ulcer. *Rev. Czech. Med. 19*, 81.
51. Lam, S.K. and Ong. G.B. (1976): Duodenal ulcers, early and late onset. *Gut 17*, 169.
52. Cohen, B.H., Diamond, E.L., Graves, C.G. et al (1977): A common familial component in lung cancer and chronic obstructive pulmonary disease. *Lancet II*, 523.

53. Bonnevie, O. (1977): Causes of death in duodenal and gastric ulcer. *Gastroenterology 73*, 1000.
54. Rotter, J.I., Monson, R.R. and Grossman, M.I. (1980): Duodenal ulcer and pulmonary disease: which comes first? (Submitted for publication.)
55. Wormsley, K.G. and Grossman, M.I. (1965): Maximal histalog test in control subjects and patients with peptic ulcer. *Gut 6*, 427.
56. Samloff, I.M., Liebman, W.M. and Panitch, N.M. (1975): Serum group I pepsinogens by radioimmunoassay in control subjects and patients with peptic ulcer. *Gastroenterology 69*, 1196.
57. Lam, S.K. and Lai, C.L. (1978): Gastric ulcers with and without associated duodenal ulcer have different pathophysiology. *Clin. Sci. Mol. Med. 55*, 97.
58. Rotter, J.I., Rimoin, D.L., Gursky, J.M. et al. (1977): HLA−B5 associated with duodenal ulcer. *Gastroenterology 73*, 435.
59. Kwitko, A. and Shearman, D.J.C. (1978): Antibodies to secretory IgA (SIgA) in duodenal ulcer disease. *Gut 19*, A437.
60. Samloff, I.M. and Liebman, W.M. (1974): Radioimmunoassay of group I pepsinogens in serum. *Gastroenterology 66*, 494.
61. Samloff, I.M. (1969): Slow moving protease and the seven pepsinogens: electrophoretic demonstration of the existence of eight proteolytic fractions in human gastric mucosa. *Gastroenterology 57*, 659.
62. Samloff, I.M. (1971): Immunologic studies of human group I pepsinogens. *J. Immunol. 106*, 692.
63. Samloff, I.M. (1979): Serum pepsinogens I and II. In: *Developments in Digestive Diseases*, pp. 1−12. Ed: J.E. Berk. Lea and Febiger, Philadelphia.
64. Rotter, J.I., Rimoin, D.L., Samloff, I.M. et al. (1977): The genetics of peptic ulcer disease − elevated serum group I pepsinogen concentrations in siblings and twins of ulcer probands. *Gastroenterology 72*, 1165.
65. Rotter, J.I., Rubin, R., Meyer, J.H. et al. (1979): Rapid gastric emptying − an inherited pathophysiologic defect in duodenal ulcer? *Gastroenterology 76*, 1229.
66. Calam, J., Taylor, I.L., Dockray, G.J. et al. (1979): Subgroup of duodenal ulcer patients with familial G-cell hyperfunction and hyperpepsinogenemia I. *Gut 20*, A934.
67. Taylor, I.L., Calam, J., Rotter, J.I. et al. (1980): Familial hypergastrinemic and hyperpepsinogenemic I duodenal ulcer. (Submitted for publication.)
68. Fodor, O., Vestea, S., Urcan, S. et al. (1968): Hydrochloric acid secretion capacity of the stomach as an inherited factor in the pathogenesis of duodenal ulcer. *Am. J. Dig. Dis. 13*, 260.

Environmental aspects of ulcer disease

A.R. Cooke
Department of Internal Medicine, Kansas University Medical Center, Kansas City, Kansas, U.S.A.

The frequent association of drug ingestion with peptic ulcer has led to a general assumption that certain drugs increase the incidence of peptic ulcer in man. This clinical impression is often a result of extrapolation of the known ulcerogenic effects in animals to human subjects. Proof of this association must rest with epidemiological studies almost all of which are retrospective. The possibility of doing a prospective study to prove an association between drug ingestion and peptic ulceration is very remote, since to prove an increased incidence would require thousands of patients in control and treatment groups. Thus, it seems likely that with many potentially-ulcerogenic drugs absolute proof will never be obtained. Therefore, in considering the associations discussed below one should remember the difficulties in proving any association. However, lack of proof should not allow one to conclude that the phenomenon does not exist.

In this brief review, those drugs for which there are enough studies to come to some conclusions will be discussed in greater detail than other drugs for which the evidence is sparse or not well documented. For a more detailed review of this topic, the reader should consult an earlier work [1].

Smoking

There is a strong association between smoking and peptic ulcer [2–5]. Smokers have more ulcers (gastric and duodenal) than nonsmokers and smokers have higher death rates from ulcers than nonsmokers [6, 7]. However, no relationship has been found between the amount smoked and the risk of ulcer. Doll and coworkers found that gastric ulcers healed faster if smoking was stopped [5] but this finding could not be confirmed in a recent study by Herrmann and Piper ([8] and Table I).

Table I: Effect of smoking and alcohol on ulcer recurrence.

Index of ulcer		Recurrence	No recurrence	Significance
Healed	(50)			
Nonsmokers	(25)	8	17	$p > 0.25$
Smokers	(25)	5	20	
Unhealed	(33)			
Nonsmokers	(17)	8	9	$p \geq 0.10$
Smokers	(16)	12	4	
Healed	(50)			
No alcohol	(25)	5	20	$p > 0.25$
Alcohol	(25)	8	17	
Unhealed	(33)			
No alcohol	(21)	14	7	$p > 0.25$
Alcohol	(12)	6	6	

Modified from [9].

Salicylates

Chronic acetylsalicylic acid usage is now well established as a cause of gastric ulcer [10–12]. This is very well documented in the report from the Boston Drug Surveillance Program [13]. In that study there was an association between hospital admissions for newly diagnosed uncomplicated benign gastric ulcer and heavy regular long-term acetylsalicylic acid ingestion (4 or more days per week). No relationship was found between acetylsalicylic acid usage (heavy or light) and duodenal ulcer. Light, regular acetylsalicylic acid use (1–3 days per week) was not associated with gastric ulcer. Factors such as age, sex and smoking habits did not obscure the associations between peptic ulceration and acetylsalicylic acid ingestion. It seems likely that patients with rheumatoid arthritis are at a greater risk. Acetylsalicylic acid has also been shown to retard the healing of gastric ulcers ([9]; Table II).

Corticosteroids

Two large reviews have examined the role of corticosteroids as a cause of peptic ulcers. In one review composed of retrospective studies, it was found that patients with rheumatoid arthritis had a prevalence varying from 0–38%

Table II: Effect of analgesics on ulcer recurrence.

Status on discharge	Total number	With recurrence (%)	Significance
Healed (50)	50	26	NS
No analgesics	30	33	NS
Daily analgesics	12	17	NS
Unhealed (33)	33	61	NS
No analgesics	16	56	NS
Daily analgesics	12	83	$p < 0.05$

Modified from [9]. NS = not significant.

Table III: Prevalence of peptic ulceration in rheumatoid arthritis and nonrheumatoid patients treated with corticosteroids.

Disease	Number of studies	Number of patients	Mean prevalence % (Range)
Asthma, ulcerative colitis, allergies, dermatoses, etc.	9	1,699	0.3 (0– 1.1%)
Rheumatoid arthritis	23	4,278	6.7 (0–38.4%)

Data from [14].

whereas a group of miscellaneous diseases (asthma, ulcerative colitis, allergies, etc.) had a prevalence of 0–1.1% ([14]; Table III). In 1967 Cooke concluded from his review of the literature that corticosteroids probably did not increase the incidence of peptic ulcer but he suggested that a firm conclusion was not justified because the studies were from selected groups of patients and no controls of any kind were studied [14].

These defects were largely remedied by the survey of Conn and Blitzer [15] who carried out a retrospective analysis of peptic ulcer prevalence in a large number of prospective case control studies of adrenocorticosteroids or adrenocorticotropic hormone therapy in a variety of diseases (Table IV). The authors concluded that the prevalence of peptic ulcer was not increased in those receiving adrenocorticosteroids. They did not find more ulcers in patients receiving a daily dose of greater than 20 mg of prednisone or its equivalent when compared to those receiving a lower dose. Total doses of greater than 1,000 mg of prednisone were associated with ulcers. Although corticosteroids retard ulcer healing in animals there are no studies in man.

Table IV: Rates of proved peptic ulcer in controlled studies of adrenocorticosteroid therapy.

Group	Number of patients	Patients with peptic ulcer (%)	Patients with hemorrhage from ulcer (%)	Patients with perforation of ulcer (%)
Control	2,346	0.8	0.2	0.1
Steroid	2,985	1.3	0.3	0.1

Modified from [15].

Indometacin

The small number of reports and lack of prospective studies of the nature outlined for acetylsalicylic acid adrenocorticosteroids make it impossible to decide whether indometacin is ulcerogenic. The evidence from 5 studies (634 patients, 35 new or reactivated ulcers) indicates a prevalence of 5.5% [16–20]. This figure is no greater than that given for the prevalence in the general population. One study, however, does raise the possibility that indometacin is ulcerogenic. Rothernich carried out a prospective study of 216 patients (mainly with rheumatoid arthritis) for periods up to 30 months [21]. Barium meals were given to 12 patients at random, all of whom had dyspepsia. Gastrointestinal symptoms occurred in 25% of the patients and about three-fourths were receiving other drugs. Ten of 216 patients receiving indometacin and other drugs developed a peptic ulcer (4 exacerbations of a preexisting ulcer), a prevalence of 4.6% and an incidence rate of 2.8%. Two of 74 patients receiving only indometacin developed an ulcer, an incidence of 2.7%. This high incidence is suggestive of an ulcerogenic role but needs confirmation by other prospective studies.

Phenylbutazone

I am unaware of any controlled prospective studies examining the relationship between phenylbutazone and peptic ulceration, and hence all data are retrospective.

In 1955, Mauer, in a survey of 23 publications containing 3,934 patients, found 40 patients in whom gastric complications occurred (1%); there were 22 patients with acute peptic ulcers (0.6%) and 18 patients with exacerbation of preexisting ulcers [22]. This evidence indicates that peptic ulceration is a doubtful complication of phenylbutazone. In a large study in 1969 of 562 patients (about 50% with rheumatoid arthritis) treated for 2–10 years with daily doses of 100–800 mg, only 3 patients were found to have a peptic ulcer [23]. This evidence indicates that peptic ulcer is probably not a complication of phenylbutazone.

Caffeine (coffee, tea, colas) and ethanol

I am unaware of any convincing epidemiological evidence implicating alcohol as a cause of peptic ulcer in man. An exception to this statement is the association of duodenal ulcer with alcoholic cirrhosis of the liver. Ethanol was found not to retard the healing of gastric ulcer [9].

Coffee, both with and without caffeine, stimulates gastric acid secretion. The evidence linking coffee drinking to ulcers is doubtful. Friedman et al. did not find any association between alcohol and coffee consumption and the prevalence of peptic ulcer [2]. In contrast, Paffenbarger et al. found in college students that ingestion of coffee and other beverages (mainly colas) increased the risk of later development of ulcers [24]. Ingestion of milk decreased the risk. Alcohol and tea drinking were not associated with an increased risk, whereas cigarette smoking was correlated with subsequent development of peptic ulcer.

Other analgesic drugs

Phenacetin and paracetamol

There is virtually no evidence of these drugs being ulcerogenic despite widespread use.

Acetylsalicylic acid substitutes

There is little epidemiological information, apart from anecdotal case reports, concerning drugs such as mefenamic acid, fenoprofen, naproxen, tolmetin, ibuprofen, to make a judgment about their possible ulcerogenic role in man.

Pathogenesis

This can be considered under the following possible mechanisms.

Stimulation of acid secretion

Of all the drugs considered above only caffeine and coffee (with or without caffeine) are moderately strong stimulants of acid secretion [25–27]. All the other agents either have no effect or cause mild inhibition or stimulation of acid secretion [1].

Mucosal resistance.

Gastric mucus   There is great doubt that mucus has any protective role on gastric mucosa apart from its lubricating properties. Mucus is a thin, unstirred layer with weak naturalizing and buffering capacity and acid diffuses rapidly through it [28].

Gastric mucosal permeability   The gastric mucosa is resistant to damage by acid and is relatively water-tight. The impermeability of the gastric mucosa has been called the 'gastric mucosal barrier'. This impermeability depends upon the integrity of the gastric mucosal cells and their tight junctions. A great number of the drugs mentioned above, including acetylsalicylic acid, alcohol and indometacin, when topically applied, will make the gastric mucosa more permeable [29–31]. This can be shown experimentally by an increased leak of hydrogen ion from the lumen of the stomach, a gain of sodium ion into the lumen and a decrease in the transmucosal electrical potential difference (PD) which reflects the electrolyte changes. When a number of these drugs were studied in man only unbuffered acetylsalicylic acid and ethanol decreased PD [32], whereas indometacin did not although it had done so in the dog [30]. Phenylbutazone and prednisone had no effect also [32].

It is believed (with good supporting evidence) that once the gastric defenses are breached, acid in the lumen diffuses into the mucosa and submucosa and sets in sequence a series of events which results in destruction of capillaries and ultimately causes gastric erosions [33, 34]. This mechanism explains very well the mechanism of gastric erosions induced by acetylsalicylic acid but this, of course, does not mean it explains the development of chronic gastric ulceration.

Inhibition by prostaglandins

Most of the anti-inflammatory drugs e.g., acetylsalicylic acid, indometacin, phenylbutazone, etc., inhibit prostaglandin synthetase and thus deplete tissues of prostaglandins [35, 36]. Prostaglandins have been found to inhibit gastric acid secretion but more importantly to be cytoprotective to the gastric mucosa [37, 38]. Robert and coworkers found that several prostaglandins of the A, E, or F type given orally or subcutaneously to rats prevented damage to gastric mucosa treated with absolute ethanol, 0.6 N HCl, 0.2 N NaOH, 25% NaCl or boiling water [37]. The effect of the prostaglandins was dose dependent. Cytoprotection by prostaglandins was unrelated to inhibition of gastric secretion since they were maximally effective at doses that had no effect on gastric secretion and antisecretory compounds e.g., cimetidine or antacids were not cytoprotective.

Thus, acetylsalicylic acid may act not only by a topical effect on the gastric mucosa but also via prostaglandin synthetase inhibition. Indirect evidence for the latter effect has been found in cats using intravenous acetylsalicylic acid [39]. In those studies, continous intravenous acetylsalicylic acid infusion caused deep gastric ulcers and these effects were not associated with any changes in sodium-hydrogen fluxes or gastric mucosal PD. Since most of the nonsteroidal anti-inflammatory drugs inhibit prostaglandins then this may be their mechanism of gastric damage. Studies need to be done in man to confirm this very interesting animal data.

Reduction of mucosal adenosine triphosphate

Studies have indicated that acetylsalicylic acid reduces mucosal adenosine triphosphate and phosphocreatine content in the gastric mucosa, probably as a result of metabolic inhibition [40]. This mechanism will result in reduced transmucosal resistance and thus mucosal damage.

Pyloric incompetence and duodenal reflux

Smoking has been found to cause reflux of duodenal contents by inhibiting the pyloric sphincter [41]. Repeated exposure to duodenal contents (bile, pancreatic juice) can cause gastritis and possibly lead to gastric ulcer. This mechanism would not explain how smoking is associated with duodenal ulcer.

Inhibition of pancreatic secretion

Smoking and nicotine inhibit pancreatic secretion and thus have been postulated to cause duodenal ulcers by this mechanism i.e., failure to neutralize acid in the duodenum [42].

Addendum

In a recent controlled clinical trial of the treatment of duodenal ulcer, it was found that whereas smoking had no effect on ulcer healing in the antacid group it did retard healing in the placebo group [43].

Summary

A number of drugs in common use in clinical medicine as well as smoking and alcohol have been implicated as causing peptic ulceration. The vast majority of the drugs cause peptic ulceration or erosions in animals but extrapolation of this data to man is fraught with difficulties. There is strong and consistent evidence that people who smoke cigarettes have more ulcers than nonsmokers, have higher mortality rates from these ulcers and may have impaired healing. Alcohol consumption is not correlated with peptic ulcer development except in those with alcoholic cirrhosis of the liver. Regular and chronic use of acetylsalicylic acid e.g., in rheumatoid arthritis, is associated with the development of gastric ulcer but not duodenal ulcer. Acetylsalicylic acid has been found to retard the healing of gastric ulcer. Corticosteroids in large doses are probably associated with the development of peptic ulcer, although this is not proven. The evidence for indometacin and phenylbutazone is inconclusive. The evidence associating coffee drinking with peptic ulceration is equivocable. The other caffeine-containing beverages (tea, colas) do not seem to be implicated. The newer nonsteroidal anti-inflammatory agents have not had sufficient widespread use to evaluate them as ulcerogenic compounds in human subjects.

The mechanism by which acetylsalicylic acid and smoking cause peptic ulceration is not proven. Acetylsalicylic acid breaks the gastric mucosal barrier and also inhibits prostaglandin synthetase. Both these mechanisms may operate in causing gastric ulceration. Reduction of mucosal adenosine triphosphate may be a further mechanism. The other new nonsteroidal anti-inflammatory compounds, if ulcerogenic, may also work via prostaglandin inhibition. Smoking inhibits pancreatic secretion and thus gastric acid is inadequately neutralized; also smoking relaxes the pyloric sphincter thereby allowing reflux of duodenal contents into gastric mucosa and thus causing damage.

From this review it would seem that only smoking (causing gastric and duodenal ulcers) and chronic acetylsalicylic acid ingestion (causing gastric ulcers) are proven to be ulcerogenic.

References

1. Cooke, A.R. (1978): Drug damage to the gastroduodenum. In: *Clinical Gastroenterology*, 2nd Edition, Vol. 1, Chapter 47, p. 807. Eds: J.S. Fordtran and M.H. Sleisenger. W.H. Saunders, Philadelphia.
2. Friedman, G.D., Siegelaub, A.B. and Seltzer, C.C. (1974): Cigarettes, alcohol, coffee and peptic ulcer. *N. Engl. J. Med. 290*, 469.
3. Monson, R.R. (1970): Cigarette smoking and body form in peptic ulcer. *Gastroenterology 58*, 337.
4. Edwards, F., McKeown, T. and Whitefield, A.G.W. (1964): Association between smoking and disease in men over sixty. *Lancet I*, 196.
5. Doll, R., Jones, F.A. and Pygott, F. (1958): Effect of smoking on the production and maintenance of gastric and duodenal ulcers. *Lancet I*, 657.
6. Doll, R. and Hill, A.B. (1964): Mortality in relation to smoking: 10 years' observation of British doctors. *Br. Med. J. 1*, 1399.
7. Hammond, E.C. (1966): Smoking in relation to the death rates of one million men and women. In: *Epidemiological Approaches to the Study of Cancer and Other Diseases*. National Cancer Institute Monograph No. 19, pp. 127–204. Ed: W. Haenszel. U.S. Public Health Service, Bethesda.
8. Herrmann, R.P. and Piper, D.W. (1973): Factors influencing the healing rate of chronic gastric ulcer. *Am. J. Dig. Dis. 18*, 1.
9. Piper, D.W., Shinners, J., Greig, M. et al. (1978): Effect of ulcer healing on the prognosis of chronic gastric ulcer. *Gut 19*, 419.
10. Gillies, M. and Skyring, A. (1968): Gastric ulcer, duodenal ulcer and gastric carcinoma: A case control study of certain social and environmental factors. *Med. J. Aust. 2*, 1132.
11. Gillies, M. and Skyring, A. (1969): Gastric and duodenal ulcer. The association between aspirin ingestion, smoking and family history of ulcer. *Med. J. Aust. 2*, 280.
12. Duggan, J.M. and Chapman, B.L. (1970): The incidence of aspirin ingestion in patients with peptic ulcer. *Med. J. Aust. 1*, 797.
13. Levy, M. (1974): Aspirin use in patients with major upper gastrointestinal bleeding and peptic ulcer disease. *N. Engl. J. Med. 290*, 1158.
14. Cooke, A.R. (1967): Corticosteroids and peptic ulcer: Is there a relationship? *Am. J. Dig. Dis. 12*, 323.
15. Conn, H.O. and Blitzer, B.L. (1976): Nonassociation of adrenocorticosteroid therapy and peptic ulcer. *N. Engl. J. Med. 294*, 473.
16. Hart, F.D. and Boardman, P.L. (1963): Indomethacin: A new non-steroid anti-inflammatory agent. *Br. Med. J. 2*, 965.
17. Lovgren, O. and Allander, E. (1964): Side effects of indomethacin. *Br. Med. J. 1*, 118.
18. Taylor, R.T., Huskisson, E.C., Whitehouse, G.H. et al. (1968): Gastric ulceration occuring during Indomethacin therapy. *Br. Med.J. 4*, 734.
19. Lockie, L.M. and Norcross, D.B. (1966): In: *Arthritis and Allied Conditions*, 7th Edition, p. 345. Ed: J.L. Hollander. Lea and Febiger, Philadelphia.
20. Katz, A.M., Pearson, C.M. and Kennedy, J.M. (1965): A clinical trial of indomethacin in rheumatoid arthritis. *Clin. Pharmacol. Ther. 6*, 25.

21. Rothernich, N.O. (1966): An extended study of indomethacin. *J. Am. Med. Assoc. 195*, 531.
22. Mauer, E.F. (1955): The toxic effects of phenylbutazone (Butazolidin). *N. Engl. J. Med. 253*, 404.
23. Sperling, I.L. (1969): Adverse reactions with long-term use of phenylbutazone and oxyphenbutazone. *Lancet II*, 535.
24. Paffenbarger, R.S., Wing, A.L. and Hyde, R.T. (1974): Chronic disease in former college students. XIII. Early precursors of peptic ulcer. *Am. J. Epidemiol. 100*, 307.
25. Roth, J.A. and Ivy, A.C. (1944): The effect of caffeine upon gastric secretion in the dog, cat and man. *Am. J. Physiol. 141*, 454.
26. Chvasta, T.E. and Cooke, A.R. (1971): Emptying and absorption of caffeine from the human stomach. *Gastroenterology 61*, 838.
27. Cohen, S. and Booth, G.H. (1975): Gastric acid secretion and lower esophageal sphincter pressure in response to coffee and caffeine. *N. Engl. J. Med. 293*, 897.
28. Heatley, N.G. (1959): Muco-substance as a barrier to diffusion. *Gastroenterology 37*, 313.
29. Davenport, H.W., Warner, H.A. and Code, C.F. (1964): Functional significance of gastric mucosal barrier to sodium. *Gastroenterology 47*, 142.
30. Chvasta, T.E. and Cooke, A.R. (1972): The effect of several ulcerogenic drugs on the canine gastric mucosal barrier. *J. Lab. Clin. Med. 79*, 302.
31. Weisbrodt, N.W., Keinzle, M. and Cooke, A.R. (1973): Comparative effects of alaphatic alcohols on the gastric mucosa. *Proc. Soc. Exp. Biol. Med. 142*, 450.
32. Murray, H.S., Strottman, M.P. and Cooke, A.R. (1974): Effect of several drugs on gastric potential difference. *Br. Med. J. 1*, 19.
33. Davenport, H.W. (1967): Salicylate damage to the gastric mucosal barrier. *N. Engl. J. Med. 276*, 1307.
34. Cooke, A.R. (1976): The role of the mucosal barrier in drug-induced gastric ulceration and erosions. *Am. J. Dig. Dis. 21*, 155.
35. Flower, R. Gryglewski, R., Herbaczynska-Cedro, K. and Vane, J.R. (1972): Effects of anti-inflammatory drugs on prostaglandin biosynthesis. *Nature 238*, 104.
36. Vane, J.R. (1971): Inhibition of prostaglandin synthesis as a mechanism of action of aspirin-like drugs. *Nature 231*, 232.
37. Robert, A., Nezamis, J.E., Lancaster, C. and Hanchar, A.J. (1979): Cytoprotection by prostaglandins in rats. *Gastroenterology 77*, 433.
38. Robert, A. (1979): Cytoprotection by prostaglandins. *Gastroenterology 77*, 761.
39. Bugat, R., Thompson, M.R., Aureas, D. and Grossman, M.I. (1976): Gastric mucosal lesions produced by intravenous infusions of aspirin in cats. *Gastroenterology 71*, 754.
40. Spenney, J.G. and Bhown, M. (1977): Effect of acetylsalicylic acid on gastric mucosa. *Gastroenterology 73*, 995.
41. Read, N.W. and Grech, P. (1973): Effect of cigarette smoking on competence of the pylorus. *Br. Med. J. 3*, 313.
42. Solomon, T.E. and Jacobson, E.D. (1972): Cigarette smoking and duodenal ulcer disease. *N. Engl. J. Med. 286*, 1212.
43. Peterson, W.L., Sturdevant, R.A.L., Frankl, H.D. et al. (1977): Healing of duodenal ulcer with an antacid regimen. *N. Engl. J. Med. 297*, 341.

Animal models of ulcer disease

H.M. Jennewein and R. Hammer
Department of Pharmacology, C.H. Boehringer, Sohn, Ingelheim; and Department of Biochemistry, Thomae/Biberach, West Germany

Introduction

The basic aim of pharmacology is the finding of compounds which are effective in human diseases. In order to achieve this aim, pharmacological research must make use of animal models, which in principle can be classified into 3 kinds of pharmacological models: the hypothesis model, the analogue model and the disease model. In the present paper the various models will be discussed with respect to their contribution to the study of the pathophysiology and therapy of human ulcer disease.

Hypothesis model

The hypothesis model is based on one or more hypotheses concerning the physiology or pathophysiology of a disease. For ulcer disease, the usual assumption is that there is an imbalance between the aggressive factors and the protective factors. There is no difficulty in measuring the aggressive factors, such as acid or pepsin secretion, in animals. But if an inhibition of acid secretion is beneficial in certain forms of ulcer disease, some further hypotheses concerning the physiology of acid secretion are necessary to achieve a concept for its inhibition by drugs.

The classical example of the use of hypothesis models is the development of H_2-receptor antagonists using certain pharmacological tests: on the isolated guinea pig atria, the electrically stimulated uterus, and models to measure gastric secretion [1]. The results obtained with these models, which were based on the hypothesis that histamine plays a crucial role in gastric secretion and ulcer disease, have contributed substantially to our knowledge of gastric physiology and pathophysiology.

Although the causal involvement of acid secretion in ulcer pathogenesis cannot be proven by such studies, there is no doubt nowadays that acid secretion is an important factor in the healing process, and perhaps in the recurrence of duodenal ulcer [2]. Using H_2-receptor antagonists and others as a tool, a complex picture of stimuli interaction emerged from a study of the physiology of gastric secretion. It could be demonstrated [3–5] that the 3 main stimuli (histamine, gastrin, acetylcholine) act differentially on the changes associated with acid secretion, namely on the fusion process of the tubulovesicles to secretory canaliculi, the oxygen consumption, and the aminopyrine accumulation as a measure of proton secretion. Various interactions of the stimuli may occur at the cellular level, indicating the importance of stimuli other than histamine, such as acetylcholine and gastrin.

The impressive long-term results obtained after selective proximal vagotomy in ulcer disease [6] particularly underline the importance of acetylcholine, although other endogenous stimuli and inhibitors may also be involved in vagal action. Drug treatment having the same effcct as proximal selective vagotomy is not available, because of the lack of specificity of classical antimuscarinic agents. Pirenzepine, however, is a novel anti-muscarinic drug which, in contrast to the classical antimuscarinic drugs, seems to differentiate clearly between inhibition of gastric secretion and, for example, blockade of smooth muscle action and tachycardia in pharmacological and human studies [7]. This differentiation has been further substantiated in various binding studies using different organs [8]. From these studies it can be concluded that using an antagonist, muscarinic receptors can be divided into subclasses with respect to the different affinities of binding sites (Fig. 1). These can be classified into high-, medium-, and low-affinity binding sites, which are distributed differentially in the various tissues and will be recognized by pirenzepine, in contrast to the situation with classical antimuscarinic drugs. It seems that secretory glands consist mainly of high- and medium-affinity binding sites, whereas heart and smooth muscle show homogeneous low-affinity binding sites.

To further elucidate the activity of the 3 main stimuli, receptor binding studies using the gastric mucosa and/or isolated gastric cell preparations are strongly needed. Such studies have been performed using H_2-receptor antagonists [9], pirenzepine [10] and gastrin [11, 12] and yielded encouraging results. In these studies, proteolytic degradation of the receptors is the main problem, and reproducibility of the results by other laboratories must follow before final conclusions can be drawn. Nevertheless, those receptor studies, and also investigations into the intracellular mechanism of gastric secretion, such as the studies on the adenosine triphosphate-driven proton pump [13], will help create a hypothesis concerning the mechanism of the aggressive factors.

With respect to the pathophysiology of ulcer disease, however, no further

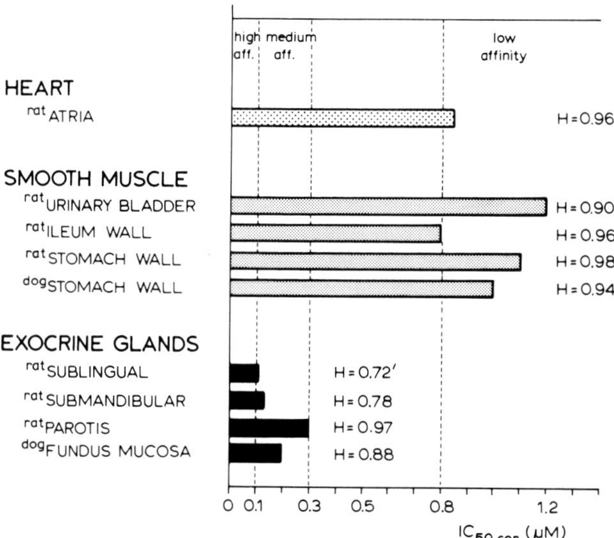

Fig. 1:   Pirenzepine binding sites with differing affinities in various peripheral organs. H = Hill coefficient. Adapted and extended from results of Hammer et al. [8].

contributions can be expected from new antisecretory compounds because powerful antisecretory drugs are now available. So future research into ulcer pathogenesis requires not work on the aggressive factor but work on the development of animal hypothesis models of the protective factors of the gastric mucosa. A fruitful hypothesis concerning superficial cells and their function as an equivalent to the protective factors is emerging. Mucus may be useful, not as a protective factor itself but as a parameter of the function of these cells. However, methodological and physiological problems seem to inhibit the development of a sensitive, rapid, and valid model. The assessment of cytoprotective factors by measurement of the protection against mucosal injury, independent of acid secretion, may be more promising. The studies of Robert [14] indicate a role of prostaglandins and the hypothesis could be put forward that the cyclic adenosine 3',5'-monophosphate content of the superficial cells may be an indicator of cell integrity. From this it remains to be clarified to what extent the prostaglandin and the adenylate cyclase system of the superficial cells are involved in ulcer pathogenesis.

Analogue model

The analogue model is based on an established drug with known clinical effect. If an unknown drug has an effect in a certain model similar to that of the known drug, then the clinical effect can be predicted by analogy. In this way neither the mechanism of action nor the clinically relevant effect need to be measured in this model.

Currently, all models used in gastroenterology for the screening of H_2-receptor antagonists are analogue models, since the H_2-receptor concept has proved to be effective. Moreover, models used in ulcer disease to measure gastric secretion are analogue models, and consequently all drugs found by these methods are analogue drugs.

As far as the relevance of analogue models in ulcer disease is concerned, it can be stated that analogue models which are based on a known and well-established drug effect in man will not improve our understanding of ulcer disease and its pathogenesis. Thus progress in drug development originating from analogue models will be marginal, and will consist of drugs with fewer side effects, lower doses and so on. If the analogue model is not based on a therapeutic mechanism of action but on a side effect, the results obtained are potentially misleading. If this is the case, then of course no progress at all can be expected from such a model.

Disease model

It is always the aim of the experimental researcher to develop models which closely resemble the disease under investigation. It is hoped that in this way further insight into the etiology, the healing process and the therapy of the disease will be gained. Unfortunately, no single ideal disease model is known. For ulcer disease, numerous attempts have been made to develop disease models corresponding to the human disease in at least some respects. Usually they are classified by the way in which the disease is induced in the animals. The 3 main groups are given in Tables I–III. These are: surgically induced ulcers or erosions; centrally induced ulcers or erosions; and chemically induced erosions.

Etiology

With respect to the etiology of ulcer disease, the influence of the central nervous system, gastric secretion and drugs can be investigated experimentally in disease models.

Central nervous system   Several models have been described which show that alterations or manipulation via the central nervous system are able to produce

Table I: Surgical induction of 'ulcers'.

1. Pylorus ligation ('Shay-ulcer') [15]

2. Local mucosal injury [16–18]
    a. Toxic
    b. Thermic
    c. Mechanic

3. Disturbed homeostasis [19–21]
    a. Mann Williamson
    b. Dragstedt
    c. Antral exclusion

Table II: Central induction of 'ulcers'.

1. Stress [22–27]
    a. Immobilization
    b. Cold
    c. Shock (bleeding, burning, etc.)

2. Hypothalamic manipulations [28]

3. Behavioral interactions [29]; i.e., executive monkey

Table III: Induction of 'ulcers' by drugs.

1. Steroidal and nonsteroidal antiphlogistics [30–34]
   a. Glucocorticoids
   b. Acetylsalicylic acid
   c. Phenylbutazone
   d. Indometacin
   e. Flufenamic acid
   f. Cinchophen
	3. Vasoactive substances [39–41]
	   a. Phenylephrine
	   b. Serotonin
	   c. Caffeine
	   d. Adenosine
	   e. Alcohol

2. Secretion stimulators [35–38]
   a. Histamine, compound 48/80
   b. Acetylcholine, carbachol
   c. Insulin
   d. Gastrin
   e. Reserpine
	4. Other substances [42–45]
	   a. Mercaptamine
	   b. Antibiotics
	   c. Nicotine
	   d. Glucose
	   e. Pantothenic acid deficiency, etc.

erosions of the gastric or duodenal mucosa. From the results obtained it is obvious that several pathophysiological interactions are responsible for the manifestation of acute gastric erosions. The complex interrelationships between pathogenetic factors are shown in Figure 2. It can be seen that various stress factors, which may be partly psychological or physical, may affect the central nervous system by producing changes in the limbic system which controls the emotions and has connections with the hypothalamus, as the control center of the autonomous and endocrine system. The hypothalamus is also interrelated with the medullary centers controlling the cardiovascular system. Alterations in these areas lead to phasic changes of gastric secretion [46], to disturbed gastrointestinal motility [47], to an increase of glucocorticoids, catecholamines and histamine [48], and, very important, to hypotension, disturbed microcirculation and consequently to mucosal ischemia [23]. All these interdependent changes decrease the vitality of the gastric mucosal and capillary cells, leading finally to necrosis, erosions, bleeding and ulcers. Obviously, these pathological events may in turn act as stress factors, thus setting up a vicious circle.

Centrally induced experimental ulcers are acute in nature, and will heal within a week. They do not therefore resemble chronic human peptic ulcer

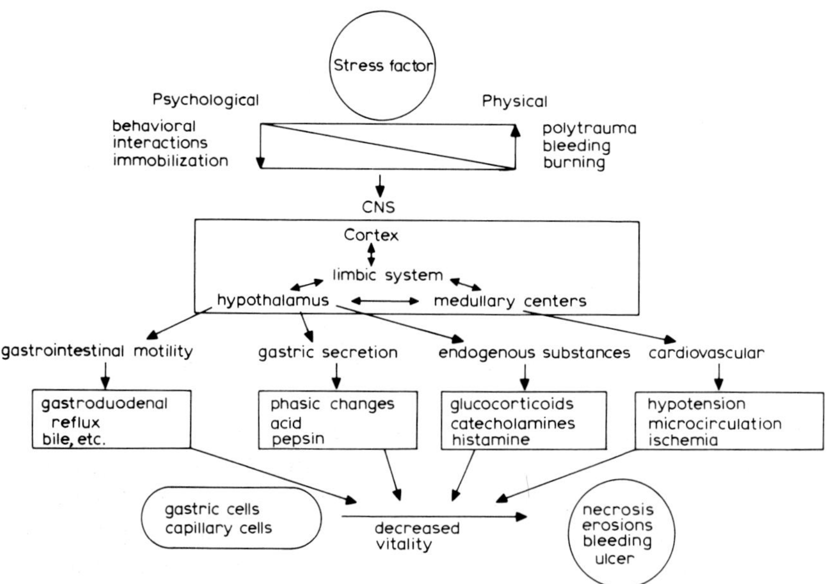

Fig. 2: Mechanisms involved in the development of stress ulcers.

disease, but are more similar to the acute stress erosions, which occur after burning (Curling's ulcer), shock, major surgery, and in intensive care units. Our knowledge in this field results primarily from these disease models, and has given rise to a specific therapy.

Acid secretion It has been demonstrated by a great number of experimental procedures that an increase in gastric secretion can cause duodenal, anastomotic or gastric ulcers (erosions) in animals. The prevalence of duodenal erosions in hypersecretion models using long-term infusions of carbachol, gastrin or histamine, or surgically induced disturbances of homeostasis, has supported the assumption that in duodenal ulcer, hypersecretion or an increase of gastric emptying could be one of the noxae.

Drugs Another factor which may play a role in ulcer disease, and an area in which the 'ulcer models' may contribute, is the effect of exogenously administered drugs. Under certain circumstances, vasoconstricting agents cause erosions, indicating a possible role of bloodflow or the microcirculation in ulcer disease. Some antiphlogistics may cause erosions by inhibiting prostaglandin synthetase. The relevance of these disease models is thus in helping to create new hypotheses, which should then be studied in more specific tests. The drug-induced erosion models can also assist in the finding of drugs better avoided in patients with ulcer disease, because they are irritant or otherwise noxious to the mucosa. In addition, it should also be emphazised that the irritant effect of the duodenal content on the gastric mucosa has led to the hypothesis of Duplessis [49], which has stimulated research in the field of gastroduodenal reflux, gastric emptying and pyloric function in health and disease.

Healing

The second area in which the disease models are hoped to contribute is the healing process of ulcers. It is well-known that in most cases of so-called ulcer models, not real ulcers but more or less acute erosions are present. These erosions have very little in common with the human chronic peptic ulcer with respect to pathomorphological appearance and healing characteristics. Therefore, attempts have been made to develop models which cover this aspect of ulcer disease as well. Only a few models for studying the healing process are available [16–18], of which the acetic acid ulcer has received wider attention. Indeed, as shown in Figure 3, the macroscopic appearance of an acetic acid ulcer in a dog and the histology of this ulcer resemble the

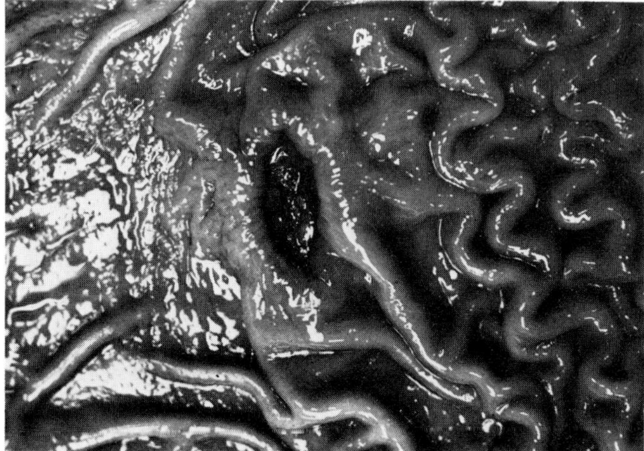

Fig. 3:   Ulcer induced by intramucosal injection of acetic acid via a gastroscope in a dog.

pathomorphological picture of the human peptic ulcer. In contrast to the erosion, the acetic acid ulcer also needs several weeks for healing [18] and it seems that aggravations do sometimes occur during the healing period (Fig. 4). The disadvantage of this model is that ulcers are induced rather artificially by necrosis of normal mucosa in otherwise healthy animals. Investigations into the healing and its influence by drugs are also handicapped by considerable variations, by lack of specificity, and by the time required for performance.

Summary

In human ulcer disease, at least 3 kinds of ulcers must be distinguished, and further subdivisions may be possible. The first are acute stress ulcers. Hypothesis models as well as the centrally induced disease models are those which have contributed essentially to our knowledge of the etiology and treatment of this disease. The second group comprises the duodenal ulcers. Disease models have helped give rise to the assumption that there may be a prevalence of aggressive factors. Consequently, various hypothesis models have led to the development of an effective drug treatment, which is based on the reduction of aggressive factors. Finally, in the gastric ulcer group, some hypothesis models are in use, but the various analogue and disease models have so far resulted in little success in studies of either the etiology or the healing process.

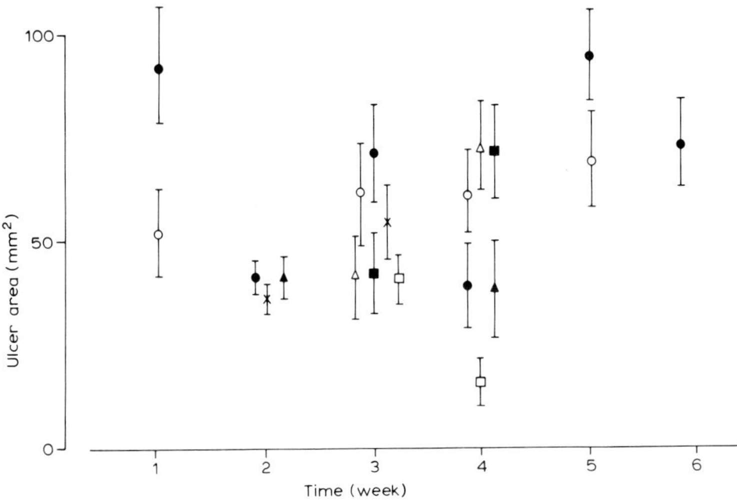

Fig. 4: Healing of acetic acid ulcer in the rat. The results of various experiments are shown: the different symbols represent the different experiments. (Mean ± SEM; n = 20.)

References

1. Black, J.W., Duncan, W.A.M., Durant, C.J. et al. (1972): Definition and antagonism of histamine H_2-receptors. *Nature (London) 236*, 385.
2. Burland, W.L. and Simkins, M.A. (Eds) (1977): *Cimetidine: Proceedings of the 2nd International Symposium on Histamine H_2-Receptor Antagonists.* Excerpta Medica, Amsterdam-Oxford.
3. Berglindh, T. (1977): Effects of common inhibitors of gastric acid secretion on secretagogue-induced respiration and aminopyrine accumulation in isolated gastric glands. *Biochem. Biophys. Acta 464*, 217.
4. Cheret, A.M., Girodet, J. and Lewin, M. (1977): Stimulation of isolated rat parietal cell by gastrin. In: *Hormonal Receptors in Digestive Tract Physiology*, p. 405. Eds: S. Bonfils, P. Fromageot and G. Rosselin. North Holland Publishing Company, Amsterdam-New York-Oxford.
5. Forte, T.M., Machen, T.E. and Forte, J.G. (1977): Ultrastructural changes in oxyntic cells associated with secretory function: a membrane-recycling hypothesis. *Gastroenterology 73*, 941.
6. Bauer, H. (1978): Therapeutisches Prinzip: Vagotomie. In: *Ulcustherapie*, pp. 159–184. Eds: A.L. Blum and J.R. Siewert. Springer Verlag, Berlin-Heidelberg-New York.
7. Blum, A.L. and Hammer, R. (Eds) (1979): *Die Behandlung des Ulcus pepticum mit Pirenzepin.* Demeter Verlag, Gräfelfing.
8. Hammer, R., Berrie, C.P., Birdsall, N.J.M. et al. (1980): Pirenzepine

distinguishes between different subclasses of muscarinic receptors. *Nature (London) 283*, 90.

9. Nielsen, S.T., Yellin, T.O., Edwards, P.N. and Large, M.S. (1979): Radioligand binding assay of H_2-receptors with [^{3}H]ICI A 5165. (Abstract). *Pharmacologist 21*, 265.

10. Hammer, R.: Unpublished results.

11. Lewin, M., Soumarmon, A., Bali, J.P. and Bonfils, S. (1976): Interaction of ^{3}H-labelled synthetic human gastrin-I with rat gastric plasma membranes. Evidence for the existence of biologically reactive gastrin receptor sites. *Febs Lett. 66*, 168.

12. Takeuchi, K., Speir, G.R. and Johnson, L.R. (1979): Mucosal gastrin receptor. I. Assay standardization and fulfillment of receptor criteria. *Am. J. Physiol. 237*, E284.

13. Sachs, G., Spenney, G.G. and Rehm, W.S. (1977): Gastric secretion. In: *International Review of Physiology: Gastrointestinal Physiology II, Vol. 12*, pp. 127–171. Ed: R.K. Crane. University Park Press, Baltimore.

14. Robert, A., Nezamis, J.E., Lancaster, C. and Hanchar, A.J. (1979): Cytoprotection by prostaglandins in rats. Prevention of gastric necrosis produced by alcohol, HCl, NaOH, hypertonic NaCl, and thermal injury. *Gastroenterology 77*, 433.

15. Shay, H., Komarov, S.A., Fels, S.S. et al. (1945): A simple method for the uniform production of gastric ulceration in the rat. *Gastroenterology 5*, 43.

16. Skoryna, S.C., Fam, F.S. and Kahn, D.S. (1971): Experience with production of experimental gastric ulcers by local thermal injury. In: *Peptic Ulcer*, pp. 138–142. Ed: C.J. Pfeiffer. Munksgaard, Copenhagen.

17. Takagi, K., Okabe, S. and Saziki, R. (1970): A new method for the production of chronic gastric ulcer in rats and the effect of several drugs on its healing. *Jpn. J. Pharmacol. 19*, 418.

18. Umehara, S., Ito, H., Tabayashi, T. et al. (1971): Studies on an experimental chronic gastric ulcer induced by the clamping-cortisone method in rats. In: *Peptic Ulcer*, pp. 118–137. Ed: C.J. Pfeiffer. Munksgaard, Copenhagen.

19. Dragstedt, L.R., Oberhelman, H.A. and Smith, C.A. (1951): Experimental hyperfunction of the gastric antrum with ulcer formation. *Ann. Surg. 134*, 332.

20. Jennewein, H.M., Ganguli, P.C., Siewert, R. and Waldeck, F. (1976): Experimental hypergastrinaemia in the dog. *Horm. Metab. Res. 8*, 455.

21. Mann, F.C. and Williamson, C.S. (1973): The experimental production of peptic ulcer. *Ann. Surg. 77*, 409.

22. Hartman, F.W. (1945): Curling's ulcer in experimental burns. *Ann. Surg. 121*, 54.

23. Hase, T. and Moss, B.J. (1973): Microvascular changes of gastric mucosa in the development of stress ulcer in rats. *Gastroenterology 65*, 224.

24. Menguy, R., Desbaillets, L. and Masters, Y.F. (1974): Mechanisms of stress ulcer: influence of hypovolemic shock on energy metabolism in the gastric mucosa. *Gastroenterology 66*, 45.

25. Rossi, G., Bonfils, S., Lieffogh, F. and Lambling, A. (1956): Technique nouvelle pour produire des ulcerations gastriques chez le rat blanc: l'ulcère de contrainte. *Compt. Rend. Soc. Biol. 150*, 2124.

26. Takagi, K. and Okabe, S. (1968): The effects of drugs on the production and recovery processes of the stress ulcer. *Jpn. J. Pharmacol. 18*, 9.

27. Watanabe, K. (1966): Some pharmacological factors involved in formation and

prevention of stress ulcer in rats. *Chem. Pharm. Bull. 14*, 101.

28. French, J.D., Porter, R.W., von Amerongen, F.K. and Raney, R.B. (1952): Gastrointestinal hemorrhage and ulceration associated with intracranial lesions. *Surgery 32*, 395.

29. Brady, J.V. (1958) Ulcers in 'executive' monkeys. *Sci. Am. 199*, 95.

30. Brodie, D.A. and Chase, B.J. (1967): Role of gastric acid in aspirin-induced gastric irritation in the rat. *Gastroenterology 53*, 604.

31. Churchill, T.P. and Van Waconer, F.H. (1932): Production of gastric and duodenal ulcers in experimental cinchophen poisoning of dogs. *Arch. Pathol. 14*, 860.

32. Djahanguiri, B. (1969): The production of acute gastric ulceration by indomethacin in the rat. *Scand. J. Gastroenterol. 4*, 265.

33. Robert, A. and Nezamis, J.E. (1958): Ulcerogenic property of steroids. *Proc. Soc. Exp. Biol. Med. 99*, 443.

34. Wax, J., Clinger, W.A., Warner, P. et al. (1970): Relationship of the enterohepatic cycle to ulcerogenesis in the rat small bowel with flufenamic acid. *Gastroenterology 58*, 722.

35. Eagleton, G.B. and Watt, J. (1965). Acute gastric ulceration in the guinea-pig induced by a single intraperitoneal injection of aqueous histamine. *J. Pathol. Bacteriol. 90*, 679.

36. Emas, S. and Grossman, M.I. (1967): Production of duodenal ulcers in cats by infusion of porcine gastrin. *Gastroenterology 52*, 959.

37. Emas, S. and Fyrö, B. (1967): Gastric and duodenal ulcers in cats following reserpine. *Acta Physiol. Scand. 71*, 316.

38. Robert, A., Stout, T.J. and Dale, J.E. (1970): Production by secretagogues of duodenal ulcers in the rat. *Gastroenterology 59*, 95.

39. Djahanguiri, B., Pousti, A. and Hemmati, M. (1969): The production of acute gastric ulceration by phenylephrine HCl in the rat. *Pharmacology 2*, 243.

40. Hedinger, C. and Veraguth, P. (1957): Magengeschwüre bei Ratten unter Behandlung mit 5-Hydroxytryptamin. *Schweiz. Med. Wochenschr. 87*, 1175.

41. Nicoloff, D.M., Peter, E.T., Leonard, A.S. and Wangensteen, O.H. (1965): Catecholamines in ulcer provocation. *J. Am. Med. Assoc. 191*, 383.

42. Berg, B.N., Zucker, T.F. and Zucker, L.M. (1949): Duodenal ulcers produced on a diet deficient in pantothenic acid. *Proc. Soc. Exp. Biol. Med. 71*, 374.

43. Robert, A. and Dale, J.E. (1971): Prevention of duodenal ulcers in rats by feeding. *Proc. Soc. Exp. Biol. Med. 136*, 439.

44. Röhm, F., Seybold, G. and Pirtkien, R. (1964): Die verschiedenen Formen des experimentellen Ulcus ventriculi bei der Ratte und seine medikamentöse Beeinflussung. *Drug Res. 14*, 47.

45. Selye, H. and Szabo, S. (1973): Experimental model for production of perforating duodenal ulcers by cysteamine in the rat. *Nature (London) 244*, 458.

46. Kitagawa, H., Fujiwara, M. and Osumi, Y. (1979): Effect of water immersion stress on gastric secretion and mucosal blood flow in rats. *Gastroenterology 77*, 298.

47. Goldman, H. and Rosoff, C.B. (1968): Pathogenesis of acute gastric ulcers. *Am. J. Pathol. 53*, 227.

48. Lorenz, W., Reimann, H.J. and Fischer, M. (1978): Pathogenese der akuten gastroduodenalen Läsion (Streßulcus). In: *Ulcus-Therapie*, pp. 50–62. Eds: A.L.

Blum and J.R. Siewert. Springer Verlag, Berlin-Heidelberg-New York.
49. Du Plessis, D.J. (1965): Pathogenesis of gastric ulceration. *Lancet I*, 974.

Discussion

Genetics and epidemiology

The discussion centered around the concept that peptic ulcer disease probably is a genetically heterogenous disease. The heterogeneity is suggested by factors like ethnic variability, associations with rare syndromes, studies using subclinical markers and other factors. Family studies have shown that duodenal ulcer disease can be separated into hyperpepsinogenemic-I and normopepsinogenemic-I types still encompassing different subgroups with characteristic functional changes such as increased gastrin release or a rapid gastric emptying pattern. Only 40% of those carrying the trait will develop clinically overt ulcer disease. It is so far unclear which other factors will play a role in the disease expression. Presumably environmental factors and perhaps additional genetic factors interact with the hyperpepsinogenemia. The elucidation of these factors which may convert a genetic predisposition into clinical disease may be conceivably of therapeutic importance and usefulness. Thus, it could be that in the future we will be able to determine subtypes of duodenal disease differing in prognosis and response to therapy.

The existence of rare, distinct genetic syndromes associated with peptic ulcer is multiple endocrine adenomatosis (Werner syndrome). The pancreatic adenomas may secrete gastrin resulting in a severe ulcer disease (Zollinger-Ellison-syndrome). That is an autosomal dominant defect, and it is clearly a genetic disease. Gastrinoma of the pancreas and associated ulcer disease may also occur as a sporadic mutation without familial aggregation and without endocrine tumors in other organs. Thus these rare disorders suggest that what we recognize as 'common' peptic ulcer may, in fact, comprise several disorders.

In relatively few epidemiologic investigations an increased frequency of ulcer disease has been elucidated since the nineteenth century. Parallel to this development there has been a change in the age incidence of the disease. Investigations from European countries within the last decades have registered incidence rates of new gastric ulcers to be nearly 0.4 per 1,000 population, and new duodenal ulcers to be between 1.0 and 2.7. The age-specific incidence rates increased with age in men and women. If there is a change in the age incidence of the disease one has to taken into consideration a dramatic change in the age-specific hospital admission rates, when compared with the general population. Age-specific hospital admission rates show that there has been a reduction of about 80% in ulcer admission, both duodenal and gastric, for younger men. This has not happened in older people, for whom there may even have been an increased hospital admission rate. Crude rates probably conceal these differences.

Environmental factors

The interpretations of the results of studies examining the association of different environmental factors with ulcer disease is often controversial due to the small number of patients studied. During the past decade numerous studies have documented that the incidence of smoking is increased in persons with ulcer disease and that both gastric and duodenal ulcers are more prevalent in smokers than in nonsmokers. In the study by Peterson et al., 78% of the antacid-treated group healed at 4 weeks as compared to 45% of the placebo group [1]. When these groups were broken down into smokers and nonsmokers, 69% of the ulcers of nonsmokers who took placebo healed, versus 32% of ulcers of smokers who took placebo ($p < 0.05$). Antacids in this study appeared to make the most difference when treating the duodenal ulcers of smokers. Smoking seems to retard ulcer healing rates in this study but other investigations in patients with gastric ulcer did not show an influence of smoking on ulcer healing [2]. The question as to whether smoking will play a role in the chances of the patient dying from his ulcer disease was examined in 4 studies [3–6]. The results show that mortality from gastric ulcer is greater in smokers than in nonsmokers except in one study including ex-smokers in the smoking group [6]. The mortality was also increased in smokers with peptic ulcer [4, 5] and duodenal ulcer disease [3].

Summarizing these epidemiologic data it appears that smokers have more than a 2-fold greater chance of dying from ulcer disease than nonsmokers. The effect of smoking on mechanisms like acid secretion, pancreatic secretion, and secretin release and pyloric reflux which are all implicated in the pathogenesis of ulcer disease has been examined by many investigators. Most studies have shown that smoking does not significantly alter acid secretion [7]. Smoking inhibits pancreatic bicarbonate secretion but there is no evidence that this is due to inhibition of secretin release [8]. The consequent lowered capacity to neutralize gastric acid in the duodenum is a plausible but yet unproven mechanism by which smoking might play a role in the occurrence of duodenal ulcer. It has been hypothesized that excessive reflux of duodenal contents through an incompetent pyloric sphincter may play a role in the pathogenesis of gastric ulcer. Manometric and radiologic studies have shown that smoking decreases basal pyloric sphincter and increases duodenogastric reflux [9, 10]. But again the relevance of these findings in the pathogenesis of gastric ulcer formation will need further investigation.

Nonsteroidal anti-inflammatory agents

The evaluation of the occurrence of peptic ulcer during the administration of anti-inflammatory drugs requires the calculation of true incidence rates. To exemplify the need for this calculation, Professor Grossman gave an estimate of the incidence of indometacin-induced ulcers based on the observation of Rothernich [11].

'In this series [11], 2 new cases of peptic ulcer among 74 patients receiving indometacin for periods of up to 30 months were observed. If we take the most conservative estimate of incidence by assuming that all patients were followed for 30 months (which was not actually the case), then the calculated annual incidence in Rothernich's study is 11 new cases per 1,000 persons per year which is to be compared with an expected incidence of 1.8 per 1,000 per year in the general population [12]. Thus, the observed rate was more than 6 times the expected rate. Furthermore, since almost all ulcers seen in persons taking anti-inflammatory drugs are gastric in location, the expected rate for this lesion is 0.13 per 1,000 per year [12] and the observed rate then becomes more than 80 times the expected rate. I have found no papers in the literature that deal correctly with the comparison of the number of observed new cases in those taking the drug with the expected number in the general population when both are expressed as new cases per 1,000 persons per year. To establish with 90% power in a one-sided test at the 5% level of significance that a certain drug doubled the incidence of gastric ulcer one would need to study more than 198,000 patients. To detect a 10-fold increase, one would need to study 7,700 patients. Among 2,200 patients taking one gram of acetylsalicylic acid per day for 3 years, the incidence of peptic ulcer diagnosed during hospitalization was 1.3% compared with 0.2% in 2,200 patients taking placebo tablets [13]'

Grossman.

Recently it has been shown that 23% of patients taking more than 3 g acetylsalicylic acid/day for more than three months will develop ulcers, confirming the high incidence of mainly prepyloric gastric ulcers in patients who receive chronic aspirin therapy [14]. Enteric-coated acetylsalicylic acid caused significantly fewer gastric ulcers than did regular or buffered acetylsalicylic acid [14]. This observation was recently confirmed by Lanza et al. [15] who evaluated endoscopically the effect of acetylsalicylic acid, buffered acetylsalicylic acid, and enteric-coated acetylsalicylic acid on gastric and duodenal mucosa. At the doses employed (those normally used to treat rheumatoid arthritis), acetylsalicylic acid and buffered acetylsalicylic acid consistently produced significantly greater mucosal damage than did enteric-coated acetylsalicylic acid or placebo in the stomach ($p < 0.01$) and duodenum ($p < 0.05$) [15]. In addition to acetylsalicylic acid, other nonsteroidal inflammatory drugs such as indometacin, ketoprofen, naproxen and others were shown to produce gastric mucosal lesions in either patients with rheumatoid arthritis or degenerative joint disease. The gastric lesions may be present in the absence of gastrointestinal symptoms [16].

In summary, the discussion of Chapter I dealt with the importance and clinical application of elevated serum pepsinogen as a marker for duodenal ulcer disease. Furthermore, the evidence for association of environmental factors and ulcer disease was discussed and critically evaluated.

Ulcer models

In the discussion Professor Lorenz and others emphasized the need for clinical scientists to look for experimental models in which ulcers are produced by mimicking circumstances that appear to be ulcerogenic in man (see Table). Some animal models have been developed along these lines [17] but the majority of animal models still rely on pharmacologic means of uncertain significance to human disease. Reasonable models exist for acute ulcerations but less so for chronic ulcer disease. Several possible models for chronic ulcer were therefore discussed. The mercaptamine model where chronic-appearing duodenal ulcers are produced by repeat administration of mercaptamine to rats is a representative example. It was pointed out that such ulcers are preventable by administration of somatostatin even though acid secretion only drops slightly. Another approach developed by Bonfils' group is antral transplantation to the colon which results in hypergastrinemia, gastric hypersecretion, and duodenal ulcerations in dogs and rats. Often it is not possible to determine whether ulcers in a given model result from an increase in aggressive factors or of a weakening of protective factors or a combination of both.

It is remarkable that even in highly artificial experimental ulcer models the same therapeutic or prophylactic agents employed in clinical medicine: antisecretory drugs, antacids, and cytoprotective agents are effective. Thus, animal models developed so far, whereas they may provide only limited

Table: Pathological states and stressful conditions associated with acute gastro-duodenal lesions.

Condition	Hypothesis tested by	
	Report or review on animal experiments	Prospective trial or reliable clinical survey
Trauma	Friesen et al.	Bowen and Fleming Glass and Stremple
Major surgery and postoperative complications	Merendino et al.	Weber et al.
Cerebral injury	Cushing	Kamada et al.
Hemorrhage shock	Menguy et al.	Goodman and Frey
Respiratory insufficiency	Mullane et al.	Skillman et al. Harris et al.
Fat embolism	Baronofsky and Wangensteen	Mears
Renal insufficiency	Mullane et al.	Fischer and Stremple
Infection (sepsis)	Rasche and Butterfield Mc Cracken et al.	Le Gall et al. Lucas et al.
Immobilization	Bonfils et al.	Holle
Psychological stress	Paré, Sawrey et al.	Wolf and Wolff
Burns	Hartman	Czaja et al. Feller
'Ulcerogenic' drugs	Robert and Nezamis Di Pasquale	Kapp et al., Welch et al. Rainford, Roth

Reproduced with permission from [17].

information as to the pathogenesis of chronic human ulcer, may be quite valuable to assess therapeutic approaches.

An intriguing feature of experimental ulcers is the progression of ulcers from one part of the stomach to another. Ulcerogenetic factors applied acutely often result in ulcers developing in the acid-secreting part of the stomach whereas chronic application of the same ulcerogenetic factors commonly results in lesions developing in the antrum and/or duodenum. There is a clinical correlate to these observations: severely burned patients or acutely-induced acetylsalicylic acid lesions tend to occur in the proximal stomach. Species differences may also determine ulcer location. Other times a slight change in the ulcerogenic insult or procedure determines a variation in the location of lesions produced. The precise reasons which determine the location of ulcers in such experimental models are unknown.

References

1. Peterson, W., Sturdevant, R.A.L., Frankl, H. et al. (1977): Healing of duodenal ulcer with an antacid regimen. *N. Engl. J. Med. 297*, 341.
2. Piper, D.W., Hunt, J. and Heap, T.R. (1980): The healing rate of chronic gastric ulcer in patients admitted to hospital. *Scand. J. Gastroenterol. 15*, 113.
3. Hammond, E.C. and Horn, D. (1958): Report on forty-four months of follow-up of 187,783 men. *J. Am. Med. Assoc. 166*, 1294.
4. Dorn, H.F. (1959): Tobacco consumption and mortality from cancer and other diseases. *Public Health. Rep. 74*, 581.
5. Doll, R. and Peto, R. (1976): Mortality in relation to smoking: 20 years' observations on male British doctors. *Br. Med. J. II*, 1525.
6. Weir, J. and Dunn, S.C. (1970): Smoking and mortality: a prospective study. *Cancer 25*, 105.
7. Debas, H., Cohen, M., Holubitsky, I. and Harrison, R. (1971): Effect of cigarette smoking on human gastric secretory responses. *Gut 12*, 93.
8. Murthy, S., Dinoso, V., Clearfield, H. and Chey, W. (1977): Simultaneous measurement of basal pancreatic, gastric acid secretion, plasma gastrin, and secretin during smoking. *Gastroenterology 73*, 758.
9. Valenzuela, J., Defilippi, C. and Csendes, A. (1976): Manometric studies on the human pyloric sphincter. *Gastroenterology 70*, 481.
10. Read, N.W. and Grech, P. (1973): Effect of cigarette smoking on competence of the pylorus: preliminary study. *Br. Med. J. III*, 313.
11. Rothernich, N.O. (1966): An extended study of indomethacin. I. Clinical pharmacology. *J. Am. Med. Assoc. 195*, 531.
12. Bonnevie, O. (1975): The incidence of duodenal ulcer in Copenhagen County. *Scand. J. Gastroenterol. 10*, 385.
13. Aspirin myocardial infarction study research group (1980): A randomized controlled trial of aspirin in persons recovered from myocardial infarction. *J. Am. Med. Assoc. 243*, 661.
14. Silvoso, G.R., Ivey, K.J., Butt, J.H. et al. (1979): Incidence of gastric lesions in patients with rheumatic disease on chronic aspirin therapy. *Ann. Intern. Med. 91*, 517.
15. Lanza, F.L., Royer, G.L. and Nelson, R.S. (1980): Endoscopic evaluation of the effects of aspirin, buffered aspirin, and enteric-coated aspirin on gastric and duodenal mucosa. *New Engl. J. Med. 303*, 136.
16. Caruso, I. and Bianchi Porro, G. (1980): Gastroscopic evaluation of anti-inflammatory agents. *Br. Med. J. I*, 75.
17. Lorenz, W., Fischer, M., Rohde, H. et al. (1980): Histamine and stress ulcer: new components in organizing a sequential trial on cimetidine prophylaxis in seriously ill patients and definition of a special group at risk (severe polytrauma). *Klin. Wochenschr. 58*, 653.

Chapter II: Pathogenesis of ulcer disease

Gastric mucus and mucosal resistance to injury

W. Domschke
Department of Medicine, University of Erlangen-Nürnberg, Erlangen, Federal Republic of Germany

In the alimentary tract, mucus is the skin of the gut. Some think of mucus as one of Nature's perfections in protection, while others consider it to be mainly a relic of our past, inherited from slippery ancestors like snails, snakes, earthworms, etc. To facilitate orientation in the field of gastric mucus, data available at present shall be compiled subsequently.

Biochemical and biophysical aspects of gastric mucus

The term 'mucosubstance' is often used synonymously with mucus. It embraces, however, at least 2 chemical terms, mucopolysaccharides and glycoproteins (Table I).

In *mucopolysaccharides*, the sugar or polysaccharide component (sulfated or nonsulfated) is the major constituent, with only a relatively small or no amino acid moiety at all. Due to the obligatory presence of L-iduronic acid and/or glucuronic acid, mucopolysaccharides show acidic reaction and, hence, may also be called acid animopolysaccharides. Gastric muco-

Table I: Gastric mucosubstances.

Mucopolysaccharides
    mostly carbohydrates
Glycoproteins
    carbohydrates plus protein core
    (a)   Neutral glycoproteins
         — fucomucins
         — dihexose-hexosamine glycoproteins
    (b)   Acid glycoproteins
         — sulfated glycoproteins
         — sialomucins

polysaccharides bear some resemblance to the glycosaminoglycans which are obviously essential for maintaining the structural integrity particularly of many connective tissues, synovial fluid, umbilical cord and cartilages [1].

In *glycoproteins*, the protein constituent is more essential. A peptide core is linked to oligosaccharide chains via O-(or N-)glycosidic bonds between serine, aspartic acid and/or threonine and N-acetylgalactosamine residues [2]. *Neutral* glycoproteins contain neutral carbohydrate groups (e.g., fucose or dihexose-hexosamines). Many of these compounds are structurally related to blood group antigens and serum glycoproteins. *Acid* glycoproteins are of 2 types: sulfated glycoproteins and mucins containing sialic acids. Sulfated glycoproteins appear to be less important quantitatively in human gastric secretion than in that of the dog. Sulfates, if detected at all in human gastric juice, mostly stem from contaminating salivary secretions [3]. In man, neutral and sialic acid containing glycoproteins form the bulk of gastric muco-substances and thus they are mainly responsible for the viscous and gel-forming properties of mucus.

Gastric mucus glycoproteins are characterized by a high carbohydrate to protein ratio, the carbohydrate usually constituting more than 65% of the dry weight. Glycoproteins typically have a 'bottle-brush' structure in that a large number of carbohydrate side-chains are attached like bristles to a protein core.

Among the different types of monosaccharide residues, sialic acids have attracted special interest. Sialic acid is the general name given to any substituted neuraminic acid. In humans, the only important sialic acid is N-acetylneuraminic acid (NANA). On glycoprotein sugar side-chains, NANA residues are always in a terminal position. This is important in that NANA bears a carboxyl group which gives the molecule a strongly negative charge. The function of these negatively-charged residues is not entirely clear, although, at least in some conditions, it is important in determining the tertiary structure of the glycoprotein. There will be mutual repulsion between negatively-charged groups residing on adjacent carbohydrate chains, resulting in an expansion of the tertiary structure of the molecule and a rise in its viscous properties. Evidence has been provided that this is a feature at least of sheep submaxillary gland mucus [4], pig gastric mucus [5], and rat intestinal mucus glycoproteins [6].

The second structural feature affecting the viscosity and gel-forming properties of gastric mucus glycoprotein, at least in the pig, is the polymerization of the classical bottle-brush shaped glycoprotein subunits into the native glycoprotein. According to the 'windmill' model of Allen and Snary [7], 4 typical but not necessarily identical glycoprotein arms (molecular weight, 5×10^5) are connected centrally via disulfide bonds between nonglycosylated peptide areas to form the native glycoprotein (molecular weight, 2×10^6). This structure is illustrated in Figure 1. The polymerized glycoprotein can be split again into the 4 subunits by disulfide-bond-breaking reagents such as mercaptoethanol or dithiothreitol, and by proteolytic enzymes such as trypsin, pepsin and pronase. The glycosylated region of each glycoprotein subunit constitutes about 75% of the protein core and consists of about 160 carbohydrate side-chains with an average of 15 sugar residues per chain [8].

The function of gastric mucus, particularly lubrication and protection, eventually depends on the formation of a water-insoluble viscogelatinous covering of the surface mucosa. Such cover is provided by gel formation, which occurs at a concentration of 30–40 mg/ml of glycoprotein. At this point of concentration, which is achieved at the mucosal surface, strong nonconvalent intermolecular interactions develop, leading to the formation of viscous, sticky mucus gel. The mucus gel can be completely resolubilized by guanidinium chloride or by homogenization in water, demonstrating that the gel is stabilized solely by noncovalent interactions between the component glycoprotein molecules [9].

In summary, the viscosity of gastric mucus glycoprotein depends: on the presence of negatively-charged groups (particularly NANA residues) in the 'bottle-brush' subunit structure; on the degree of subunit polymerization to result in 'windmill'-shaped molecules; and on the gel-forming properties of the 'windmill'-stuctured glycoproteins.

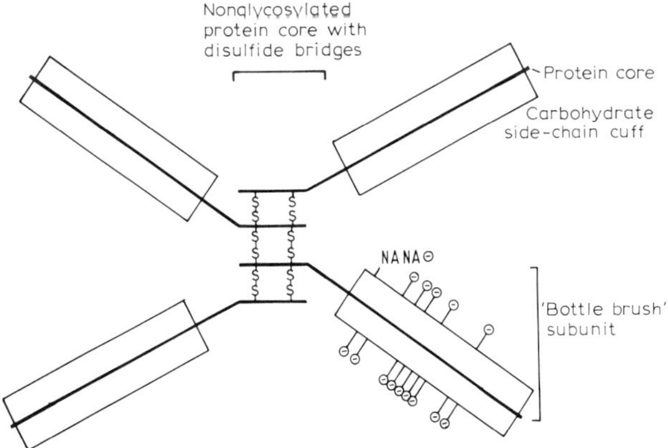

Fig. 1: Quaternary structure of gastric mucus glycoprotein, the 'windmill' model (adapted from [5]). NANA⁻ = negatively-charged N-acetylneuraminic acid residue.

Regulation of gastric mucus secretion

Knowledge of the mechanisms and control of gastric mucus secretion is meager and mostly somewhat circumstantial. It seems, however, unanimously accepted that mucus is secreted continuously in healthy man, even during resting conditions. There is no evidence that usual stimulants of gastric acid output (e.g., feeding, gastrin or histamine) exert any appreciable influence on mucus secretion (Table II) [10]. With respect to the effects of secretin, parasympathetic and sympathetic neurotransmitters, general conclusions are difficult to reach at present. Acetylcholine, for example, was thought to provide the major physiologic stimulus to gastric mucus discharge [11]. However, these studies were so designed that the effect of vagally-stimulated gastric acid secretion per se on the mucus glands could not be eliminated as a possible cause of the increase of mucus secretion after vagal stimulation. With vagally innervated and denervated antral pouches in dogs, the administration of pilocarpine or acetylcholine proved to be entirely ineffective as to stimulation of mucus secretion [12]. More positive results have been obtained with serotonin and prostaglandins. Serotonin has been shown to stimulate mucus production in the gastrointestinal tract of dogs [10]. As entero-chromaffin cells produce serotonin and lie in close vicinity to mucus-producing cells, it is tempting to assume that local serotonin production might normally influence mucus production by paracrine action. The same may be

Table II: Stimuli of gastric mucus release.

Feeding	−
Gastrin	−
Histamine	−
Secretin	?
Acetylcholine	?
Epinephrine	?
Serotonin	+
Prostaglandins	+
Ethanol	+
Mechanical irritation	+
Acid	+

− = no apparent influence on secretion.
? = questionable influence on secretion.
+ = positive influence on secretion.

true for endogenous prostaglandins, as the oral administration of E_1- and, even more, E_2-type prostaglandins has been demonstrated to significantly enhance gastric mucus production in man [±13–15]. Finally, convincing evidence has been reported that local irritants such as ethanol [16] and even mechanical irritation appear to trigger gastric mucus discharge. So, increase in mucus secretion may be interpreted to occur, at least in part, as a response to aggressive forces. Accordingly, acidification of the gastric mucosa in dogs has been demonstrated to be the most potent stimulus to mucus secretion [10]. In man, gastric acid secretory rates and mucus output data seem to be linearly related. In gastric ulcer patients, however, acid secretion prevails over mucus release.

It is also in keeping with the concept of mucus stimulation by acid that, in patients with duodenal ulceration known for supranormal gastric acid secretory rates, the viscosity of gastric mucus has been shown to be significantly greater than in control subjects [17]. A surplus in gastric mucus production in duodenal ulcer patients can be interpreted in different ways. Firstly, it could be the consequence of an enhanced driving force common for both acid and mucus secretion (cholinergic stimulation, however, is still a matter of debate in the regulation of mucus production). Secondly, it could represent the protective reaction of the mucosa to the acid irritant. Thirdly, increased mucus release could be an inborn error of metabolism which might be causative for the acid hypersecretion, in that the presence of thick tenacious mucus covering the antral mucosa may block the pH receptors and, in so doing, prevent the normal mechanism of inhibition of acid secretion from taking place [18].

Mucus and gastric disease

As to the role of mucus in the pathogenesis of gastric disease, a good deal of controversy still exists. For instance, the incrimination of mucus as being potentially involved in ulcerogenesis is essentially based on a lack of evidence indicating that any other substance plays a dominant role.

Investigations of the pathogenetic significance of gastric mucus should aim at clarification of the following points: quantitative changes in mucus concentration and output; qualitative changes in mucus composition; altered desquamation rates of mucus-containing surface epithelial cells; and abnormalities of mucus glycoprotein biosynthesis. Changes in mucus concentration, output and composition can be detected by the biochemical techniques referred to earlier in the present paper. Epithelial cell shedding rates can be measured using the DNA assay in gastric washings [19].

Glycoprotein biosynthesis can be estimated best in biopsy particles by the incorporation of radioactive glucose into glucosamine, galactose into galactosamine, and of radioactive glucosamine or N-acetylneuraminic acid into glycoproteins [20].

In studies along these lines beginning in 1950, the problem of the deficiency of mucus in gastric ulcer has repeatedly been taken up [21]. So far, however, it has not been solved conclusively. Most of the studies in man have dealt with gastric aspirates (that is to say, mainly with the water-soluble mucus). Studies of this kind allow for quantitative estimation of mucus being released into the gastric lumen. Fortunately enough, biochemical and physical analysis of the water-soluble mucus from aspirates in comparison with the water-insoluble mucus sticking to the stomach wall gave identical results after the insoluble mucus gel had been completely solubilized by means of proteolytic enzyme treatment [22]. In other words, the carbohydrate side-chain composition of soluble mucus directly reflects that of the insoluble one, and thus can be used as an index of the latter. In addition to mucus analysis in gastric aspirates, gastric mucosal biopsy particles can be employed for determination of the stationary mucosal mucus concentration and composition, as well as for estimation of mucosal glycoprotein biosynthesis activity. Viewing the data available at present, the picture arising seems not entirely uniform; it presents, however, with some characteristic lines.

Gastric juice mucus analysis has revealed that, at least during histamine stimulation, the mucus production of gastric ulcer patients is frequently too low to compensate for their enhanced acid secretion, while in healthy subjects both gastric acid and mucus outputs were reported to increase in a more balanced ratio [23]. On the other hand, Roberts-Thomson et al. were unable to find significant differences between the carbohydrate composition of glycoproteins from patients with chronic gastric ulcer and that of gastric glycoproteins from control subjects [24]. It deserves mention, however, that these authors used a more drastic hydrolysis procedure for the determination of sialic acids than is usually recommended. Employing mild hydrolysis conditions, which ensure conservation of NANA residues [25, 26], Domschke et al. [27] and Gheorghiu et al. [28] demonstrated that, in gastric ulcer patients, the gastric output of glycoprotein-bound NANA is significantly lower than in healthy controls. These results are in keeping with data reported by Johnston et al. who, in gastric mucosal biopsies from patients with gastric ulcer disease, were able to show glycoprotein biosynthesis to be markedly reduced from normal [29]. Stationary concentrations of total glycoprotein sialic acids, however, were found unchanged in the ulcer condition as compared to controls [30].

In studies in patients with gastric ulceration, the rate of exfoliation of gastric epithelial cells was determined to be markedly elevated over normal, concomitant with the defective secretion of gastric mucus glycoproteins [31]. In other words, there seems to be an inverse correlation between gastric mucus secretory rates and epithelial cell turnover, suggesting that the longer the lifespan of the cell, the more mucus is produced. In gastric ulcer, the shortened life-cycle of gastric epithelial cells results in a shorter period during which synthesis and secretion of mucus can occur.

Drugs and gastric mucus

There are a number of drugs which may cause inhibition or stimulation of gastric mucus secretion. Knowledge of this data should improve understanding of the mode of action of both drugs with noxious side effects and therapeutic agents exerting beneficial effects.

In general, it appears that drugs which inhibit gastric glycoprotein production, when administered to patients for the treatment of various disorders, are capable of causing upper gastrointestinal injuries such as erosions or ulceration. Drugs of this kind particularly include anti-inflammatory agents such as salicylates, phenylbutazone, indometacin, cortisone and adrenocorticotropin (Table III). These drugs may also delay ulcer healing and favor perforation and hemorrhage.

The mechanism of the gastrointestinal irritation induced by the drugs mentioned above (namely, impairment of mucus synthesis and loss of

Table III: Drugs affecting synthesis and/or secretion of gastric mucosubstances.

Inhibition
    Salicylates
    Phenylbutazone
    Indometacin
    Corticosteroids

No Effect
    Estrogens
    Gestagens
    H_2-receptor antagonists

Stimulation
    Papaverine
    Prostaglandins
    Carbenoxolone

integrity of the gastric mucus barrier) has been studied most intensively with acetylsalicylic acid. Contrary to phenylbutazone and indometacin, which do not pass from the blood to the gastric secretion, salicylates pass easily into the stomach from the circulation. When dogs with vagally-denervated gastric-antral pouches received acetylsalicylic acid, the rate of mucus secretion from the pouches decreased substantially [32]. Following acetylsalicylic acid, the mucus was altered biochemically in that the concentration of protein-bound carbohydrates, particularly sialic acids and hexosamines, was significantly reduced. Reduction of gastric mucus biosynthesis by oral acetylsalicylic acid was demonstrated in rats, exhibiting a significant decrease in the rate of incorporation of N-acetyl(^{3}H)glucosamine into gastric glycoproteins [33]. Similar studies on the effects of phenylbutazone, indometacin and corticosteroids on the synthesis of gastric mucus have been carried out in the rat and ferret [33]; the rates of incorporation of both N-acetyl-(^{3}H)-glucosamine and ^{14}C-galactose into rat gastric mucosal glycoprotein were inhibited by administration of any of these 3 drugs. Acetylsalicylic acid and phenylbutazone also diminished the hexose content of the gastric mucus glycoprotein, from which it may be inferred that those drugs inhibit the synthesis of mucus glycoprotein by impairment of glycosylation. Menguy and Desbaillets reported a reduction of the antral mucus during the administration of phenylbutazone, indometacin, cortisone and adrenocorticotropin to dogs, with a considerably lower carbohydrate proportion in mucus glycoproteins than that determined during control and recovery periods [34]. Finally, a decreased gastric mucus release, as indicated by glycoprotein-bound NANA output, has been established following glucocorticoid treatment in man [35, 36]. Anti-inflammatory drugs not only reduce gastric mucus production but also enhance the exfoliation of gastric epithelial mucous cells, as was observed in dog Heidenhain pouches. The same was true in man in that the gastric DNA loss, taken as a measure of the degree of shedding of mucosal cells into the gastric lumen, was markedly increased. On the other hand, following cortisone or adrenocorticotropin, the rate of cell exfoliation fell significantly.

As a matter of fact, there are many drugs which do not exert any appreciable effect on gastric mucus properties. However, in some of these (Table III), the noneffect is unexpected or deserves special mention. Estrogens, for instance, greatly stimulate production of endocervical mucus of the thin, watery type while, on the other hand, synthesis of the viscous luteal phase type of cervical mucus is essentially enhanced by gestagens. Interestingly enough, neither estrogens nor gestagens, though administered in high dosage for 4 weeks, were able to convert gastric mucus properties in man [unpublished results]. The same held true for histamine H$_2$-receptor antagonists studied in both the cimetidine [37] and the ranitidine formulations [38].

The pronounced gastric acid inhibitory property of certain prostaglandins prompted investigations as to whether these compounds also exert an anti-ulcer influence. Indeed, it was found that antisecretory prostaglandins could heal gastric and duodenal ulcers in man and prevent experimental ulcers produced by various methods in rats, cats, and guinea pigs. Later on, however, it became clear that the prevention of gastrointestinal ulcers by prostaglandins was not only a consequence of reduced acid secretion, but that many prostaglandins and prostaglandin analogues exhibit anti-ulcer activity irrespective of their ability to inhibit acid secretion [39]. This additional property of prostaglandins has been termed 'cytoprotection', and it might be due, at least in part, to stimulation of gastric mucus secretion, as has been established in rat [40], dog [41] and man [42].

Carbenoxolone, a pentacyclic triterpene related to an extract from liquorice root, is a particularly interesting drug because of its unique effect in accelerating the healing of peptic ulcer without an appreciable effect on acid or pepsin secretion. This drug, however, enhances the synthesis and output of gastric mucus in both human patients [43] and experimental animals, and markedly enhances the rates of incorporation of a number of radioactively-labelled sugar moieties [29]. These effects were not seen with preparations of human duodenal mucosa. It has consequently been suggested that one mode of action of carbenoxolone is to enhance the synthesis of gastric mucus by increasing the activities of the microsomal glycosyl transferases, and thus to strengthen the protection of the gastric mucosa against the corrosive actions of acid, pepsin, and bile. As shown in Figure 2, the gastric secretion of glycoprotein-bound NANA in gastric ulcer patients is indeed increased after 4 weeks' carbenoxolone therapy, while there is only a slight and insignificant elevation of mucus output following 4 weeks of cimetidine. Conversely, the gastric DNA loss rates, which were markedly higher than normal at the time of diagnosis, fell significantly towards normal in these same patients after treatment with carbenoxolone, while gastric epithelial shedding rates remained almost unchanged after cimetidine (Fig. 3). Hence, some relationship between cell turnover (as measured by DNA loss into the gastric juice) and mucus secretion (as expressed in terms of glycoprotein-bound NANA output) is apparent. When the mucosa is normal and the epithelial cells survive their full lifespan to produce normal adult cells, they also produce a full complement of mature mucus. When the loss and turnover is high (as in the gastric ulcer condition), the cells survive a short time, they are immature and the amount of mucus produced is smaller. This state of affairs

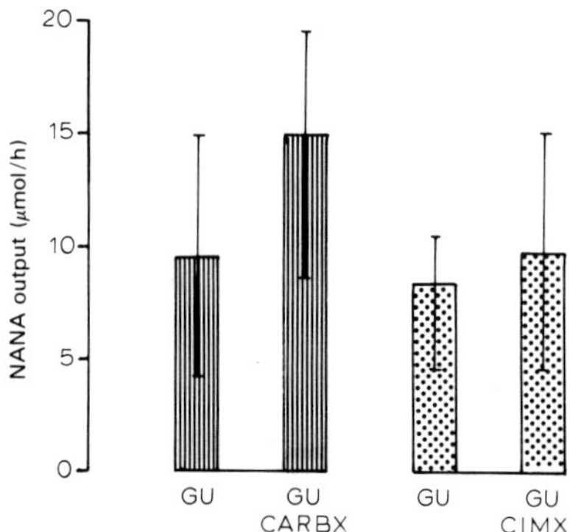

Fig. 2:   Gastric NANA (mucus) output. Paired data from 17 patients (GU and GU-CARBX) and 9 patients (GU, GU-CIMX) with gastric ulcer (GU) before and after 4 weeks' treatment with either carbenoxolone (CARBX) or cimetidine (CIMX; 1 g/day). GU-CARBX vs. GU:p<0.01. Means ± SD and medians with 95% confidence limits.

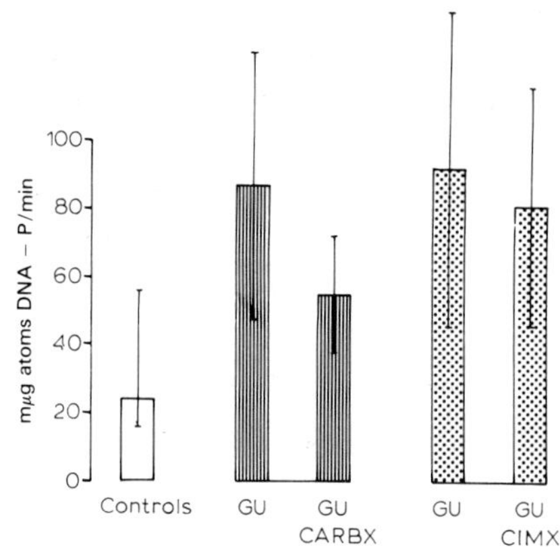

Fig. 3:   Rate of gastric DNA (cell) loss in 19 control subjects, and 17 patients (GU, GU-CARBX) and 9 patients (GU, GU-CIMX) with gastric ulcer (GU) before and after 4 weeks' therapy with either carbenoxolone (CARBX) or cimetidine (CIMX; 1 g/day). GU-CARBX vs. GU: p<0.01. DNA = deoxyribonucleic acid, P = phosphorus. Means± SD and medians with 95% confidence limits.

obviously is returned towards normal by carbenoxolone [31].

Interestingly enough, some relationship between carbenoxolone and endogenous prostaglandin metabolism has been detected, in that the drug inhibits gastric prostaglandin dehydrogenase and Δ13 reductase, enzymes which usually deactivate the prostaglandins (Fig. 4; [43]). Consequently, prolongation of endogenous prostaglandin activity may be assumed, and it is tempting to speculate that stimulation of gastric mucus secretion by carbenoxolone is mediated through increased endogenous prostaglandins. On the other hand, inhibition of mucus secretion by salicylates, indometacin and glucocorticoids may be referred to decreased levels of endogenous prostaglandins as being the consequence of diminished synthesis (Fig. 4) [44].

In summary, a review of the presently available data reveals that some evidence has accumulated that, in a considerable number of drug effects on gastric mucus secretion, the endogenous prostaglandins play a role as common mediators.

Function of gastric mucus

Despite widely-held assumptions about the function of secreted mucus (such as lubrication, water-proofing, interaction with bacteria and protection of surface epithelial cells), direct evidence of an in-vivo function for mucus does not exist. The time-honored concept that mucus protects mucosal surfaces from potentially injurious acids and proteolytic enzymes is based on circumstantial evidence, in that it generally appears that drugs which inhibit gastric glycoprotein synthesis (e.g., salicylates, indometacin, phenylbutazone, steroids) aggravate ulceration, while those which stimulate glycoprotein production and secretion (e.g., carbenoxolone, prostaglandins) promote ulcer healing. In an attempt to substantiate what gastric protection is, a differentiation between the 'gastric mucus barrier' and the 'gastric mucosal

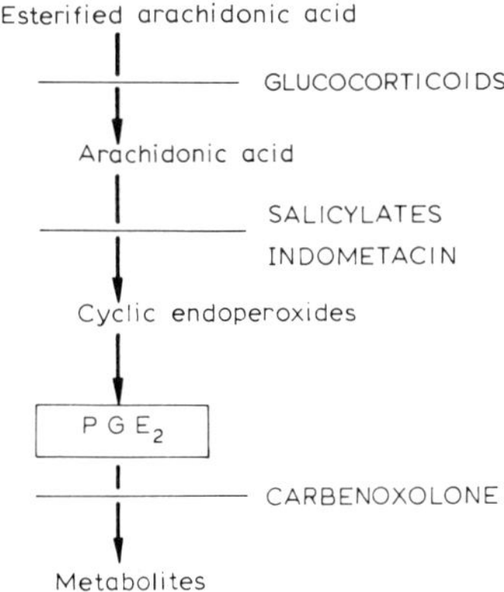

Fig. 4:   Interference of various drugs with prostaglandin (PG) metabolism.

barrier' should be made. The *mucus* barrier is provided by the mucus layer adherent to the stomach wall, and this layer has been postulated as the 'first line of defense' [45]. As a 'second line of defense', the epithelial cells themselves have been thought to play a part in constituting the *mucosal* barrier. The mucosa was assumed to have the ability to prevent diffusion of hydrogen ions from the gastric lumen into the interstitial space and the passage of sodium ions in the opposite direction. This hypothesis of 'back-diffusion of acid' was systematically tested by Teorell in the early 1950s [46] and, consequently, has been further extended to explain the increased disappearance of acid in various pathological states of the stomach. However, this concept has been repeatedly questioned since the publication of Teorell's data and, hence, gastric acid back-diffusion is at present still a matter of debate [47]. It might rather be that disappearance of acid from the stomach lumen is due to neutralization of hydrogen ions by bicarbonate ions secreted from epithelial cells.

As to the role of the gastric mucus barrier (i.e., the thin layer of mucus that is adherent to the surface of epithelial cells), this was best explained by Heatley, who suggested that the mucus barrier represents some 'unstirred layer' which can be freely penetrated by H^+ ions from the luminal side and by HCO_3^- ions from the cell surface plane [48]. In other words, the mucus layer may function as a 'mixing barrier' in which hydrogen and bicarbonate ions meet, resulting in a pH gradient with low pH levels existing on the luminal side and alkaline levels on the cell surface side. Consequently, the epithelial cells should under normal circumstances be protected from the highly acid gastric content, while they should be more closely exposed to acid in states of reduced mucus layer thickness.

Summary

In gastric ulceration, but not in the duodenal ulcer condition, the gastric mucosal glycoprotein biosynthesis and mucus secretion have been demonstrated by several authors to be characteristically reduced. Similar reductions have been reported in patients following administration of a number of anti-inflammatory drugs, such as salicylates, phenylbutazone, indometacin and corticosteroids, which are capable of causing upper gastrointestinal injury. The decrease in mucus production is inversely related to enhanced gastric epithelial cell turnover, suggesting that, in disease states, cell proliferation prevails over maturation. It has been speculated that impairment of mucus production may entail ill-functioning of the gastric mucus barrrier, which normally serves as an 'unstirred layer'-like mixing compartment for luminal hydrogen and epithelial bicarbonate ions. Consequently, it is assumed that, in disease states, the gastric mucosa is more closely exposed to the noxious acid-pepsin content of the stomach lumen. It must be admitted, however, that the changes in mucus secretion may not be a critical causal factor of gastric mucosal injury, but rather another manifestation of the causal factor. In either case, therapy with drugs such as carbenoxolone or prostaglandins improves the situation in patients with gastric ulcer by allowing the epithelial cells to mature to adulthood and to increase mucus production towards normal levels. Whether or not this effect causes or is just concomitant to drug-induced healing of gastric ulceration awaits further clarification.

References

1. Lindahl, U. and Höök, M. (1978): Glycosaminoglycans and their binding to biological macromolecules. *Ann. Rev. Biochem. 47*, 385.
2. Spiro, R.G. (1969): Glycoproteins. Their biochemistry, biology and role in human disease. *N. Engl. J. Med. 281*, 991.
3. Lambert, R., André, C. and Bérard, A. (1971): Origin of the sulfated glycoproteins in human gastric secretions. *Digestion 4*, 234.
4. Gottschalk, A. (1960): Correlation between composition, structure, shape, and function of a salivary mucoprotein. *Nature (London) 186*, 949.
5. Clamp, J.R., Allen, A., Gibbons, R.A. and Roberts, G.P. (1978): Chemical aspects of mucus. *Br. Med. Bull. 34*, 25.
6. Forstner, J.F., Jabbal, I. and Forstner, G.G. (1973): Goblet cell mucin of rat small intestine. Chemical and physical characterization. *Can. J. Biochem. 51*, 1154.
7. Allen, A. and Snary, D. (1972): The structure and function of gastric mucus. *Gut 13*, 666.
8. Starkey, B.J., Snary, D. and Allen, A. (1974): Characterization of gastric mucoproteins isolated by equilibrium density gradient centrifugation in caesium chloride. *Biochem. J. 141*, 633.
9. Allen, A., Pain, R.H. and Robson, T.R. (1976): Model for the structure of the gastric mucus gel. *Nature (London) 264*, 88.
10. Menguy, R. and Thompson, A.E. (1967): Regulation of secretion of mucus from the gastric antrum. *Ann. N.Y. Acad. Sci. 140*, 797.
11. Bottin, C., Zeitoun, P. and Lehy, T. (1973): Excrétion des mucines des glandes pyloriques chez le rat après stimulation cholinergique. *Biol. Gastroenterol. 6*, 307.
12. Menguy, R. (1969): Gastric mucus and the gastric mucous barrier. *Ann. J. Surg. 117*, 806.
13. Domschke, W., Domschke, S., Hornig, D. and Demling, L. (1978): Prostaglandin-stimulated gastric mucus secretion in man. *Acta Hepato-Gastroenterol. 25*, 292.
14. Johansson, C. and Kollberg, B. (1979): Stimulation by intragastrically

administered E_2 prostaglandins of human gastric mucus output. *Eur. J. Clin. Invest. 9,* 229.

15. Ruppin, H., Person, B., Robert, A. and Domschke, W. (1979): Zytoprotektive Wirkungen von Prostaglandin E_2 auf die Magenschleimhaut beim Menschen. *Dtsch. Med. Wochenschr. 104,* 1457.

16. Florey, H. (1955): Mucus and the protection of the body. *Proc. R. Soc. (London) Ser. B. Biol. Sci. 143,* 144.

17. Pringle, R. (1977): Gastric mucus viscosity and peptic ulcer. In: *Mucus in Health and Disease*, p. 227. Eds: M. Elstein and D.V. Parke. Plenum Press, New York.

18. Curt, J.R.N. and Pringle, R. (1969): Viscosity of gastric mucus in duodenal ulceration. *Gut 10,* 931.

19. Croft, D.N., Pollock, D.J. and Coghill, N.F. (1966): Cell loss from human gastric mucosa measured by the estimation of deoxyribonucleic acid in gastric washings. *Gut 7,* 333.

20. Lukie, B.E. and Forstner, G.G. (1972): Synthesis of intestinal glycoprotein. Incorporation of $(1-^{14}C)$glucosamine in vitro. *Biochim. Biophys. Acta 261,* 353.

21. Glass, G.B.J., Barowsky, H. and Schwartz, S.A. (1950): Correlation of secretory patterns of gastric mucous substances with gastroscopic findings in humans; their significance for the diagnosis of 'atrophic gastritis'. *Gastroenterology 19,* 829.

22. Snary, D. and Allen, A. (1972): Studies on gastric mucoproteins: The production of radioactive mucoproteins by pig gastric mucosal scrapings in vitro. *Biochem. J. 127,* 577.

23. Carlborg, L., Dahlgren, S. and Nordgren, B. (1970): Gastric secretion of hydrochloric acid and sialic acid in patients with peptic ulcer and gastric cancer during intravenous infusion of histamine. *Scand. J. Gastroenterol. 5,* 427.

24. Roberts-Thomson, I.C., Clarke, A.E., Maritz, V.M. and Denborough, M.A. (1975): Gastric glycoproteins in chronic peptic ulcer. *Aust. N. Z. J. Med. 5,* 507.

25. Warren, L. (1959): The thiobarbituric acid assay of sialic acids. *J. Biol. Chem. 234,* 1971.

26. Warren, L. (1959): Sialic acid in human semen and in the male genital tract. *J. Clin. Invest. 38,* 755.

27. Domschke, W., Domschke, S., Classen, M. and Demling, L. (1972): Some properties of mucus in patients with gastric ulcer. Effect of treatment with carbenoxolone sodium. *Scand. J. Gastroenterol. 7,* 647.

28. Gheorghiu, Th., Frotz, H., Klein, H.J. and Hübner, G. (1973): *Das hepatogene Ulkus. Magenschleim und Ulzerogenese.* Witzstrock Verlag, Baden-Baden.

29. Johnston, B., Lindup, W.E., Shillingford, J.S. et al. (1975): The pharmacological biochemistry of carbenoxolone. Its effects on gastric mucus. In: *Fourth Symposium of Carbenoxolone*, p. 3. Eds: F. Avery-Jones and D.V. Parke. Butterworths, London.

30. Roberts, S.H., Heffernan, C. and Douglas, A.P. (1975): The sialic acid and carbohydrate content and the synthesis of glycoprotein from radioactive precursors by tissues of the normal and diseased upper intestinal tract. *Clin. Chim. Acta 63,* 121.

31. Domschke, W., Domschke, S., Hagel, J. et al. (1977): Gastric epithelial cell turnover, mucus production, and healing of gastric ulcers with carbenoxolone. *Gut 18,* 817.

32. Menguy, R. and Masters, Y.F. (1965): Effects of aspirin on gastric mucous secretion. *Surg. Gynecol. Obstet. 120,* 92.

33. Dekanski, J.B., MacDonald, A., Sacra, P. and Parke, D.V. (1975): Effects of fasting, stress and drugs on gastric glycoprotein synthesis in the rat. *Br. J. Pharmacol. 55*, 387.

34. Menguy, R. and Desbaillets, L. (1968): The gastric mucous barrier: influence of protein-bound carbohydrate in mucus on the rate of proteolysis of gastric mucus. *Ann. Surg. 168*, 475.

35. Kuhn, D. (1974): Kohlenhydratreiche Proteine des Magensaftes und Magenschleims unter dem Einfluß von Cortisonderivaten. *Med. Klin. 69*, 694.

36. Domschke, W., Domschke, S., Huber, W. and Demling, L. (1977): Glucocorticoid and mineralocorticoid actions on gastric secretion in man. *Acta Hepato-Gastroenterol. 24*, 34.

37. Domschke, W., Domschke, S., Lux, G. et al. (1976): Wirksame Cimetidin-Therapie beim Ulcus duodeni. Ergebnisse einer Doppelblindstudie. *Dtsch. Med. Wochenschr. 101*, 1752.

38. Domschke, S., Lux, G. and Domschke, W. (1980): Effect of ranitidine on pentagastrin-induced gastric secretion of pepsin and N-acetylneuraminic acid (NANA) in man. *Gastroenterology 78*, 1158.

39. Robert, A. (1976): Antisecretory, antiulcer, cytoprotective and diarrheogenic properties of prostaglandins. In: *Advances in Prostaglandin and Thromboxane Research*, Vol. II, p. 507. Eds: B. Samuelsson and R. Paoletti. Raven Press, New York.

40. Bolton, J.P., Palmer, D. and Cohen, M.M. (1976): Effect of the E_2 prostaglandins on gastric mucus production in rats. *Surg. Forum 27*, 402.

41. Bolton, J.P. and Cohen, M.M. (1978): Stimulation of non-parietal cell secretion in canine Heidenhain pouches by 16,16-dimethyl prostaglandin E_2. *Digestion 17*, 291.

42. Domschke, W., Domschke, S., Hornig, D. and Demling, L. (1978): Prostaglandin-stimulated gastric mucus secretion in man. *Acta Hepato-Gastroenterol. 25*, 292.

43. Domschke, W., Domschke, S., Classen, M. and Demling, L. (1972): Some properties of mucus in patients with gastric ulcer. Effect of treatment with carbenoxolone sodium. *Scand. J. Gastroenterol. 7*, 647.

44. Peskar, B.M. (1977): On the synthesis of prostaglandins by human gastric mucosa and its modification by drugs. *Biochim. Biophys. Acta 487*, 307.

45. Hollander, F. (1954): The two-component mucous barrier. *Arch. Int. Med. 93*, 107.

46. Teorell, T. (1953): Transport processes and electrical phenomena in ionic membranes. *Prog. Biophys. Chem. 3*, 305.

47. Thjodleifsson, B. and Wormsley, K.G. (1977): Back-diffusion — fact or fiction? *Digestion 15*, 53.

48. Heatley, N.G. (1959): Mucosubstance as a barrier to diffusion. *Gastroenterology 37*, 313.

Prostaglandins as cytoprotective factors

A. Robert
Department of Experimental Biology, The Upjohn Company, Kalamazoo, Michigan, U.S.A.

Peptic ulcer and various forms of gastritis are likely to result from the interaction of 2 factors: the contact of the gastroduodenal mucosa with noxious agents on the one hand, and a decreased resistance of the mucosa to these agents. Examples of noxious agents include the acid-pepsin complex, certain drugs such as nonsteroidal anti-inflammatory compounds including acetylsalicylic acid, corticosteroids, and chemotherapeutic agents, and antiparietal cell antibodies. Agents and conditions capable of increasing gastroduodenal mucosal resistance are not well identified. I will describe here the role of prostaglandins (PG) as cytoprotective agents.

Definition of cytoprotection

This term refers to the property of several PG to protect the mucosa of the stomach and the intestine against becoming inflamed and necrotic, when this mucosa is exposed to noxious agents.

Examples of cytoprotection

Animals

Chemicals such as absolute ethanol, 0.6 N HCl, 0.2 N NaOH, 25% NaCl solution, 80 mM of taurocholic acid, 200 mg/kg of acetylsalicylic acid, as well as boiling water, when given orally to fasted rats produce extensive necrosis of the gastric mucosa. By giving very small amounts of certain PG, either orally or subcutaneously, just a few minutes before the necrotizing agents, the stomach remains intact [1–3]. Some of the PG that were found to be cytoprotective and their potency are shown in the Table.

The gastric mucosal barrier constitutes a natural protection against the

Table: Cytoprotection by various prostaglandins.

Prostaglandin	Oral ED_{50} (μg/kg)	Subcutaneous ED_{50} (μg/kg)
16,16-dimethyl PGE_2	0.05	0.15
16,16-dimethyl PGA_2	10	—
PGE_2	25	75
15(S)-15-methyl $PGF_{2\beta}$	50	—
15(R)-15-methyl $PGF_{2\beta}$	75	—

The ED_{50} is the minimum dose which reduces the number of gastric lesions produced by oral administration of absolute ethanol by 50%.

back-diffusion of acid already secreted into the gastric lumen. Strong irritants, however, when placed in the stomach, can break this barrier and allow acid back-diffusion. Chemicals such as ethanol, bile acids and acetylsalicylic acid are barrier breakers [4]. In the dog, the breaking of the gastric mucosal barrier by various agents was prevented by administration of several PG, including PGE_2 [5], 16,16-dimethyl PGE_2 [6, 7], and PGI_2 [8]. These PG prevented H^+ back-diffusion and efflux of Na^+ into the lumen, changes characteristic of a broken mucosal barrier. Similar protection was found for 15(S)-15-methyl PGE_2 in rats given taurocholic acid and indometacin [9].

Humans

Nonsteroidal anti-inflammatory compounds are known to damage the gastric mucosa. Lesions ranging from erosive gastritis to hemorrhagic gastritis as well as frank ulcers have been reported. One consequence of the gastric injury is to increase the amount of occult blood lost in the feces, from less than 1 ml/day (which is normal) to 8 ml or more [10]. Administration of PGE_2 (1 mg) 30 minutes before taking either acetylsalicylic acid (666 mg or 2 tablets 4 times a day) or indometacin (50 mg 3 times a day) prevented this increase in occult blood by protecting the stomach against damage caused by the NOSAC [11–13].

In another study the amount of deoxyribonucleic acid (DNA) present in gastric washings was measured as an indication of cell desquamation (since DNA comes from cell nuclei). DNA was increased 3-fold by oral administration of 50 ml of 40% ethanol. Treatment 15 minutes earlier with PGE_2 (1 mg) prevented this rise in DNA in gastric washings [14]. This result indicates that in spite of the presence of ethanol, gastric mucosal cells were held together by treatment with PGE_2.

Are antisecretory agents cytoprotective?

Histamine H_2-receptor antagonists such as cimetidine, and antacids are widely used in the treatment of peptic ulcer, the mode of action being reduction in gastric acidity. In a broad sense, this antiulcer property can be called a form of cytoprotection. However, there are important differences between the antiulcer effect of antisecretory drugs and antacids on the one hand, and cytoprotective PG on the other:

a. Certain cytoprotective PG are not antisecretory. PG such as $PGF_{2\beta}$ and 16,16-dimethyl PGA_2 are cytoprotective (e.g., they protect the stomach against necrotizing agents) although they do not affect gastric secretion.

b. PG that inhibit gastric secretion are cytoprotective at nonantisecretory doses. Thus, 16,16-dimethyl PGE_2 protects the stomach against absolute ethanol or boiling water in rats at a dose of 0.5 μg/kg whereas the oral antisecretory ED_{50} in the same species is 250 μg/kg.

c. Neither cimetidine, scopolamine methyl bromide (an anticholinergic) nor antacids prevent gastric necrosis produced by agents such as absolute ethanol [2].

The conclusion is that cytoprotection is a property of PG that is independent from any effect on gastric secretion. Certain studies have suggested that cimetidine and propantheline bromide (another anticholinergic) can inhibit acetylsalicylic acid-induced gastric lesions in rats through cytoprotection [15, 16]. The fact that the gastric lesions were reduced even when the acetylsalicylic acid was suspended in HCl was given as evidence that the protection could not be due to acid inhibition, since in these studies exogenous acid was placed in the stomach. Other studies, however, led to a different conclusion. It was found that cimetidine and propantheline bromide can indeed reduce acetylsalicylic acid-induced gastric damage, but only when HCl is given at concentrations of 0.15 N or less. When the concentration is raised to 0.35 N, neither of the 2 drugs is protective anymore, whereas a PG such as 16,16-dimethyl PGE_2 remains fully protective, even when given at doses as low as 2.5 μg/kg [17]. Similar results were obtained in rats in which another analogue of PGE_2, 15(R)-15-methyl PGE_2 methyl ester, inhibited gastric mucosal erosions produced by acetylsalicylic acid, whereas cimetidine was inactive [18]. This PG analogue and 16,16-dimethyl PGE_2 also prevented the formation of gastric lesions produced by taurocholic acid [19, 20]. It appears that cimetidine and propantheline bromide can inhibit acid secretion sufficiently to reduce the ulcerogenicity of acetylsalicylic acid; this would be the case when only a low concentration of HCl is given together with the acetylsalicylic acid. Administration of a higher concentration of HCl (e.g.

0.35 *N*) with the acetylsalicylic acid overcomes the antisecretory effect of these drugs, which then are no longer protective. These studies stress the fact that cytoprotection by PG is a property independent of inhibition of acid secretion, and a property not shared by antisecretory drugs.

Mechanism of cytoprotection

The mechanism is unknown. The following hypotheses have been proposed:

Stimulation of mucus secretion

Cytoprotection could be explained by the secretion of a mucus layer acting as a physicochemical barrier against noxious substances present in the gastric lumen. Cytoprotective PG do indeed stimulate mucus secretion in rats [21, 22], dogs [23], and humans [14, 24]. In these studies, mucus was expressed as hexosamines, N-acetyl neuraminic acid, or in terms of alcian blue binding capacity. In one study, the aminosalicylic acid-positive granules in mucus cells obtained through biopsy were increased following oral administration of 15(R)-15-methyl PGE_2 [25].

Tightening of the gastric mucosal barrier

Cytoprotection could be mediated through a strengthening of the mucosal barrier. Such an effect has been reported in dogs and rats for PGE_2, 16,16-dimethyl PGE_2, and PGI_2 [5–9].

Stimulation of the gastric sodium pump

In-vitro studies with isolated canine gastric mucosa showed that indometacin reverses sodium transport from mucosa to serosa (which is normal) to serosa to mucosa (which is abnormal). This effect was counteracted by application of a PG (16,16-dimethyl PGE_2) [26]. This effect seems to be mediated through stimulation of cyclic adenosine monophosphate in the mucosa. It was proposed that the ulcerogenic effect of an agent such as indometacin could be due to the lack of transport of sodium and that PG would be cytoprotective by restoring the proper direction of sodium transport.

Possible clinical applications of cytoprotection

Cytoprotective PG might be used in the treatment of various gastrointestinal diseases characterized by inflammation and/or necrosis. Such diseases include peptic ulcer and various forms of gastritis (spontaneous as well as drug induced). The reports that PGE_2 prevents gastric bleeding produced by acetylsalicylic acid and indometacin [11–13] and cellular exfoliation produced by ethanol [14] are the first examples of gastric cytoprotection in humans.

Summary

Several PG protect the mucosa of the gastrointestinal tract against necrosis produced by agents such as absolute ethanol, a strong acid or a strong base, acetylsalicylic acid and even boiling water. This protective property is called cytoprotection; the effect is independent of inhibition of gastric secretion, and it takes place after minute amounts of PG are given orally or parenterally. The presence of PG within the cells appears to be necessary for maintaining the cellular integrity of the gastric mucosa.

The mechanism of cytoprotection is unknown. Prostaglandins may be cytoprotective by stimulating mucus secretion, or by tightening the gastric mucosal barrier, or by regulating sodium transport. Cytoprotective PG are expected to be beneficial in the treatment of peptic ulcer and gastritis. Prostaglandin E_2 has been reported to prevent gastric bleeding induced in humans by nonsteroidal anti-inflammatory compounds.

References

1. Robert, A., Nezamis, J.E., Lancaster, C. and Hanchar, A.J. (1977): Gastric cytoprotective property of prostaglandins. *Gastroenterology 72*, 1121.
2. Robert, A., Nezamis, J.E., Lancaster, C. and Hanchar, A.J. (1979): Cytoprotection by prostaglandins in rats: prevention of gastric necrosis produced by alcohol, HCl, NaOH, hypertonic NaCl, and thermal injury. *Gastroenterology 77*, 433.
3. Robert, A. (1979): Cytoprotection by prostaglandins. *Gastroenterology 77*, 761.
4. Davenport, H.W. (1969): Gastric mucosal hemorrhage in dogs. Effects of acid, aspirin, and alcohol. *Gastroenterology 56*, 439.
5. Cohen, M.M. (1975): Prostaglandin E_2 prevents gastric mucosal barrier damage. *Gastroenterology 68*, 876.
6. Tepperman, B.L., Miller, T.A. and Johnson, L.R. (1978): Effect of 16,16-dimethyl prostaglandin E_2 on ethanol-induced damage to canine oxyntic mucosa. *Gastroenterology 75*, 1061.
7. Bolton, J.P. and Cohen, M.M. (1979): Effect of 16,16-dimethyl prostaglandin E_2 on the gastric mucosal barrier. *Gut 20*, 513.
8. Konturek, S.J., Bowman, J., Lancaster, C. et al. (1979): Cytoprotection of the canine gastric mucosa by prostacyclin: possible mediation by increased mucosal blood flow. *Gastroenterology 76*, 1173.

9. Whittle, B.J.R. (1977): Mechanisms underlying gastric mucosal damage induced by indomethacin and bile salts, and the actions of prostaglandins. *Br. J. Pharmacol. 60*, 455.

10. Grossman, M.I., Matsumoto, K.K. and Lichter, R.J. (1961): Fecal blood loss produced by oral and intravenous administration of various salicylates. *Gastroenterology 40*, 383.

11. Cohen, M.M. (1978): Mucosal cytoprotection by prostaglandin E_2. *Lancet II*, 1253.

12. Johansson, C., Kollberg, B., Nordeman, R. and Bergström, S. (1979): Mucosal protection by prostaglandin E_2. *Lancet I*, 317.

13. Johansson, C., Kollberg, B., Nordeman, R. et al. (1980): Protective effect of prostaglandin E_2 in the gastrointestinal tract during indomethacin treatment of rheumatic diseases. *Gastroenterology 78*, 479.

14. Ruppin, H., Person, B., Robert, A. and Domschke, W. (1980): Cytoprotection in man by prostaglandin E_2. *Proc. Soc. Exp. Biol. Med.* (In press.)

15. Guth, P.H., Aures, D. and Paulsen, G. (1978): Topical aspirin + HCl lesions: protection by prostaglandin and cimetidine. *Gastroenterology 74*, 1126.

16. Guth, P.H., Aures, D. and Paulsen, G. (1979): Topical aspirin plus HCl gastric lesions in the rat. Cytoprotective effect of prostaglandin, cimetidine and probanthine. *Gastroenterology 76*, 88.

17. Robert, A., Hanchar, A.J., Nezamis, J.E. and Lancaster, C. (1979): Cytoprotection against acidified aspirin: comparison of prostaglandin, cimetidine and probanthine. *Gastroenterology 76*, 1227.

18. Carmichael, H.A., Nelson, L.M. and Russell, R.I. (1978): Cimetidine and prostaglandin: evidence for different modes of action on the rat gastric mucosa. *Gastroenterology 74*, 1229.

19. Carmichael, H.A., Nelson, L., Russell, R.I. et al. (1977): The effect of the synthetic prostaglandin analog 15(R)-15-methyl-PGE_2 methyl ester on gastric mucosal hemorrhage induced in rats by taurocholic acid and hydrochloric acid. *Am. J. Dig. Dis. 22*, 411.

20. Chaudhury, T.K. and Robert, A. (1980): Prevention by mild irritants of gastric necrosis produced in rats by sodium taurocholate. *Dig. Dis. Sci.* (In press.)

21. Bolton, J.P., Palmer, D. and Cohen, M.M. (1976): Effect of the E_2 prostaglandins on gastric mucus production in rats. *Surg. Forum 27*, 402.

22. Bolton, J.P., Palmer, D. and Cohen, M.M. (1978): Stimulation of mucus and nonparietal cell secretion by the E_2 prostaglandins. *Am. J. Dig. Dis. 23*, 359.

23. Bolton, J.P. and Cohen, M.M. (1978): Stimulation of non-parietal cell secretion in canine Heidenhain pouches by 16,16-dimethyl prostaglandin E_2. *Digestion 17*, 291.

24. Ruppin, H., Person, B., Robert, A. and Domschke, W. (1979): Gastric cytoprotection by prostaglandins (PG): possible mediation by mucus secretion. *Physiologist 22*, 110.

25. Fung, W.P., Lee, S.K. and Karim, S.M.M. (1974): Effect of prostaglandin 15(R)-15-methyl E_2-methyl ester on the gastric mucosa in patients with peptic ulceration. An endoscopic and histologic study. *Prostaglandins 5*, 465.

26. Chaudhury, T.K. and Jacobson, E.D. (1978): Prostaglandin cytoprotection of gastric mucosa. *Gastroenterology 74*, 58.

Experimental studies on gastric cytoprotection by prostaglandins, antisecretory agents and epidermal growth factor

S.J. Konturek, T. Radecki, T. Brzozowski, I. Piastucki, A. Dembińska-Kieć and A. Zmuda

Institute of Physiology and Department of Pharmacology, Medical Academy, Kraków, Poland

Introduction

Acetylsalicylic acid and other nonsteroidal anti-inflammatory compounds (NOSAC) can produce gastric mucosal lesions in laboratory animals [1, 2] and in man [3]. Since NOSAC inhibit the biosynthesis of prostaglandins [4] and exogenous prostaglandins effectively prevent the formation of NOSAC-induced lesions [2], it has been postulated that these lesions result from a deficiency of mucosal prostaglandins. The withdrawal of normal protection, provided by endogenous prostaglandins, has been suggested to be the major factor in the pathogenesis of NOSAC-induced gastric mucosal damage [5].

Recently, Robert and his colleagues reported that prostaglandins possess a remarkable property for protecting gastric and intestinal mucosa against damaging agents and this phenomenon has been called 'cytoprotection' [6]. They found that prostaglandins, and not other antisecretory agents, are cytoprotective and that this effect is completely independent of the inhibition of gastric secretion. Robert suggested that gastric cytoprotection against damaging agents is mediated by endogenous formation of cytoprotective prostaglandins [5] but no study was undertaken to demonstrate the changes in mucosal prostaglandins during gastric cytoprotection.

This study was designed to assess the capability of gastric mucosa to generate prostaglandins in intact and acetylsalicylic acid-treated rats and to compare the effects of prostaglandins and other gastric inhibitory agents on the formation of acetylsalicylic acid-induced gastric ulcers and the generation of mucosal prostaglandins.

Methods

Two series of experiments were performed on Wistar rats, weighing 120–150 g. In one series, the generation and bioassay of gastric mucosal prostaglandins was carried out and in the other series, the effects of prostaglandins and other gastric inhibitory compounds on acetylsalicylic acid-induced gastric ulcers were compared. The animals were fasted but had free access to water for 36 hours before the study. They were housed before and during the experiments in cages with wide mesh wire bottoms to prevent coprophagy.

Generation and bioassay of prostaglandins

All rats were first anesthetized with ether and intubated with a polyethylene tube (outer diameter 0.75 mm) one end being placed in the stomach through a small incision in the forestomach and the other end brought through the abdominal wall to the shoulder region. This tube was used for the intragastric (i.g.) instillation of acetylsalicylic acid, HCl (0.15 *M* HCl), or saline. After surgery, each animal was placed in a Bollman cage under light restraint and allowed to recover from anesthesia for a one-hour period.

Groups of 8–10 rats then received one of the following treatments: 1. i.g. saline + subcutaneous (s.c.) saline (control); 2. i.g. acetylsalicylic acid + i.g. HCl; 3. i.g. acetylsalicylic acid + i.g. HCl + s.c. ranitidine (0.5 mg/kg/hr); 4. i.g. acetylsalicylic acid + i.g. HCl + s.c. propantheline bromide (2 μg/kg/hr); and 5. i.g. acetylsalicylic acid + i.g. HCl + s.c. epidermal growth factor (EGF) (1 μg/kg/hr).

A solution of acetylsalicylic acid was freshly prepared at the start of each test by dissolving 3 g of $NaHCO_3$ and 3 g of acetylsalicylic acid in 100 ml of distilled water giving a stock solution containing 30 mg/ml of acetylsalicylic acid. This was given i.g. as a bolus of 60 mg/kg followed by a constant i.g. infusion of 40 mg/kg/hr. This dose was used recently by Kauffman and Grossman to produce gastric ulcers in rats [2]. Ranitidine, propantheline bromide and EGF were dissolved in saline just before administration and infused s.c. in a dose that was found, in separate tests with chronic gastric fistula rats, to be without any influence on basal gastric acid and pepsin secretion. Instillation of i.g. acetylsalicylic acid and HCl or saline was carried out at a rate of 4 ml/hr for a 3-hour period.

At the end of the experiment, each animal was removed from the restraining cage and again lightly anesthetized with ether. The abdomen was opened, and the stomach quickly removed and opened along the greater curvature and then the animals were killed. Gastric mucosal tissue was prepared for the generation of PGs according to the method described by Whittle [7]. Gastric mucosa was carefully removed, the antral and fundic portions separated, and then plunged in ice-cold 0.05 M trometamol buffer (pH 9.0). Tissue samples of approximately 300 mg were chopped, washed of blood and debris for 5 seconds with 1 ml of ice-cold trometamol buffer and centrifuged at 9,000 g for 10 seconds. After removal of the supernatant, fresh trometamol buffer was again added to the residual tissue in the proportion 0.5 ml/150 mg of tissue weight. This sample was shaken for 60 seconds at room temperature using a steady speed of a vortex stirrer and centrifuged at 9,000 g for 15 seconds. Supernatant was used for assay of generated prostacyclin (PGI_2) immediately after centrifugation and then again after 30 minutes' storage at room temperature to destroy PGI_2 for assay of generated PGE_2.

Assay of PGI_2   The anti-aggregatory properties of PGI_2 were used to determine its concentration in supernatants [8]. Rabbit blood was withdrawn by heart puncture and added to a 3.8% solution of sodium citrate (9:1 v/v). Platelet rich plasma (PRP) was prepared by centrifugation of citrated blood at 200 g for 10 minutes at room temperature. PRP was aggregated at 37° Ci in a Born aggregometer with threshold pro-aggregatory concentrations of 2–5 μM of adenosine diphosphate (ADP). The anti-aggregatory potency of standard PGI_2 was measured by instillation of PGI_2 at concentrations of 0.4–10 ng/ml one minute before ADP was added. The percentage inhibition of the ADP-induced aggregation was plotted against the effective concentrations of PGI_2, so as to obtain a standard curve. To measure the amount of PGI_2 synthetized by mucosa, 5–50 μl of the supernatant from the incubation samples were instilled into PRP one minute before ADP addition. The content of a PGI_2-like activity in tested samples was calculated by comparison of their anti-aggregatory potency with that of synthetic PGI_2. Results are expressed in nanograms of generated PGI_2/g of tissue weight.

Assay of PGE_2   Rat stomach strips (RSS) and rat colon (RC) superfusion technique was used to determine the PGE_2-like activity [9]. RSS and RC were superfused in cascade with pregased (95% O_2 and 5% CO_2) Krebs solution containing such pharmacological antagonists as: phenoxybenzamine (2 μg/ml), propranolol (4 μg/ml), atropine sulfate (0.1 μg/ml), methysergide (0.1 μg/ml), diphenhydramine (0.1 μg/ml) and indometacin (1 μg/ml). The tone of RSS and RC were recorded with auxotonic levels (2–4 g initial load) using Harvard Transducers, type 386, connected to a Watanabe multirecorder. Calibration doses of PGE_2, $PGF_{2\alpha}$ or 25–200 μl of supernatant were infused alternately over the assay organs. Results are expressed as nanograms of generated PGE_2/g of tissue weight.

Acetylsalicylic acid-induced gastric ulceration

As in the study on the generation and assay of mucosal prostaglandins, the animals were intubated under light anesthesia. One hour after recovering from anesthesia the animals were placed in Bollman cages and an i.v. bolus injection of 60 mg/kg of acetylsalicylic acid followed by a constant infusion of 40 mg/kg/hr for a 3-hour period was performed. Simultaneous gastric perfusion with 0.15 M HCl was carried out at a rate of 4 ml/hr.

Groups of 8–10 animals received one of the following treatments: 1. i.g. acetylsalicylic acid + i.g. HCl + s.c. saline (control); 2. i.g. acetylsalicylic acid + i.g. HCl + s.c. PGE$_2$ (20 μg/kg/hr); 3. i.g. acetylsalicylic acid + i.g. HCl + s.c. PGI$_2$ (10 μg/kg/hr); 4. i.g. acetylsalicylic acid + i.g. HCl + s.c. ranitidine (0.5 mg/kg/hr); 5. i.g. acetylsalicylic acid + i.g. HCl + s.c. propantheline bromide (10 μg/kg/hr); and 6. i.g. acetylsalicylic acid + i.g. HCl + EGF (1 μg/kg/hr). Each of the substances tested was used in a dose that was found in separate experiments to be without any influence on gastric secretion in chronic gastric fistula rats. The infusion was given s.c. starting 30 minutes before and throughout the 3-hour infusion experiment. Solutions of ranitidine, propantheline bromide and EGF were prepared and infused as in the previous tests with prostaglandins. Prostaglandin solutions were freshly prepared just before the experiment; PGE$_2$ was dissolved in saline and kept at room temperature whereas PGI$_2$ was dissolved in isotonic trometamol solution and kept in ice throughout the infusion.

At the end of the experiment, each animal was removed from the restraining cage and anesthetized again. The sample of blood was taken from the inferior vena cava for salicylate determination and then the animals were killed. The stomach was removed and opened along the greater curvature. The surface of each gastric ulcer was measured planimetrically and the total surface of all gastric ulcers was summated in each animal and expressed in square millimeters.

Serum salicylate determination   Serum salicylate concentrations were measured by the method of Saltzman [10] and the results are expressed in micrograms per milliliter.

Results

Effects of acetylsalicylic acid and ranitidine, propantheline bromide and EGF on the generation of prostaglandins in gastric mucosa.

In control rats receiving only i.g. and s.c. infusions of saline, the PGE_2-like activity was generated in large quantities both in antral and fundic mucosa (Fig. 1). PGE_2 averaged 230 ±45 and 143 ± 29 ng/g of tissue weight of antral and fundic mucosa, respectively. The corresponding values for PGI_2 were 388 ± 48 and 274 ± 36 ng/g of tissue weight (Fig. 2). The difference in the amounts of generated PGI_2 and PGE_2 between antral and fundic mucosa was statistically significant ($p < 0.05$).

Acetylsalicylic acid given in combination with i.g. 0.15 M HCl resulted in a reduction in the amounts of generated PGE_2 by about 82% in the antrum and 73% in the fundus. This treatment completely abolished PGI_2 activity both in antral and fundic mucosa. The amounts of generated PGE_2 and PGI_2 activity in rats receiving acetylsalicylic acid + HCl + ranitidine, propantheline bromide or EGF were not different from those obtained in animals getting acetylsalicylic acid + HCl without these agents (Figs 1 and 2).

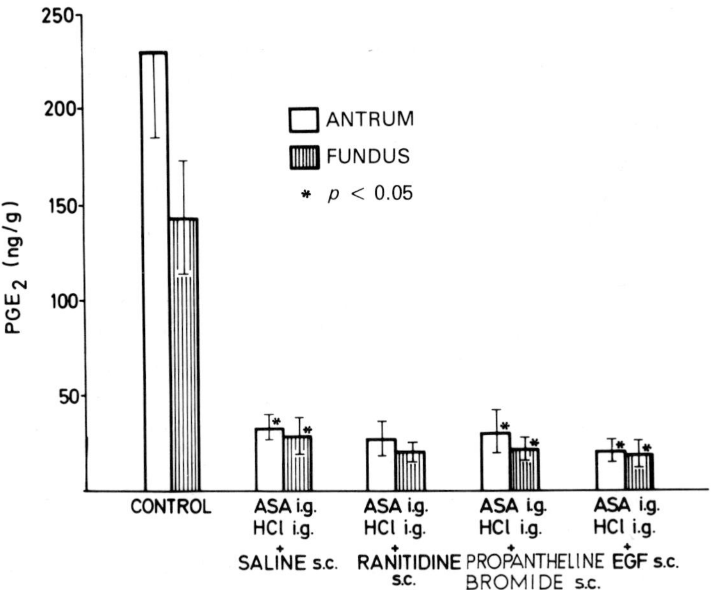

Fig. 1:   *PGE₂-activity generated by the fundic and antral mucosa of the stomach in intact rats treated with i.g. acetylsalicylic acid + HCl alone or in combination with a s.c. infusion of ranitidine, propantheline bromide or EGF. In this and subsequent figures each column shows the mean ± SEM of 8–10 determinations in 8–10 rats. Asterisk indicates significant (p < 0.05) decrease below the control value.*

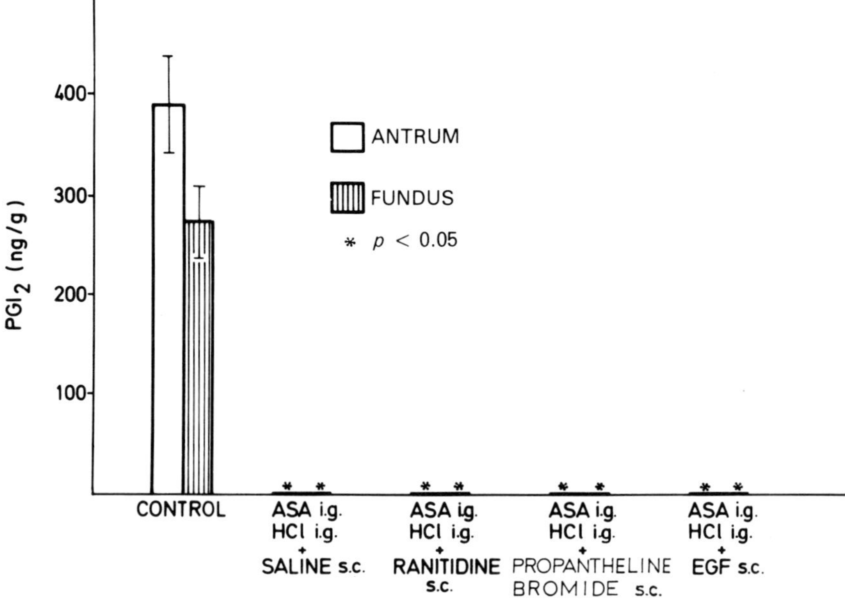

Fig. 2: PGI$_2$-activity generated by the fundic and antral mucosa of the rat stomach in intact rats treated with i.g. acetylsalicylic acid + HCl alone or in combination with a s.c. infusion of ranitidine, propantheline bromide or EGF.

Effects of prostaglandins, ranitidine, propantheline bromide and EGF on gastric ulcer formation in the gastric mucosa.

All rats treated with i.g. acetylsalicylic acid + i.g. HCl developed gastric ulcers occurring mainly in the fundic gland area. The mean ulcer area was 25.8 ± 3.15 mm^2. Plasma salicylate concentrations in this group of rats was about 320 ± 47 μg/ml (Fig. 3). PGE$_2$, PGI$_2$, ranitidine, propantheline bromide or EGF infused s.c. in a nonantisecretory dose resulted in almost complete prevention of ulcer formation by i.g. acetylsalicylic acid + HCl. The difference in the degree of the reduction in the mean ulcer area between groups of rats receiving prostaglandins, ranitidine, propantheline bromide or EGF was not significant. The plasma salicylate levels in groups treated with these agents were not different from those receiving acetylsalicylic acid + HCl alone.

Discussion

This study provides evidence that intact gastric mucosa of the rat is capable of

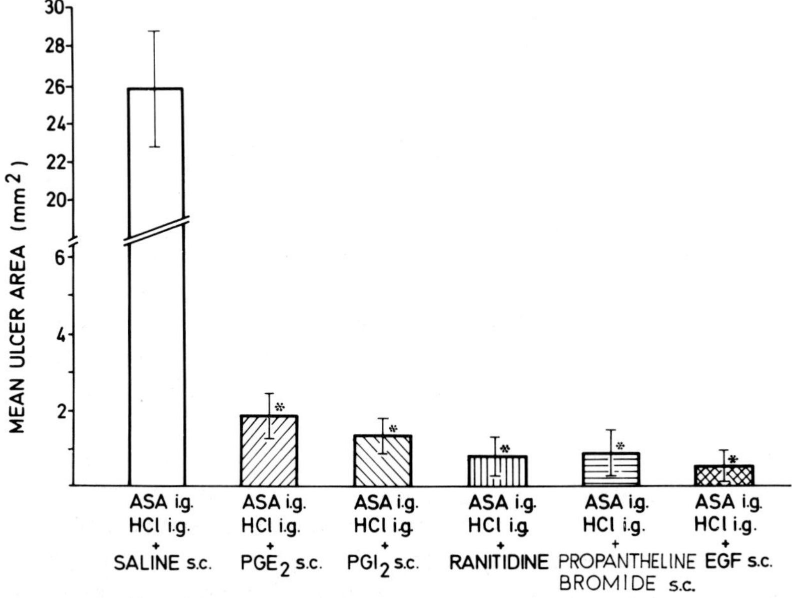

Fig. 3:   Mean ulcer area in rats treated with i.g. acetylsalicylic acid + HCl alone or in combination with PGE₂, PGI₂, ranitidine, propantheline bromide or EGF.

generating large quantities of PGE$_2$ and PGI$_2$ and that i.g. instillation of acetylsalicylic acid and HCl greatly reduces the PGE$_2$ and completely abolishes PGI$_2$ biosynthetizing capability of the mucosa, resulting in the formation of mucosal lesions. Replacement therapy with PGE$_2$ or PGI$_2$ given in nonantisecretory doses prevents acetylsalicylic acid-induced gastric lesions. These results lend support to the concept that normal generation of prostaglandins is essential for protecting the gastric mucosa against chemical injury by the action of these prostaglandins, other than by inhibition of gastric secretion [5].

Although gastric cytoprotection was claimed to be a unique property of prostaglandins [5, 6], our study shows conclusively that a number of other substances , such as H$_2$-receptor antagonists (ranitidine) and anticholinergics (propantheline bromide) are also cytoprotective when administered at a non-antisecretory dose. Thus, it appears that the cytoprotection is not an unique property of prostaglandins and this agrees with previous findings in this respect [2].

The mechanism of gastric cytoprotection by H$_2$-receptor antagonists or anticholinergics is unknown. Several hypotheses have been suggested [5], but one of them postulated the mediation of endogenous mucosal prostaglandins. The possibility existed that the pretreatment with other cytoprotective substances such as ranitidine, propantheline bromide or EGF, somehow prevented the usual deficiency of prostaglandins occurring in the gastric mucosa exposed to acetylsalicylic acid and HCl. Direct measurement of prostaglandin biosynthesizing capability showed, however, that under conditions when cytoprotection against acetylsalicylic acid-induced gastric damage can be demonstrated, the capability of gastric mucosa to generate prostaglandins is negligible and not different from that occurring after treatment with acetylsalicylic acid alone without cytoprotective substances. Thus, it appears that gastric cytoprotection observed with ranitidine or propantheline bromide, is not mediated by mucosal prostaglandins and further studies are needed to explain this phenomenon.

This study demonstrates that EGF, a peptide bearing a marked structural relationship to urogastrone is also cytoprotective [11]. Since the peptide was used at a nonantisecretory dose, its cytoprotective effect cannot be explained by simple inhibition of gastric secretion. EGF is known to have a potent mitogenic effect upon many types of cell in culture [12] and to increase the rate of cellular proliferation in gastric mucosa [13]. It is likely, therefore, that the cytoprotective effect of EGF is directly related to the alterations of in-mucosal cell metabolism and trophic action on the gastric mucosa. Other trophic substances such as growth hormone [14] and pentagastrin [15] were also reported to increase gastric mucosal resistance and to prevent the formation of peptic ulceration in rats.

Summary

Rat gastric mucosa is capable of generating both PGE_2 and PGI_2-activity in significantly higher concentrations in the antrum than in the fundus. I.g. instillation of acetylsalicylic acid + HCl results in almost complete suppression of prostaglandin biosynthesizing capability of the gastric mucosa and in the formation of mucosal lesions. Exogenous prostaglandins, ranitidine, propantheline bromide and EGF, given s.c. in a nonantisecretory dose almost completely prevented the formation of acetylsalicylic acid-induced ulcers indicating that all these substances are cytoprotective. This prevention was not accompanied by any significant increase in prostaglandin biosynthesizing capability of gastric mucosa, indicating that gastric cytoprospective effects of tested substances are not mediated by the generation of mucosal prostaglandins.

References

1. Brodie, D.A. and Chase, B.J. (1967): Role of gastric acid in aspirin-induced gastric irritation in the rat. *Gastroenterology 53*, 604.
2. Kauffman, G.L. and Grossman, M.I. (1978): Prostaglandin and cimetidine inhibit the formation of ulcers produced by parenteral salicylate. *Gastroenterology 75*, 1099.
3. Levy, A. (1974): Aspirin use in patients with major upper gastrointestinal bleeding and peptic ulcer disease. *N. Engl. J. Med. 290*, 1158.
4. Vane, J.T. (1971): Inhibition of prostaglandin synthetase as a mechanism of action for aspirin-like drugs. *Nature 231*, 232.
5. Robert, A. (1979): Cytoprotection and prostaglandins. *Gastroenterology 77*, 761.
6. Robert, A., Nezamis, J.E., Lancaster, C. and Hanchar, A.J. (1979): Cytoprotection by prostaglandins in rats: prevention of gastric necrosis produced by alcohol, HCl, NaOH, hypertonic NaCl and thermal injury. *Gastroenterology 77*, 433.
7. Whittle, B.J.R. (1978): Potential endogenous inhibitor of prostaglandin synthetase in plasma failure to inhibit cyclo-oxygenase in platelets and gastric mucosa. *J. Pharmacol. Pharmac. 30*, 467.
8. Gryglewski, R.J., Bunting, S., Moncada, S. et al. (1976): Arterial walls are protected against deposition of platelets thrombi by a substance (Prostaglandin X) which prevents platelet aggregation. *Prostaglandins 12*, 685.
9. Vane, J.R. (1964): The use of isolated organs for detecting active substances in the circulating blood. *Br. J. Pharmac. Chemother. 23*, 360.
10. Saltzman, A. (1948): Fluorophotometric method for the estimation of salicylate in blood. *J. Biol. Chem. 174*, 399.
11. Gregory, H. (1975): The isolation and structure of urogastrone and its relationship to epidermal growth factor. *Nature 257*, 325.
12. Hollenberg, M.D. and Gregory, H. (1977): Human urogastrone and mouse epidermal growth factor share a common receptor in cultured human fibroblasts. *Life Sci. 20*, 267.
13. Gospodarowicz, D. and Moran, J.S. (1976): Growth factors in mammalian cell culture. *Ann. Rev. Biochem. 45*, 521.
14. Vanamee, P., Winawer, S.J. and Sherlock, P. (1970): Decreased incidence of restraint-stress induced gastric erosions in rats treated with bovine growth hormone. *Proc. Soc. Exp. Biol. Med. 135*, 259.
15. Takeuci, K. and Johnson, L.R. (1979): Pentagastrin protects against stress ulceration in rats. *Gastroenterology 76*, 327.

Lysosomal stability and mucosal resistance to injury

D. Waldron-Edward* and L. Greenberg
*Laboratoire de Biochimie du Tissu Conjonctif, Faculté de Médecine,
Université Paris-Val de Marne, Creteil, France; and Department of Surgery,
McGill University, Montreal, Canada*

Postulated activity of lysosomes and lysosomal enzymes in gastric mucosal breakdown

Gastric ulcers, experimentally induced, are associated with changes in
lysosomal stability. Thus, changes in lysosomal acid hydrolase activity have
been implicated, not only in the liver during endotoxemic shock [1, 2], but
also in mucosal lesions. Ferguson et al. have shown that serotonin-induced
ulcers can be prevented by prostaglandin PGE_1 which stabilizes the lysosomal
membrane [3, 4], while dramatic changes in mucosal enzyme levels [5] and,
more importantly, in their relative latency [6] are associated with the topical
application of ulcerogens. Although lysosomes undoubtedly play a major role
in tissue breakdown, the precise step in which they participate in ulcerogenesis
is not known. As it is felt that such knowledge would greatly help in the
development of efficient methods of prophylaxis or of therapy applied to
mucosal resistance, several postulated mechanisms of action must be
considered.

Acid hydrolases, within the acid environment provided by the lumen of the
lysosomal sac, are known to break down soluble macromolecules as well as
structural elements of other intracelluler organelles, or of material introduced
into the cell by endocytosis. This latter step is brought about by fusion,
leading to the development of large secondary lysosomes. It can be postulated
that these physiologically-active processes, or autophagy, may be accelerated
by ulcerogenic stimulation.

Alternatively, the lysosomal membranes may be ruptured or disorganized in
such a way that all, or perhaps some, specific enzymes may be released into

* D. Waldron-Edward is on sabbatical leave from the Department of Surgery, McGill
University, Montreal, Canada.

the cytosol. This step would be unlikely to cause any deleterious result within the cells, unless the well-buffered intracellular pH was reduced to the extent that the acid hydrolases became active. This possibility exists in the gastric mucosa where H^+ ion is known to be insorbed under ulcerogenic conditions.

A third possibility is the export or exocytosis of lysosomal enzymes by fusion of the vesicular membranes with the plasma membrane. This phenomenon has been much studied in cultured fibroblasts, which are also known to endocytose these enzymes [7, 8]. In the case of the gastric mucosal cells, it can be postulated that export to the external cell wall could perhaps cause a suitable microenvironment for the breakdown of the cell membrane, in particular, the many glycoproteins and glycolipids which are an integral part of the overall lipid membrane structure.

Any of these 3 procedures may take place. However, it is also possible that 2 or all 3 may occur, especially in view of the rather unusual features of the epithelial mucosa of the mammalian stomach.

In many of the experiments reported hereafter, we have worked with scrapings of canine gastric mucosa, removed immediately after sacrifice and chilled. Biopsies were taken in certain cases and treated in the same way. This mixed cell population with which we worked made it impossible to ascertain the exact location of the bound acid hydrolases. Many workers have observed lysosomal vesicles, by means of electron microscopy, only within the parietal cells [9, 10] and rarely in the mucin-bearing cells. Working with both dogs and rats, however, we have found sedimenting particle-bound acid hydrolases both in the nonparietal cell-bearing area in the case of the canine antrum [11] as well as in the fundus, giving evidence that in these species at least the organelles are present at quite high levels in the regions where mucin-bearing cells predominate.

As the second mechanism of lysosomal action postulated above seemed most open to investigation, we have initiated studies using several approaches to this problem.

Direct investigation of the stability of the lysosomal membrane before and after ulcerogenic stimulation can be carried out by subjecting the isolated organelles to certain tests. The lysosomes may be isolated intact with their occluded enzymic contents, by careful homogenization of the tissue followed by differential centrifugation. The latent enzymes within the organelles may then be released into the surrounding medium by applying known stresses or tests, such as those discussed below. Any enzyme labilized in this manner can be assayed in the supernatant. Although certain acid hydrolases may remain bound, even to the ruptured vesicular membrane and thus sediment on recentrifugation, it was found that the major part of the canine mucosal lysosomal enzymes were released when using the most severe conditions of test. On the other hand, an ulcerogenic stimulus appears to render the membrane unstable, so that the potentially latent enzymes are released under the mildest conditions.

The following tests of the stability of the isolated lysosome can be applied:
A. Preincubation of isolated organelle preparations at 37°C for 240 minutes.
A1. Preliminary manipulation during preparation of the lysosome-enriched fraction under strictly controlled routine conditions is known to cause the breakdown of a certain amount of enzyme-organelle binding: ulcerogenic stimuli in vivo were found to increase enzyme lability during lysosomal isolation.
B. Mechanical stress: mild stress is applied by prolonged or repeated homogenization of the mucosa or of the lysosome-enriched fraction.
C. Osmotic lysis: suspension of the lysosome-rich fraction in hypoosmolal solution.
By these means, one can make a comparison of the effect of topically applied ulcerogen in vivo on the lability of the lysosome-bound acid hydrolases subsequently isolated or alternatively the effect of application of the ulcerogen to lysosomal suspension isolated and prepared from untreated tissue.

Three forms of experimental ulcerogenic stimuli have been applied in our studies on lysosomal stability. Both dilute ethanol (20%) and bile are recognized ulcerogens in the canine antrum, but only in the presence of luminal acid do visibly discernible lesions appear. A third form of acute gastric mucosal damage which develops in the canine fundus, accompanying endotoxin-induced shock, also occurs only in the presence of luminal acid. For this reason, in all the experiments reported here, acid saline (HCl 120 mEq/l plus NaCl 40 mEq/l) used in all earlier experiments was applied to the luminal mucosa, as described by the authors [5, 6, 11–13], by direct application to mucosal lucite chambers or by instillation. In some cases, saline (NaCl, 160 mEq/l) was used.

Ethanol-induced lesions

For topical application of ulcerogens, lucite chambers were mounted on the exposed antral mucosa, with vascular supply intact, as previously described [5, 6]. Ethanol (20% v/v) in acid saline very rapidly causes a visible whitening in localized areas on the mucosal surface. After 30 minutes, at least one hemorrhagic lesion appears. On the other hand, no lesion appears when a neutral ethanolic saline solution is applied. Ethanol acid saline also causes damage when observed histologically whereas neutral ethanol has little effect.

Labilization of lysosome-bound acid hydrolases in vivo. Isolation of lysosome-rich fractions

Test A – preincubation   The effect of ethanol, topically applied to the mucosa, on the stability of lysosomes during preincubation for 4 hours, is illustrated in Table I. Saline and acid saline treatment of the mucosa in vivo effected the same degree of enzyme lability: of the acid hydrolases assayed, 10–18% was released into the medium. Some differentiation seems to take place in that α-L-fucosidade, pH 6.0, is more labile in both cases (average

Table I: Lysosome preincubation test, 4 hours at 37°C.

Ethanol	Saline		Acid saline	
	0	+	0	+
	% released during incubation			
Cathepsin D	18 ± 2 (8)	60 ± 3*(3)	17 ± 1 (3)	49 ± 1* (3)
β-N-Acetylglucosaminidase	11 ± 2 (8)	54 ± 2*(3)	11 ± 2 (3)	44 ± 1* (3)
β-Galactosidase	14 ± 1 (8)	40 ± 8*(3)	13 ± 1 (3)	43 ± 2* (4)
α-Galactosidase	10 ± 3 (7)	42 ± 1*(3)	11 ± 3 (3)	29 ± 3**(2)
α-L-Fucosidase (pH 3.0)	11 ± 2 (8)	ND	ND	48 ± 3 (2)
α-L-Fucosidase (pH 6.0)	30 ± 2 (5)	50 ± 3*(3)	28 ± 4 (3)	29 ± 1 (4)

$*p < 0.001$, $**p < 0.05$.

A single lucite chamber was introduced onto the antral mucosa of anesthetized dogs, taking care to use the same experimental conditions as previously described [6]. The mounted mucosa were treated with either acid saline 20 ml, acid saline containing absolute ethanol (20%), neutral saline or neutral saline with absolute ethanol (20%). After 30 minutes, the mucosae were removed, homogenized, divided into several equal parts and centrifuged at high speed to prepare particulate lysosome-rich fractions as described earlier [6]. The pellets were resuspended in a solution of 0.25 M sucrose and 5 mM Tris (hydroxymethyl aminomethane) hydrochloride and an aliquot was immediately centrifuged at 3.6 x 10^6 g average minutes: the remaining suspensions were incubated at 37°C for 240 minutes and centrifuged at 3.6 x 10^6 g average minutes. Enzyme activity was assayed both in the pellets and in the supernatants as previously described. All assays were carried out in triplicate. The results are expressed as percentage of the total enzyme, which was released during incubation, $\overline{X}$ ± SD. + Refers to saline and acid saline containing absolute ethanol. Numbers in parentheses refer to number of dogs. ND = no determination.

29%). Application of ethanol in either neutral saline or in acid solution significantly increased enzyme lability.

Test A1   The preliminary manipulation required during the preparation of these lysosome-enriched fractions followed by resuspension in 0.25 M sucrose before preincubation inevitably increases the fragility of the lysosomal membranes (Table II).

In general, particulate enzymes from control mucosae vary considerably in the stability of their binding to the subcellular organelles: α-L-fucosidase pH 6.0 in particular remains bound to a large extent, whereas α-galactosidase appears to be more labile. Ethanol treatment of the mucosa, whether in neutral or in acid solution, significantly increases the destabilization of the lysosome-binding of all the enzymes assayed.

Table II: The destabilizing effect of topically applied ethanol during preparative isolation of the lysosome-rich fraction.

Ethanol	Saline		Acid saline	
	0	+	0	+
	% total lysosomal enzyme released			
Cathepsin D	32 ± 1 (8)	38 ± 3**(3)	33 ± 3 (3)	60 ± 3*(3)
β-N-Acetylglucosamin-idase	31 ± 1 (8)	35 ± 1* (3)	33 ± 1 (3)	59 ± 5*(3)
β-Galactosidase	33 ± 1 (8)	40 ± 2* (3)	34 ± 2 (3)	55 ± 2*(4)
α-Galactosidase	50 ± 1 (7)	60 ± 1* (3)	51 ± 1 (3)	79 ± 6*(2)
α-L-Fucosidase (pH 3.0)	39 ± 4 (8)	ND	ND	55 ± 3 (2)
α-L-Fucosidase (pH 6.0)	25 ± 2 (5)	48 ± 3* (3)	25 ± 3 (3)	75 ± 2*(4)

* $p < 0.001$, **$p < 0.01$.

Experimental conditions were as described in Table I. In each experiment, one lysosome-rich pellet was resuspended in 0.25 M sucrose, and centrifuged immediately at 3.6×10^6 g average minutes at 0°C. Enzymes were assayed in the resulting pellets and in the supernatants (S). A second lysosome-rich pellet was homogenized in 0.9% NaCl-Triton X-100 (1%), to assay total enzyme activity (T) in the lysosomal fraction. The results are expressed as $\frac{S}{T} \times 100$. All assays were carried out in triplicate. Student's t-test was applied to compare the results obtained between mucosae treated with saline in the absence and presence of ethanol, and mucosae treated with acid saline in the absence and presence of ethanol. Numbers in parentheses refer to number of dogs. ND = no determination.

Application of the ulcerogen to the lysosome-enriched fraction in vitro

A more marked differentiation of membrane destabilization by ethanol in acid solution appeared when the ulcerogen was applied directly to the lysosomes in vitro. The lysosome-enriched fractions from untreated mucosae were resuspended in 0.25 M sucrose containing either ethanol (10%) or ethanol 10% + HCl (120 mEq/l) and subjected to the preincubation test. After 240 minutes the lysosomal organelles in neutral ethanolic sucrose suspension had released 54% vs 45% (sucrose only) of their total acid phosphatase, and 44% vs 39% (sucrose only) of their total β-N-acetylglucosaminidase, compared with lysosome-rich fraction incubated in sucrose alone (control). Suspension in 0.25 M sucrose containing ethanol plus acid, as described above, however, released significantly more acid phosphatase (76%) and β-N-acetylglucosaminidase (85%) (n = 3; $p < 0.001$).

It can be concluded from the foregoing evidence that ethanol even at this low concentration can disrupt lipid membranes, with a potential leakage of acid hydrolases from their organelle binding. Only if H^+ ion becomes accessible, however, thus increasing intracellular acidity, can the acid hydrolases so released assume their destructive capacity.

Bile-induced lesions

Biliary reflux has often been postulated as playing a role in the etiology both of human gastritis and of gastric ulcers. Altimirano and Martinoya [14] and Birkett and Silen [15] have suggested that mucosal membranes are rendered permeable by the lipophilic components of bile. It seemed possible that this effect on membrane stability could be extended to intracellular organelle membranes. However, Waldron-Edward et al. found that bile alone has rather little direct effect on the binding or latency of acid hydrolases [6]. Fresh canine bile, applied directly to antral mucosa mounted in lucite chambers, can be seen to cause precipitation of adherent gastric mucin but no well-defined lesions appear. Only when most of the bile is removed by aspiration and rapid washing, and replaced by acid saline, do hemorrhagic lesions appear. A simple direct assay of free, nonsedimenting enzymes, in mucosal homogenates demonstrated that their levels of activity were higher in the bile-acid treated mucosae than in the corresponding controls, but only to a marginal degree. Further studies have also shown that there is no change in the nonlysosomal enzyme, alkaline phosphatase, in the bile-acid treated mucosa. On the other hand, increased organelle fragility is much more markedly illustrated by submission of the isolated lysosome-rich fraction to mechanical stress and to osmotic lysis (Fig. 1).

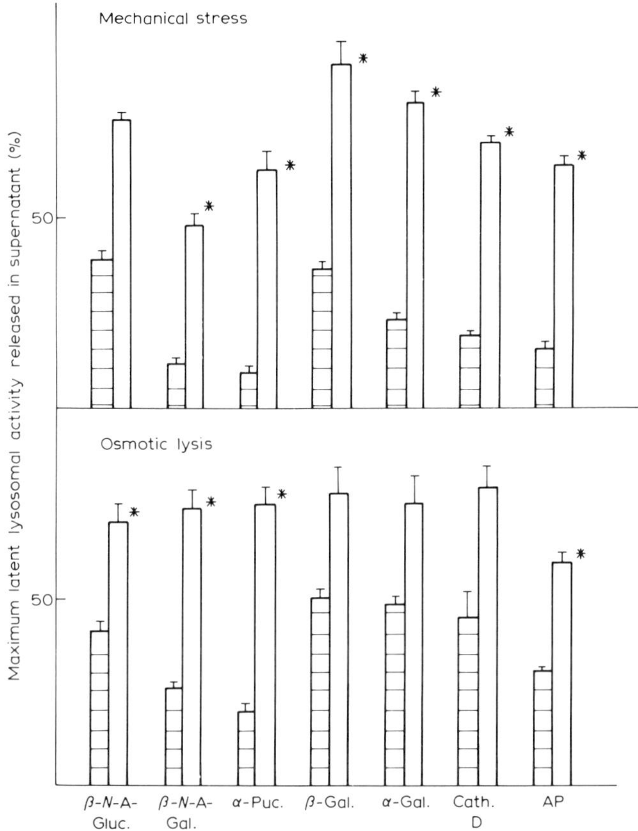

*Fig. 1: Fragility of lysosomal membranes in bile + acid-treated mucosa in 4 dogs. Canine antral mucosa, mounted in lucite chambers, was treated with either acid saline for 60 minutes (barred), or with canine gallbladder bile for 30 minutes followed by acid saline for 30 minutes (blank) using the same techniques as described previously [6]. Lysosome-enriched fractions were prepared as described in Table I. Their stability was submitted to tests of mechanical stress and osmotic lysis. Each assay was carried out in triplicate. *p < 0.001 (paired Student's t-test).*

It was concluded therefore that the detergent, lipid-disrupting qualities of the bile acids alone do not disturb the organelle-membrane structures very profoundly. With the influx of insorbed H^+ion, the latent acid hydrolases are released into an active acidic environment, exposing the mucosal cell structure to biodegradation and breakdown.

Indirect investigation of lysosomal stability or membrane-binding can also be carried out by differentiating 'free' acid hydrolase activity, presumably in the cytosol, found in tissues homogenized in a solution of 0.25 M sucrose in 5 mM tris HCl (pH 7.4), from the 'total' activity, including that released from membrane-binding by the detergent, Triton-X-100. Latent or lysosome-bound activity is thus defined as the difference: total activity − free activity.

Lesions induced by endotoxic shock

Lysosomal acid hydrolases have been implicated in the acute gastrointestinal damage induced by stress [3], but no report so far has been made of their significance in the gastric mucosal lesions during endotoxemia. Shock was produced in male, fasting dogs by i.v. injection of *Escherichia coli* endotoxin. Arterial blood pressure was continously monitored throughout the experiment (5−120 minutes). Gastric mucosal blood flow was also monitored.

Endotoxin shock results in severe fundic mucosal ischemia, with the suppression of H^+ ion secretion. The gastric luminal contents therefore remain neutral for up to the total time interval covered (120 minutes); no visible lesion appears. However, if acid saline is instilled into the lumen of the pylorus ligated stomach, immediately before shock is induced, hemorrhagic lesions develop quite rapidly in the fundic area, that is, within the first 15 minutes. Prolonging the period of shock did not appear to alter the number of lesions observed (18 dogs, 15−120 minutes).

To find some measurable correlation between lysosomal stability or latency on the one hand, and the extent of tissue damage in these dogs on the other, at least 2 different series of experiments were required. In Series I, after induction of shock, a mid-line abdominal incision was made, the stomach was exposed and sequential biopsies were made by means of a biopsy forceps (6 mm). The abdomen was covered and kept warm during the experiment. In Series II, when acid saline was instilled into the lumen, no sequential biopsies could be taken. Within certain time intervals after the induction of shock, the stomach was removed: the biopsy forceps was used to obtain multiple mucosal samples.

One or more samples were set aside for histological examination (hematoxylin and eosin). The remaining were immediately chilled and homogenized for the assay of free and total α-L-fucosidase activity at pH 3.0 and 6.0, β-N-acetylglucosaminidase and acid phosphatase whenever possible. Protein was assayed on all samples: the methods of assay are described elsewhere [12].

The tissue damage score is given in Table III. Histological examination showed that minor damage was always apparent, even in sections from control mucosae. No ulcers or subsurface lesions were seen, and it must be

Table III: Tissue damage score after treatment with endotoxin or endotoxin with luminal acid saline, compared with control anesthetized dogs.

	No. of dogs	Interstitial bleeding	Surface damage	Subsurface damage	No. of dogs with ulceration
Control	37	0.49 ± 0.74	1.08 ± 0.78	0	0
Endotoxin shock	27	0.87 ± 1.07	1.63 ± 0.99***	0.19 ± 0.58	0
Endotoxin shock + luminal acid	18	0.72 ± 1.02	2.28 ± 0.88*	0.83 ± 1.20**	9

$*p < 0.001$, $**p < 0.01$, $***p < 0.02$.

Shock was induced by i.v. injection of endotoxin at a rate of 3 mg/kg. The shock state was assumed to have been reached when the arterial blood pressure had dropped to at least 40 mm Hg; arterial blood pressure thereafter fluctuated, sometimes ranging from 40–170 mm Hg. Visible ulceration was scored on inspection of the entire mucosa on completion of the experiment. Sections of fundic mucosa, stained by hemotoxylin and eosin, were examined by an outside examiner and graded as follows: no damage = 0; capillary breakdown or interstitial bleeding = 0.5–3; damage to surface epithelial cells = 0.5–3; damage extending below the surface epithelial cells = 1–3. Time of shock ranged from 5–120 minutes. Duration of shock appeared to bear little or no relationship to lesion severity or number. Student's *t*-test of significance was applied.

assumed that superficial damage was due to experimental artefact. After endotoxin shock, however, extensive damage appeared in the connective tissues of the mucosal capillaries, that is there was interstitial bleeding which probably relates to the massive fundic ischemia. In Series II, severe surface damage and damage to deeper cells in the mucosa (not defined here) appeared in the shocked mucosae, treated with luminal acid. Gross visible ulceration was observed in 9 of these dogs, including 3 dogs with multiple erosions. Ulcers observed in 19 dogs (not recorded) were observed to develop within 5–15 minutes; but no correlation appeared to exist between the number of ulcers and the duration of shock, ranging from 5–120 minutes. Under the conditions used in these experiments, no ulcers were observed in the antral region.

Enzyme activities in the mucosae of endotoxin-shocked dogs is shown in Table IV. A preliminary overall analysis of the results of assays for lysosomally bound or latent activity, compared with free α-L-fucosidase activity, is given in Table IVa, showing striking differences in both forms of acid hydrolase in the insulted tissue. There is a wide variation from the mean values in each group of dogs, however, confirming earlier experiences [5].

Table IV: *Enzyme activities in mucosae of endotoxin-shocked dogs.*

Enzyme	Control	Endotoxin	Endotoxin + luminal HCl
a.		nM/min/g wet tissue	
α-L-Fucosidase	(17)	(57)	(16)
Latent	78 ± 53	69 ± 48	90 ± 34***
Free	101 ± 48	107 ± 50	219 ± 50*
b. Cell preincubation test	Percentage latent activity remaining after 240 minutes at 37°	∓	∓
α-L-Fucosidase	32.0 ± 7 (7)	28.3 ± 1.5 (4)	85.8 ± 17.2 (5)*
β-*N*-Acetylglucosaminidase	7.1 ± 1 (4)	23.5 ± 4.5 (4)	64.3 ± 14.5 (4)*
Acid phosphatase	38.3 ± 9 (3)	23.7 ± 19 (3)	100 ± 20 (2)**

Test of significance vs endotoxin: *$p < 0.001$, **$p < 0.01$, ***$p < 0.05$. Numbers in parentheses refer to number of dogs investigated. ∓ = endotoxemia; 15 minutes. Endotoxemia was induced as described in Table III. Free enzyme activity was assayed im mucosa homogenized in a solution of 0.25 *M* sucrose in 5 m*M* tris HCl, pH 7.4. Latent activity (total minus free) was determined by assaying total enzyme activity in mucosa homogenized in 0.9% NaCl-Triton X-100 (1%). The upper part of the Table (a) shows free and latent enzymes in gastric mucosa with and without luminal acid saline. The lower half (b) shows the cell preincubation test: mucosal scrapings were prepared and suspended in MEM for 4 hours as previously described [13]. All enzyme activity assayed as described previously [12]. Percentage latent activity present at $t = 0$, remaining bound after incubation is given, $\overline{X} ±$ SD. Recovery values are not included: in control experiments, recovery reached 85−103%, including free activity secreted into the supernatant. This was not true in the shocked mucosae. Much enzyme activity was destroyed (or inhibited) during the test.

Even in control mucosa, where $t = 0$, the differences are great, ranging from 33 to 171 units (nM/min/g of wet tissue) with a mean $\overline{X} ±$ SD, 78 ± 53, when $n = 14$. This range was not due to swelling with imbibation of water: determination of wet weight/dry weight in a very large number of canine mucosae showed a ratio of 100 : 22.5 ± 0.4. The difference in the state of shock mucosa did not exceed ± 1.35%.

Further analysis of the results to determine the effect of the duration of shock on membrane stability indicated that after 90 minutes the amount of latent activity fell by 49%. In spite of their large range (SD), the mean values from 10 dogs, 90 to 120 minutes' endotoxemia, were 40 ± 36 units, significantly less, $p < 0.05$, than control values at $t = 0$. The free and latent activities for one typical dog in Series I are illustrated in Figure 2a. Bound or latent activity is seen to fall during the first 60 minutes of shock, thereafter remaining below the value at $t = 0$. Free activity on the other hand doubles in value then falls later to control levels. This pattern was frequently observed.

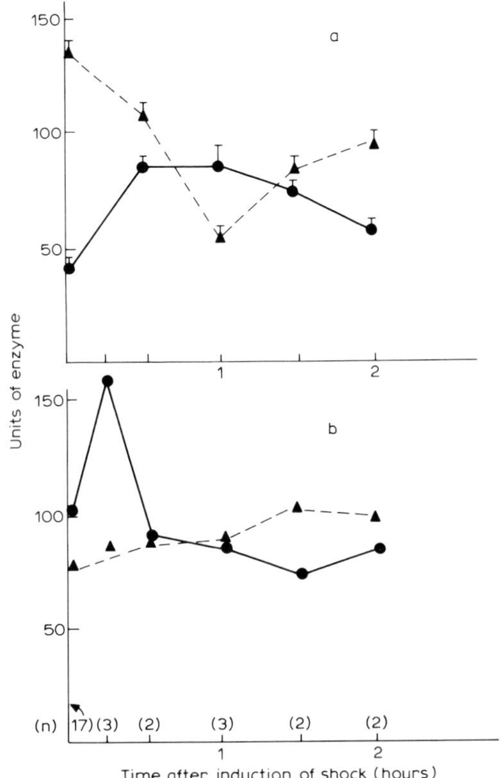

Fig. 2: Response of mucosal lysosomal latency of α-L-*fucosidase to endotoxemia, with and without luminal acid, as described in Table III. Free enzyme activity:* ●*, latent or bound lysosomal activity:* ▲*. All analyses carried out in triplicate. (a) Analysis of sequential biopsies, Series I from a single dog, mean* ± *SEM are given. (b) Series II dogs subjected to shock, with acid saline instilled into the stomach (100–150 ml). The analytical results were pooled for each time interval. (n) = number of dogs. No control values at t = 0 were assayed for these dogs, as explained in the text. Values at t = 0 were those obtained from Series I controls. A comparison of these control values (n = 17) with the average* α-L-*fucosidase in the mucosae from all the dogs in this series (n = 12) irrespective of the duration of shock showed a significant increase in latency or lysosome bound enzyme, p = >0.005, by Student's t-test.*

In Series II, endotoxemia with luminal acid caused much histologically-observed damage as well as visible lesions. The average values of acid hydrolase activity obtained at different time intervals is given in Figure 2b. As sequential biopsies could not be taken in this series, the control values of

Series I, taken at t = 0, taken immediately before induction of shock, were assumed to be equivalent in this experiment. The presence or absence of luminal acid is known to make little or no difference to mucosal acid hydrolase activities (see Table I, II and reference 6).

Although few dogs were examined at each time interval in Series II, the results indicate that the presence of acid in the lumen appears to increase the amount of latent α-L-fucosidase throughout the period of observation of shock. Free enzyme, on the other hand, soars in the first 15 minutes and then diminishes to control levels.

A further test of the stability of enzyme latency or lysosome binding during endotoxemia was developed using cell culture, or preincubation of mucosal tissue obtained from shocked animals compared with controls. This was carried out by measuring the amount of bound, latent enzyme before and after culture for 4 hours. The results, given in Figure 2b, emphasize the greatly increased stability of enzyme-membrane binding in the residual, still-viable cells.

It can be concluded therefore that although endotoxemia causes little change in total enzyme activity and little visible tissue damage, there is a slow breakdown of latency, inferring a gradual disturbance of the strength of the lysosomal enzyme binding in the fundic mucosa. Plasma membrane destabilization also occurs as there is an overall loss of mucosal lactic dehydrogenase (58%, not illustrated). If no luminal acid is present, this disturbance appears to have little effect on the mucosal structures. In the presence of luminal acid, however, even a temporary release of the lysosomal enzyme binding causes the prompt development of tissue damage and visible but localized lesions. However, as lysosomally bound α-L-fucosidase, β-N-acetylglucosaminidase and acid phosphatase are found to increase in the surrounding, noneroded areas of mucosa, it would appear that the tissue is responding to insult by increased neosynthesis of products essential to repair. This implies that accelerated autophagy is taking place within those mucosal cells which remain viable: the repair mechanism sets to work.

Summary

The topically applied ulcerogens, ethanol and bile as well as endotoxemic shock were shown to cause gastric erosions, but only in the presence of gastric acid on the lumen of the mucosa. Standard, direct tests of lysosomal stability have been applied to lysosome-enriched fractions obtained from canine gastric mucosae, subjected to ethanol or bile. Both acid and neutral ethanolic solutions disrupt membrane binding whereas fresh, slightly alkaline gallbladder bile has little effect. Latent, bound enzymes, however, were released in the presence of luminal acid on the bile-treated mucosa. It can be postulated therefore that as a probable step in ulcerogenesis, the ulcerogenic agent causes a disturbance in the intercellular membrane structure so that latent acid hydrolases become accessible for release and activation. Under such conditions, it is possible that if H^+ ion is insorbed, enzymic hydrolysis and intracellular degradation takes place outside the lysosomal sac.

Indirect tests for changes in lysosomal membrane binding, accompanying endotoxemia also suggest a 'leakage' of enzymes from their organelles. In the presence of luminal acid, H^+ ion insorption may occur in certain areas, perhaps due to localized ischemia, yielding an environment inducive to macromolecular breakdown, resulting in discernible lesions. All cells, not imbalanced by the primary insult, and in the presence of the normal extracellular environment of luminal acid, respond by neosynthesis. Increased levels of lysosomally-bound acid hydrolases thus give rise to the accelerated autophagy, necessary for repair.

References

1. Janoff, A., Weissmann, G., Zweifach, B.W. and Thomas, L. (1962): Pathogenesis of experimental shock. IV. Studies on lysosomes in normal and tolerant animals subjected to lethal trauma and endotoxaemia. *J. Exp. Med. 116*, 451.

2. Weissmann, G. and Thomas, L. (1962): Studies on lysosomes. I. The effects of endotoxin, endotoxin tolerance and cortisone on the release of acid hydrolases from a granular fraction of rabbit liver. *J. Exp. Med. 116*, 433.

3. Ferguson, W.W., Starling, J.R. and Wangensteen, S.L. (1972): Role of lysosomal enzyme release in the pathogenesis of stress ulcer-induced gastric ulceration. *Surg. Forum 23*, 380.

4. Ferguson, W.W., Edmonds, A.W., Starling, J.R. et al. (1973): Protective effect of prostaglandin E_1 (PGE_1) on lysosomal release in serotonin-induced gastric ulceration. *Ann. Surg. 177*, 648.

5. Himal, H.S., Greenberg, L., Boutros, M.I.R. and Waldron-Edward, D. (1975): Effect of aspirin on ionic movement and acid hydrolase activity of explants of canine antral and duodenal mucosae. *Gastroenterology 69*, 439.

6. Waldron-Edward, D., Boutros, M.I.R. and Himal, H.S. (1977): Effect of bile on lysosomal stability in the mucosa of the canine gastric antrum. *Gastroenterology 73*, 980.

7. Hickman, S. and Neufeld, E.E. (1972): A hypothesis for I-cell disease: defective hydrolases that do not enter lysosomes. *Biochem. Biophys. Res. Commun. 49*, 992.

8. Neufeld, E.E., Lim, T.W. and Shapiro, L.J. (1975): Inherited disorders of lysosomal metabolism. *Ann. Rev. Biochem. 44*, 357.

9. Hingson, D.J. and Ito, S. (1971): Effect of aspirin and related compounds on the fine structure of mouse gastric mucosa. *Gastroenterology 61*, 156.

10. Hahn, K.J., Krischkofski, D., Weber, E. and Morgenstern, E. (1975): Morphology of gastrointestinal effects of aspirin. *Clin. Pharmacol. Ther. 17*, 330.

11. Boutros, M.I.R., Gourgi, M.M., Himal, H.S. and Waldron-Edward, D. (1976): Establishment of the integrity of lysosomes in a glycoprotein-rich matrix. Distribution pattern of seven lysosomal enzymes in gastric mucosa. *Biochim. Biophys. Acta 444*, 508.

12. Boutros, M.I.R. and Waldron-Edward, D. (1977): Acid hydrolases: assay of activity and latency in the varied mixed cell populations of the canine gastric mucosa. *Lab. Invest. 36*, 436.

13. Waldron-Edward, D., Decaëns, C., Bader, J.P. et al. (1976): Biosynthesis of secretable glycoproteins or mucins of the G.I. tract of the rat. *Path. Biol. (Paris) 24*, 531.

14. Altimirano, M. and Martinoya, C. (1966): The permeability of the gastric mucosa of the dog. *J. Physiol. (London) 184*, 771.

15. Birkett, D. and Silen, W. (1974): Alteration of the physical pathways through the gastric mucosa by sodium taurocholate. *Gastroenterology 67*, 1131.

Gastric mucosal blood flow and resistance to injury

P.H. Guth
Medical and Research Services, Wadsworth V.A. Hospital and UCLA School of Medicine, Los Angeles, California, U.S.A.

During the past 15 years there has been a marked increase in our knowledge of the gastric microcirculation and the role of mucosal blood flow in gastric physiology and pathophysiology. Improved techniques to study the gastric microcirculation and to quantitatively measure mucosal blood flow have played a major role in this advance. The purpose of this paper is to very briefly review the anatomy and regulation of the microcirculation of the stomach and then present evidence of the role of mucosal blood flow in gastric mucosal resistance to injury.

Anatomy and regulation of the gastric microcirculation

Injection techniques [1, 2] and in vivo microscopic studies [3] have provided good descriptions of the gastric microvascular anatomy. This is diagrammatically presented in Figure 1. A supplying artery pierces the external muscle layer of the stomach and sends a branch to this layer. This branch divides into smaller arterial vessels, which supply the capillaries of the muscle layer. The main artery continues into the submucosa, where it enters an extensive submucosal arterial plexus. Mucosal arterioles from this plexus pierce the muscularis mucosae to supply blood to mucosal capillaries. The capillaries run between and parallel to the glands, but interconnect by short channels at right angles to the axis of the gland tubules. At the mucosal surface they form loops around the gland openings and then drain into collecting veins. These course perpendicularly from the superficial mucosa to the submucosa, where they enter an extensive submucosal venous plexus. Veins from this plexus pierce the external muscle layer to carry blood away from the stomach. As they go through the muscle layer they are joined by smaller venous branches draining the muscle capillaries. Contrary to early reports [1], no submucosal arteriovenous anastomoses have been found in the stomach of man [2], rat [3], dog [5] or cat [6].

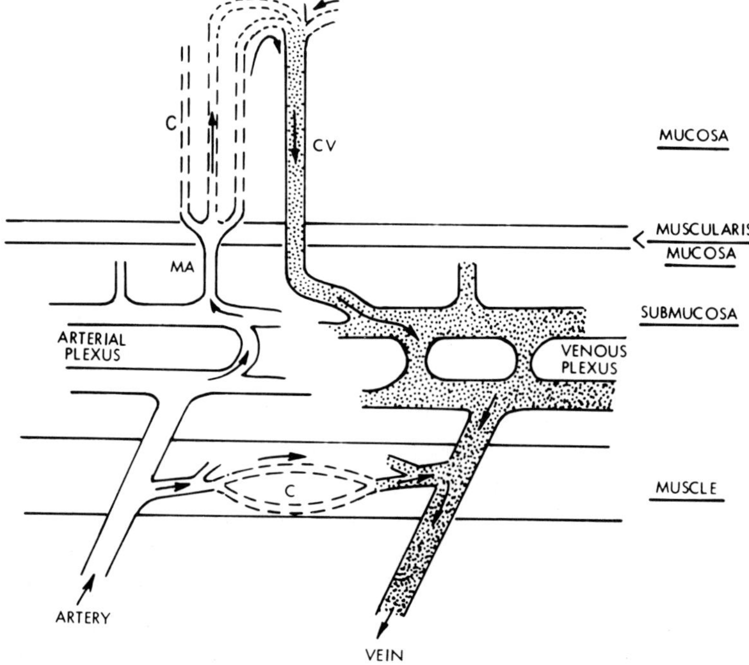

*Fig. 1:   Diagrammatic representation of the gastric microcirculation. MA = mucosal
arteriole; C = capillary; CV = collecting vein. Reproduced by permission from Guth,
P.H. (1977): The gastric microcirculation and gastric mucosal blood flow under normal
and pathological conditions. In: Progress in Gastroenterology, Vol. III, pp. 323–347.
Ed: G.B.J. Glass. Grune and Stratton, Inc., New York.*

The submucosal arterioles control blood flow to the mucosa. Constriction
of these vessels, including their mucosal arteriolar branches, decreases blood
flow to the mucosa; dilatation increases mucosal blood flow [6, 7]. The
influence of various agents on gastric blood flow has been studied using the
aminopyrine clearance technique [8] or the radiolabelled microsphere technique [9] to measure gastric mucosal blood flow, as well as electromagnetic
flow probes [10] and in-vivo microscopy [3]. Splanchnic nerve stimulation
decreases [6, 7, 11] and vagal nerve stimulation increases [6, 7, 12] blood flow.
Alpha-adrenergic agents decrease [13] and beta-adrenergic agents increase [8]
blood flow. Indometacin, an inhibitor of prostaglandin synthesis, decreases
[14], and prostaglandins of the E, A and I_2 types increase blood flow [15, 16].
Gastrin increases blood flow, but this is secondary to the increase in acid
secretion (which calls forth an increase in mucosal blood flow) and not to a
direct effect on the gastric microvessels [17, 18].

Mucosal blood flow and resistance to injury

In recent years, experimental evidence has accumulated that mucosal blood flow plays an important role in the prevention of injury to the gastric mucosa. Two lines of evidence have been developed in support of this concept.

Decreased mucosal blood flow is needed for gastric mucosal injury

Mersereau and Hinchey used an ex vivo gastric chamber technique to study acute gastric mucosal lesions induced by hemorrhagic shock in the rat [19]. This permitted direct observation of lesion development. Immediately after induction of hemorrhage, the glandular mucosa blanched rather uniformly. As the blood pressure stabilized at 20 mm Hg, some color returned to the mucosa and, under stereomicroscopic observation, sluggish flow was observed in mucosal collecting veins. Small white superficial areas were then seen, and these slowly enlarged. With retransfusion of blood, bleeding began in the base of these lesions. In the normotensive rat superfusion with 150 mM HCl caused no gastric damage, while in the hypotensive rat as little as 50 mM HCl produced lesions in all animals. In the totally ischemic stomach (clamping of the blood supply for 10 minutes), as little as 25 mM HCl produced mucosal lesions. These studies led to the hypothesis that 'at adequate hydrogen ion concentration, ulceration occurs at pre-existing focal breaks in the mucosa when the mucosal blood flow is so reduced that it cannot prevent the build up of toxic concentrations of hydrogen ions' [19].

Using a lucite gastric chamber technique in dogs, Ritchie studied the effect of topical 100 mM HCl alone, HCl + 5 mM sodium taurocholate, and HCl + sodium taurocholate topically + close intra-arterial vasopressin infusion [20]. Mucosal blood flow was measured by the aminopyrine clearance technique. No lesions were observed in the mucosae exposed to HCl or

Table I: Effect of acid test solution (ATS), ATS + sodium taurocholate (TC), and ATS + TC + vasopressin (VP) on lesion index, aminopyrine clearance (AC) and hydrogen ion flux ($\triangle H^+$).

	ATS	ATS + TC	ATS + TC + VP
Lesion index	0	0	3.5 ± 0.2[a,b]
$\triangle H^+$ (μEg/0.5 hour)	$+70 \pm 48$	-444 ± 28[a]	-504 ± 48[a]
AC (ml/min)	1.72 ± 0.19	3.28 ± 0.21[a]	0.56 ± 0.15[a,b]

a = significant difference vs. ATS.
b = significant difference vs. ATS + TC.
Adapted from [20].

HCl + taurocholate (Table I). However, mucosal blood flow was almost doubled by the combination of HCl + sodium taurocholate. Vasopressin infusion markedly reduced blood flow, but lesion formation in the presence of HCl was minimal. However, when taurocholate in acid was applied to the mucosa and vasopressin infused, there was a marked reduction in blood flow and marked gross mucosal damage occurred. Ritchie also measured hydrogen ion back diffusion and found a similar H^+ loss whether taurocholate was applied with or without the vasopressin infusion. He postulated that the increased blood flow during HCl + taurocholate application might be a compensatory mechanism to protect against the increased back-diffusion of H^+, and that under ischemic conditions lesion formation was the result of the inability to effectively clear or neutralize H^+, which entered the mucosa as a consequence of permeability changes induced by the bile salts.

Whittle performed analagous studies in the rat using ^{14}C-aniline clearance to measure gastric mucosal blood flow [21]. Indometacin 20 mg/kg i.v. over 10 minutes decreased mucosal blood flow, but had no effect on acid back-diffusion. Gastric perfusion with 2 mM sodium taurocholate in 100 mM HCl increased acid back-diffusion. This was accompanied by an increase in mucosal blood flow and few lesions developed. However, administration of indometacin during acid-taurocholate perfusion reduced this elevated mucosal blood flow without changing acid back-diffusion, and extensive mucosal damage occurred. These results suggest that, although a decrease in mucosal blood flow or an increase in acid back-diffusion can lead to a low incidence of erosions, a combination of both produces extensive mucosal damage.

Cheung and Chang studied the role of gastric mucosal blood flow and H^+ back-diffusion in the pathogenesis of acute gastric lesions due to the topical application of the barrier breaker p-chloromercuribenzene [22]. They used a dog gastric chamber technique and measured blood flow to the mucosa with radiolabelled microspheres. Exposure of the mucosa to p-chloromercuribenzene resulted in a significant increase in H^+ back-diffusion, which was accompanied by a rise in mucosal blood flow. Hemorrhagic shock alone caused a marked mucosal ischemia without disruption of the permeability barrier. The severest mucosal injury occurred under experimental conditions, where ischemia and increased back-diffusion were induced simultaneously.

These independent studies indicate that, under experimental conditions in which the gastric mucosal barrier to acid back-diffusion is broken and mild mucosal injury may or may not occur, decreasing mucosal blood flow results in marked lesion formation.

Increased mucosal blood flow protects against gastric mucosal injury

The thesis that the pathogenesis of acute mucosal lesions was the result of bile salt-induced H^+ back-diffusion plus gastric mucosal ischemia was further tested by Ritchie and Shearburn [23]. They repeated the previously-described studies by Ritchie [20], with the addition of the close intra-arterial infusion of the beta-adrenergic agonist isoprenaline. Their results are presented in Table II. Animals subjected to HCl + taurocholate + shock but receiving isoprenaline still demonstrated an increased H^+ loss, but mucosal blood flow returned to near normal levels and there was a significant decrease in lesions. These findings suggest that increased blood flow protects against lesion-formation under these experimental conditions. In a similar dog gastric chamber study, McGreavy and Moody investigated the effect of the close intra-arterial infusion of isoprenaline on acetylsalicylic acid-induced gastric mucosal lesions [24]. Topical acetylsalicylic acid increased H^+ loss and produced gross lesions. Isoprenaline did not affect acetylsalicylic acid-induced H^+ loss, but did increase blood flow and decrease lesions, suggesting that a marked increase in blood flow may prevent or ameliorate experimentally-produced erosive gastritis. Whittle, in studies in the rat, observed that the administration of (15S)−15 methyl prostaglandin E_2 decreased the acid back-diffusion, increased the mucosal blood flow and significantly reduced the lesions formed by topical sodium taurocholate + HCl during indometacin infusion [21].

These independent studies indicate that, under experimental conditions with topical barrier breakers in which marked mucosal lesions develop, increasing mucosal blood flow protects against lesion formation.

Table II: Effect of acid test solution (ATS), 5 mM of sodium taurocholate (TC), hemorrhagic shock (S) and isoprenaline (I) on lesion index, aminopyrine clearance (AC) and hydrogen ion flux ($\triangle H^+$).

	ATS	ATS + TC + S	ATS + TC + S + I
Lesion index	0.3 ± 0.2	4.4 ± 0.3^a	$1.6 \pm 0.5^{a,b}$
$\triangle H^+$ ($\mu Eg/0.5$ hour)	-71 ± 46	-700 ± 202^a	-921 ± 55^a
AC (ml/min)	2.85 ± 0.25	0.79 ± 0.13^a	$2.01 \pm 0.37^{a,b}$

a = significant difference vs. ATS.
b = significant difference vs. ATS + TC + S.
Adapted from [23].

How does blood flow protect the gastric mucosa?

Two hypotheses have been presented concerning how mucosal blood flow protects the gastric mucosa against injury: by maintaining adequate tissue oxygenation and energy sources, and by removing or buffering back-diffusing acid.

Tissue oxygenation and energy sources

Menguy and his colleagues reported a profound reduction in gastric mucosal adenosine triphosphate levels within 15 minutes after the induction of hemorrhagic shock in rats [25]. This severe deficit in energy metabolism coincided with the development of epithelial cell necrosis; gross erosions were present within 60 minutes after the induction of shock. They proposed that stress ulcers related to hemorrhagic shock might result from a mucosal energy deficit severe enough to cause cellular necrosis. The observed small glycogen reserve of the gastric mucosa and the absence of a prompt increase in lactate-pyruvate in response to complete ischemia suggested that the gastric mucosa is a tissue with an aerobic type of metabolism. It would appear that the integrity of the gastric mucosa requires a minute-by-minute supply of glucose and oxygen and cannot tolerate the anaerobic state. In subsequent studies, Menguy and Masters found that the antral mucosa tolerates the 'partial ischemia' of hemorrhagic shock and 'complete ischemia' (complete severance of gastric vascular connections) far better, with respect to maintenance of energy metabolism, than the corpus mucosa [26, 27]. This might explain why stress ulceration involves mainly the corpus of the stomach and spares the antrum, a feature of this condition noted in both human beings [28] and animals [29].

Removal of back-diffusing acid

Kivilaakso, Fromm and Silen studied the pH of the lamina propria of the fundus and the antrum in both rabbits and dogs during hemorrhagic shock [30]. A small area of the gastric wall was denuded of its seromuscular coat and, using a micromanipulator, an antimony microelectrode was advanced vertically into the mucosa so that its tip was in the mid-portion of the mucosa. The millivoltage was recorded continuously by a high-input impedance pH/electrometer. In the rabbit fundic mucosa, a relatively permeable membrane, pH rapidly and profoundly decreased (from 7.35 to 6.62), and this was associated with severe lesion formation. In canine fundic mucosa, a less permeable membrane, intramural pH decreased much more slowly. However, when the mucosal barrier was disrupted by the addition of 5 mM taurocholate to the acidic mucosal solution, a more rapid and profound decrease in intramural pH to 6.50 occurred, with severe and extensive mucosal lesion formation. These findings suggest that the critical determinant of lesion development during shock is not tissue anoxia, but an impaired capacity of the mucosa to remove or buffer the influx of acid. Moody et al., based on their studies cited above and their findings that carbenoxolone markedly increased H^+ back-diffusion but also greatly increased blood flow without a concomitant development of lesions [22, 24], came to a similar conclusion [31].

Summary

The various studies described above indicate that gastric mucosal blood flow plays an important role in protecting the gastric mucosa against injury. This concept is diagrammatically presented in Figure 2. When disruption of the gastric mucosal barrier to acid back-diffusion occurs and H^+ enters the interstitial tissue, there is a compensatory increase in mucosal blood flow. When this increased flow is sufficient to dilute, buffer and remove this excess H^+, tissue injury is minimized or may not occur at all. If, under the same conditions, mucosal blood flow is decreased (e.g., by hemorrhagic shock or

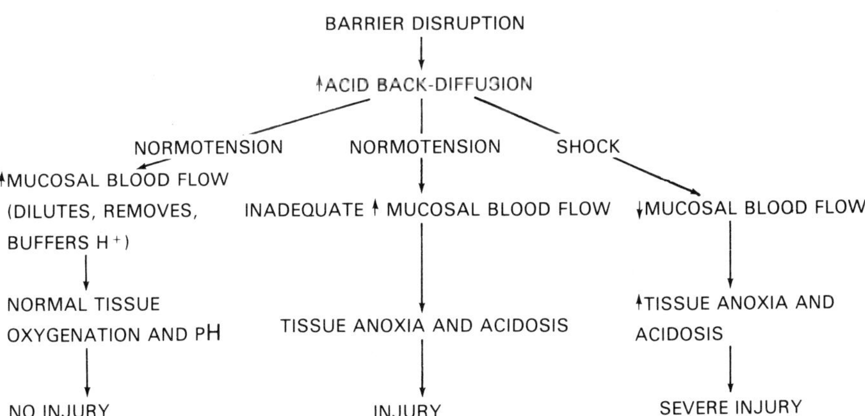

Fig. 2: Diagrammatic representation of the interrelation between mucosal blood flow and disruption of the gastric mucosal barrier to acid back-diffusion in mucosal lesion formation.

vasoconstrictor agents), marked lesion formation results. Conversely, increasing blood flow by vasodilating agents under these latter conditions will protect against mucosal injury. The mechanism of this protective effect probably involves both removal of influxing H^+ and maintenance of adequate tissue oxygenation and energy sources.

References

1. Barlow, T.E., Bentley, F.H. and Walder, D.N. (1951): Arteries, veins and arteriovenous anastomoses in the human stomach. *Surg. Gynecol. Obstet. 93*, 657.
2. Piasecki, C. (1974): Blood supply to the human gastroduodenal mucosa with special reference to the ulcer-bearing areas. *J. Anat. 118*, 295.
3. Guth, P.H. and Rosenberg, A. (1972): In vivo microscopy of the gastric microcirculation. *Am. J. Dig. Dis. 17*, 391.
4. Guth, P.H. (1977): The gastric microcirculation and gastric mucosal blood flow under normal and pathological conditions. In: *Progress in Gastroenterology*, Vol. III, pp. 323–347. Ed: G.B.J. Glass. Grune and Stratton, Inc., New York.
5. Shoemaker, C.P. Jr. and Powers, S.R. Jr. (1966): The absence of large functional arteriovenous shunts in the stomach of the anesthetized dog. *Surgery 60*, 118.
6. Guth, P.H. and Smith, E. (1977): Nervous regulation of the gastric microcirculation. In: *Nerves and the Gut*, pp. 365–373. Eds: F.P. Brooks and P.W. Evers. Charles B. Slack, Inc., Thorofare.
7. Guth, P.H. and Smith, E. (1975): Neural control of gastric mucosal blood flow in the rat. *Gastroenterology 69*, 935.
8. Jacobson, E.D., Linford, R.H. and Grossman, M.I. (1966): Gastric secretion in relation to mucosal blood flow studied by a clearance technique. *J. Clin. Invest. 45*, 1.
9. Archibald, L.H., Moody, F.G. and Simons, M. (1975): Measurement of gastric blood flow with radioactive microspheres. *J. Appl. Physiol. 38*, 1051.
10. Kolin, A. (1960): Blood flow determination by electromagnetic method. In: *Medical Physics*, Vol. 3, pp. 141–155. Ed: O. Glasser. Yearbook Publishers, Inc., Chicago.
11. Reed, J.D., Sanders, D.J. and Thorpe, V. (1971): The effect of splanchnic nerve stimulation on gastric acid secretion and mucosal blood flow in the anesthetized cat. *J. Physiol. (London) 214*, 1.
12. Martinson, J. (1965): The effect of graded vagal stimulation on gastric motility, secretion and blood flow in the cat. *Acta Physiol. Scand. 65*, 300.
13. Zinner, M.J., Kerr, J.C. and Reynolds, D.J. (1975): Adrenergic mechanisms in canine gastric circulation. *Am. J. Physiol. 229*, 977.
14. Main, I.H.M. and Whittle, B.J.R. (1975): Investigation of the vasodilator and antisecretory role of prostaglandins in the rat gastric mucosa by use of non-steroidal anti-inflammatory drugs. *Br. J. Pharmacol. 53*, 217.
15. Main, I.H.M. and Whittle, B.J.R. (1973): The effects of E and A prostaglandins on gastric mucosal blood flow and acid secretion in the rat. *Br. J. Pharmacol. 49*, 428.

16. Whittle, B.J.R., Boughton-Smith, N.K., Moncada, S. and Vane, J.R. (1978): Actions of prostacyclin (PGI$_2$) and its product 6-oxo-PGF$_1$ on the rat gastric mucosa in vivo and in vitro. *Prostaglandins 15*, 955.

17. Guth, P.H. and Smith, E. (1976): The effect of gastrointestinal hormones on the gastric microcirculation. *Gastroenterology 71*, 435.

18. Jacobson, E.D. and Chang, A.C.K. (1969): Comparison of gastrin and histamine on gastric mucosal blood flow. *Proc. Soc. Exp. Biol. Med. 130*, 484.

19. Mersereau, W.A. and Hinchey, E.J. (1973): Effect of gastric acidity on gastric ulceration induced by hemorrhage in the rat, utilizing a gastric chamber technique. *Gastroenterology 64*, 1130.

20. Ritchie, W.P. Jr. (1975): Acute gastric mucosal damage induced by bile salts, acid, and ischemia. *Gastroenterology 68*, 699.

21. Whittle, B.J.R. (1977): Mechanisms underlying gastric mucosal damage induced by indomethacin and bile salts, and the actions of prostaglandins. *Br. J. Pharmacol. 60*, 455.

22. Cheung, L.Y. and Chang, N. (1977): The role of gastric mucosal blood flow and H$^+$ back-diffusion in the pathogenesis of acute gastric erosions. *J. Surg. Res. 22*, 357.

23. Ritchie, W.P. Jr. and Shearburn, E.W. III (1977): Influence of isoproterenol and choleystyramine on acute gastric mucosal ulcerogenesis. *Gastroenterology 73*, 62.

24. McGreavy, J.M. and Moody, F.G. (1977): Protection of gastric mucosa against aspirin-induced erosions by enhanced blood flow. *Surg. Forum 28*, 357.

25. Menguy, R., Besbaillets, L. and Masters, Y.F. (1974): Mechanism of stress ulcer: influence of hypovolemic shock on energy metabolism in the gastric mucosa. *Gastroenterology 66*, 46.

26. Menguy, R. and Masters, Y.F. (1974): Mechanism of stress ulcer. II. Differences between the antrum, corpus, and fundus with respect to the effects of complete ischemia on gastric mucosal energy metabolism. *Gastroenterology 66*, 509.

27. Menguy, R. and Masters, Y.F. (1974): Mechanism of stress ulcer. III. Effects of hemorrhagic shock on energy metabolism in the mucosa of the antrum, corpus, and fundus of the rabbit stomach. *Gastroenterology 66*, 1168.

28. Lucas, C., Sugawa, C. and Walt, A. (1971): Natural history and surgical dilemma of 'stress' gastric bleeding. *Arch. Surg. 102*, 266.

29. Harjola, P.T. and Sivula, A. (1966): Gastric ulceration following experimentally induced hypoxia and hemorrhagic shock. *Ann. Surg. 163*, 21.

30. Kivilaakso, E., Fromm, D. and Silen, W. (1978): Relationship between ulceration and intramural pH of gastric mucosa during hemorrhagic shock. *Surgery 84*, 70.

31. Moody, F.G., McGreavy, J., Zalewsky, C. et al. (1977): The cytoprotective effect of mucosal blood flow in experimental erosive gastritis. *Acta Physiol. Scand. Special Sup.*, 35.

Morphological phases in the development and healing of ulcers

T. Miyake
First Department of Internal Medicine, Faculty of Medicine, Kyoto University, Kyoto, Japan

Factors influencing location of ulcers: What are the mucosal defensive factors of the stomach?

It is well known that the potent digestive action of gastric juice plays a very important role in the development of peptic ulcers, judging from the fact that the sites where ulcers develop are limited to those areas that are influenced by gastric juice. As regards the etiology of peptic ulceration, Shay and Sun reported that ulcers develop as the result of an imbalance between an increase in aggressive factors and a decrease in mucosal defensive factors [1]. Therefore, the treatment of peptic ulcer should be basically oriented to the suppression of aggressive factors and the enhancement of mucosal defensive factors. Although acid and pepsin have been clearly established as the chief aggressive factors, the exact mechanism of mucosal defensive factors is as yet unknown.

In order to find out what the mucosal defensive factors of the stomach are, it is necessary to consider those factors which have been shown to be related to the healing of ulcers in clinical comparative studies between acute gastric mucosal lesions (AGML) and chronic ulcers, and between easily-curable ulcers and intractable ulcers.

Acute gastric mucosal lesions and chronic gastric ulcer: clinical and endoscopic observations

The recent advance and spread of emergency endoscopy has enabled us to take pictures of ulcers at very early stages in their development. In most cases, the causes of such AGML are relatively apparent. Such manifestations develop quite suddenly and, in most cases, are accompanied by severe epigastric pains, vomiting, hematemesis and melena and patients sometimes fall into hemorrhagic hypovolemic shock. Endoscopic findings often reveal irregular multiple and shallow ulcers or erosions, which in many cases are healed within a very short period (2–3 weeks). On the other hand, the ordinary chronic ulcers which are often clinically encountered and are without any subjective symptoms are mostly single and round-shaped, deep, and take long clinical courses before healing.

Sakita and Fukutomi [2] and Miwa [3] have reported a useful classification of the 3 stages of gastric ulcer, based on endoscopic findings. The 3 stages they suggest are the active stage, the healing stage and the scarring stage, each of which can be further divided into 2 substages.

Active stage

A1   The surrounding mucosa is edematously swollen, and no regenerating epithelium seen endoscopically.

A2   The surrounding edema has decreased, the ulcer margin is clear and a small amount of regenerating epithelium is seen in this margin. A red halo (marginal zone) and a white slough circle (ulcer margin) are frequently seen. Usually, converging mucosal folds can be followed right up to the ulcer margin.

Healing stage

H1   The white coating has become thin and the regenerating epithelium extends into the ulcer base. The gradient between the ulcer margin and the ulcer floor is becoming flat. The ulcer crater is still evident, and the ulcer margin is sharp. The diameter of the mucosal defect is about one-half to two-thirds of that seen in A1.

H2   The defect is smaller than in H1 and the regenerating epithelium covers most of the ulcer floor. The area of white coating is about one-quarter to one-third of that seen in A1.

Scarring stage

S1   The regenerating epithelium now completely covers the floor of the ulcer. The white coating has disappeared. Initially, the regenerating region is markedly red, and on close observation, many capillaries are seen. This is called the 'red scar'.

S2   In several months to a few years, the redness is reduced to the color of the surrounding mucosa. This is called the 'white scar'.

While we have employed this system of classification and have found it useful, we have long felt the need for a clearer understanding of the relation between endoscopic appearance and histological findings. Previous reports have shown that the recurrence rate of gastric ulcer is closely correlated with the endoscopic scarring stage present at the time of termination of therapy [4, 5]. If the red scar is covered by a thin and flat surface epithelial layer and mucous secretory function is still poor and immature histologically, it may not be competent to diagnose the case as a 'recovery', although endoscopic demonstration of ulcer healing in the red scar stage (S1) is allowed.

As previously mentioned, acute ulcers are multiple at the level of U1-I (within the mucosa) or U1-II (up to the submucosa); chronic ulcers, on the other hand, often develop singly at the level of U1-III (up to the muscular layer) or U1-IV (up to the subserosa). It is clear, statistically, that healing time is in proportion to the depth of ulceration. The following 3 conditions in the healing of ulcers may be indicated: reduction of ulcer diameter; purification of ulcer bottom; and shallowing of ulcers. The healing of ulcers involves the covering of the defected site with regenerated epithelium, followed by the filling of the site with proliferated connective tissue, since the proper muscular layer itself is not regenerated.

Morphological phases in the development and healing of ulcers: endoscopic, histological and dissecting (stereoscopic) microscope studies

Endoscopic observation of the development of ulcers

In many cases it has been observed that at emergency endoscopy, just after the development of an ulcer, multiple mucosal bleedings can be seen. Administration of hematin hydrochloride will cause these bleedings to change to a darker color which at follow-up appear fused and expanded. Meanwhile, after about 3 days, these dark spots will be exfoliated and digested by gastric juice and become white-coated erosions or ulcers.

Histological comparative studies between easily-curable ulcers and intractable ulcers

In order to see what factors would be involved in the length of the ulcer healing period, a comparative histochemical study was performed on easily-curable ulcers and intractable ulcers [6].

Materials and methods Sulpiride, (*N*-(1-ethylpyrrolidin-2-yl-methyl)-2-methoxy-5-sulfamoylbenzamide) which improves the blood flow of the gastric mucosa, was given to 21 patients hospitalized for surgical operations because of intractable gastric ulcers. While 11 patients (52.4%) were healed by sulpiride therapy, 50 mg intramuscularly twice a day for 4 weeks, gastrectomy was carried out on schedule in 10 cases where complete healing could not be demonstrated by the X-ray and endoscopic examinations. Histochemical examinations were conducted on the resected stomachs.

As a control group, 10 operated patients of chronic intractable ulcers with clinical courses similar to those of sulpiride group were selected from another group of 98 gastrectomized patients. Healing conditions of the resected stomachs in both groups were compared, in particular from the standpoint of the connective tissue. These selected patients satisfied the following conditions:
– Patients who had undergone continuous treatment since being correctly diagnosed as suffering from gastric ulcer with either X-ray or by endoscopic examination more than 6 months previously but who still suffered from recurrences.
– Patients who had relapsed despite continuous treatment after correct diagnosis within the previous 3 months.
– Patients meeting both aforesaid conditions without any findings of healing.
– Patients who had been hospitalized.

The resected stomachs of both groups were immediately fixed in formalin and carnoy, and the following histochemical methods were applied:
Hematoxylin-eosin stain; Van Gieson's solution; Azan stain; De Oliveira's silver stain; Phosphortungstic acid-hematoxylin stain; Alucian blue stain; Toluidine blue stain (pH 4.1, 7.0); Periodic acid Schiff reaction (PAS); Saunder's acridine-orange fluorescence microscopy [7] (Orthoplan (Leiz), exciting filter 3 mm, BG 12, suppression filter K 530, acridine-orange 1/10,000, pH 7.2, 1/15 M PBS); and hyaluronidase digestion method (hyaluronidase HSE 5342, pH 6.0, acetic acid buffer solution, 38°C, 2 hours' incubation).

Results and discussion   From the generative zone present at the gastric glandular neck, proliferation occurs at the ulcer margin, and at the bottom of the ulcer a single layer of regenerated epithelium extends toward the ulcer center. This regenerated epithelium suspends its growth just before fibrinoid necrosis, if any exists in the direction of its extension. A white coating covers and protects the thin regenerated epithelial layer, beneath which a basement membrane forms; below this membrane granulated tissue, abundant in blood vessels, proliferates.

Histological study of the tissue in the intractable ulcer group, showed that proliferation of the regenerated epithelium was not sufficient. Fibrinoid necrosis remained for a long time and proliferation of the granulated tissue was incomplete.

The decrease in blood flow, the quantitative and qualitative deficiency of acid mucopolysaccharides in the connective tissue, the delayed formation of collagen fibers and the presence of extensive scar in the muscular layer, owing to poor capillarization and the formation of intravascular thrombosis, seem characteristic of the histopathological findings of intractable ulcers. On the other hand, in the sulpiride group very favorable histopathological findings of the resected stomachs were observed compared with those in the intractable ulcer group (e.g., marked epithelization, remarkable regeneration of the granulated tissue and a higher development of the capillary system without any thrombus, corresponding to the histological findings of the easily curable ulcers).

Dissecting (stereoscopic) microscope study on ulcer healing process

Over the past 13 years we have used the dissecting microscope to close-up magnifying studies on finer lesions of the mucosal surface in 338 resected stomachs [5, 8]. This method was employed in order to link together the endoscopic and histological findings. This method is also of significant importance as a basis research tool in the development of close-up magnifying endoscopy [9].

Materials and methods   Three hundred and thirty-eight fresh resected stomachs with various lesions were utilized. After the entire mucosal surface of the stomach had been prewashed with physiologic saline, the portions subject to microscopic observation were soaked in a chymotrypsin solution, followed by exposure to spoutings of saline solution to clear away the adherent mucus from the mucosal surface. Sometimes, 0.1% methylene blue was sprayed onto the cleaned surface in order to permit observation of lightly stained mucous membrane through a dissecting microscope Olympus model X-Tr (Magnification: 16× or 25×). At the same time, histological examinations were used for scrutinizing the location observed by dissecting-microscope, and the endoscopic classification of the ulcer stages were recorded.

Results and discussion   Figure 1 shows a comparison of the fundic and pyloric areas of the normal mucosa, based on the dissecting-microscope findings. The outstanding differences between these 2 areas are in the gland openings and the capillary meshwork; in addition, the blood vessels distributed in the mucosa are more sparse in the pyloric area than in the fundic area. Numerous areae gastricae can be seen; the gland openings in the fundic area appear round or oval, and surrounded with capillaries, which form a meshwork.

On the other hand, while can be observed around the gland openings in the pyloric area, they do not encircle these completely, as in the fundic area. The openings themselves are cleft-like. In the continuous slice sample made parallel to the surface, it can be seen that several pyloric glands are open at the bottom of this cleft.

It is interesting to note that a thin colloidal mucinoid layer, not stained with methylene blue, remains just above the epithelial layer even after wash-out of the mucus by digestion with chymotrypsin.

The mucous barrier may certainly prevent H^+ ion back-diffusion. As Silen has pointed out, it is some dynamic variable state [10]. Under dissecting-microscopic observation, the superficial and middle parts of the mucous layer appear liquid and fluffy, and are easily dissolved by chymotrypsin and washed out by physiological saline solution. The underlayer of mucus, namely

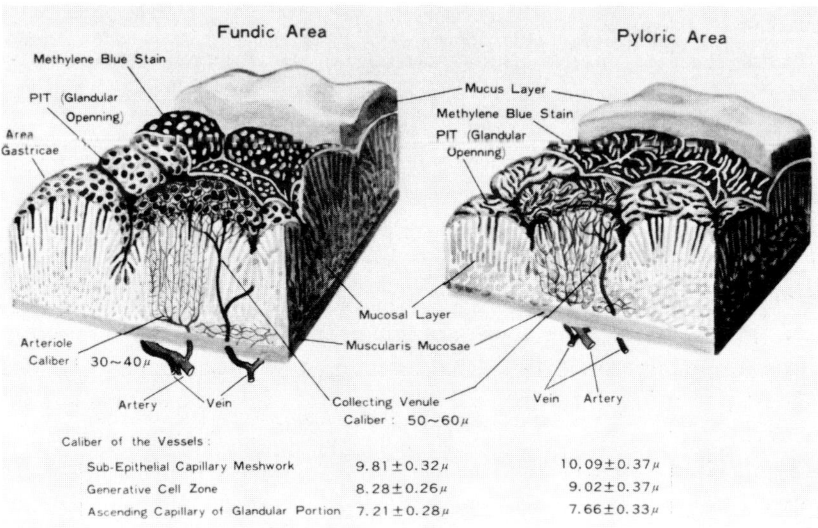

Fig. 1: A comparison of the fundic and pyloric areas of the normal human gastric mucosa based on the dissecting-microscope findings.

mucinoid substance just above the epithelium, which may consist of mucin and glycoprotein freshly secreted by the surface epithelial cells, protects the mucosal surface and the epithelium.

Even in the normal gastric mucosa, H^+ back diffusion occurs to some extent slowly into the mucous barrier from its surface. It may be supposed that H^+ back diffusion is related to the speed of production and secretion of mucus by the surface epithelial cells.

Of the 338 cases studied, 86 specimens were found to be benign. When observed under the dissecting microscope, these 86 specimens could be arranged in a sequence of gradually-proliferating epithelization and concomitant tissue maturation, confirmed by the staging of endoscopic classification. The following 4 stages were classified by dissecting-microscopic observations, and correlated with endoscopic and histologic findings on the same portion of the specimens:

Stage I (Initial stage)   This phase of the healing process corresponds to Sakita's A2 stage. A single layer of flat regenerated epithelium can be observed in the ulcer margin, extending toward the center of the ulcer. From the ulcer margin in which the generative zone is located, spindle-shaped protuberances, like a pen-point, ascend to the extended regenerated epithelium (Fig. 2). Histologically, a white coating covers the thin layer of regenerated epithelium and fibrinoid necrosis exists under the white coating.

Stage II (Growing stage)   This corresponds to Sakita's H1-H2 stage. Under the dissecting microscope, the regenerated cells produced at the pen-point shaped location are seen growing in a long papilla-form or a low palisade-like appearance, reddish in tone, and extending radially toward the center of the ulcer (see Fig. 2) The diameter of the ulcer is reduced. Histologically, the ulcer is covered by a single layer of epithelium near the center of the ulcer, while the palisade-like regenerated epithelium shows a papilla-form on the cut surface (see Fig. 5). The ulcerated tissue, to which India ink had been infused intravascularly (the continous slice sample) shows numerous new proliferated capillaries intertwined and extending towards the generative zone and papilla-form regenerating epithelium, seen in reddish tone endoscopically.

Stage III (Palisade scar)   This phase of epithelial regeneration corresponds to the major part of Sakita's red-scar (S1) stage. The palisade-like regenerated radial epithelium from ulcer margin develops ditches crossing obliquely or rectangulary (see Fig. 5). Those separated small portions can be recognized as

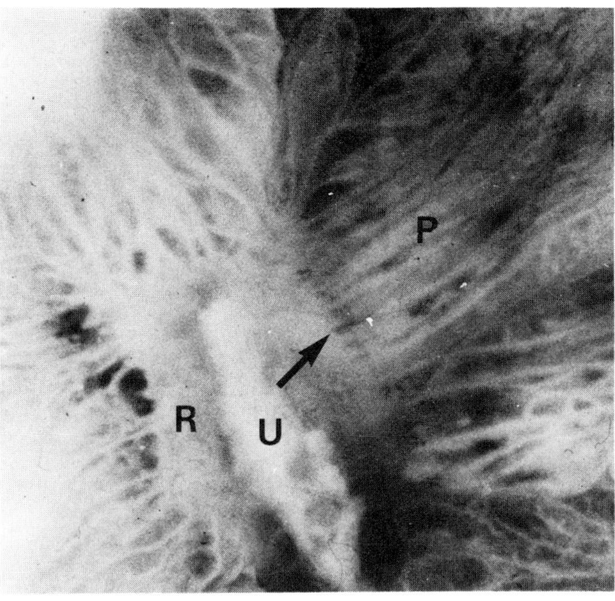

Fig. 2:   Dissecting-microscopic picture of Stage II (Growing Stage) corresponding to Sakita's endoscoping healing stage (H1-H2). The ulcer (U) is seen to be surrounded by regenerated thin epithelium (R) and the latter by pen-point shaped protuberances (arrow) which result in the characteristic palisade-like regenerated epithelium (P). Magnification: 16×. Reproduced with permission from [5].

small red spots. The white coating has already disappeared. Gradually, the palisade-shaped regenerated mucosa is separated by the ditches to form squares in the center of the healing ulcer. The color tone of the mucosa is hyperemic in intense redness, which after India ink infusion, proved to be a large number of new blood vessels. Histologically, the surface epithelial cells have infiltrated the tissue and begun to form an immature gland structure, namely the pseudo-pyloric gland. The cave surface is deep and the regenerated mucosa is tufted. The mucin-producing function of the surface epithelial cells has not yet matured (Fig. 5).

Stage IV (Cobblestone scar)   This corresponds to Sakita's white-scar (S2) stage, and also slightly overlaps his red-scar (S1) stage. Under the dissecting microscope, the square reddish form described above has matured to a round cobblestone-like regenerated mucosa (Fig. 5.) Capillaries have receded and the redness has disappeared. Maturation of the mucosa into a round shape,

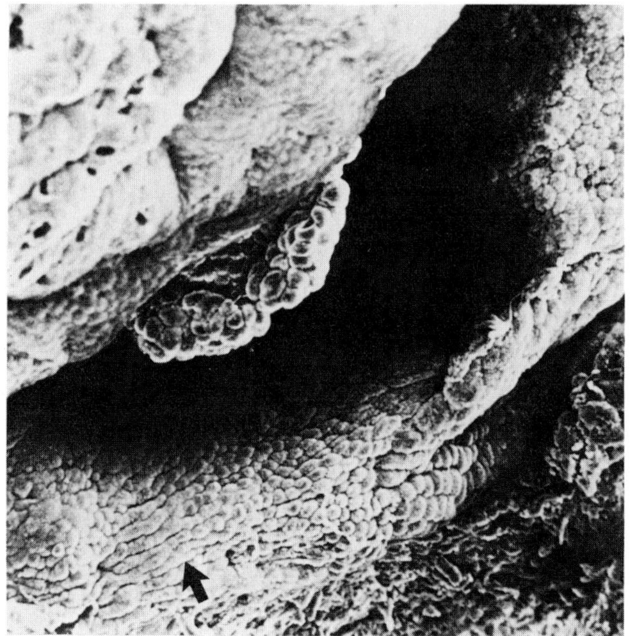

Fig. 3:   Scanning electron microscopic picture of Stage II (Growing Stage) classified by dissecting-microscope findings. The palisade-like regenerated epithelium becomes thin and a pen-point shaped. Though the cells at the pen-point shape region are isolated individually, the rosary-like or syncytium-like arrangement of the cell lines which are occasionally bifurcated are seen (arrow). Magnification: 330×. Reproduced with permission from [11].

separate from the palisade-form, is considered to be a result of the increase of its dimensions by proliferation of epithelial cells. Histologically, the outstanding feature of the cobblestone-like regenerated epithelium is its rich supply of pseudo-pyloric glandular structures. The cobblestone-like regenerated mucosa further continues its differentiation, and at the time the gland openings are formed on the top of each cobblestone, the formation of the proper tubular gland is completed in the mucosa. Histologically, this stage represents complete recovery.

Our study of gastric ulcer recurrence has revealed that the recurrence rate is significantly higher in patients treated until the attainment of the red-scar stage (palisade-scar stage) than in those treated until the white-scar stage (cobblestone-scar stage) [4]. This indicates that the treatment of ulcer disease should be continued to the cobblestone-scar stage, even after endoscopically-demonstrated disappearance of a spot-like white coating.

Cell regeneration and electron microscopic studies: scanning electron microscopic observation

In order to support the findings of the dissecting-microscopic observations, a scanning electron microscopic study was also performed [11].

Materials and methods

Six freshly resected stomachs with benign ulcers (U1-II, U1-III, and U1-IV) were utilized. The adherent mucus was washed out with saline solution from the surface of the samples. Specimens were fixed in 2.5% glutaral for 2 hours, were then washed in phosphoric acid buffer solution, and then dehydrated in a graded solution of ethanol. They were then dried, using amyl acetate and liquid CO_2 as the exchange solution. The samples were thin-coated on a 100 Å layer of gold paladium or a vacuum evaporator and then viewed on the JSM-U_3 scanning electron microscope using an accelerating voltage of 15 kv. Histological examinations were also performed, and the endoscopic classification of ulcer stages as recorded.

Results and discussion

Under the scanning electron microscope, gland openings in the normal fundic area are round or oval as was also seen with the dissecting microscope. The epithelial cells forming the openings are clearly visible and on their surface sparse and short micro-villi are observed. On the other hand, most openings in the pyloric area are cleft-like. Unlike those in the fundic area, tall and dense micro-villi are observed on the cell surface. These micro-villi are similar to those in the duodenum and small intestine, and seem to be related to absorption.

Figure 3 shows a scanning electron microscopic picture of the growing stage of the ulcer healing process (classified by dissecting microscope). The innumerable cells, as a sheet of cell layer, extend toward the center of the ulcer from the pen-point shaped regenerative zone. Though the cells at the pen-point shape region were isolated individually, the rosary-like or syncytium-like arrangement of the cell lines, which are occasionally bifurcated, are seen. The regenerated epithelial cells seem not only to be produced by and sent out passively from the generative zone, but also to carry out mitosis and maturation actively. Figure 4 is a photograph of a cut surface of the cobble-stone-like regenerated mucosa. The round-shaped cobblestone mucosa is more mature than the palisade-like mucosa or squared-form cobblestone

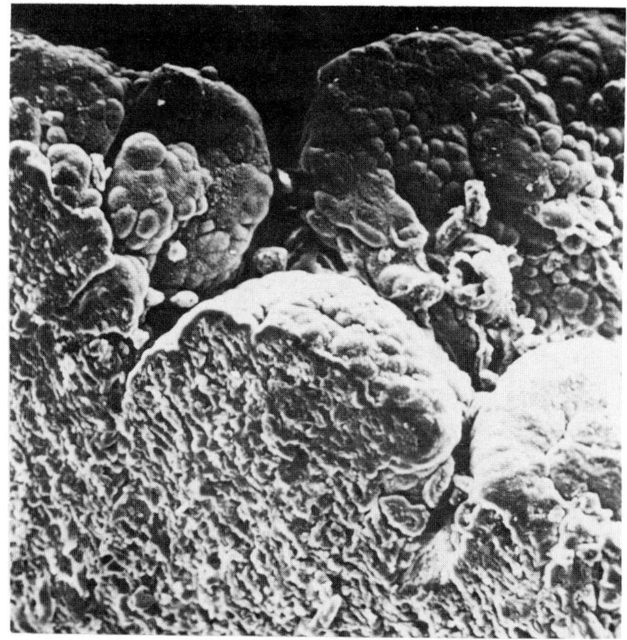

Fig. 4:   Cut surface of the cobblestone-like regenerated mucosa. The regenerated epithelial cells creep further into the granulation tissue from the bottom of the caved region to form the tubular gland structures. Scanning electron microscopy. Magnification: 330×. Reproduced with permission from [11].

mucosa and has invaded the tissue from the bottom of the caved region and so is differentiated from the tubular gastric glands.

In a shallow ulcer of U1-II, the muscularis mucosa contract upward. In U1-III and U1-IV, the pen-point shaped generative zone grows actively by cell proliferation and produces the palisade-like form. Thereafter, the regenerated mucosa gradually matures from the square form to the round-shaped cobblestone-like form after being separated by crossing ditches from the marginal region (Fig. 5).

Summary

The results and discussions so far presented are summarized in Figure 6. Ultimately, the surface structure of the mucosa depends upon the equilibrium between the cell production and the cell loss of the epithelial cell [12]. The mucus as a mucous barrier performs a dynamic metabolism, which certainly

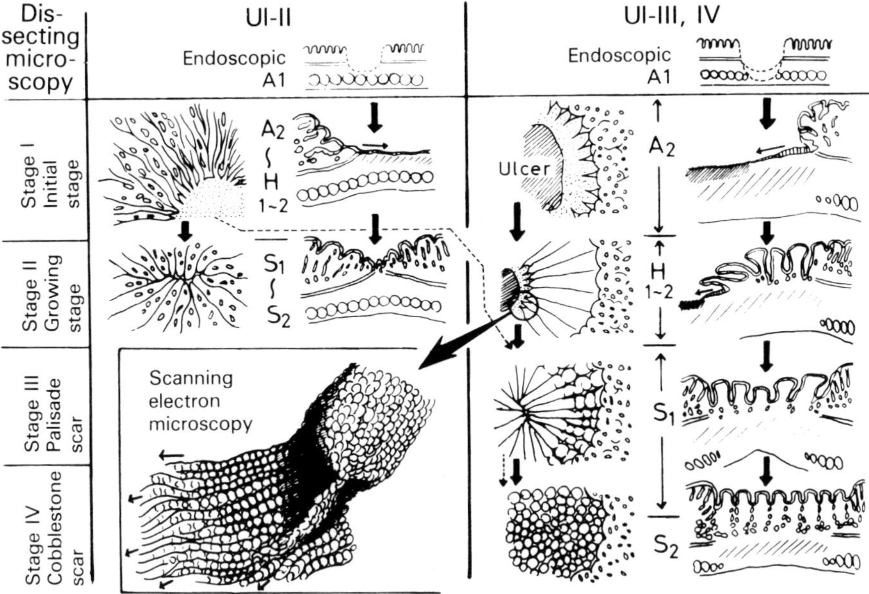

Fig. 5: Healing process of gastric ulcer (Ul-II, Ul-III, and Ul-IV). Correlation of gastric ulcer healing features by endoscopy, dissecting-microscopy, scanning electron microscopy and histology. Reproduced with permission from [11].

seems to inhibit H^+ back-diffusion, protecting the surface epithelial cells and relating to such hormones as secretin, prostaglandin [13, 14], glucagon [15] etc. Moreover, it may also be assumed that the thin colloidal mucinoid layer observed with the dissecting microscope just above the surface epithelium is an active mucosal barrier.

The regenerated epithelium continues its growth, protected from aggressive factors by being sandwiched between the white coating which extends like the eaves of a house and the basement membrane which consists of acid mucopolysaccharides and reticular fibrils. The cell activities of the stem cells in the generative zone and the regenerated epithelial cells hold a vital significance. The synthesis of acid mucopolysaccharides and collagen are also important factors, and among them capillary blood flow may be the most important factor. These factors are complexly interrelated and, together, may be referred to as the mucosal defensive factors.

Acknowledgments

The author is grateful to Professor Haruto Uchino, Kyoto University, and to

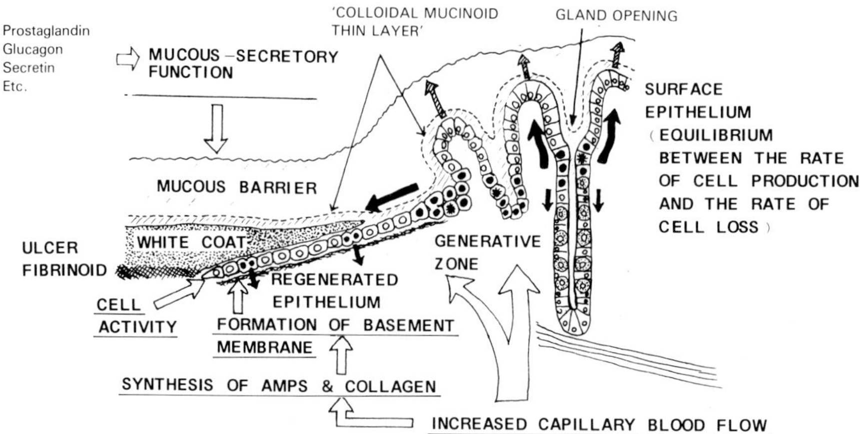

Fig. 6: A scheme showing the mucosal defensive factors of the stomach.

his co-researchers, Dr. Akio Todo, Kobe Municipal Hospital, Dr. Masami Oishi, Shingu Municipal Hospital, and Dr. Takeshi Suzaki, Tenri Hospital.

References

1. Shay, H. and Sun, D.C.H. (1953): Etiology and pathology of gastric and duodenal ulcer. In: *Gastroenterology, 2nd Edition,* p. 420. Ed: H.L. Bockus. Saunders Co., Philadelphia-London-Toronto.
2. Sakita, T. and Fukutomi, H. (1971): Endoscopic diagnosis in ulcers of stomach and duodenum. In: *Endoscopic Diagnosis* (in Japanese), p. 197. Ed: Y. Yoshitoshi. Nankodo Co., Tokyo.
3. Miwa, T. (1972): Chronic ulcer of the stomach. In: *Gastroenterology*, Chapter 5, p. 49. Ed: T. Sakita. International Medical Foundation of Japan, Tokyo.
4. Miyake, T., Ariyoshi, J., Suzaki, T. et al. (1980): Endoscopic evaluation of the effect of Sucralfate therapy and other clinical parameters on the recurrence rate of gastric ulcers. *Dig. Dis. Sci. 25,* 1.
5. Miyake, T., Suzaki, T. and Oishi, M. (1980): Correlation of gastric ulcer healing features by endoscopy, stereoscopic microscopy, and histology, and a reclassification of the epithelial regenerative process. *Dig. Dis. Sci. 25,* 8.
6. Miyake, T., Yamamoto, Y., Suzaki, T. et al. (1970): Clinical and experimental studies on the anti-ulcer effect of Sulpiride. Part III. Histopathological study on intractable ulcer of the stomach with special reference to the connective tissue (in Japanese). *Jpn. Arch. Intern. Med. 17,* 113.
7. Saunders, A.M. (1962): Histochemical identification of acid mucopolysaccharides with acridine orange. *J. Histochem. Cytochem. 10,* 683.

8. Suzaki, T. and Miyake, T. (1975): Dissecting-microscope study of the gastric mucosa. Capillary picture visualized by India ink infusion and gland opening pattern. II. Adenomatous polyp, atypical epithelium and benign ulcer (in Japanese). *Gastroenterol. Endosc. 17*, 532.

9. Suzaki, T., Miyake, T., Yamamoto, Y. et al. (1970): Microgastrofiberscope − A new device in diagnosis of gastric cancer based on dissecting-microscope findings. *Jpn. Arch. Intern. Med. 17*, 27.

10. Silen, W. (1977): New concept of the gastric mucosal barrier. *Am. J. Surg. 133*, 8.

11. Todo, A., Miyake, T., Suzaki, T. et al (1976): Scanning electron microscopic observation of the regenerated epithelium in gastric ulcer in various healing stages (in Japanese). *Jpn. J. Gastroenterol. 73*, 35.

12. Croft, D.N. (1977): Cell turnover and loss and the gastric mucosal barrier. *Am. J. Dig. Dis. 24*, 383.

13. Dousa, T.P. and Dozois, R.R. (1977): Interrelationships between histamine, prostaglandins, and cyclic AMP in gastric secretion: A hypothesia. *Gastroenterology 73*, 904.

14. Robert, A., Nezamis, A.E., Lancaster, C. and Hanchar, A.J. (1979): Cytoprotection by prostaglandins in rats. Prevention of gastric necrosis produced by alcohol, HCl, NaOH, hypertonic NaCl, and thermal injury. *Gastroenterology 77*, 433.

15. Tarnawski, A., Krause, W.J. and Ivey, K.J. (1978): Effect of glucagon on aspirin-induced gastric mucosal damage in man. *Gastroenterology 74*, 240.

Discussion

The discussion of papers in this Chapter centered around mechanisms which determine mucosal resistance to injury.

Bicarbonate secretion by gastric mucosa

The potential protective role of gastric bicarbonate secretion against mucosal injury, not dealt with in depth by any of this Chapter's contributors, was then debated. Bicarbonate is actively secreted by the gastric mucosa. Only recently, however, have accurate techniques been available for quantification of gastric bicarbonate production in experimental animals. Cholinergic agents, calcium, and prostaglandin derivatives stimulate bicarbonate secretion by the gastric epithelium whereas ischemia, acetylsalicylic acid and indometacin reduce it [1, 2, 3].

In discussing the potential protective role of bicarbonate secretion against acid-injury it was pointed out that, for a given area of gastric mucosa, bicarbonate production is only one-tenth or less of maximal acid output. However, it is possible that the main neutralizing effect of bicarbonate occurs close to the apical membrane of gastric epithelial cells, within an 'unstirred layer' which allows a stable pH gradient to be developed [1]. It is possible that one of the roles of mucus (whose production is, incidentally, also enhanced by prostaglandins) is to increase and stabilize this unstirred layer. At this time, however, there is no direct evidence that surface epithelial secretion of bicarbonate plays an important role in mucosal defense. It is certain that breakdown of the 'mucosal barrier' with diffusion of plasma bicarbonate into the gastric lumen is not the mechanism of increased bicarbonate production under some conditions. Therefore, whether increased bicarbonate secretion represents a protective mechanism that can be modulated according to requirements or simply a consequence of injury has not been totally ascertained.

Prostaglandins

Present evidence suggests a central role for prostaglandins in the mechanisms which determine mucosal protection. Some questions remain, however, as to whether prostaglandins play a causative role or simply reflect metabolic transformation nonspecifically associated with the phenomenon of increased mucosal resistance to injury. Indeed, whereas studies by Robert indicate that mucosal resistance to injury can be enhanced by mild 'irritation' and that this effect can be blocked with drugs inhibiting prostaglandin synthesis [4], there is little or no direct evidence that prostaglandin synthesis is increased in the mucosa exposed to the same irritants. Further, as Konturek et al. describe in their contribution (pages 78–86), a variety of antisecretory drugs (H_2-blockers, anticholinergics) administered at nonantisecretory doses can enhance mucosal resistance in experimental models without a measurable increase in tissue prostaglandin activity measured by bioassay. These are intriguing results which need to be confirmed and expanded. However, they also can be criticized in that nonantisecretory doses of active inhibitors (defined by a lack of measurable effect on luminal acid secretion) do not exclude a local change in pH enhancing mucosal resistance. Other investigators have shown that, in the presence of luminal hydrochloric acid instilled exogenously, H_2-blockers do not exhibit significant protective activity whereas exogenous prostaglandin derivatives do [5].

Mucosal blood flow

The regulation of mucosal blood flow is still being sorted out. However, an increase in mucosal blood flow and oxygen supply may be one of the mechanisms by which the gastric mucosa becomes more resistant to injury. Prostaglandins and H^+-back-diffusion may play an important role. Dr. Rudolf Schiessel of Vienna, Austria presented a summary of his studies performed at Dr. W. Silen's laboratory in Boston, Massachusetts, where it was found that H^+-back-diffusion stimulates gastric mucosal blood flow. When they perfused rabbit fundus with increasing intraluminal (H^+) they found a linear correlation to mucosal blood flow measured by the microsphere method (Fig. 1).

Changing the perfusate from buffer (pH = 7) to 80 mM HCl (isosmolar with NaCl) gave a significant rise of blood flow and no change of the pH in the lamina propria measured with a microelectrode. When vasopressin was infused under these conditions, the blood flow, and the pH in the lamina propria dropped and ulceration occurred (Fig. 2). From this experiment it was concluded that there is an autoregulation of blood flow in fundic mucosa similar to the brain where the extracellular pH regulates blood circulation. These studies indeed open the path for further investigation of the mechanisms which decrease or enhance resistance in response to conditions and requirements prevailing locally at a particular time.

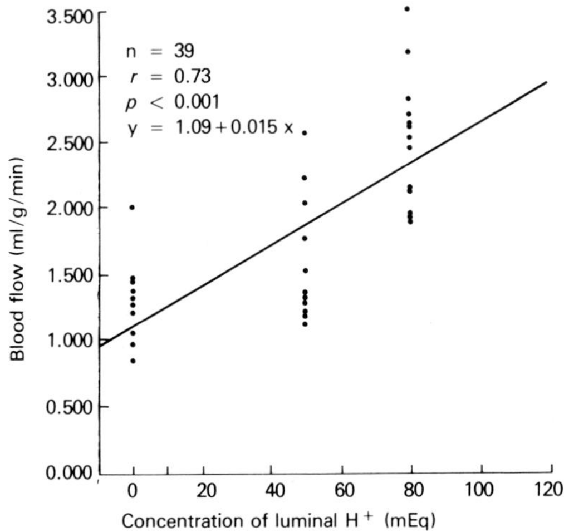

Fig. 1: Relation of H^+ in the gastric lumen to mucosal blood flow at 60 minutes after the start of pouch perfusion (3 samples per stomach). The regression line was calculated by the least square method.

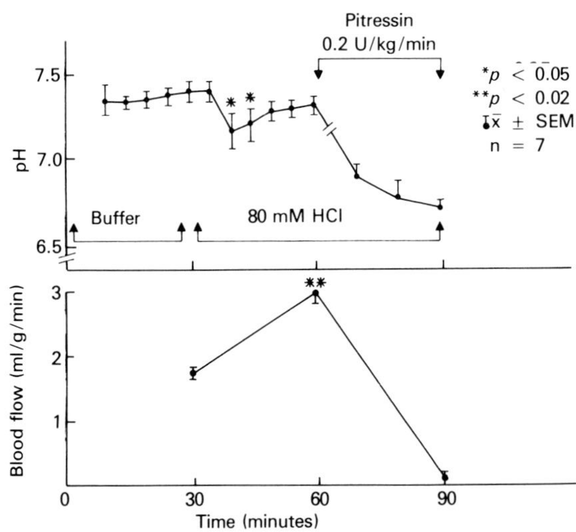

Fig. 2: Effect of perfusion with 80 mM HCl on intramural pH and mucosal blood flow. The infusion of pitressin significantly decreased both intramural pH and mucosal blood flow (Duncan's test).

Morphology

As Dousa points out in his review (pages 128–136), Miyake's work on stages of ulcer healing provides a tentative anatomic localization of protective and repair mechanisms: mucus, epithelial regeneration and blood flow. It should be pointed out, however, that much of this work was performed on acute erosions whose pathogenesis and pattern of healing may differ from chronic ulcerations. Indeed, depth of ulceration is one of the most important factors determining speed and pattern of healing. In superficial erosions the generating zone of epithelial growth occurs at the bottom of the lesion whereas in deeper ulcers the generating zone is around the neck. The anatomic healing pattern of duodenal ulcers appears to be similar to that of gastric ulcers.

References

1. Kauffman, G.L. (1980): Gastric bicarbonate secretion: an update. *Brain Res. Bull. 5*, 15.
2. Allen, A. and Garner, A. (1980): Progress report: mucus and bicarbonate secretion and their possible role in mucosal protection. *Gut 21*, 249.
3. Kivilaakso, E. and Silen, W. (1979): Pathogenesis of experimental gastric mucosal injury. *New Engl. J. Med. 301*, 364.
4. Robert, A. (1979): Cytoprotection by prostaglandins. *Gastroenterology 77*, 761.
5. Carmichael, H.A., Nelson, L.M. and Russell, R.I. (1978): Cimetidine and prostaglandin: evidence for different models of action on the rat gastric mucosa. *Gastroenterology 74*, 1229.

Pathogenesis of ulcer disease: comments and perspectives

T.P. Dousa
Mayo Clinic and Foundation, Rochester, Minnesota, U.S.A.

The least risky comment one could make concerning the topic of this chapter, would be a statement that the pathogenesis of ulcer disease is a complex multi-factional process, that no single factor was identified and that no single solution is at hand; and also that much more information should be gathered and more investigations conducted. Fortunately, there is no necessity to hide behind such generalities, since it appears that the mainstream of current investigative work in this field, many findings of which are presented here, naturally converges to the several specific points which may prove to be the cellular basis for gastric mucosa resistance to ulcerogenic attacks of very diverse origins. These main factors of interest, which are dealt with directly or indirectly by virtually all contributed papers, include the potential roles of glycoproteins (GP) and glycosaminoglycans (GAG)*, within cells of gastric mucosa or secreted by mucosal cells, and the role of prostaglandins (PG); the role of lysosomes and mucosal blood flow may well also directly or indirectly be related to these 2 preceding factors.

In his extensive contribution Professor Miyake analyzes, from many diverse points, the development and healing of ulcers mainly in humans. The pervading impression which offers itself from his analysis is the potentially prominent role of GAG and GP in cytologically defined entities − in the form of 'mucous barrier', 'colloidal mucinoid thin layer', and mucosal basement membrane which all potentially participate in, or are involved in cellular processes in mucosal cytoprotection. These processes include regeneration of mucosal epithelium, synthesis of mucosal basement membrane as well as synthesis of GP and GAG which are other extracellular constituents of the

* Glycosaminoglycans (GAG) were formerly more frequently named mucopoly-saccharides and the term prostaglandin(s) (PG) in a broader sense describes any product of PG cyclooxigenase in general.

gastric mucosal layer. GP and GAG are implicated in many factors contributing to the resistance of tissue to noxious influences and in the processes of tissue regeneration.

Gastric mucosal GAG and GP are discussed in more specific detail by Professor Domschke. Unique biochemical properties of GP and GAG which apparently make these compounds suitable for the cytoprotective functions are briefly reviewed. While the importance of sialic acid (*N*-Acetylneuraminic acid) as a major exoglycosidase, and hence critical point for initiation of GP and GAG catabolism, cannot be underestimated [1], opinion about the contribution of sialic acid component to overall acidity of GP and GAG should be guarded. Conceivably, sulfated GP and GAG could contribute equally or even more to the acidic properties of GP and GAG than was believed some time ago, and their presence and role in gastric mucosa may deserve reappraisal with the use of updated biochemical methodology. In this context it is useful to recall that, until very recently, sialic acid was considered to be a major source of negative charges of GP and GAG in renal glomerulus [2], while most recent investigations indicate that previously unsuspected sulfated GP and GAG, such as heparan sulfate, play a major role as an electronegative barrier [3–5].

In this observer's opinion, analysis of composion as well as studies on the biosynthesis and catabolism of specific GP and GAG of gastric mucosa (both extracellular and intracellular) deserve much more vigorous attention than has been attracted in the past several years. This effort should include also the study of cytotopic localization of GP and GAG and careful distinction has to be made between integral cellular GP and GAG (e.g. components of membranes), and those which are constituents of extracellular substances. Such research, focused on specific GP and GAG in distinct sites of mucosal structure, may reveal subtle specific deficiencies of GP and GAG in gastric mucosa tissue prone to ulceration; such deficiencies were indeed suggested by global and not always strictly quantitative studies reported in the past.

Numerous observations, many of these recounted by Professor Domschke, point to one important (and perhaps major) regulatory factor in the metabolism of GAG and GP – prostaglandins (PGs). Many observations show that drugs which are PG synthesis inhibitors (namely glucocorticoids and nonsteroidal anti-inflammatory agents [NSAIA]) are also frequently ulcerogenic and were also observed to reduce gastric production of GAG and GP. PG, on the other hand, has been shown to promote GP and GAG synthesis in some nongastric tissues, e.g., in fibroblasts [6, 7] or in synoviocytes [8, 9]. It is thus plausible that NSAIA and glucocorticoids, through their action to diminish PG synthesis, may block formation of GP and GAG in gastric mucosa and, consequently, make it more vulnerable to ulcerogenic attacks. Observation that carbenoxolone, a drug which has potential to decrease PG breakdown and thus accumulate endogenous PG, also promotes gastric mucous secretion, may serve as a good reminder that not only biosynthesis but also biodegradation of PG determines PG tissue levels and consequently their putative regulatory action on GP and GAG metabolism in gastric mucosa.

A clear and succinct recount of the evidence that PGs indeed have a cytoprotective effect on gastric mucosa against ulcer formation in both clinical and experimental situations is provided by Professor Robert. Professor Robert summarizes and emphasizes evidence for a critically important point: that cytoprotective PG effect is distinct from the frequently reported ability of PG (PG and/or PG-like compounds) to inhibit gastric acid (HCl) secretion and to antagonize the action of histamine and other HCl secretagogues [10]. Mechanisms by which PG (which one of the numerous PGs is specifically relevant here we do not know) antagonizes HCl secretion still remains unknown, in spite of the fact that numerous hypotheses were proposed. The cytoprotective action of PG, unrelated directly to modulation of HCl secretion, may well be related to the regulatory effect of PG on the biosynthesis and catabolism of GP and GAG which are components of the gastric mucosa defense system.

In view of the potentially pivotal role of GP and GAG in the genesis and healing of gastric mucosa ulcers, it is useful to recall that lysosomal hydrolases are the only known metabolic pathway for catabolism of extracellular GAG and GP [1]. The cytodigestive function of lysosomal enzymes may be expressed in the process of autophagy-release of hydrolytic enzymes from lysosomes within the cells, in response to noxious stimuli and extracellular digestion, as well as in digestion of phagocytosed material in 'secondary lysosomes' [11]. Professor Waldron-Edward reports an observation which indicates that indeed lysosomal hydrolases are released from association with lysosomes, to a greater extent than normal under experimental pathologic conditions which impair gastric mucosa.

While this mechanism of increased lysosomal injury − more ready leak of lysosomal enzymes into the intracellular environment − could certainly contribute to damage of intrinsic gastric mucosa cells, it is in order to consider the potential pathogenic role of lysosomal enzymes actively released (by exocytosis) from otherwise undamaged gastric mucosal cells into extracellular space. It is of note that while lysosomal hydrolases are maximally active only at acidic pH (pH 4−5), such extracellular pH conditions might be expected to prevail in, or on the surface of, gastric mucosa. Not only secretion of HCl into the lumen renders gastric juice acidic, but also the presence of negatively charged extracellular GP and GAG is expected to create the acidic colloid environment favorable for the action of lysosomal hydrolases exocytosed from gastric mucosal cells. Exocytosed lysosomal hydrolases may thus catalyze the degradation of GAG and GP extracellular material of gastric mucosa: mucosal coating, mucus itself and even GAG and GP of cell surface membranes. A possibility should also be considered that some GAG and GP of mucous material could be endocytosed (phagocytosed) and then digested within secondary lysosomes [11, 12]. Internalization of GAG seems to be an important feature of GAG metabolism [13]. Therefore, examination of the total activity of lysosomal enzymes and stability of lysosomes isolated from gastric mucosa towards ulcerogenic conditions and factors could be considered as the first, very important step in the exploration of digestive function of lysosomes in gastric mucosa. The dynamics of lysosomes in gastric musoca, however, may turn out to be very complex and important for the pathogenesis of ulcer disease.

Analogies from nongastric tissues suggest that a connection exists between PG and the dynamic function of lysosomes. PGs, mainly PGE_2, were reported to increase stability of isolated lysosomes towards diverse noxious influences [12, 14]. Perhaps even more importantly, PG was shown to inhibit lysosomal enzyme release – exocytosis of lysosomal hydrolases [12, 15]. One can then envision that besides PGs' action to *increase synthesis* of GAG and GP, mentioned above, PG may *decrease the catabolic breakdown* of GAG and GP of gastric mucosa by inhibiting lysosomal hydrolases release from cells and by increasing the stability of lysosomes within gastric cells.

Dr. Guth's presentation on the role of blood supply for the resistance of gastric mucosa towards injury underlines not only the importance of this factor per se, but in addition, it could be considered that the supply of oxygen and nutrients to gastric mucosa could relate to and determine some regulatory factors which have been discussed above. Adequately supply of oxygen is, in general, necessary for PG synthesis from arachidonic acid at peroxidation and also intermediary metabolism could determine the level of nicotinamide adenine dinucleotide – NAD – a coenzyme in the major catabolic pathway of PG. Oxygen supply could determine cellular levels of adenosine triphosphate (ATP), which has a key role as a substrate for adenosine 3',5'-cyclic monophosphate (cAMP) synthesis catalyzed by adenylate cyclase and as an inhibitor of cAMP phosphodiesterase.

This leads us to cAMP. The potential role of this intracellular regulating factor cAMP, which was not discussed at this session, may be worth mentioning. It is not only because of cAMP importance in general, or because cAMP was implicated in the modulation of tissue response to injury [12], but because cAMP may actually be a common denominator of those cellular components involved in ulcer formation and cytoprotection which are outlined and discussed in the presented papers.

There is an abundant evidence that PGs stimulate adenylate cyclase and increase cAMP accumulation in many tissues. In gastric mucosa, PGs, namely PGE_2 and its metabolically stable analogues, as well as some other PGs were shown to stimulate, markedly, adenylate cyclase in both the fundus and antrum of the stomach and to elevate cAMP levels [16–19]. Indirect [17], and recently, more direct evidence [19] suggest that PG stimulates cAMP accumulation in mucosal cell populations which are distinct from oxyntic cells containing a cAMP system sensitive to histamine [10, 17, 19]. Moreover, PG stimulates adenylate cyclase and cAMP accumulation not only in mucosa of the stomach but also in duodenum and other portions of the small intestine. From analogy obtained in experiments on tissues other than gastric mucosa, it may be expected that cAMP may influence both GAG and GP biosynthesis [6, 7, 20–26] as well as GAG and GP catabolism through action on lysosomes [1, 14, 15], mentioned above. Exogenous cAMP (or cAMP chemical analogues) has been shown to enhance synthesis of GAG and GP in several diverse cell systems [6, 7, 20–26]. Not only PG [6–9, 25], but also some other hormones which stimulate cAMP accumulation were shown to increase incorporation of precursors into GAG and GP and thus enhance biosynthesis of these compounds [6, 7, 20, 22, 23].

Assuming that lysosomal enzymes are a major factor in catabolism of GAG and GP it should be recalled that in the majority of studies cAMP was observed to inhibit release of lysosomal enzymes (exocytosis) from diverse cell population [12, 15]. In addition, cAMP was shown to decrease phagocytosis [27], and fusion of phagocytic vacuoles into 'secondary lysosomes' [28]. PG and cAMP were reported to increase stability of lysosomes in lysosomal fractions and consequently to diminish the leak of lysosomal enzymes from these organelles [14]. Providing that these actions of cAMP are applicable also to the cells of gastric mucosa, one can imagine that at least some cytoprotective function, associated with PG action as well as metabolism of GAG and GP, could be regulated by cAMP levels. Increased cAMP would thus promote biosynthesis and decrease biodegradation of GAG and GP in gastric mucosa (Figure). Humoral agents and drugs, mainly PG, which promote cAMP synthesis and accumulation would thus stimulate GAG and GP synthesis within gastric mucosa and thereby exert their cytoprotective action. If PG would be considered a major agonist of cAMP then either insufficient content of PG in gastric mucosa or some defects, including those caused by drugs, in a PG-sensitive cAMP system may be related to failure of

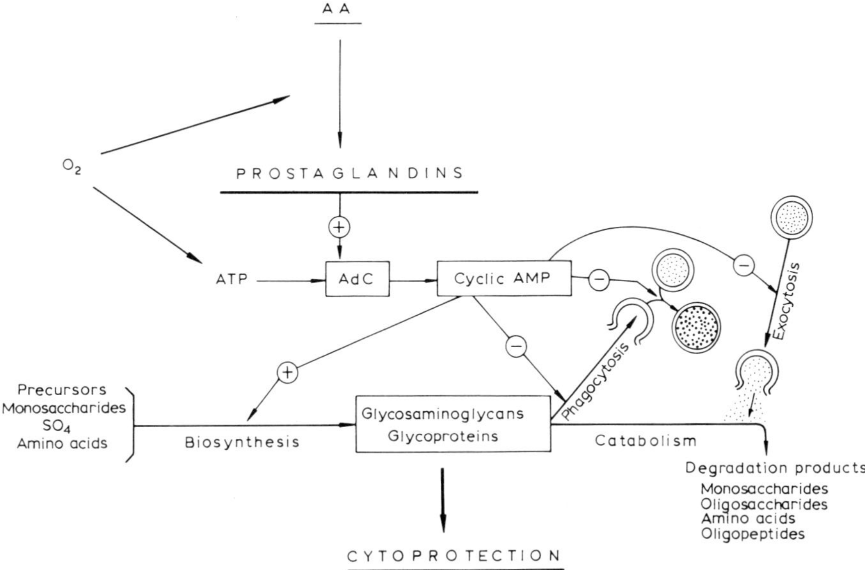

Figure: Hypothetical relationship between prostaglandins (PG), cyclic AMP, glyco-saminoglycans (GAG) and glycoprotein (GP) metabolism within the gastric mucosa. AA = arachidonic acid; AdC = adenylate cyclase; O_2 = oxygen supplied by arterial blood; —⊕→ denotes positive regulatory influences (stimulation, enhancement); —⊖→ denotes negative regulatory influences (inhibition, decrease); ◯ = lyso-some ('primary lysosome'); and ◉ = 'secondary lysosome'. PG stimulates cAMP formation and accumulation; cAMP stimulates biosynthesis of GAG and GP which are involved in cytoprotection. Also, cAMP modulates functions of lysosomes and other elements of cellular digestion in direction towards decrease of GAG and GP cata-bolism. Adequate supply of O_2 by perfusing blood is necessary for synthesis of PG, supply of ATP for cAMP formation, GAG and GP biosynthesis, and other metabolic events.

GAG and GP metabolism and consequently to the pathogenesis of gastric ulcer lesions. In this connection it should be considered that some treatment regimens reported by Professor Konturek − other than supply of exogenous PG − may very well be acting not only on the PG-cAMP-GAG system (Figure), but on one (or more) steps subsequent to PG biosynthesis [29, 30]. If some agent should, e.g., stabilize by direct action lysosomes or directly stimu-late GAG and PG biosynthesis it may conceivably exhibit its anti-ulcerogenic effect even when PG synthesis is suppressed.

Drs. Simon and Kather's report [29] is a good reminder that NSAIA should not be automatically presumed to only inhibit PG synthesis, but that they also sometimes act on steps in the outlined sequence distal to PG formation (see Figure).

The observation that at least in some situations exogenous, long-acting analogues of PG which are known to stimulate cAMP formation in gastric mucosa [16, 31] have an antiulcerogenic effect suggests that deficiency of PG alone may be the main factor in decreased resistance of the gastric tissue. PG deficiency could be caused by yet unknown factors and/or by drugs which block PG formation: mainly glucocorticoids and NSAIA; however, as mentioned above, NSAIA could inhibit not only PG synthesis but also directly, e.g., on adenylate cyclase [29]. In any case, a decreased level of cAMP in the population of gastric mucosal cells which is involved in GAG and GP synthesis and in cells which contain GAG and GP catabolizing lysosomal system, would tip the metabolic balance towards depletion of GAG and GP, lesser cytoprotection and hence an ulcerogenic state. As briefly mentioned above, a lack of oxygen and nutrients supply due to diminished blood perfusion could have an adverse effect both on PG and cAMP accumulation.

Levels of cAMP, in certain populations of gastric mucosa cells, may thus represent a vital regulatory link between several single important factors studied and reported in this chapter.

References

1. Gregoriadis, G. (1975): Catabolism of glycoproteins, In: *Lysosomes in Biology and Pathology*, Vol. 4, pp. 265–302. Eds: J.T. Dingle and R.T. Dean. American Elsevier Publ. Co., New York.
2. Mohos, S.C. and Skoza, L. (1970): Histochemical demonstration and localization of sialoproteins in glomerulus. *Exp. Mol. Pathol. 12*, 316.
3. Kanwar, Y.S. and Farquhar, M.G. (1979): Isolation of glycosaminoglycans (heparan sulfate) from glomerular basement membranes. *Proc. Natl. Acad. Sci. U.S.A. 76*, 4493.
4. Kanwar, Y.S. and Farquhar, M.G. (1979): Presence of heparan sulfate in the glomerular basement membrane. *Proc. Natl. Acad. Sci. U.S.A. 76*, 1303.
5. Brown, D.M., Michael, A.F. and Oegema, T.R. (1980): Glycosaminoglycan (GAG) synthesis by glomeruli. *Clin. Res. 28*, 531A.
6. Peters, H.D., Peskar, B.A. and Schonhofer, P.S. (1977): Glucocorticoids: Effects on prostaglandin release, cyclic AMP levels and glycosaminoglycan synthesis in fibroblast tissue cultures. *Naunyn-Schmied. Arch. Pharmacol. 296*, 131.
7. Schonhofer, P.S., Peters, H.D., Wasmus, A. et al. (1978): Prostaglandins, cyclic nucleotides and glycosaminoglycan biosynthesis in cultured fibroblasts. *Pol. J. Pharmacol. Pharm. 30*, 183.
8. Castor, C.W. (1974): Connective tissue activation. VI. The effects of cyclic nucleotides on human synovial cells in vitro. *J. Lab. Clin. Med. 83*, 46.
9. Castor, C.W. (1975): Connective tissue activation. VII. Evidence supporting a role for prostaglandins and cyclic nucleotides. *J. Lab. Clin. Med. 85*, 392.
10. Dousa, T.P. and Dozois, R.R. (1977): Interrelationships between histamine, prostaglandins, and cyclic AMP in gastic secretion: A hypothesis. *Gastroenterology 73*, 904.

11. de Duve, C. (1980): The role of lysosomes in cellular pathology. *Triangle 9*, 200.

12. Ignarro, L.J. (1977): Regulation of polymorphonuclear leukocyte, macrophage, and platelet function. In: *Comprehensive Immunology, Vol. 3, Immunopharmacology*, pp. 61–86. Eds: J.W. Hadden, R.G. Coffey and F. Spreafico. Plenum Medical Book Co., New York.

13. Lindahl, U. and Hook, M. (1978): Glycosaminoglycans and their binding to biological macromolecules. *Annu. Rev. Biochem. 47*, 385.

14. Ignarro, L.J., Oronsky, A.L. and Perper, R.J. (1973): Effects of prostaglandins on release of enzymes from lysosomes of pancreas, spleen and kidney cortex. *Life Sci. 12, Part I*, 193.

15. Ignarro, L.J. (1975): Regulation of lysosomal enzyme release by prostaglandins, autonomic neurohormones and cyclic nucleotides. Lysosomes in Biology and Pathology V. *Frontiers Biology 43*, 481.

16. Dozois, R.R., Kim, J.K. and Dousa, T.P. (1978): Interaction of prostaglandins with canine gastric mucosal adenylate cyclase cyclic AMP system. *Am. J. Physiol. 235*, E546.

17. Wollin, A., Code, C.F. and Dousa, T.P. (1976): Interaction of prostaglandins and histamine with enzymes of cyclic AMP metabolism from guinea pig gastric mucosa. *J. Clin. Invest. 57*, 1548.

18. Simon, B. and Kather, H. (1978): Distribution of prostaglandin-sensitive adenylate cyclase in human upper gastrointestinal tract. *Digestion 17*, 264.

19. Wollin, A., Soll, A.H. and Samloff, I.M. (1979): Actions of histamine, secretin, and PGE_2 on cyclic AMP production by isolated canine fundic mucosal cells. *Am. J. Physiol. 237*, E437.

20. Forstner, G., Shih, M. and Lukie, B. (1973): Cyclic AMP and intestinal glycoprotein synthesis: The effect of β-adrenergic agents, theophylline, and dibutyryl cyclic AMP. *Can. J. Physiol. Pharmacol. 51*, 122.

21. LaMont, J.T. and Ventola, A. (1977): Stimulation of colonic glycoprotein synthesis by dibutyryl cyclic AMP and theophylline. *Gastroenterology 72*, 82.

22. Mueller, P.L., Schreiber, J.R., Lucky, A.W. et al. (1978): Follicle-stimulating hormone stimulates ovarian synthesis of proteoglycans in the estrogen-stimulated hypophysectomized immature female rat. *Endocrinology 102*, 824.

23. Ax, R.L. and Ryan, R.J. (1979): FSH stimulation of ^{3}H-glucosamine-incorporation into proteoglycans by porcine granulosa cells in vitro. *J. Clin. Endocrinol. Metab. 49*, 646.

24. Drezner, M.K., Neelon, F.A. and Lebovitz, H.E. (1976): Stimulation of cartilage macromolecule synthesis by adenosine 3',5'-monophosphate. *Biochim. Biophys. Acta 425*, 521.

25. Tomida, M., Koyama, H. and Ono, T. (1977): Effects of adenosine 3'5'-cyclic monophosphate and serum on synthesis of hyaluronic acid in confluent rat fibroblasts. *Biochem. J. 162*, 539.

26. Goggins, J.F., Johnson, G.S. and Pastan, I. (1972): The effect of dibutyryl cyclic adenosine monophosphate on synthesis of sulfated acid mucopolysaccharides by transformed fibroblasts. *J. Biol. Chem. 247*, 5759.

27. Bergman, M.J., Guerrant, R.L., Murad, F. et al. (1978): Interaction of polymorphonuclear neutrophils with Escherichia coli. Effect of enterotoxin on phagocytosis, killing, chemotaxis and cyclic AMP. *J. Clin. Invest. 61*, 227.

28. Lowrie, B.D. (1978): Tubercle bacilli in infected macrophages may inhibit

phagosome-lysosome fusion by causing increased cAMP concentrations. In: *Molecular Biology and Pharmacology of Cyclic Nucleotides*, p. 311. Eds: G. Folco and R. Paoletti. North-Holland Biomedical Press, Amsterdam.

29. Simon, B. and Kather, H. (1979): Prostaglandin-sensitive adenylate cyclase in human gastric mucosa. Inhibition by nonsteroid antiinflammatory agents. *Pharmacology 19*, 96.

30. Peters, H.D., Dinnendahl, V. and Schonhofer, P.S. (1975): Mode of action of antirheumatic drugs on the cyclic 3',5'-AMP regulated glycosaminoglycogen secretion in fibroblasts. *Naunyn-Schmied. Arch. Pharmacol. 289*, 29.

31. Simon, B., Kather, H. and Krommerell, B. (1978): Effects of prostaglandins and their methylated analogues upon human adenylate cyclase in the upper gastrointestinal tract. *Digestion 17*, 547.

Chapter III: Regulation of gastric secretory function: relevance to ulcer disease

Intracellular mechanisms of acid secretion*

G. Sachs, T. Berglindh, E. Rabon and G. Saccomani
Laboratory of Membrane Biology, University of Alabama, Birmingham, Alabama, U.S.A.

In this brief survey of parietal cell biology we will attempt to summarize some of the more recent findings relating to process of acid secretion, which is the main function of this cell.

Stimulation

The major stimulant of acid secretion is histamine, and the effect is mediated by a receptor adenylate cyclase complex with a guanidine triphosphatase regulatory subunit [1, 2]. As shown in Figure 1, there is no requirement for extracellular Ca^{++} in terms of histamine-stimulated acid secretion, at least in rabbit gastric glands. In contrast, gastrin stimulation in this system is dependent on the presence of the phosphodiesterase inhibitor IMX. Moreover, the gastrin stimulation is critically dependent on extracellular Ca^{++}. An essential histaminic component is also involved in the gastrin + IMX response, since it also can be blocked by the H_2-receptor antagonist cimetidine [3]. Cholinergic stimulation of gastric glands is transient, but is potentiated and normalized by histamine [4]. It may be assumed that the cyclic adenosine monophosphate (cAMP) pathway predominates, but there is modulation of the cAMP response by, perhaps, another second messenger system. In the case of cholinergic stimulation, Ca^{++} removal inhibits even the transient cAMP independent response. These data are summarized in Figure 2, which synthesizes some of the data on stimulation. The rest of this paper will involve aspects of the cellular response to stimulus.

* This work was supported by the following grants: NIH AM 15878, 21588; NFS PCM 78–09208.

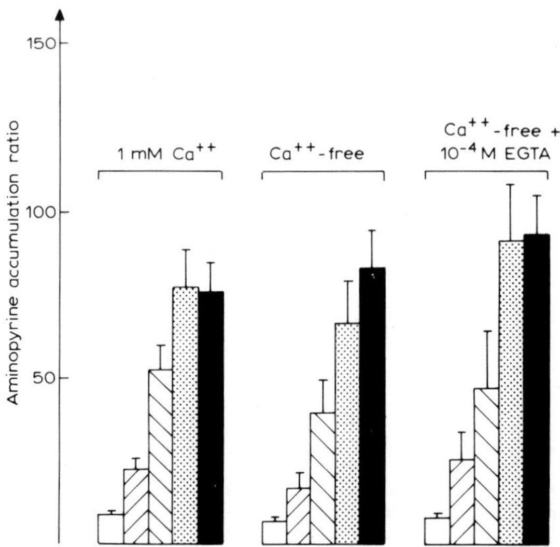

Fig. 1:   The aminopyrine accumulation ratio of gastric glands due to varying concentrations of added histamine (10^{-6}, 3×10^{-6}, 10^{-5} and 10^{-4} M) in regular medium (1 mM Ca^{++}), Ca^{++} −free medium, and Ca^{++} −free medium with 10^{-4} M EGTA. Control glands were washed in normal medium and the others in Ca^{++} −free medium. (Bars show ± SEM, n = 4). ▢ control, ▨ 10^{-6} M, ▧ 3×10-₆ M, ▨ 10^{-5} M, ■ 10^{-4} M. Reproduced with permission from [3].

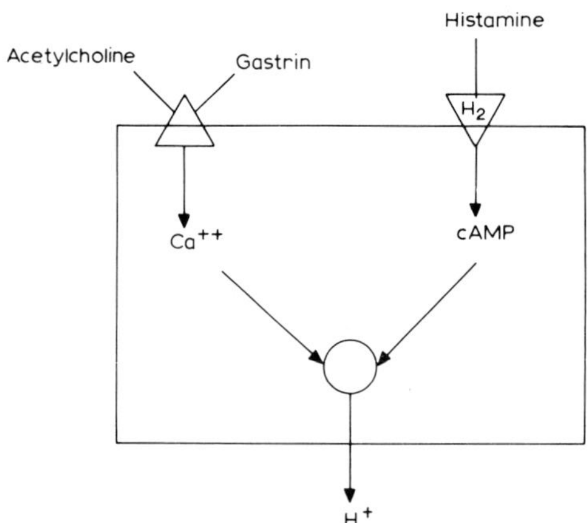

Fig. 2:   A model illustrating the external Ca^{++} requirement for gastrin or cholinergic stimulation of acid secretion, and the cAMP mediation of histamine stimulation. The gastrin and acetylcholine sites are not intended to be identical.

A hypothetical model of the parietal cell

The parietal cell has certain special structural features. It is conical, protrudes from the surface of the gastric gland, contains numerous mitochondria and a specialized smooth surfaced tubulovesicular system which, upon stimulation, is transformed to a microvillus lining of secretory canaliculi. At least 2 active transport systems are present in the cell: the transport of Cl^- and the transport of HCl.

There are convincing data that Cl^- transport is not a primary active process. Either Na^+ removal [5] or ouabain will block Cl^- secretion in the in-vitro frog and piglet gastric mucosa [6, 7]. This suggests the model as presented in Figure 3. The basal-lateral membrane is visualized as containing a NaCl symport coupled to the $(Na^+ + K^+)$ adenosine triphosphatase (ATPase). Since the latter transports 3 Na^+ per ATP, the symport is illustrated as moving 3 NaCl per cycle. Extrusion of 3 Na^+ results in the accumulation of 3 Cl^- and 2 K^+. In the resting cell, at steady state, there must be efflux of 2 KCl by a leak pathway, also illustrated as a symport pathway. It

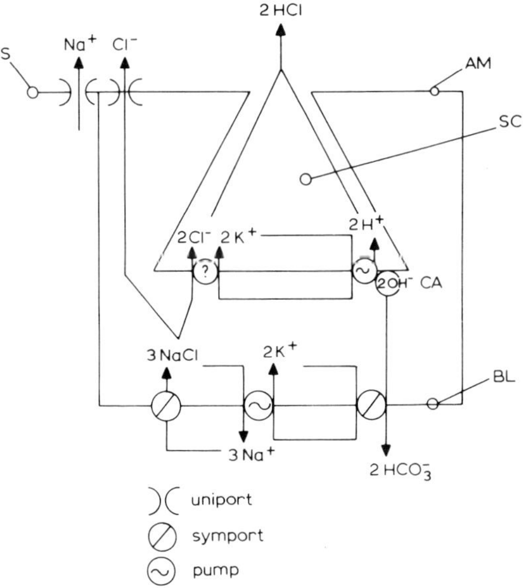

Fig. 3: A conceptual model of gastric parietal cell showing the location of the $(Na^+ + K^+)$-ATPase, the ion cycle associated with these enzymes, the secondary active Cl^- transport and HCO_3^- efflux present in the acid secretory cell. AM = apical membranes, SC = secretory canaliculus, CA = carbonic anhydrase, BL = basal lateral membranes, S = paracellular shunt.

should be pointed out that the symport is not a necessary assumption. It is however likely that this K^+ leak is somehow coupled to the $(Na^+ + K^+)$-ATPase, since loss of K^+ upon K^+ removal from the bathing medium is less severe than the loss of K^+ resulting from pump inhibition either by ouabain or Na^+ removal, indicating a tightly coupled K^+ recycling.

There remains an additional Cl^- in the cell, and a need to satisfy the circuit requirements of the electrogenic pump. This is modeled as exit of Cl^- from the apical surface of the cell electrogenically, with, under open circuit conditions, Na^+ moving paracellularly. Thus, in the parietal cell Cl^- is not at electrochemical equilibrium and the additional Cl^- conductance across the apical cell membrane will result in a relative depolarization of the cell surface facing luminally, with therefore a net negative potential difference across the tissue.

The secreting cell requires 2 additional processes. Firstly, the process of acid secretion results in the development of HCO_3^- secretion equal to the acid rate. It is necessary to remove the anion from the cell, and this is modeled as a $KHCO_3$ symport. The driving force for this is the combination of the chemical gradients for both ions, if electroneutral. There is considerable evidence for a lack of HCO_3^- conductance on the basal surface of the cell.

The process of acid secretion involves the entry of KCl across the membrane of the secretory canaliculus, followed by exchange of the luminal K^+ for H^+ by the gastric ATPase. This will be justified later, but the way the cell is modeled, it appears that there are 3 cation cycles, 2 coupled to anion transport and 1 coupled to the transport of HCl.

Proof of the site of acid secretion

Recently optical techniques have been able to resolve the question of the cellular site of acid secretion. Thus, Nomarski optics show the expansion of the secretory canaliculus with onset of secretion. Fluorescence optics show the accumulation of acridine orange in the space bounded by the membrane of the secretory canaliculus due to a pH gradient. Finally, high concentrations and therefore hypertonic accumulation of the weak base aminophenazone results in swelling of the canalicular space due to trapping of this weak base [7].

K^+ requirement for acid secretion

The essential nature of intracellular K^+ for acid secretion has been confirmed repeatedly using in-vitro frog mucosa, or isolated rabbit glands [8, 9]. Particularly in the latter, it is possible to define the level of intracellular K^+ that supports acid secretion rather strictly. Since acid secretion into an intracellular compartment occurs as a function of cellular K^+ concentration, either with or without secretagogue, knowing cell K^+ it is possible to measure the apparent K_a for K^+. It seems now quite clear that the K_a for K^+ falls with the addition of histamine, i.e. when the parietal cell is stimulated, from ca. 60 to 30 mM in the presence of 30 mM Na^+.

ATP requirement for acid secretion

Opposing theories for the energy source for acid secretion have classically suggested ATP or redox sources [10]. A simple way to resolve this question would be to inhibit mitochondrial oxidation using CN^- or N_3^- and then add ATP to the cell, provided ATP could enter. This latter can actually be achieved by subjecting the gland suspension to high-voltage discharge. Following such an induced permeability it is readily shown that ATP can indeed restore the acid secretory properties of the mitochondrially-blocked parietal cell [11]. Accordingly, using intact cells it has been possible to establish that acid secretion depends on activation of adenylate cyclase which in turn through several unknown steps affects the K^+ dependent ATPase. Therefore it is of importance to identify this enzyme and determine its properties and regulation.

Isolation of the K^+ ATPase

The first description of this ATPase was in frog gastric mucosa [12]. It was, however, in hog gastric mucosa that the purification of the enzyme was achieved and also in this species that most of the transport and kinetic features were elicited [13]. The relatively high purity of the enzyme allowed direct demonstration of its presence in the parietal cell by showing anti-ATPase binding to the parietal cell specifically, and by peroxidase methods further localizing the enzyme to the microvilli of the secretory canaliculus [14].

Transport properties of the ATPase

It was shown in dog microsomes that the addition of ATP in the presence of K^+ resulted in uptake of H^+ by the gastric vesicles [15]. These data were further extended by demonstrating that the mechanism of action of the enzyme was the electroneutral exchange of H^+ for K^+, and that the rate-limiting step in intact fresh vesicles was the penetration of K^+ into the vesicle interior [13]. It is presumably this step that is regulated in the intact cell since the apparent affinity for K^+ is increased by histamine. From this, a KCl entry pathway must be available at the secretory surface, and then the K^+ is exchanged for H^+ by the ATPase. A model is illustrated in Figure 4.

Catalytic properties of $(H^+ + K^+)$ ATPase

The enzyme consists of a group of peptides of molecular weight 100,000. The catalytic subunit is phosphorylated by ATP during the reaction and kinetic measurements show that is is phosphorylated and dephosphorylated rapidly enough to act as an intermediate in the overall ATPase reaction [16]. More detailed studies show the following reaction steps [17]:

$$E - K^+_{out} + ATP + H^+_{out} \longleftrightarrow E - ATP - H^+_{out} + K^+_{out};$$
$$E - ATP - H^+_{out} + Mg^{++} \longleftrightarrow E - P - H^+_{out} + ADP;$$
$$E - P - H^+_{out} \longleftrightarrow E - P - H^+_{in};$$
$$E - P - H^+_{in} + K^+_{in} \longleftrightarrow E - P - K^+_{in} + H^+_{in}; \text{ and}$$
$$E - P - K^+_{in} \longleftrightarrow E - K^+_{out} + P, \text{ etc.}$$

This is consistent with the model presented in Figure 5. Predictions of the model that are borne out by experiments are that: the decrease of external pH increases phosphorylation in the presence or absence of external K^+; external K^+ inhibits ATPase and transport; internal K^+ accelerates transport and phosphorylation; decreasing internal pH inhibits catalytic rate; and K^+ is transported towards the ATP (cytosolic) side of the enzyme, H^+ towards the

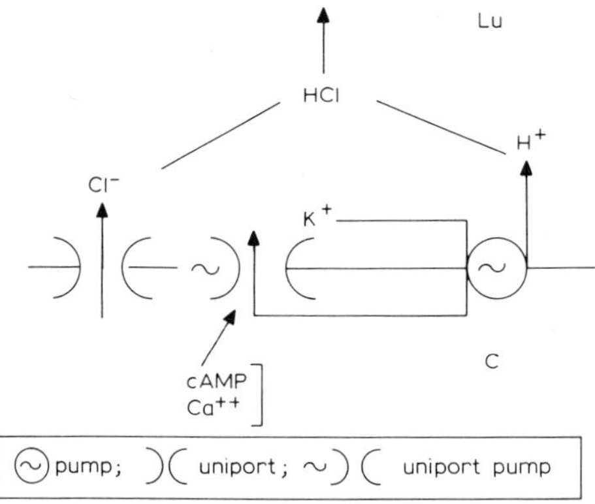

Fig. 4:   A model for the requirement of K^+ and Cl^- entry into the luminal face of the gastric ATPase, with a possible Cl^- conductance and K^+ 'pump' as well as the H^+ pump. Lu = lumen, C = cytoplasm.

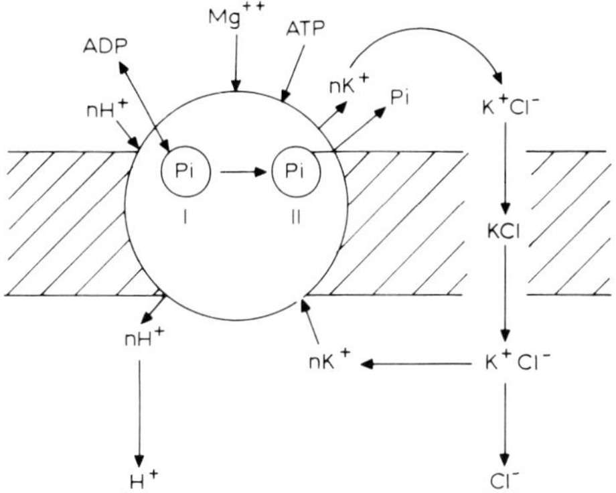

Fig. 5:   A model of the reaction sequence of the gastric ATPase starting with the ATP-dependent displacement of K^+ from the cytosolic face of the pump, followed by phosphorylation, H^+ transport, K^+ binding and dephosphorylation accompanied by K^+ translocation.

luminal surface. It is also possible to tentatively identify the K^+ binding sites internal and external to the enzyme by site specific reagents [18]. The internal site is a hydrophobically located carboxyl group, the external site, which may also act as a proton acceptor, is probably a histidine group.

Summary

It seems that at present a fairly cohesive picture of the mechanism of H^+ transport by the parietal cell is emerging. Stimulation of secretion results in the relaxation of actin filaments allowing the development of microvilli in the expanding secretory canaliculus. In the microvilli of the canaliculus a $H^+:K^+$ exchange ATPase resides and activation of this enzyme requires supply of ATP to the catalytic site, and K^+ as KCl to the K^+ activating site on the luminal surface. Although the general picture is comprehensible many of the details are not understood. It seems, however, that the parietal cell has developed a highly specific system for H^+ secretion, making the development of drugs to inhibit acid secretion by the gastric mucosa by inhibiting the proton pump a distinct possibility.

References.

1.   Sung, C.P., Jenkins, B.C., Burns, L.R. et al. (1973): Adenyl and guanyl cyclase in rabbit gastric mucosa. *Am. J. Physiol. 225*, 1359.

2. Chew, K., Hersey, S.D., Sachs, G. and Berglindh, T. (1980): Histamine responsiveness of isolated gastric glands. *Am. J. Physiol. 238,* G312.

3. Berglindh, T., Takeguchi, N. and Sachs, G. (1980): Ca^{++} dependent secretagogue stimulation in isolated gastric glands. *Am. J. Physiol. 239,* G90.

4. Berglindh, T. (1977): Potentiation by carbachol and aminophylline of histamine and db-cAMP induced parietal cell activity of isolated gastric glands. *Acta Physiol. Scand. 99,* 75.

5. Sachs, G., Shoemaker, R. and Hirschowitz, B. (1965): Effect of Na^+ removal from in vitro frog mucosa. *Proc. Soc. Exp. Biol. Med. 120,* 702.

6. Forte, J.G. and Machen, T.E. (1975): Transport and electrical phenomena in resting and secreting piglet mucosa. *J. Physiol. 244,* 33.

7. Berglindh, T., DiBona, D.R., Ito, S. and Sachs, G. (1980): Probes of parietal cell function. *Am. J. Physiol. 238,* G165.

8. Harris, J.B., Frank, H. and Edelman, I.S. (1958): Effect of K^+ in ion transport and bioelectric potential of frog gastric mucosa. *Am. J. Physiol. 195,* 499.

9. Berglindh, T. (1978): Effects of K^+ and Na^+ on acid secretion in isolated gastric glands. *Acta Physiol. Scand. Spec. Sup.,* 55.

10. Hersey, S.J. (1974): Interactions between oxidative metabolism and acid secretion in gastric mucosa. *Biochim. Biophys. Acta 244,* 157.

11. Berglindh, T., DiBona, D.R., Pace, C.S. and Sachs, G. (1980): The ATP dependence of H^+ secretion. *J. Cell. Biol. 85,* 392.

12. Ganser, A.L. and Forte, J.G. (1973): K^+ stimulated ATPase in purified microsomes of bullfrog oxyntic cell. *Biochim. Biophys. Acta 307,* 169.

13. Sachs, G., Chang, H.H., Rabon, E. et al. (1976): A non-electrogenic H^+ pump in plasma membranes of hog stomach. *J. Biol. Chem. 251,* 7690.

14. Saccomani, G., Helander, H.E., Crago, S. et al. (1979): Immunological studies of gastric $(H^+ + K^+)$-ATPase. *J. Cell Biol. 23,* 271.

15. Lee, J., Simpson, E. and Scholes, P. (1974): Change of outer pH in suspensions of microsomal vesicles accompanying ATP hydrolysis. *B. Biophys. Res. Comm. 60,* 825.

16. Wallmark, B. and Mardh, S. (1979): Phosphorylation and dephosphorylation kinetics of K^+ stimulated phosphohydrolase from hog gastric mucosa. *J. Biol. Chem. 254,* 11, 899.

17. Wallmark, B., Stewart, H.B., Rabon, E. et al. (1980): The catalytic cycle of $(H^+ + K^+)$-ATPase. *J. Biol. Chem. 255,* 5313.

18. Saccomani, G., Barcellona, M.L. and Sachs, G. (1980): Evidence for K^+ site in gastric H^+ pump. *Fed. Proc. 39,* 778.

Parietal cell receptors of acid secretion*

M.J.M. Lewin
Unité de Recherches de Gastroentérologie, INSERM U.10, Hôpital Bichat, Paris, France

In this report I briefly review the general and methodological aspects of parietal cell receptors focussing particularly on the biochemical evidence presently available for some candidate receptors. Physiological and pharmacological approaches can be found in detail elsewhere [1, 2].

General aspects of parietal cell control in vivo

In-vivo studies on parietal cell receptors are especially difficult because of the multiplicity of pathways participating in the control of gastric acid secretion (Fig. 1). Furthermore, this control involves a variety of chemical messengers which can combine their effects [3].

Acetylcholine is likely to be the major mediator of the neuronal stimulation of gastric acid secretion by the postganglionic fibers of the vagus nerve. However, this nerve is known to also stimulate gastrin release from storage G cells according to a mechanism which may not be cholinergic in nature. Moreover, so-called peptidergic fibers that are suggested to secrete various peptides effective in gastric secretion as either activators or inhibitors have recently been described. These peptides include gastrin, somatostatin and vasointestinal peptide (VIP) [4, 5].

As far as gastrin is concerned, the classical hormonal feed-back inhibition pathway does play a major role in the stimulation of acid secretion. Blood transportation is also required in order for the duodenal gastrin inhibitory peptide (GIP), and perhaps secretin as well, to exert a negative feed-back [6, 7]. In the case of somatostatin this pathway is unlikely to be of significant importance because of this peptide's short half-life in blood. Rather, somatostatin is believed to diffuse across intercellular space, paracrinally,

* This work was partially supported by INSERM grant No. ATP 74 79 106.

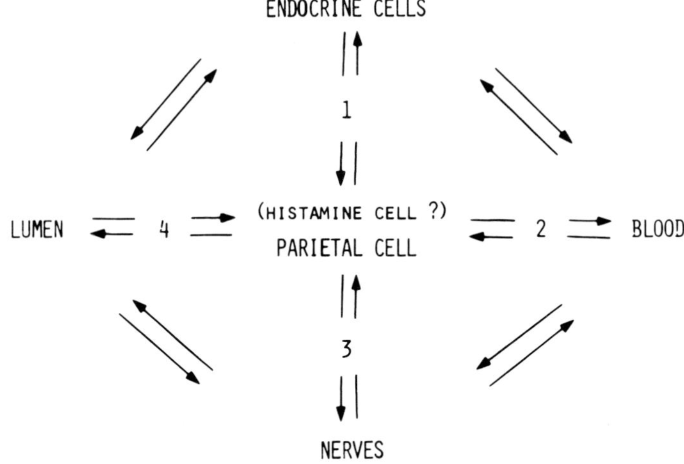

Fig. 1:   A diagrammatic view of parietal cell control in vivo. Paracrine (1), endocrine (2), neurocrine (3) and luminal (4) pathways. For reason of clarity putative direct interactions between nerves and endocrine cells are not represented. Possible involvement of histamine cells is also indicated.

with the possible aid of cellular processes [8]. Paracrine pathways are likely to be used also by VIP and other putative inhibitors of gastric acid secretion such as glucagon, prostaglandins, dopamine and serotonin.

It is not presently known whether physiological stimulation of acid secretion by histamine involves hormonal or paracrine pathways, or both. There is scant evidence for mucosal histamine release by gastrin. It has even been suggested that histamine could be the final common mediator for all stimuli of acid secretion; evidence for or against this is still controversial [3].

Various agents are capable of effecting gastric acid secretion via the luminal pathways. H^+ ions and aminoacids are 2 well-known examples of agents exerting an indirect effect as inhibitor and activator, respectively, by means of a primary action on antral G cells. Direct effects of aminoacids and other, as yet unidentified, agents on the parietal cells have also been suggested. It has even been suggested that luminal secretion of gastrin and other 'endocrine' products should occur which could contribute to the control of parietal cell function [9]. However, unless it is admitted that the luminal membrane of parietal cells contains hormone receptors, it appears unlikely that such luminal secretions could play a significant physiological role.

In spite of this puzzling situation, important information has emerged from in-vivo secretory studies with the aid of the Michaelis Menten analysis of dose-response curves as a mathematical model [3]. These studies have provided indirect evidence for gastric receptors to gastrin, histamine and acetylcholine. Furthermore, they have suggested that most of the known inhibitors react directly with these receptors. However, in-vivo studies were unable to provide any comprehensive model for receptor control of gastric acid secretion because of uncertainties as to the cellular location of the sites and because of the possible cell-to-cell interaction as suggested above.

In-vitro models

As an alternative to these difficult in-vivo approaches, a great deal of effort has been devoted to the study of parietal cell receptors under in-vitro conditions. Indeed, such conditions compound the problem because they make it possible to control all extracellular factors.

Those in-vitro preparations of entire gastric mucosa that have been extensively used for electrophysiological studies in the Ussing chamber have proved to be of limited interest in the study of parietal cell receptors because of their restricted functional competence in mammalian species. Mucosal fragments, isolated cells and tubules, as well as subcellular preparations like homogenates or membrane fractions, have proven more helpful [10]. Admittedly, these materials cannot provide any direct evidence for in-vitro H^+ secretion because they do not retain any cell or tissue polarity; furthermore, in the case of acellular systems, the secretory mechanism is found decomposed into separate elements. Indirect indices of parietal cell activity have, however, been proposed and these may be used to monitor acid secretion in in-vitro intact cell systems, i.e., oxygen consumption, morphological transformation and ^{14}C-aminopyrine uptake [11–19]. On the other hand, in-vitro preparations of gastric mucosa offer the advantage of their suitability for biochemical investigation. Direct approaches may then be attempted by studying the binding of appropriate radioligands to the putative receptors, and the effect of stimuli on the production of adenosine $3'5'$-cyclic monophosphate (cAMP) or of other possible intracellular messengers [20].

It should be borne in mind, however, that in-vitro systems, with the exception of isolated cells, are of no aid in solving the problem of cellular heterogeneity. In effect, metabolic as well as biochemical response of intact mucosal fragments, isolated tubules and acellular preparations cannot be ascertained to reflect direct action of stimuli on the parietal cell because indirect action on this cell is possible through primary activation of another cell type. With respect to this problem, isolated cell systems do represent a special interest. In isolated cell suspensions there is indeed no possibility of direct cell-to-cell coupling, and cell-to-cell interaction by means of a chemical mediator appears to be very unlikely because of dilution. Furthermore, suitable centrifugation methods are now available that permit separation of parietal cells from other cell types in isolated cell suspensions (Fig. 2; [20]).

One must, however, be aware that parietal cell isolation, and gastric tubule isolation as well, could to some extent alter cell responsiveness. This could be a consequence of the use of proteolytic enzymes to dissociate the connective tissue or a consequence of the very absence of this connective tissue in isolated cells or tubules [17]. Thus, carbachol responses in isolated parietal cell preparations are suspected to be exaggerated with regard to cAMP, and aminopyrine uptake whereas histamine responses appear rather weak, at least in the dog [13, 14]. The question of whether responsiveness of isolated tubules is more 'physiological' than that of isolated cells has not yet been documented in com-

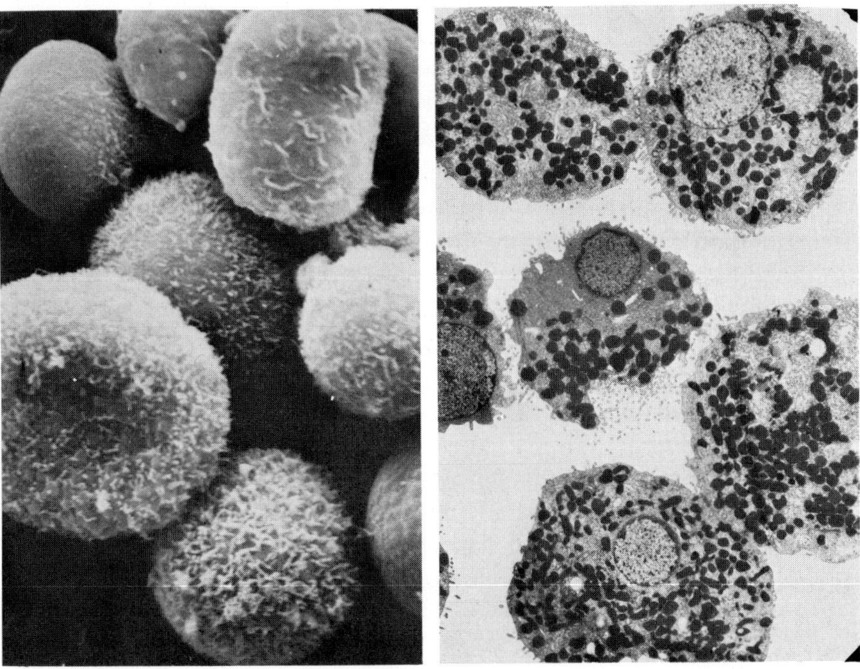

Fig. 2:   Electron microscopic appearance of rat isolated gastric cells. On the left, the various cell types present in crude preparations are shown by scanning microscopy. Parietal cells correspond to the large cells lined with microvilli. On the right, transmission microscopy view of a 95% purified population of parietal cells as characterized by their abundant mitochondria and their intracellular canaliculi.

parative studies carried out on the same animal species. In both types of preparation there exist evidence that functional activation, as assessed by ^{14}C-aminopyrine uptake or O_2 consumption, can correlate with the biochemical (cAMP) response [14–16].

Biochemical evidence for some candidate receptors

Gastrin receptors

In our laboratory we have demonstrated gastric binding sites for gastrin with the aid of ^{3}H-gastrin as a radioligand. These binding sites were shown to occur in plasma membranes [21] and isolated cells [22, 23] from rat fundic mucosa. They were suggested to be specific because native gastrin competed with ^{3}H-gastrin for occupancy, and binding was a saturable function of hormone concentration. The apparent equilibrium dissociation constant (K_D) was estimated to be 5 x $10^{-9}M$ and maximum capacity to be 10,000 sites/cell. In agreement with a possible role in the mediation of gastrin stimulation of acid secretion, the sites were found to copurify with parietal cells by iterative centrifugation [23]. Moreover, site occupancy by ^{3}H-gastrin was competitively antagonized by NPS-gastrin (an analogue of synthetic human gastrin I bearing a nitrophenylsulphenyl group in 14-tryptophan) whereas NPS-gastrin competitively antagonized stimulation of gastric acid secretion by gastrin [3, 24].

Further documentation on gastrin binding sites in rat fundic mucosa were obtained by subsequent studies from other laboratories with the use of ^{125}I-gastrin as a radioligand. These provided evidence for competitive antagonism of the binding by peptides of the gastrin family such as pentagastrin and cholecystokinin [25, 26], while secretin did not produce any such effect [26]. This hormone specificity strengthens the likelihood of a physiological role of the sites. In one of these studies, however, binding was localized to particles sedimenting with mitochondria rather than with plasma membranes [25]. This might reflect differences in subcellular fractionation techniques or would alternatively suggest that the sites have more than one location, either on, or within, the cell. It is also to be noted that the use of ^{125}I-gastrin led to K_D values markedly lower than those reported from studies with ^{3}H-gastrin (these values were below $10^{-11}M$ in one instance and close to 4 x $10^{-10}M$ in the other). However, this variance is likely to have no specific meaning since it could result from the different experimental conditions used, especially as regards temperature of the assays, and from possible errors in the estimation of specific activity of the tracers.

Firm evidence for a physiological role of gastrin binding sites as true receptors has not yet been provided [27], however, some authors have reported that gastrin does stimulate gastric adenylate cyclase in Necturus [28], rat [29, 30] and man [31]. This could be regarded as a strong argument in favor of the participation of the sites in the process of acid secretion since this is strongly suggested to involve cAMP as an intracellular mediator. Such a view, however, is challenged by several other studies which have controversially shown a lack of effect of gastrin and related peptides on gastric cyclase [3, 32]. This discrepancy might be linked to the technical difficulties in attempting to preserve intactness and entireness of gastrin receptors in vitro. Furthermore, it is possible that maintainance of subtle and fragile coupling with other receptors is crucial in order for the gastrin receptors to stimulate the cyclase.

Histamine receptors

Over the years a large number of observations have been made in favor of the presence of specific histamine receptors on the parietal cell.

Pure pharmacological evidence will not be discussed here, as this can briefly be summarized as follows: histamine stimulation of gastric acid secretion is not affected by classical antihistamines (i.e. now referred to as H_1-type antagonists) whereas it is strongly and competitively inhibited by the so-called H_2-antagonists such as metiamide, burimamide, cimetidine [33], the recently reported ranitidine [34] and ICI 125,211 [35]; gastric acid secretion is strongly stimulated by specific H_2-agonists such as 4-methylhistamine [36], Dimaprit [37] and Impromidine [38, 39] whereas it is poorly, if at all, stimulated by specific H_1-agonists such as 2(2-pyridyl)ethylamine (PEA) [40]; and it is suggested that these effects reflect direct interaction at a common receptor site because of the structural similarities occurring between histamine and H_2-antagonists (Fig. 3; [3, 36]).

Biochemical evidence, primarily concerned with the stimulatory effect of histamine on gastric mucosal adenylate cyclase and cAMP, has been recently obtained. Preliminary observations on histamine binding sites have also been reported [41].

Histamine stimulation of gastric adenylate cyclase has been documented in several animal species, in particular the guinea pig [42, 43]. Histamine stimulation of cAMP production in biopsy and surgical specimens from the human stomach has been documented [44], although this has been invalidated by other studies [45]. Such findings support the proposal of a gastric histamine receptor coupled to adenylate cyclase as a catalytic unit. It should

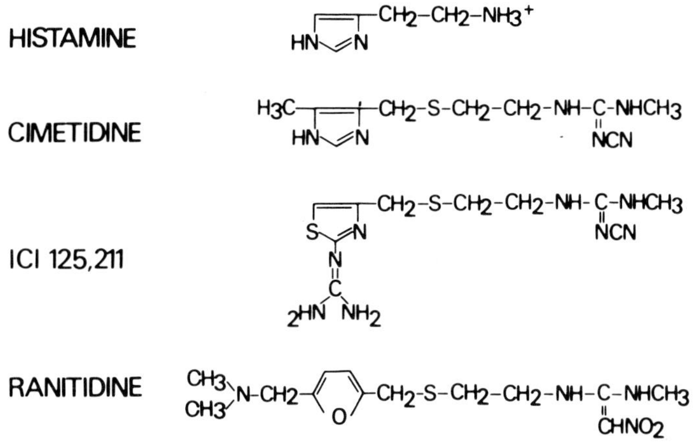

HISTAMINE

CIMETIDINE

ICI 125,211

RANITIDINE

Fig. 3: Structural similarities between histamine and specific H_2-antagonists cimetidine, compound ICI 125,211 and ranitidine.

be pointed out, however, that direct evidence for stimulation of gastric acid secretion by exogenous cAMP is still lacking. Furthermore, specific location of the histamine-sensitive cyclase on parietal cells has been demonstrated in only 2 studies and 2 animal species, i.e. the dog [14, 46, 47] and the rat [48]. On the other hand, investigations directed to ascertain the H_2-type specificity of the gastric histamine-sensitive cyclase led to striking results. Thus, in guinea-pig gastric microsomes, the H_1-antagonist mepyramine was nearly as potent as burimamide in antagonizing histamine stimulation of adenylate cyclase [42]. One explanation for this unexpected finding could be that in acellular preparations H_1-antagonists can gain access to sites which are not accessible in vivo because these are located on the inner side of the plasma membrane or even deeply within the cell. Of possible interest in this respect is the recent report of an Na^+-dependent histamine-uptake system in isolated tubules and microsomal fractions from the rabbit stomach [49].

Conclusive evidence for this has been searched for in studies carried out on intact isolated cells. In gastric mucosal cells in the dog, the stimulation of cAMP production caused by histamine and 4-methylhistamine was competitively inhibited by low concentrations of burimamide and metiamide (apparent K_D $2.3 \times 10^{-6}M$ and $3.7 \times 10^{-7}M$, respectively) while the H_1-antagonists tested produced no comparable effect [46]. These were, however, used at a unique and relatively low ($5 \times 10^{-5}M$) concentration. In the guinea pig, isolated gastric cells were shown to produce cAMP in response to histamine and 4-methylhistamine, and also to the H_1-agonists 2-

methylhistamine and PEA at higher concentrations [43]. Furthermore the increase in cAMP caused by histamine and these analogues was inhibited competitively by metiamide and cimetidine as well as by classical H_1-type antihistamines. These findings are in agreement with those obtained on H_2-receptors from other tissues, such as brain [50] and heart [51].

Our own studies on isolated guinea-pig gastric cells have resulted in very similar data although, in our hands, inhibition by H_1-antagonists was only partially competitive in nature. Furthermore, we were able to compare, on the same material, the degree of specificity for H_2- versus H_1-antagonists of adenylate cyclase (non-intact cells) to that of cAMP production (intact cells) and found no marked difference.

From such results, one is led to conclude that the intactness of the plasma membrane is unlikely to be a determinant for the selective sensitivity of acid secretion to H_2-agonists and antagonists. As an alternative explanation, one may propose that in-vitro preparations lack a cofactor that is critically required for preventing the action of H_1-type molecules to non-H_2 sites of action, in vivo. One may also suggest that cAMP production involves several compartments among which only one is of physiological importance for the activation of acid secretion. In agreement with this suggestion are recent findings from our laboratory showing that histamine and H_2-agonists, Dimaprit and Impromidine, stimulate cAMP-dependent protein kinase activity in isolated guinea-pig gastric cells. However, apparent K_D for histamine was about 10 times lower than that for activation of adenylate cyclase or cAMP production. Furthermore, cAMP-dependent protein kinase activation caused by histamine and H_2-agonists was competitively inhibited by micro-molar concentrations of cimetidine while it was not by up to millimolar concentrations of the H_1-antagonist, diphenhydramine [52].

Direct evidence for binding of histamine and its analogues to the putative receptor sites has been recently proposed with the use of ^{14}C-histamine as a radioligand [41]. Specific histamine binding was demonstrated in rat as well as guinea-pig isolated gastric cells. Furthermore in the latter material, concentration dependence of binding was found to be consistent with that for activation of adenylate cyclase, of cAMP production and activation of kinases (Fig. 4). In accord with the conclusions drawn from the above discussion, 2 main classes of specific sites were demonstrated. High affinity sites were suggested to be coupled with an adenylate cyclase system as an intracellular effector and to represent H_2-type receptors. Low affinity sites were suggested to be more sensitive to H_1-type antagonists. These sites, however, are unlikely to represent typical H_1-receptors, as occurring in ileum for instance, because of their relatively low affinity. They could represent the non-H_2 sites discussed

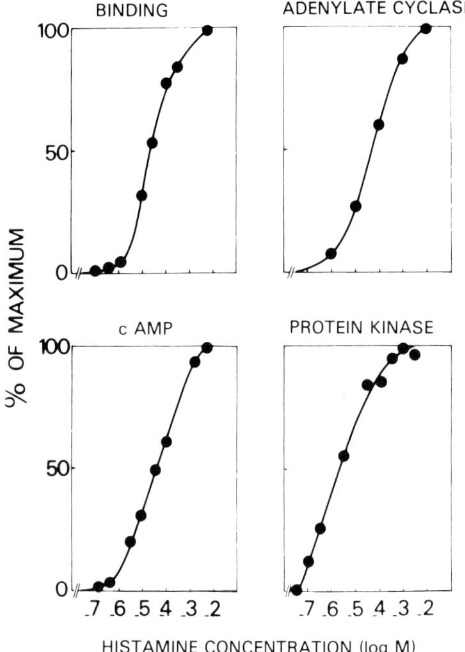

Fig. 4: Histamine H₂-receptor on isolated guinea-pig gastric cells. Concentration dependence for 'binding', activation of adenylate cyclase, activation of cAMP formation and activation of cAMP-dependent protein kinases.

above (Fig. 5). However, these binding studies are greatly hindered by 2 problems; one is that histamine metabolism is suggested to proceed at a high rate due to the presence of methyltransferases in the parietal cell, and secondly is the likely presence of a selective histamine transport system on this cell [49]. Therefore, firm evidence for H_2-receptor labeling in the gastric mucosa has probably to wait till more specific radioligands are available.

In addition to these observations, and possibly in connection with them, recent reports have suggested the possibility that there might exist different subclasses of H_2-receptors [53, 54].

Somatostatin receptors

We have recently reported preliminary evidence for the presence of specific binding sites for somatostatin on parietal cells [55, 56]. Studies were carried out using ^{125}I-Tyr$_1$-somatostatin, as an analogue of the naturally-occurring tetradecapeptide, and purified populations of isolated mucosal cells from rat

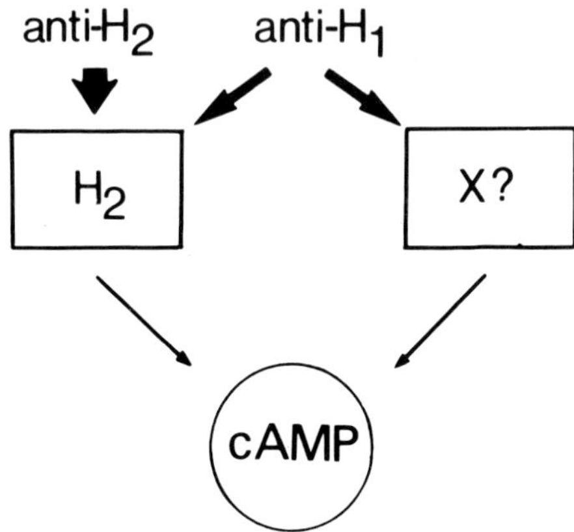

Fig. 5:   A 2-site model for gastric histamine H₂-receptor. H₂-receptor sites selectively respond to H₂-agonists and antagonists and are coupled to adenylate cyclase as a catalytic unit. Non-H₂, non-H₁ sites also occur, are relatively more specific for H₁-type molecules and can inhibit cAMP formation upon occupancy by H₁-antagonists.

fundus. Two main classes were identified corresponding to K_D values of $4.5 \times 10^{-9}M$ and $7.0 \times 10^{-8}M$ and to maximum capacity of 4,000 and 70,000 sites/cell, respectively. Sites of higher affinity $(0.8 \times 10^{-10}M)$ were also demonstrated but these were shown to be associated with cells distinct from parietal cells. The precise subcellular location of the sites remains to be ascertained. Indirect evidence suggests, however, that they should be located at least partly within the parietal cell, in agreement with previous demonstration of a cytosolic somatostatin-binding protein [57]. In addition to their location on, or within, the parietal cells, other observations argue for a potential role of such binding sites in the regulation of gastric acid secretion. Thus, acetamido-methyl-dihydrosomatostatin did not compete with somatostatin for site occupancy, suggesting that cyclization of the molecule is as crucial for binding as it is for its effectiveness in vivo. Furthermore, secretin and glucagon behaved as weak partial antagonists of binding, in agreement with the reported interactions of these peptides with somatostatin at liver and pancreas receptors [58, 59]. Unexpectedly, however, gastrin was found to have no evident effect on somatostatin binding (Fig. 6). To conciliate this finding with the reported competitive antagonism of gastrin stimulation of acid secretion by somatostatin in vivo, one may propose that somatostatin sites are distinct from, and sequential with, the putative gastrin receptors. It should be pointed out, however, that the present lack of evidence for a

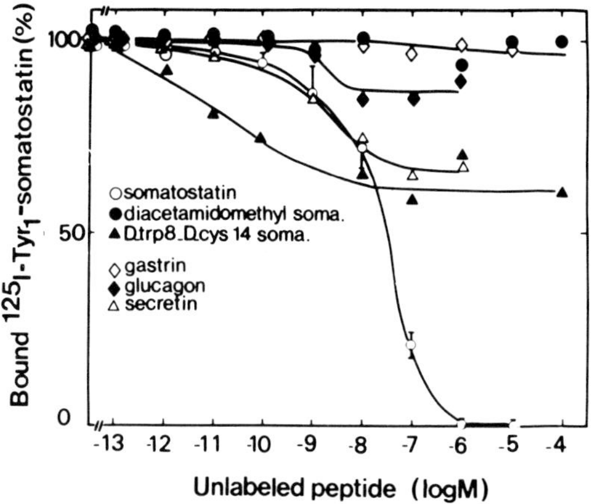

Fig. 6: Displacement of ^{125}I-Tyr$_1$-somatostatin bound to purified rat isolated parietal cells by native somatostatin, chemically modified analogues of somatostatin and some gastrointestinal hormones. In agreement with in-vivo observations, diacetamidomethyl somatostatin (which cannot undergo cyclization) is apparently uneffective and D-Trp 8-D Cys 14-somatostatin shows a high, although partial, affinity for the sites. Secretin and glucagon are weak antagonists of somatostatin binding. Gastrin shows no evident effect.

biological event associated with somatostatin binding introduces a strong note of caution in interpreting the sites as being putative receptors.

Other candidate receptors

The probable occurrence of muscarinic receptors on parietal cells is suggested by studies using indirect indices to monitor gastric acid secretion in vitro [13], but direct biochemical evidence is still lacking. Stimulation by secretin and catecholamine of rat gastric mucosal adenylate cyclase has been suggested [60], but the specificity of this effect to parietal cells has not been proven. VIP receptors have been extensively documented, both in terms of binding characteristics and of stimulation of adenylate cyclase in the pancreas and intestine, but to date, not in the stomach. However, stimulation by nanomolar concentrations of VIP of human gastric adenylate cyclase has been recently suggested [44]. There is presently no biochemical evidence for parietal cell receptors for GIP. The occurrence of parietal cell receptors for prostaglandins has been suggested to account for the inhibitory effect of these agents on acid secretion. Furthermore, studies on gastric mucosal homogenates have shown a stimulatory effect of prostaglandins on cAMP production [60]. These striking results (in view of a second messenger role of cAMP) can be explained by evidence that prostaglandins stimulate cAMP formation in nonparietal cells while they inhibit histamine-stimulated cAMP formation in parietal cells [47,48].

Conclusion and prospects

So far, there seems to exist reasonable evidence for a specific histamine receptor on parietal cells coupled to acid secretion mechanisms through an adenylate cyclase-cAMP-protein kinase pathway. The presence of other receptors on the parietal cells is far from being firmly stated. Gastrin and somatostatin receptors have been suggested, on the basis of binding studies. However, to date there is no evidence for a biological event associated with binding. Only circumstantial evidence has been provided for cholinergic and VIP receptors. There is no doubt that future investigations will clear up some of these point. However, substantial progress has been achieved in the general biochemistry of gastric mucosa with the development of cellular and sub-cellular fractionation techniques [19]. Also, in a large number of laboratories concerned with gastric physiology or related fields, the 'know how' of receptor demonstration has been considerably improved. Thus, one may think that the problem of parietal cell receptors for cholinergics on isolated cell systems with the use of (^{3}H)-quinuclidinyl benzilate as a marker according to the method used in the pancreas [61] is already virtually solved. Also, one may anticipate that parietal cell receptors for VIP will soon be documented with the method used for VIP receptors in the intestine [62]. Much more difficult to elucidate appears to be the question of interactions between the various putative parietal cell receptors. One must realize that no clear insight into this question has been brought about by the above biochemical studies on binding or on adenylate cyclase activation. In this respect, it is possible that significant advances must await further understanding of receptor and adenylate cyclase control especially regarding the role of guanylic nucleotides, ions and phospholipids, and further knowledge of the metabolic requirements of the secretory machinery. Finally, one may suggest that future studies on parietal cell receptors could also discover the presence of unexpected receptors (for instance for opioïds) or even receptors for so far unidentified hormone or hormone-like factors that play a significant but discreet role in the control of gastric acid secretion.

Summary

In-vivo approaches to parietal cell receptors are faced with difficulties linked to the multiplicity of control pathways, the occurrence of various interactions between different mediators and the cellular heterogeneity of the gastric mucosa. These difficulties can, however, be overcome using in-vitro models such as membrane fractions and, especially, purified isolated cells. Direct investigations have been attempted on these models to characterize binding sites and intracellular messengers for a number of known activators and inhibitors of acid secretion. So far, on the grounds of pharmacological and biochemical evidence, only histamine receptors appear to be demonstrated. Gastric cells bind ^{14}C-histamine with an apparent K_D around $10^{-5}M$. Binding is apparently associated with an increase in adenylate cyclase activity and in cAMP formation which in turn activates a cAMP-dependent protein kinase system with a K_D around $10^{-6}M$. To account for the effects of H_1- and H_2-agonists and antagonists on these events, a 2-site model was proposed which suggested the occurrence of 'non-H_2, non-H_1' sites in addition to true H_2-receptor sites. Evidence for gastric gastrin-binding sites was provided by 3 separate laboratories, however, studies failed to demonstrate any biological signal as a consequence of site occupancy. The same is true for somatostatin receptors, recently suggested on the basis of binding studies. Gastric receptors for VIP, secretin, glucagon and prostaglandins have been postulated to explain the stimulatory effect of these agents on cAMP formation in fundic mucosal homogenates. However, in agreement with the probable second messenger role of cAMP in acid secretion, cAMP formation in response to these inhibitors is likely to relate to non-parietal cells. To date, cholinergic receptors have not been documented on biochemical grounds.

References

1. Konturek, S.J. (1980): Gastrointestinal hormones and gastric acid, pepsin and mucus secretion. In: *Gastrointestinal Hormones*, pp. 529–564. Ed: G.B.J. Glass. Raven Press, New York.
2. Soll, A.H. (1979): Hormonal control of parietal cell function. *World J. Surg. 3*, 441.
3. Lewin, M.J.M., Soumarmon, A. and Bonfils, S. (1977): Gastrin and histamine receptors in gastric mucosa. In: *Progress in Gastroenterology*, Vol. III, p. 203–240. Ed: G.B.J. Glass. Grune and Stratton, New York.
4. Uvnäs-Wallensten, K. and Effendic, S. (1979): Similarities between the release of peptides induced from endocrine cells and nerves. In: *Hormone Receptors in*

Digestion and Nutrition, p. 493. Eds: G. Rosselin, P. Fromageot and S. Bonfils. Elsevier/North Holland, Amsterdam.

5. Polak, J.M. and Bloom, S.R. (1979): Neuropeptides of the gut: a newly discovered major control system. *World J. Surg. 3*, 393.

6. Brown, U.C., Dryburgh, J.R., Frost, J.L. et al. (1978): Properties and actions of GIP. In: *Gut Hormones*, p. 277–282. Ed: S.R. Bloom. Churchill Livingstone, Edinburgh.

7. Johnson, L.R. and Grossman, M.I. (1971): Intestinal hormones as inhibitors of gastric secretion. *Gastroenterology 60*, 120.

8. Larsson, L.I., Goltermann, N., De Magistris, L. et al. (1979): Somatostatin cell processes as pathways for paracrine secretion. *Science 205*, 1393.

9. Uvnäs-Wallensten, K. (1977): Occurrence of gastrin in gastric juice in antral secretion and in antral perfusates of cats. *Acta Physiol. Scand. 96*, 19.

10. Haffen, K., Lewin, M.J.M. and Robberecht, P. (1979): Intérêt du modèle de cellules isolées du pancréas exocrine, de l'estomac et de l'intestin grêle pour la recherche en gastroentérologie. *Gastroentérol. Clin. Biol. 3*, 267.

11. Cheret, A.M., Girodet, J. and Lewin, M.J.M. (1977): Stimulation of isolated rat parietal cell by gastrin. In: *Hormonal Receptors in Digestive Tract Physiology*, p. 405. Eds: S. Bonfils, P. Fromageot and G. Rosselin. Elsevier/North Holland, Amsterdam.

12. Sachs, G., Spenney, J.G. and Lewin, M.J.M. (1978): H^+ transport: regulation and mechanism in gastric mucosa and membrane vesicles. *Physiol. Rev. 58*, 106.

13. Soll, A.H. (1978): The actions of secretagogues on oxygen uptake by isolated mammalian parietal cells. *J. Clin. Invest. 61*, 370.

14. Soll, A.H. (1979): Secretagogue stimulation of (^{14}C) aminopyrine accumulation by isolated canine parietal cells. *Am. J. Physiol. 238*, G366.

15. Berglindh, T., Helander, H.F. and Obrink, K.J. (1976) Effects of secretatogues on oxygen consumption, aminopyrine accumulation and morphology in isolated gastric glands. *Acta Physiol. Scand. 97*, 401.

16. Chew, C.S., Hersey, S.J., Sachs, G. and Berglindh, T. (1980): Histamine responsiveness of isolated gastric glands. *Am. J. Physiol. 238*, G312.

17. Sachs, G., Rabon, E., Helander, H.F. et al. (1979): Role of K^+ in parietal cell biology. In: *Hormone Receptors in Digestion and Nutrition*, pp. 327–336. Eds: G. Rosselin, P. Fromageot and S. Bonfils. Elsevier/North Holland, Amsterdam.

18. Sonnenberg, A., Berglindh, T., Lewin, M.J.M. et al. (1979): Stimulation of acid secretion in isolated gastric cells. In: *Hormone Receptors in Digestion and Nutrition*, pp. 337–348. Eds: G. Rosselin, P. Fromageot and S. Bonfils. Elsevier/North Holland, Amsterdam.

19. Soll, A.H. (1976): The physiology of the isolated mammalian parietal cell: actions and interactions of secretagogues. In: *Hormonal Receptors in Digestive Tract Physiology*, p. 406. Eds: S. Bonfils, P. Fromageot and G. Rosselin. Elsevier/North Holland, Amsterdam.

20. Lewin, M.J.M. (1980): Hormone receptor control of electrolyte secretion in the gastrointestinal tract. In: *Gastrointestinal Hormones*, pp. 477–504. Ed: G.B.J. Glass. Raven Press, New York.

21. Lewin, M.J.M., Soumarmon, A., Bali, J.P. et al. (1976): Interaction of ^{3}H synthetic human gastrin I with rat gastric plasma membranes. Evidence for the existence of biologically reactive gastrin receptor sites. *Febs Lett. 66*, 168.

22. Lewin, M.J.M., Soumarmon, A. and Bonfils, S. (1977): Gastrin receptors sites in rat gastric mucosa. In: *Hormonal Receptors in Digestive Tract Physiology*, pp. 379–387. Eds: S. Bonfils, P. Fromageot and G. Rosselin. Elsevier/North Holland, Amsterdam.

23. Soumarmon, A., Cheret, A.M. and Lewin, M.J.M. (1978): Localization of gastrin receptors in intact isolated and separated rat fundic cells. *Gastroenterology 73*, 900.

24. Lewin, M.J.M., Soumarmon, A., Morgat, J.L. and Bonfils, S. (1977): Characterization of gastrin receptor sites in rat gastric mucosa. *Gastroenterology 72*, A8/818.

25. Brown, J. and Gallagher, N.D. (1978): A specific gastrin receptor site in the rat stomach. *Biochim. Biophys. Acta 538*, 42.

26. Johnson, L.R., Takeuchi, K. and Speir, G.R. (1979): Mucosal gastrin receptor. In: *Hormone Receptors in Digestion and Nutrition*, pp. 401–412. Eds: G. Rosselin, P. Fromageot and S. Bonfils. Elsevier/North Holland, Amsterdam.

27. Lewin, M.J.M. and Bonfils, S. (1978): From gastrin receptor occupancy to H^+ secretion: a missing link? *Acta Hepato-Gastroenterol. 25*, 504.

28. Nakajima, S., Hirschowitz, B.I. and Sachs, G. (1971): Studies on adenylate cyclase in Necturus gastric mucosa. *Arch. Biochem. Biophys. 143*, 123.

29. Bali, J.P., Soumarmon, A., Lewin, M.J.M. and Bonfils, S. (1977): A gastrin sensitive adenylate cyclase system in rat gastric mucosa. In: *Hormonal Receptors in Digestive Tract Physiology*, pp. 401–402. Eds: S. Bonfils, P. Fromageot and G. Rosselin. Elsevier/North Holland, Amsterdam.

30. Nafrady, J. and Wollemann, M. (1977): Direct stimulatory action of pentagastrin on the adenylate cyclase of rat stomach mucosa. *Biochem. Pharmacol. 26*, 2083.

31. Becker, M. and Ruoff, H.J. (1979): Pentagastrin activation of adenylate cyclase in human gastric biopsy specimen. *Sep. Exp. 35*, 781.

32. Domschke, W., Domschke, S., Classen, M. and Demling, L. (1974): Failure of pentagastrin to stimulate cyclic AMP accumulation in human gastric mucosa. *Scand. J. Gastroenterol. 9*, 467.

33. Brimblecombe, R.W., Duncan, W.A.M., Durant, G.J. et al. (1975): Cimetidine – a non thiourea H_2-receptor antagonist. *J. Int. Med. Res. 3*, 86.

34. Bradshaw, J. Vrittain, R.T., Clitherow, J.W. et al. (1979): AH 19065: a new potent, selective histamine H_2-receptor antagonist. *Br. J. Pharmacol. 66*, 464P.

35. Yellin, T.O., Buck, S.H., Gilman, D.J. et al. (1979): ICI 125,211: a new gastric antisecretory agent acting on histamine H_2-receptors. *Life Sci. 25*, 2001.

36. Durant, G.J., Ganellin, C.R. and Parsons, M.E. (1975): Chemical differentiation of histamine H_1- and H_2-receptor agonists. *J. Med. Chem. 18*, 905.

37. Parsons, M.E., Owen, D.A.A., Ganellin, C.R. and Durant, G.J. (1977): Dimaprit, a highly specific histamine H_2-receptor agonist. *Agents Actions 7*, 31.

38. Durant, G.J., Duncan, W.A.M., Ganellin, C.R. et al. (1978): Impromidine (SK&F 92676) is a very potent and specific agonist for histamine H_2 receptors. *Nature (London) 276*, 403.

39. Hunt, R.H., Mills, J.G., Beresford, J. et al. (1980): Gastric secretory studies in humans with Impromidine (SK&F 92676) – A specific histamine H_2 receptor agonist. *Gastroenterology 78*, 505.

40. Levi, R., Ganellin, C.R., Allan, G. and Willens, H.J. (1975): Selective impairment of atrioventricular conduction by 2-(2-pyridyl)-ethylamine and 2-(2-

thiazolyl)-ethylamine, two histamine H_1-receptor agonists. *Eur. J. Pharmacol. 34*, 237.

41. Lewin, M.J.M., Grelac, F., Cheret, A.M. et al. (1979): Demonstration and characterization of histamine H_2-receptor on isolated guinea pig gastric cell. In: *Hormone Receptors in Digestion and Nutrition*, pp. 383–390. Eds: G. Rosselin, P. Fromageot and S. Bonfils. Elsevier/North Holland, Amsterdam.

42. Perrier, C.V. and Griessen, M. (1976): Action of H_1 and H_2 inhibitors on the response of histamine sensitive adenylyl cyclase from guinea pig mucosa. *Eur. J. Clin. Invest. 6*, 113.

43. Batzri, S. and Gardner, J.D. (1979): Action of histamine on cyclic AMP in guinea pig gastric cells: inhibition by H_1 and H_2 receptor antagonists. *Mol. Pharmacol. 16*, 406.

44. Simon, B. and Kather, H. (1979): Human gastric mucosal adenylate cyclase. Modulation of enzyme activity by histamine, vasoactive intestinal peptide and prostaglandins. In: *Hormone Receptors in Digestion and Nutrition*, pp. 419–429. Eds: G. Rosselin, P. Fromageot and S. Bonfils. Elsevier/North Holland, Amsterdam.

45. Levine, R.A., Schwartzel, E.H., Bachman, S. and Talev, J.N. (1977): Gastric cyclic nucleotide concentration in health and disease: response to secretagogues and role of circulating gastrin and intragastric acid secretion. *Gastroenterology 73*, 737.

46. Scholes, P., Cooper, A., Jones, D. et al. (1977): Characterization of an adenylate cyclase system sensitive to histamine H_2 receptor excitation in cells from dog gastric mucosa. *Agents Actions 6*, 677.

47. Major, J.S. and Scholes, P. (1978): The localization of a histamine H_2-receptor adenylate cyclase system in canine parietal cells and its inhibition by prostaglandins. *Agents Actions 8*, 324.

48. Sonnenberg, A., Hunziker, W., Koelz, H.R. et al. (1978): Stimulation of endogenous cyclic AMP (cAMP) in isolated gastric cells by histamine and prostaglandin. *Acta Physiol. Scand. Spec. Suppl.*, 307.

49. Berglindh, T. and Sachs, G. (1979): Histamine uptake and release from isolated gastric glands. In: *Hormone Receptors in Digestion and Nutrition*, pp. 373–381. Eds: G. Rosselin, P. Fromageot and S. Bonfils. Elsevier/North Holland, Amsterdam.

50. Green, J.P., Johnson, C.L, Weinstein, H. and Maayani, S. (1977): Antagonism of histamine-activated adenylate cyclase in brain by D-lysergic acid diethylamide. *Proc. Nat. Acad. Sci. U.S.A. 74*, 5697.

51. Johnson, C. L., Weinstein, H. and Green, J.P. (1979): Studies on histamine H_2 receptors coupled to cardiac adenylate cyclase. *Mol. Pharmacol. 16*, 417.

52. Mangeat, P., Marchis-Mouren, G., Cheret, A.M. and Lewin, M.J.M. (1980): Specific activation of cyclic AMP-dependent protein kinase(s) by histamine H_2 agonists in isolated gastric mucosal cells from guinea pig. *Biochim. Biophys. Acta. 629*, 604.

53. Fjalland, B. (1979): Evidence for the existence of another type of histamine H_2 receptor in guinea pig ileum. *J. Pharmacol. 31*, 50.

54. Bertaccini, G., Molina, E., Zappia, L. and Zseli, J. (1979): Histamine receptors in the guinea pig ileum. *Arch. Pharmacol. 309*, 65.

55. Reyl, F., Silve, C. and Lewin, M.J.M. (1979): Somatostatin receptors on isolated

gastric cells. In: *Hormone Receptors in Digestion and Nutrition,* pp. 391–400. Eds. G. Rosselin, P. Fromageot and S. Bonfils. Elsevier/North Holland, Amsterdam.

56. Reyl, F. and Lewin, M.J.M. (1980): Specific binding sites for somatostatin on isolated gastric parietal and non-parietal cells. *Am. J. Physiol.* (Submitted for publication).

57. Ogawa, N., Thompson, T. and Friesen, H.G. (1978): Characteristics of a somatostatin binding protein. *Can. J. Physiol. Pharmacol. 56,* 48.

58. Olivier, J.R., Long, K., Wagle, S.R. and Allen, D.O. (1975): Somatostatin inhibition of glucagon stimulated cAMP accumulation in isolated hepatocytes. *Biochem. Biophys. Res. Commun. 62,* 772.

59. Robberecht, P., Deschodt-Lanckman, M., De Neef, P. and Christophe, P. (1975): Effects of somatostatin on pancreatic exocrine function. Interaction with secretion. *Biochem. Biophys. Res. Commun. 67,* 315.

60. Thompson, W.J., Chang, L.K., Rosenfeld, G.C. and Jacobson, E.D. (1977): Activation of rat gastric mucosal adenylate cyclase by secretory inhibitors. *Gastroenterology 72,* 251.

61. Larose, J., Lanoe, J., Morisset, J. et al. (1979): Rat pancreatic muscarinic cholinergic receptors. In: *Hormone Receptors in Digestion and Nutrition,* pp. 229–238. Eds: G. Rosselin, P. Fromageot and S. Bonfils. Elsevier/North Holland, Amsterdam.

62. Laburthe, M., Prieto, J., Amiranoff, B. et al. (1979): VIP receptors in intestinal epithelial cells: distribution throughout the intestinal tract. In: *Hormone Receptors in Digestion and Nutrition,* pp. 241–253. Eds: G. Rosselin, P. Fromageot and S. Bonfils. Elsevier/North Holland, Amsterdam.

Regulation of parietal cell function*

A. H. Soll and M.I. Grossman
Center for Ulcer Research and Education, Medical and Research Services, UCLA School of Medicine; and Wadsworth VA Hospital Center, Los Angeles, California, U.S.A.

Introduction

What can we learn about the physiology of isolated parietal cells from in vitro studies? The complex series of manipulations involved introduces a considerable risk of perturbing the patterns of parietal cell function, and yet this approach appears to have shed light on certain aspects of the physiology of acid secretion that have been difficult to study in vivo. This review considers the rationale for the study of dispersed parietal cells and the information that has been gained from this approach.

Parietal cell function appears to be regulated in vivo by the effects of 3 classes of chemical transmitters: those delivered via the blood (endocrine), those released from mucosal nerve terminals (neurocrine), and those released within the mucosa and diffusing to the parietal cell via the extracellular space (paracrine). The specific chemical transmitters that are recognized to be acting through these pathways are respectively gastrin, acetylcholine and histamine. Furthermore, these transmitters are *inter*dependent in their actions on the parietal cell in vivo. This interdependence is most readily appreciated from the lack of specificity in the actions of histamine H_2-receptor antagonists [1, 2] and anticholinergic agents [1, 3, 4] in vivo. These 2 agents, in contrast to their pharmacologic selectivity in other tissues, block chemically unrelated transmitters in their actions on acid secretion. This lack of specificity of the H_2-receptor blockers has been related to the theory that gastrin and acetylcholine exert their stimulation of acid secretion by releasing histamine from mucosal stores [5, 6]. However, this theory fails to explain the ability of anticholinergic

* Supported in part by NIAMDD grants Nos. AM-19984 and AM-17328 and by the Research Service of the Veterans Administration.

agents to block the action of histamine and gastrin [1, 4], and furthermore, there are no convincing data demonstrating that acetylcholine and gastrin release histamine from mammalian gastric mucosa [7, 8]. A second theory proposes that the apparent nonspecificity of antagonists is a consequence of the interdependence between secretagogues in their action on acid secretion and results from direct potentiating interactions between these agents at the parietal cell itself [9]. Although direct potentiating interactions have been found in vivo, this theory was not widely accepted, largely because of the difficulty of sorting out actions and interactions of stimulants in vivo. The development of techniques to allow isolation of the parietal cell from the effects of endogenous paracrine, neurocrine and hormonal transmitters therefore held promise for resolving this problem. The key question was whether it was possible to disperse fundic mucosa into single cells or glands with preservation of 'physiologic' responses to stimulation.

Techniques for cell preparation

Parietal cells have been dispersed by a variety of techniques using primarily either crude collagenase or pronase (see [10] for review). Canine parietal cells have been prepared from mucosa bluntly separated from submucosa and then sequentially treated with collagenase and edetic acid [11]. Cells are then washed free of enzymes and then for most experiments enriched by use of the elutriator rotor [11–13]. The elutriator rotor operates on the principle of counterflow centrifugation and serves to separate cells by sedimentation velocity, which for practical purposes reflects cell size. Since we have not been able to prepare pure parietal cell fractions, fractions of varying parietal cell content have been studied, and the several indices of parietal cell response have been correlated with the parietal cell content of the fractions.

Measures of response for studying isolated parietal cells

In intact mucosa, hydrogen ions are secreted at the apical surface of the parietal cells and an equimolar number of bicarbonate ions are secreted at the basal surface. With isolation, both of these products are released into the medium, therefore making it difficult to study the secretion of acid per se. However, Michaelangeli was able to measure acid secretion by acidification of the medium in which amphibian oxyntic cells were suspended [14], but this effect was transient and not easily suited for extensive dose-response studies. Several indirect measures have been developed for studying parietal cell function in vitro.

Oxygen consumption serves as a useful measure of parietal cell response since the secretion of acid is a highly energy-dependent process. Oxygen consumption is closely correlated with acid secretion in systems such as the ex vivo canine stomach preparation [15]. Oxygen consumption can be determined by either a Clark-type electrode [11, 16] or by respirometer [17].

In vivo, parietal cells undergo morphological transformation characterized by the coalescence of tubulovesicles into secretory canaliculi that drain at the apical surface into the lumen. A similar phenomenon occurs with the isolated parietal cell with stimulation [16–18], a finding which indicates that at least some complex and specific functions are preserved after cell isolation.

The accumulation of ^{14}C-aminopyrine (AP) by isolated parietal cells serves as a very useful index of parietal cell function. AP is a weak base that is secreted into gastric juice by a pH partition phenomenon [19]. The accumulation of AP by stimulated parietal cells probably reflects a similar process, in that AP with a pKa of 5.0 will be largely in the unionized form as it crosses the plasma membranes and enters the cell cytoplasm. However, when AP enters an acid space, such as the parietal cells secretory canaliculi, it becomes ionized and thus locked in by the surrounding lipophilic barriers. As was found in studies with oxygen consumption, AP accumulation stimulated by histamine, carbachol or gastrin correlates well with the parietal cell content of the fractions examined, thus lending support to the view that this process reflects parietal cell function. [11].

Specifity of receptors for stimulants

The isolated parietal cell, which has been removed from the influences of endogenous stimulants, provides a system to which agents can be added either alone or in combination. Studying either oxygen consumption [11] or AP accumulation [12], the receptors for histamine, gastrin, and acetylcholine appear to be pharmacologically specific. This conclusion was drawn from the effects of anticholinergic agents and H_2-receptor antagonists, which specifically inhibit carbachol and histamine, respectively, while neither blocker altered the action of gastrin (Fig. 1; [11, 12, 20]). Cimetidine, at concentrations between 3.2 and 100 μM, produced a parallel rightward shift of the histamine dose-response relationship indicating competitive inhibition, while atropine (10 μM) failed to inhibit the response to histamine. Atropine, at concentrations between 3.2 and 100 nM, produced a parallel rightward shift of the dose-response relationship for carbachol, while cimetidine (10 μM) failed to alter carbachol stimulation. The dissociation constants calculated for atropine

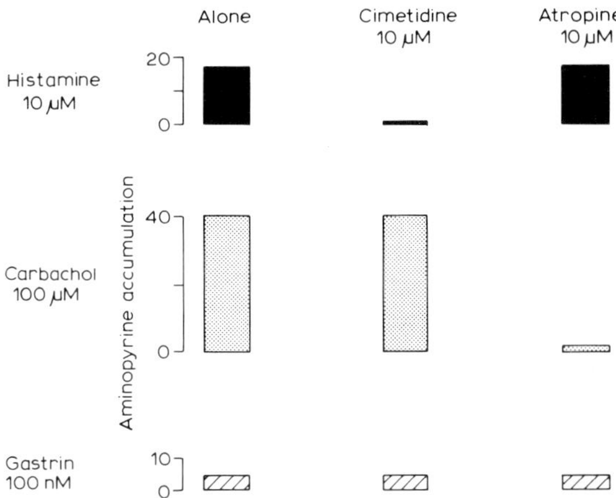

Fig. 1:   Effects of cimetidine and atropine on secretagogue stimulation of AP uptake by isolated canine parietal cells. Cells stimulated by histamine, carbachol and gastrin were treated with atropine or cimetidine and the AP accumulation ratio determined as previously described [12]. Data are the mean of 4–6 cell preparations and are adapted from previous studies [12]. Note that cimetidine only inhibits histamine action, and that atropine only blocks carbachol effects, while the small response to gastrin is not blocked by either agent.

inhibition of carbachol action and for cimetidine inhibition of histamine action were 1 nM and 1 μM, respectively [12]. Since these constants are similar to those found in other tissues, they indicate that the parietal cell possesses typical histamine H_2-receptors and typical muscarinic cholinergic receptors and that the pharmacologic properties of these receptors are not grossly altered by the rigors of tissue dispersion and cell separation.

Gastrin as a single stimulant, produces only small increases in oxygen consumption [11] and AP accumulation [12], and these effects are not blocked by either atropine or cimetidine, indicating action at a separate and presumably specific receptor.

Interdependence between stimulants

The findings that atropine and cimetidine are specific against stimulation of the function of isolated parietal cells by carbachol and histamine, respectively, are at apparent odds with the in-vivo observations such as the ability of cimetidine to block all forms of acid secretion. This apparent contradiction may reflect the existence of potentiating interactions between secretagogues at the parietal cell itself. Data obtained with studies of both oxygen consumption [21] and AP accumulation [22] indicate that potentiating interactions occur between histamine and gastrin and between histamine and carbachol [23], but not between carbachol and gastrin, in that the responses to these former 2 combinations are greater than the sum of the individual responses. However, a 3-way interaction may exist between histamine, carbachol and gastrin, although the present data do not establish that this 3-way combination produces significantly greater stimulation than the sum of the 2-way potentiating interactions between histamine and carbachol and histamine and gastrin [22].

In the presence of these potentiating interactions, the actions of cimetidine and atropine display an apparent nonspecificity reminiscent of that found in vivo. Thus, for example, when gastrin action on isolated parietal cells was enhanced by potentiating interaction with histamine, cimetidine caused an apparent inhibition of the response to gastrin, which presumably reflected withdrawal of histamine's enhancement of gastrin's action [21].

In order to fit these observations into a model explaining regulation of acid secretion in vivo, one must assume that the parietal cell in vivo in the basal state receives inputs from cholinergic and histaminic pathways sufficient to support potentiating interaction with superimposed stimuli. This possibility seems reasonable since basal acid secretion is inhibited by both H_2-blockers [24] and anticholinergic agents [25], indicating that both pathways contribute to baseline modulation of parietal cell function. Exposure to a superimposed stimulus would thus represent interaction with the effects of the endogenous histamine and acetylcholine, and thus to some extent the superimposed stimulus would be inhibited by blocking either of these endogenous stimulants. Whether atropine inhibition of gastrin action in vivo [1,4] represents a true potentiating interaction between gastrin and cholinergic inputs at the parietal cell remains unclear. These 2 stimulants may have interdependent action at some other step in the integrated response to the fundic mucosa to stimulation, such as release of histamine, but there remains no direct evidence for such a possibility.

Gastrin, as a single stimulant, produces only a small effect on the function of isolated canine parietal cells. Studies with isolated gastric glands from rabbit [17, 23] and isolated oxyntic cells from amphibian mucosa [16] fail to detect a response to gastrin. These findings either indicate that gastrin is intrinsically a weak direct stimulus for the parietal cell or that parietal cells during isolation lose their ability to respond to gastrin. The former possibility gains some credibility from the in-vivo findings that gastrin causes little stimulation of parietal cell function in the absence of endogenous histamine [1, 2], as is the case during simultaneous cimetidine administration. However, cimetidine does not totally block gastrin action in vivo and therefore gastrin alone may also have a weak action on parietal cell function in vivo independent of potentiation by or release of endogenous histamine. The findings with isolated parietal cells of a weak gastrin effect as a single agent and marked potentiation by histamine may thus be an accurate reflection of the pattern of gastrin action in vivo.

Second messengers possibly mediating secretagogue action

Since isolated parietal cells are responsive to stimulation, they provide a system allowing the study of the potential role of secondary mechanisms that may be involved in parietal-cell activation. The involvement of cyclic AMP and calcium in activation by secretagogues has been studied.

Cyclic AMP

Histamine, but neither carbachol nor gastrin, increased cyclic AMP production by this preparation of isolated parietal cells [13, 24]. In cell fractions separated by velocity techniques, histamine's effects on cyclic AMP production appeared to be localized to the parietal cell itself [24–26]. Several findings indicate that histamine's action is closely linked to stimulation of cyclic AMP production. The dose response for stimulation of cyclic AMP production [24] and of oxygen consumption [11] occur over a similar concentration range of histamine. The action of histamine on cyclic AMP production and on oxygen consumption is enhanced in a parallel fashion by the phosphodiesterase inhibitor isobutyl methyl xanthine (IMX) [24]. There is a high overall degree of correlation between stimulation of cyclic AMP production and stimulation of oxygen comsumption by histamine and IMX ($r = 0.88$, $p < 0.05$). The cyclic AMP analogue dibutyryl cyclic AMP (dbcAMP), but not the corresponding cyclic GMP analogue, stimulated both oxygen consumption [24] and AP accumulation [12].

Secretin and prostaglandin E_2 both inhibit acid secretion and yet increase cyclic AMP production in intact mucosa. Thus before one can seriously entertain the concept that cyclic AMP mediates the response of the parietal cell to stimulation, the cellular localization for the effects of secretin and prostaglandin E_2 (PGE_2) on cyclic AMP production must be determined. Secretin at concentrations above 1 nM also stimulated cyclic AMP production by isolated mucosal cells and this effect was highly correlated with the distribution of pepsinogen in various cell fractions ($r = 0.98$, $p < 0.05$) [13]. PGE_2 at concentrations above 1 μM also stimulated cyclic AMP production by isolated mucosal cells [13]. This effect, however, was not correlated with a single cell marker such as pepsinogen or the distribution of mucous cells staining with periodic acid Schiff. However, PGE_2 stimulation of cyclic AMP production was negatively correlated with the parietal-cell content of the fractions ($r = -0.79$, $p < 0.05$), indicating, at most, a minor stimulatory effect of PGE_2 on parietal-cell adenylate cyclase [13].

The above findings with PGE_2 did not clarify the mechanism by which prostaglandins inhibit acid secretion. However, we found that PGE_2, in concentrations much lower than those needed to stimulate cyclic AMP production in nonparietal cells, inhibited histamine stimulation of AP accumulation by parietal cells, with 50% inhibition found at a PGE_2 concentration of 10 nM [27]. In contrast, PGE_2 at concentrations up to 100 μM failed to inhibit stimulation of AP accumulation by carbachol, gastrin or dbcAMP. When, however, the response to carbachol was enhanced by potentiating interaction with histamine, PGE_2 did cause an apparent inhibition, presumably due to interference with histamine enhancement of carbachol action (Fig. 2). A similar apparent inhibition of gastrin action was found when the response to gastrin was potentiated by interaction with histamine, but not when gastrin action was potentiated by dbcAMP (Fig. 2). Thus PGE_2 appeared to be specific for histamine stimulation of parietal cell function and these effects corresponded with PGE_2 inhibition of histamine-stimulated cyclic AMP production, with 50% inhibition found at a PGE_2 concentration of 10 nM [25, 27] the same as for 50% inhibition of AP accumulation. It therefore appeared that the specific inhibition by PGE_2 of histamine-stimulated AP accumulation reflected inhibition of histamine activation of parietal cell adenylate cyclase.

The potential role of calcium in cell activation

There are many instances in which calcium plays a major role in coupling activation of a cell by chemical transmitters to the final cell response. The exact pattern for activation of cell processes by calcium varies among tissues [28–30]. The concentration of free calcium in the cytosol of most resting cells is very low (about 0.1 μM) but with activation calcium is delivered to the cytosol where it activates secondary cellular events. There are several mechanisms by which cytosol calcium concentrations may be increased. These include increased permeability across the plasma membrane, as reflected by an enhanced uptake of $^{45}Ca^{++}$ and dependence of the response on extracellular calcium concentrations. Alternatively, cell activation may cause a release of calcium from intracellular sites such as mitochondria or, in the case of skeletal muscle, sarcoplasmic reticulum [31]. Calcium-dependent cell acti-

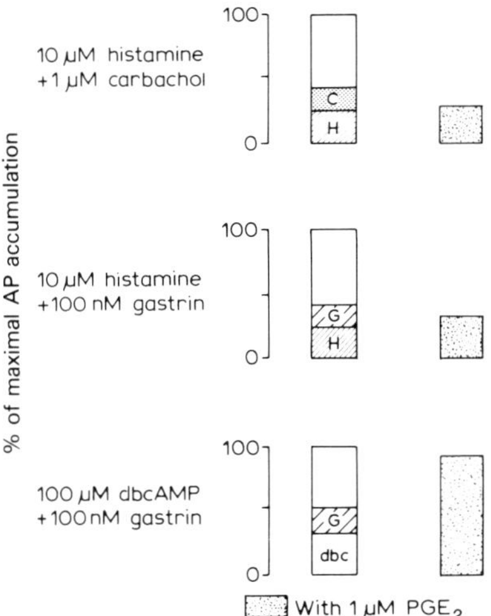

Fig. 2:   The effects of PGE$_2$ on potentiating interactions involving histamine. Parietal cell-enriched fractions were treated with histamine (H), carbachol (C), gastrin (G), and dbcAMP (dbc) alone and in combination at the indicated concentrations. AP accumulation was determined as previously described [12, 27] and presented as the percentage of the maximal AP accumulation ratio. On the left, the total height of the columns represent the response to the indicated combination of agents, while the designated portions of the columns indicate the response to the agents alone. The open portions of the columns therefore reflect the degree of potentiation. On the right, the stippled bars represent the response to these combinations of agents plus PGE$_2$ (1 μM). Note that the responses to histamine plus carbachol and histamine plus gastrin are markedly inhibited, whereas the response to gastrin plus dbcAMP is not impaired by PGE$_2$. This pattern of responses reflects the specificity of PGE$_2$ for histamine in that PGE$_2$ produces no inhibition of gastrin, dbcAMP or cholinergic agents, unless the action of these agents is enhanced by potentiating interaction with histamine. The data are the mean of 4 preparations of cells and are adapted from previous studies [27].

vation therefore either may or may not require extracellular calcium. Cholinergic, but not histaminic, stimulation of parietal cell function represents an example of cell activation being associated with an enhanced influx of extracellular calcium. Cholinergic stimulation is markedly impaired by decreasing the extracellular calcium from the normal 1.8 mM to 0.1 mM, while, under similar conditions, histamine stimulation is only minimally impaired [32]. This impairment of cholinergic stimulation by calcium removal is rapidly and completely reversed by restoration of the extracellular calcium concentration indicating that the calcium pool involved is rapidly exchangable with extracellular calcium. Lanthanum, which inhibits calcium movement across plasma membranes, provides an additional tool for studying the role of calcium. Lanthanum (100 μM) inhibits carbachol action, but does not block histamine stimulation of AP accumulation. These data point to the possibility that cholinergic stimulation of parietal cell function is related to enhanced calcium influx. In studies with $^{45}Ca^{++}$, carbachol, but not histamine, enhanced calcium influx into parietal cells [32]. In cell fractionation studies, this effect of carbachol corresponded to the parietal cell content of the fractions examined. Furthermore, the dose response for carbachol stimulation of calcium influx [32] correlated with carbachol stimulation of oxygen uptake [11], providing further evidence suggesting a close link between cholinergic stimulation of parietal cell function and the enhanced influx of calcium. In contrast to the clear data indicating that cholinergic but not histaminic action is closely linked to enhanced calcium influx, the data with gastrin effects are not definitive. Gastrin action is only moderately impaired by either removal of extracellular calcium or by treatment of cells with lanthanum [32]. Furthermore, gastrin action is not associated with enhanced influx of calcium [32]. Further studies will be necessary to elucidate the secondary mechanisms involved in gastrin action on isolated parietal cells.

Summary

The available studies with isolated parietal cells suggest a model in which the parietal cell has specific receptors for histamine, acetylcholine and gastrin and in which potentiating interactions exist between histamine on one hand and cholinergic agents and gastrin on the other. These potentiating interactions may be of great importance in modulating parietal cell response to stimulation and may underlie the apparent nonspecificity of H_2-receptor antagonists and anticholinergic agents in vivo. This apparent nonspecificity may reflect the importance of endogenous cholinergic and histaminic influence on the parietal cell in the basal state, so that the in-vivo actions of these 2 antagonists results not only from direct inhibition of histamine and acetylcholine, respectively, but also from interference with their role in potentiating interactions with superimposed stimuli. These data with isolated cells do not, however, exclude the possibility that gastrin or acetylcholine may also act through other mechanisms, such as release of endogenous histamine. However, there is little direct evidence to support these other possibilities.

Histamine's action on the isolated parietal cell appears to be closely linked to stimulation of cyclic AMP production, while cholinergics appear to activate parietal cell function by opening the gates to allow extracellular calcium to cross the plasma membrane. The secondary effector mechanisms involved in gastrin action have not been elucidated, although these mechanisms appear to be at least in part calcium dependent. The potentiating interactions that have been observed appear to require the convergence of calcium dependent and cyclic AMP dependent pathways, although the mechanisms accounting for the potentiation have not been worked out. From the present data it does not appear likely that amplification occurs either at the step of generation of cyclic AMP or at the step involving entry of extracellular calcium, since combinations of agents do not increase the rates of these processes over those found respectively, with histamine or cholinergic agents singly. The important problem of the mechanism of potentiation remains to be solved by future research.

References

1. Grossman, M.I. (1979): Control of gastric secretion. In: *Gastrointestinal Disease*, pp. 640–659. Eds: M.H. Sleisenger and J.S. Fordtran. W.B. Saunders, Philadelphia.
2. Richardson, C.R. (1978): Effect of H_2-receptor antagonists on gastric acid secretion and serum gastrin concentration. A review. *Gastroenterology 74*, 366.
3. Code, C.F., Hightower, N.C. and Hallenbeck, G.S. (1951): Comparison of the effects of methantheline bromide (Banthine) and atropine on the secretory responses of vagally innervated and vagally denervated gastric pouches. *Gastroenterology 19*, 254.
4. Hirschowitz, B.I. and Sachs, G. (1969): Atropine inhibition of insulin, histamine, and pentagastrin stimulated gastric electrolyte and pepsin secretion in the dog. *Gastroenterology 56*, 693.
5. Code, C.F. (1965): Histamine and gastric secretion: a later look, 1955–1965. *Fed. Proc. 24*, 1311.
6. Black, J.W., Duncan, W.A.M., Durant, C.J. et al. (1972): Definition and antagonism of histamine H_2-receptors. *Nature 236*, 385.
7. Beaven, M.A. (1978): Histamine: its role in physiological and pathological processes. In: *Monographs in Allergy*, Vol. 13, p. 114. S. Karger, Basel.
8. Code, C.F. (1977): Reflections on histamine, gastric secretion and the H_2 receptor. *N. Engl. J. Med. 296*, 1459.
9. Grossman, M.I. and Konturek, S.J. (1974): Inhibition of acid secretion in dog by metiamide, a histamine antagonist acting on H_2 receptors. *Gastroenterology 66*, 517.
10. Soll, A.H. (1980): Physiology of isolated canine parietal cells: receptors and effectors regulating function. In: *Physiology of the Digestive Tract*. Ed: L.R. Johnson. Raven Press, New York (In press).
11. Soll, A.H. (1978): The actions of secretagogues on oxygen uptake by isolated mammalian parietal cells. *J. Clin. Invest. 61*, 370.
12. Soll, A.H. (1980): Receptor specificity for secretagogue stimulation of ^{14}C-aminopyrine accumulation by isolated canine parietal cells. *Am. J. Physiol.* (In press).
13. Wollin, A., Soll, A.H. and Samloff, I.M. (1979): Actions of histamine, secretin,

and PGE$_2$ on cyclic AMP production by isolated canine fundic mucosal cells. *Am. J. Physiol. 237*, E437.

14. Michelangeli, F. (1978): Acid secretion and intracellular pH in isolated oxyntic cells. *J. Membr. Biol. 38*, 31.

15. Kowalewski, K. and Kolodej, A. (1972): Relation between hydrogen ion secretion and oxygen consumption by ex vivo isolated canine stomach, perfused with homologous blood. *Can. J. Physiol. Pharmacol. 50*, 955.

16. Michelangeli, F. (1976): Isolated oxyntic cells: physiological characterization. In: *Gastric Hydrogen Ion Secretion*, p. 212–236. Eds: D.K. Kasbekar, W.S. Rehm and G. Sachs. Marcel Dekker, New York.

17. Berglindh, T., Helander, H.F. and Obrink, K.J. (1976): Effects of secretagogues on oxygen consumption, aminopyrine accumulation, and morphology in isolated gastric glands. *Acta Physiol. Scand. 97*, 401.

18. Soll, A.H., Lechago, J. and Walsh, J.H. (1976): The isolated mammalian parietal cell: Morphological transformation induced by secretagogues (Abstract). *Gastroenterology 70*, 975.

19. Shore, P.A., Brodie, B.B. and Hogben, C.A.M. (1957): The gastric secretion of drugs: a pH partition hypothesis. *J. Pharmacol. Exp. Ther. 119*, 361.

20. Berglindh, T. (1977): Effects of common inhibitors of gastric acid secretion on secretagogue-induced respiration and aminopyrine accumulation in isolated gastric glands. *Biochim. Biophys. Acta 464*, 217.

21. Soll, A.H. (1978): The interaction of histamine with gastric and carbamylcholine on oxygen uptake by isolated mammalian parietal cells. *J. Clin. Invest. 61*, 381.

22. Soll, A.H. (1978): Three-way interactions between histamine, carbachol, and gastrin on aminopyrine uptake by isolated canine parietal cells (Abstract). *Gastroenterology 74*, 1146.

23. Berglindh, T. (1977): Potentiation by carbachol and aminophylline of histamine- and db-cAMP-induced parietal cells activity in isolated gastric glands. *Acta Physiol. Scand. 99*, 75.

24. Soll, A.H. and Wollin, A. (1979): Histamine and cyclic AMP in isolated canine parietal cells. *Am. J. Physiol. 237*, E444.

25. Major, J.S. and Scholes, P. (1978): The localization of a histamine H$_2$-receptor adenylate cyclase system in canine parietal cells and its inhibition by prostaglandins. *Agents Actions 8*, 324.

26. Sonnenberg, A., Hunziker, W., Koelz, H.R. et al. (1978): Stimulation of endogenous cyclic AMP (cAMP) in isolated gastric cells by histamine and prostaglandin. *Acta Physiol. Scand. Special Sup.*, 307.

27. Soll, A.H. (1980): Specific inhibition by prostaglandins E$_2$ and I$_2$ of histamine-stimulated ^{14}C-aminopyrine accumulation and cyclic AMP generation by isolated canine parietal cells. *J. Clin. Invest. 65*, 1222.

28. Berridge, M.J. (1975): The interaction of cyclic nucleotides and calcium in the control of cellular activity. In: *Advances in Cyclic Nucleotide Research*, Vol. 6, pp. 1–98. Eds: P. Greengard and G.A. Robison. Raven Press, New York.

29. Rasmussen, H. and Goodman, D.B.P. (1977): Relationships between calcium and cyclic nucleotides in cell activation. *Physiol. Rev. 57*, 421.

30. Douglas, W.W. (1976): The role of calcium in stimulus-secretion coupling. In: *Stimulus-Secretion Coupling in the Gastrointestinal Tract*, pp. 17–29. Eds: R.M. Case and H. Goebell. MTP Press Limited, Lancaster.

31. Langer, G.A. (1976): Events at the cardiac sarcolemma: localization and movement of contractile-dependent calcium. *Fed. Proc. 35*, 1274.

32. Soll, A.H. (1979): The dependence of carbachol stimulation of ^{14}C-aminopyrine accumulation of isolated canine parietal cells upon extracellular calcium (Abstract). *Gastroenterology 76*, 1251.

Intramucosal mechanisms: relevance of the mast cell concept*

W. Lorenz*, K. Mohri****, H.-J. Reimann**, H. Troidl***, H. Rohde* and H. Barth*
*Division of Experimental Surgery and Pathological Biochemistry, Department of Operative Medicine I, University of Marburg/Lahn; ** Department of Internal Medicine, Technical University, Munich; *** Department of Surgery, University of Kiel, Federal Republic of Germany; and **** Department of Surgery, Kyoto University Medical School, Kyoto, Japan

Some earlier and one recently developed concept on the interaction between histamine, gastrin and the vagus nerve

In the work of Babkin histamine was already considered as a physiological stimulant of gastric acid secretion [1]. MacIntosh [2] and Emmelin and Kahlson [3], in the first, lengthy era of histamine, postulated that this amine was released by vagal stimulation and crude gastrin preparations. Reviewing the experimental evidence available in the early fifties, Code proposed the hypothesis that histamine should be considered as the 'final chemostimulator of gastric acid secretion' [4]. However, following the isolation and chemical analysis of several gastrins by Gregory and Tracy [5] histamine appeared to lose much of its claim to be a physiological mediator of gastric secretion [6–8]. Finally, when histamine was detected in enterochromaffin and enterochromaffin-like cells in rat gastric mucosa, the possibility of physiological functions other than gastric secretion in the gastric mucosa was raised (Table I), and when a rather short-lived [20] 'evidence against histamine as final chemostimulator of gastric acid secretion' was presented [21], there was no longer 'room for histamine' in acid secretion [11].

The discovery of the histamine H_2-receptor antagonists by Black et al. has put histamine back into the reckoning [22]. Many of the earlier ideas and

* Supported by a grant from the Deutsche Forschungsgemeinschaft (Lo 199/9).

Table I: Some of the earlier concepts concerning a physiological function of histamine in gastric mucosa.

Function	Study
Final common chemostimulator of acid secretion	Code [4, 9]; Lorenz and Pfleger [10]
Regulator of metabolic processes in the mucosa	Johnson [11]
General function in polypeptide-secreting endocrine cells	Håkanson [12]
Control of microcirculation around the parietal cell	Waton [13]
Mediator of gastrin-stimulated acid secretion	Black [14]
Potentiation of gastrin-stimulated acid secretion	Troidl et al. [15]
Effector at the gastrin and acetylcholine receptors via the H_2-receptor	Grossman and Konturek [16]
Mediator and/or potentiator of gastrin release in the antrum	Lorenz et al. [17]; Fielding et al. [18]

Reproduced with permission from [19].

findings collected and evaluated in several reviews [9, 10, 19, 23, 24] had now to be granted greater recognition by gastroenterologists than in the preceding decade. But there still remained some important difficulties and problems which complicated the interpretation of the physiological role of histamine in gastric secretion: a difficulty in measuring histamine concentrations specifically in gastric juice and blood in several mammals: a difficulty in demonstrating histamine release in gastric mucosa, and in defining its role in the stimulation of acid secretion; discrepancies between several working groups concerning the formation of histamine in gastric mucosa; and a difficulty in evaluating the physiological function of methylated histamines in gastric secretion.

To illustrate present views and to stimulate experimental work for further proof or refutation of the various hypothetical mechanisms, the concept shown in Figure 1 was developed in 1976 in order to combine the major speculations about the interrelationship between the stimulatory intramucosal mechanisms for regulating gastric acid secretion.

Acetylcholine, liberated from vagal fibers or from nerve endings of the autonomous plexus, may either act directly at the receptors on the parietal cell or release histamine from the mast cell. However, why it should not have both

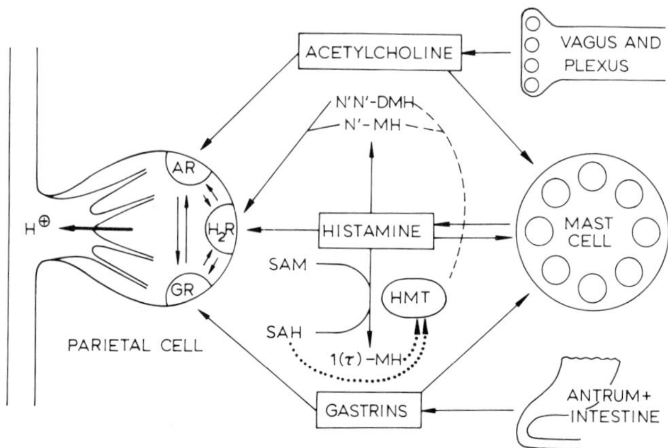

Fig. 1:   A concept of the interrelationship between the stimulatory intramucosal mechanisms for regulating gastric acid secretion. AR = acetylcholine receptor; H₂R = H₂-receptor; GR = gastrin receptor; N'N'-DMH = Nᵅ,Nᵅ-methylhistamine; N'-MH = Nᵅ-methylhistamine; SAM = S-adenosyl-L-methionine; SAH = S-adenosyl-L-homocysteine; 1 (τ)-MH = τ-methylhistamine; HMT = histamine methyltransferase (EC 2.1.1.8); → acting as an agonist or releaser; · · · ▸ acting as an inhibitor; --- ▸ acting either as an activator or inhibitor depending on the conditions used. Reproduced with permission from [25].

effects can be questioned. The various gastrins may either directly stimulate the parietal cell or release histamine from the mast cell − but why should they not have both actions? The methylated histamines may either be bound to the H₂-receptor on the parietal cells, like histamine itself, or may regulate, in combination with N-methylhistamine and S-adenosyl-L-homocysteine, the activity of the histamine-inactivating enzyme histamine methyltransferase and in this way control the actual concentration of histamine around the parietal cell. Finally there may be a re-uptake mechanism for histamine in the mast cell which may contribute significantly to the elimination of free histamine.

It seems remarkable that none of the hypothetical mechanisms in Figure 1 could be *definitely* excluded till now. There is reasonable evidence that side-chain methylated histamines do not occur in measurable quantities in the gastric mucosa of several species [26]. However, the metabolism of these compounds does not exclude the possibility that they are catabolized prior to their detection [27, 28].

Studies on mucosal histamine stores and gastric acid secretion in man: support for the concept in duodenal ulcer disease

In a prospective clinical trial mucosal histamine concentrations were determined and related to other attributes and variables such as age, sex, various gastric diseases, operations, basal and peak acid output (BAO and PAO) and pepsin output [29–32].

First of all, a fluorometric-fluoroenzymatic assay was developed for measuring mucosal histamine concentrations in endoscopic biopsies with sufficient reliability [29, 30]. Using this method and including the special precautions that have to be taken into consideration during sample-taking and preparation, astonishingly high histamine concentrations of about 40 μg/g have been found in normal subjects [19, 25, 31].

In duodenal ulcer patients, however, less stored histamine was detected than in control persons, since their mucosal histamine contents were significantly reduced by about 30% (Fig. 2; [31]). In other gastric diseases – except a case with Zollinger-Ellison syndrome! – no significant decrease in mucosal histamine levels could be observed in the same clinical trial (Table II).

Duodenal ulcer patients after selective gastric vagotomy and drainage showed a remarkable increase (about 60%) of their stored histamine in the

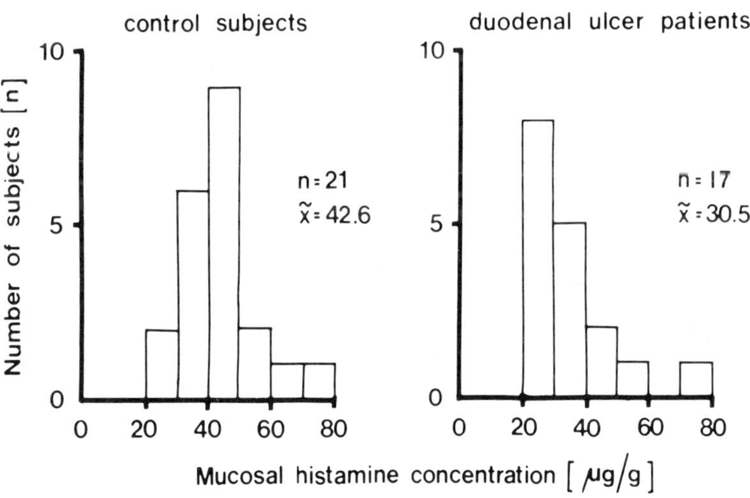

Fig. 2: Histograms of histamine concentrations in human corpus mucosa of control subjects and duodenal ulcer patients. Only male subjects were included. $\tilde{x}$ = median. Statistical significance (Mann-Whitney test) between the 2 groups of individuals p < 0.025. Reproduced with permission from [31].

Table II: Histamine concentrations in human corpus mucosa of patients suffering from various gastrointestinal diseases.

Diagnoses	n	Histamine content (μg/g)	
		Median or single values	Range
Gastric ulcer	10	37.2	15.5 – 98.8
Hiatal hernia	6	37.2	13.4 – 66.8
Cholecystitis	4	48.0	31.7 – 71.0
Gastric erosions	3	43.0	28.7 – 61.7
Zollinger-Ellison syndrome	1	13.3	–
Atrophic gastritis	1	95.8	–
Pancreatitis	1	40.3	–
Esophageal varices	1	63.0	–
Obesity	2	40.9, 45.7	–

Male and female subjects were included. Due to the small number of individuals in the groups, only for histamine values of male gastric ulcer patients could statistical significance be calculated in comparison to control subjects and duodenal ulcer patients. Using the Mann-Whitney test, in none of the 2 cases were the differences significant which should not be expected from the small number of patients (cf. those for control subjects and duodenal ulcer patients) in Figure 2. Reproduced with permission from [31].

corpus mucosa (Fig. 3). Patients with recurrent ulcer, however, had histamine contents which were as low as those in duodenal ulcer patients before or without operation [32].

Acid secretion (BAO and PAO) in normal subjects and duodenal ulcer patients before operation did not show any relation to the mucosal histamine levels [19, 25], and neither did the acid secretion in patients after vagotomy if only a *single* secretory test was used to establish any relationship. If, however, a series of stimulations was performed in each individual subject, and so defining the individual PAO after pentagastrin stimulation, an astonishingly good inverse relationship was found between the secretory response and the mucosal histamine level (Fig. 4). Furthermore, there existed a direct relationship between the reduction in acid output after vagotomy and the increased mucosal histamine level (Fig. 5.) These findings were considered as valuable for suspecting a relationship between the mucosal histamine content and the secretory capacity in man [29]. Since similar results as those obtained for mucosal histamine contents were also found for gastric histamine methyltransferase activity [33], the following scheme was developed from Figure 1 for explaining hypersecretion in duodenal ulcer patients as well as the

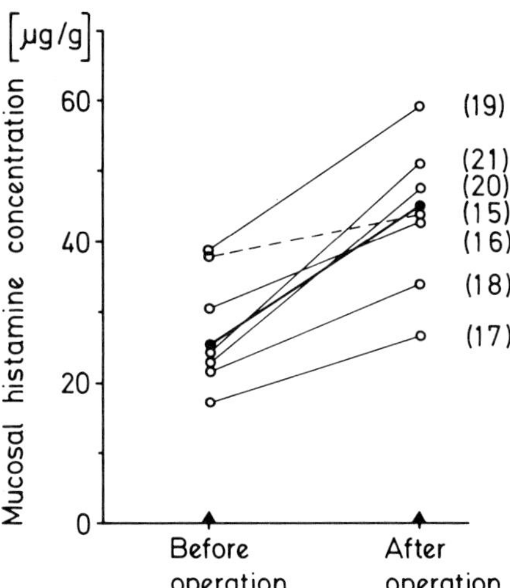

Fig. 3:   Histamine concentrations in the corpus mucosa of duodenal ulcer patients before and after selective gastric vagotomy with drainage. Histamine values for each patient represent the arithmetic means of 3 determinations. In case 16 the insulin test was omitted because of severe diabetes, but the reduction in PAO was 40%. ○————○ = single subjects; ●————● = median; – – – = positive Hollander test. Rank number of patients given in parentheses.

effect of vagotomy and of the H_2-receptor antagonist cimetidine on this hypersecretion in man (Fig. 6):

– An increased vagal drive, an augmented histamine release, and a diminished histamine inactivation cause gastric hypersecretion and hyperchlorhydria.
– Vagotomy abolishes the vagal drive, decreases histamine release and enhances histamine inactivation. This causes the reduction in basal and pentagastrin-stimulated acid secretion.
– Histamine H_2-receptor antagonists block the effects of the released histamine at the H_2-receptors of the parietal cells and increase histamine inactivation. By this action they also cause reduction in acid secretion.

The role of gastrins in this concept is either characterized by histamine release or by direct effects on the parietal cells. There is, however, little evidence that the latter are changed under the conditions of peptic ulcer, vagotomy and administration of histamine H_2-receptor antagonists.

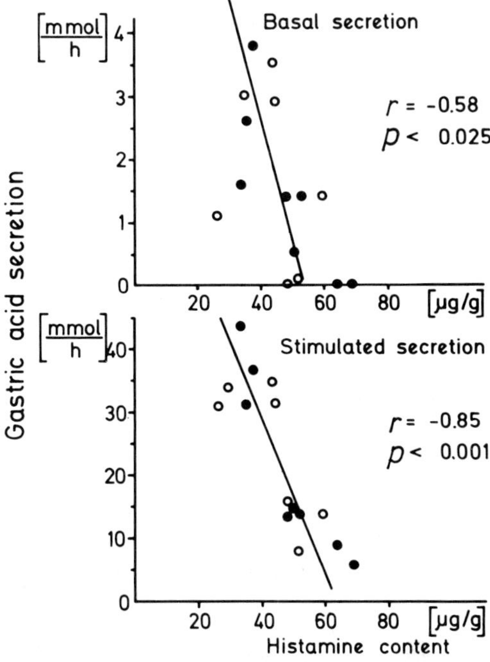

Fig. 4: Correlation between PAO and mucosal histamine content in duodenal ulcer patients after vagotomy. ○ = concept I, ● = concept II. For explanation of concepts I and II see [32].

Mast cells and other histaminocytes – a question of varying views and definitions

Several assumptions underly the hypothesis that mast-cell histamine is involved in gastric acid secretion and peptic ulcer pathogenesis. One of these assumptions postulates that in human gastric mucosa mast cells are predominantly the histamine stores which release the histamine that stimulates the parietal cells to secrete hydrochloric acid.

Many pharmacologists and physiologists do not accept this hypothesis for reasons which often are related to views of highly specialized scientists. Histamine stores in general, and mast cells in particular, have other functions which in our rather sophisticated subdiscipline, the study of gastric acid secretion, are not considered. Speculations and definitions have to include more general morphological, biochemical, pharmacological and immunological data since, otherwise, the already existing confusion will be enhanced.

Mast cells were defined for the first time by Paul Ehrlich in 1879 and, as

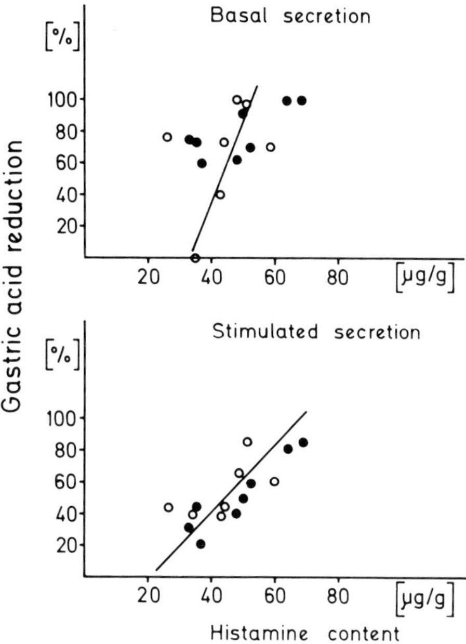

Fig. 5: Correlation between acid reduction and mucosal histamine content in patients after vagotomy. Coefficient of correlation r = 0.48 (p < 0.1) for basal secretion, r = 0.80 (p < 0.001) for pentagastrin stimulated secretion. ○ = concept I, ● = concept II. Reproduced with permission from [29].

Selye has pointed out, it seems reasonable to follow Ehrlich's description, as regards several items at least [34]. When Selye wrote his fundamental book *The Mast Cells* (please note the plural already in the title!) — in the section on Terminology he collected 25 definitions for these cells. In our opinion it is impossible to create new names for these cells, resembling mast cells in the gastric mucosa, without referring to the arguments given in the Classification section of Selye's book.

Definitions of mast cells, taken from Selye's book, by Ehrlich and Selye, respectively, are as follows:

Since metachromatic granule-containing cells are particularly numerous in tissues which proliferate as a result of inflammation or stasis, they presumably represent overfed (gemästete) elements. From this point of view, the granular cells may, in a sense, be considered products of over-feeding of connective-tissue cells and, hence, designated as "Mastzellen". A mast cell is a connective-tissue element which possesses cytoplasmatic granules that stain metachromatically under ordinary conditions.

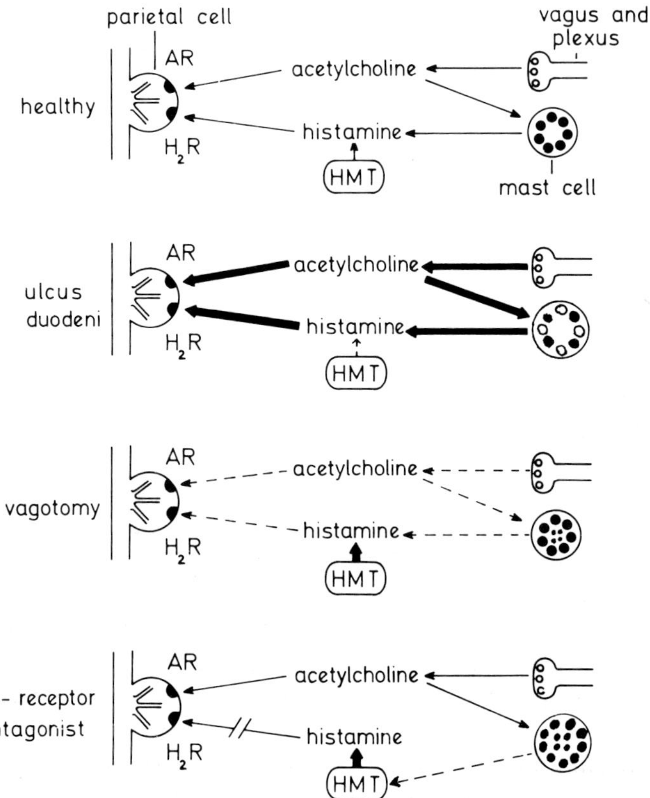

Fig. 6:   Mechanisms for stimulation of gastric acid secretion in normal subjects, duodenal ulcer patients, after vagotomy and during histamine H$_2$-receptor antagonist treatment. ⟶ enhanced effect, → normal effect, − − → diminished effect. AR = acetylcholine receptor, H$_2$R = histamine H$_2$-receptor. For further conditions see [29], Figure 1 and [53].

In human gastric mucosa there are quite numerous cells which stain metachromatically after toluidine blue treatment under ordinary conditions [35–40]. These cells were identified as mast cells on the basis of several criteria including those given in Selye's definition [39]: they stained metachromatically, showed granules with characteristic ultrastructural features, did not possess a basement lamina and were normally found in connective tissue. Their morphological features resemble strongly those described in more detail for the 'atypical' mucosal mast cells in rats which by all morphological and cytochemical, but also by functional, criteria can be classified as mast cells [41].

These mucosal mast cells which in human subjects have a preferential location in the parietal cell area [35, 39] or are at least uniformly distributed over the whole oxyntic mucosa [37, 38] contain histamine as shown by the histochemical o-phthaldialdehyde technique [37, 38, 40].

Other cells were not found to be 'histaminocytes' by this method. Histamine in these mast cells was identified by microspectrofluorometry [37, 40].

However, several questions may arise from these findings which have to be answered before it can be accepted that in human subjects histamine in the acid-producing corpus mucosa is stored predominantly in mast cells.

Do the findings in human gastric mucosa concerning histamine content and mast cell density correspond to the actual state in vivo or are they more or less artifacts?

Our group has spent a great deal of time investigating this question by testing the precision and accuracy of taking and preparing biopsies via the endoscope [29, 30]. It became apparent that the different time intervals between start of ischemia or trauma in the mucosal sample and the fixation of the tissue as they occur in postmortem specimens, surgical preparations or uncontrolled biopsies made estimations of the mucosal histamine content irrelevant. Thus the question whether histamine was localized in mast cells could not be answered reliably in those studies because histamine pools may just have disappeared after removal of the tissue. The same argument, of course, can be used when isolated 'histaminocytes' are prepared from an intact mucosa sample. However, in our studies [29] we could show for our technique of biopsy taking and preparing [30] that within a time period of 7 seconds to 7 minutes after closing the jaws of the biopsy forceps the histamine content of human corpus mucosa stayed constant. Thereafter, histamine disappeared rather quickly and nobody knows which fraction of the mucosal histamine was measured in the various earlier studies [29], or whether histamine had changed from one store into another. To achieve a shorter time than 7 seconds for sample taking and fixation was impossible for technical reasons. Tests on biopsies prepared by our technique, however, showed that histamine was localized only in cells defined as mast cells by the previously mentioned criteria [40].

Can the identity of o-phthaldialdehyde cells with toluidine blue metachromatically staining mast cells be demonstrated not only qualitatively, but really quantitatively?

Again our group has spent some time studying this question. First of all, in 7 patients with gastric diseases 6 biopsies were taken from the corpus mucosa using the technique described earlier [29, 30]. Three were used for histamine determinations, 3 for histochemical studies and pathological examinations. The histochemical identification of histamine and of the metachromatically staining cells was successful in all of the patients. For counting the o-phthaldialdehyde staining (fluorescing) cells and the toluidine blue staining cells a transcription technique was developed. The section of the biopsy specimen was first treated by o-phthaldialdehyde and photographed. Then the same section was stained by toluidine blue and was photographed again. The same area (about 2–4 mm^2) of the tissue section was taken in the 2 photographs and its square dimension was calculated by an integrator. Then the o-phthaldialdehyde cells and the mast cells were marked in this area on a sheet of transparent paper (Fig. 7). From these 2 documents the cells were counted and their number expressed in cells/mm^2 of tissue section. In 7 patients with gastric diseases 3–5 sections per biopsy were obtained from 2 biopsy specimens per patient.

In tissue sections of the human corpus mucosa the o-phthaldialdehyde cells were identical to mast cells in more than 95% of the comparisons (Table III). The very small differences were within the variation of the method, but it should be noticed that a trend as shown in Table III led to slightly higher numbers of o-phthaldialdehyde cells than those of mast cells (especially in the 2 carcinoma patients). Whether this was the consequence of the staining procedure (first o-phthaldialdehyde, second toluidine blue) or an actual biological difference (immature mast cells or cells, other than mast cells, containing histamine) should be studied in more detail. The differences, however, were considered to be too small to have a physiological significance.

Does the regression line for the mucosal histamine content and the density of the toluidine blue staining mast cells in the gastric mucosa cross the origin of the Cartesian coordinates?

Unfortunately this problem has so far not been investigated in humans, only in dogs (Fig. 8). In the dog, however, as in man, gastric histamine could be demonstrated by histochemical techniques in mast cells only and not in any other cell of the oxyntic mucosa [43]. In the gastric tissues, as in the tongue, a typical muscular tissue with mast cells sensitive to compound 48/80, the histamine content was directly related to the number of mast cells and the regression line runs through the origin (Fig. 8). Within the confidence limits of about ± 5% this finding indicates: *No mast cell, no histamine in gastric tissues* [42].

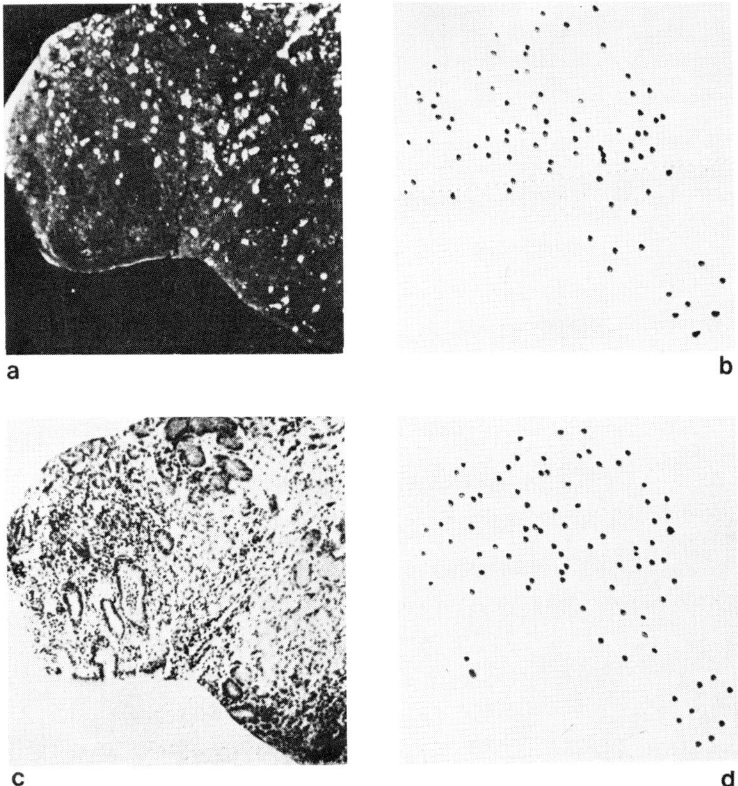

Fig. 7: o-Phthaldialdehyde staining cells (histamine cells) and toluidine blue staining cells (mast cells) in a biopsy specimen of human corpus mucosa (transcription technique). Patient H.H. (see Table III). Histamine shown by o-phthaldialdehyde vapor was identified by microspectrofluorometry (a). Mast cells were stained by toluidine blue in the same section (c). The result of transcription for o-phthaldialdehyde cells is demonstrated in b, that for mast cells in d. The cells were counted with the aid of a screen. Magnification: 120×. For further conditions see [40].

From these results the histamine content of a single mucosal mast cell could be calculated (Table IV), and was found to vary between fundus and corpus mucosa (2–4 pg/cell). It was interesting to note that Soll et al. [44, 45] found a histamine content of 2.8 pg/cell in isolated canine 'mast-like cells' which was in excellent agreement with our observations. In addition, in these mast cells the histamine content was increased considerably following repeated treatment with compound 48/80 (see Table IV).

Table III: Comparison of the density of o-phthaldialdehyde cells and toluidine blue staining mast cells in the same sections of human corpus mucosa.

Patient				Number of cells/mm²	
Name	Sex	Age (years)	Diagnosis	Histamine o-phthaldialdehyde	Toluidine blue
K.E.	♂	36	Normal	87 ± 11	87 ± 9
S.H.	♂	20	Normal	99 ± 6	97 ± 6
S.F.	♂	67	Duodenal ulcer	56 ± 7	56 ± 5
S.R.	♂	64	Gastric ulcer	92 ± 2	90 ± 3
P.K.	♀	41	Gastric ulcer	87 ± 4	86 ± 8
J.H.	♂	67	Antral carcinoma	100 ± 19	95 ± 7
H.H.	♂	56	Antral carcinoma	101 ± 5	96 ± 8

Mean values ± SD from 3–5 sections per biopsy obtained from 2 biopsy specimens per patient. The 2 normal subjects showed nonspecific gastrointestinal complaints in the definition of Troidl et al. [31], the 2 patients with gastric ulcer were allocated to type Johnson I. Staining of the mast cells with toluidine blue at pH 4.0 according to Lorenz et al. [42]. The Table was reproduced from Mohri et al. [40] and completed by adding several attributes of the patients.

In 2 of the human subjects (S.F. and H.H.) shown in Table III histamine assays and mast cell counting could be performed in the biopsy samples obtained during the same endoscopy. Using the same experimental conditions as described by Lorenz et al. [42] and the same counting and calculation procedure, *2.7 pg histamine/mast cell* were estimated for the duodenal ulcer

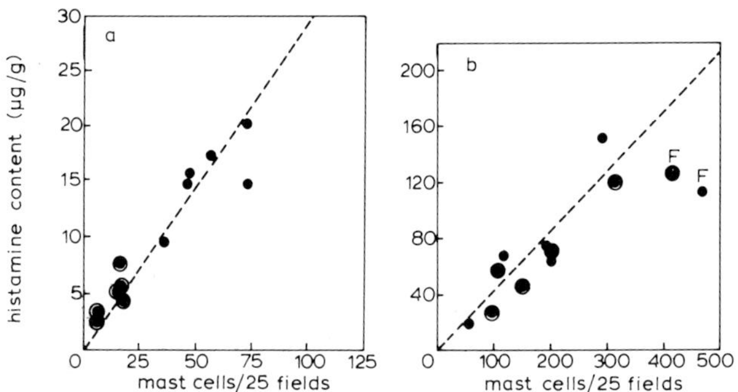

Fig. 8:   Correlation between histamine content and mast cell density of tongue and gastric mucosa in dogs (control animals and those treated by compound 48/80). Twenty-five fields correspond to an area of 1 mm². Each point in the graph represents a mean value from determinations in 5 control animals (•) or those treated by 48/80 (◉). F = fundic mucosa. a = tongue: r = 0.97, p < 0.001. b = stomach: r = 0.86, p < 0.001. Reproduced with permission from [42].

Table IV: Histamine content of the single mast cell in different tissues of the dog with and without treatment of compound 48/80.

Tissue	No.	Histamine content (pg/cell)		Increase (%)	Significance
		Untreated	Treated		
Stomach mucosa					
Fundus 1	9	1.9 ± 0.8	3.5 ± 1.0	85	$p < 0.005$
Body 2	9	4.0 ± 1.8	6.2 ± 2.0	55	$p < 0.05$
Antrum 2	9	3.8 ± 2.2	4.0 ± 1.3	—	—
Stomach musculature					
Fundus 1	5	4.5 ± 2.7	5.3 ± 2.5	18	$p < 0.2$
Body 2	5	4.1 ± 2.1	5.4 ± 0.9	32	$p < 0.1$
Antrum 2	5	4.2 ± 2.3	3.8 ± 2.1	—	—
Tongue					
Mucosa (strip 3)	5	2.5 ± 0.8	2.5 ± 1.6	—	—
Musculature (strip 3)	5	3.6 ± 2.3	3.6 ± 1.4	—	—

Mean values ± SD. Tissue pieces named according to Figure 1 and 2 in Lorenz et al. [42]. Calculation of the histamine content of the single mast cell from the histamine content/g and the number of mast cells/cm^3 = number of mast cells/25 fields x 100,000 (thickness of the section 0.01 mm, area of 1 mm^2). Reproduced with permission from [42].

patient S.F., for the carcinoma patient H.H. *3.2 pg/cell* (histamine calculated as dihydrochloride). These values for the corpus mucosa correspond very well to those obtained for mast cells of the canine gastric mucosa [44, 45].

Does the existence of at least 2 different mast cell histamine stores ('typical' and 'atypical' mast cells) in the gastric mucosa influence the validity of the hypothesis that mast cell histamine is predominantly involved in gastric acid secretion and peptic ulcer pathogenesis?

It has been suggested that the histamine assay in biopsy specimens of human gastric mucosa is a reliable biochemical test if properly performed [30], but that it is of limited value for studying the physiology and pathophysiology of acid secretion since it cannot differentiate between the various histamine stores in the gastric mucosa.

When we introduced the histamine and histamine methyltransferase assay into biopsy specimens of human gastric mucosa for investigating gastric regulatory functions and gastroduodenal disorders [33, 46] we were well aware of this idea. However, since about 90% of histamine in the human and canine corpus mucosa is stored in only one cell type, the *atypical mast cell* [39, 40, 42, 47], it is reasonable to suggest that alterations in tissue histamine of more than 10% reflect alterations of histamine stored in these special mucosal histamine pools which are considered to be involved in gastric secretion. Only about 10% of histamine in the mucosa of these 2 species is localized in the *typical mast cells* which are ubiquitously distributed in the body. Their reaction to certain stimuli and pharmacological agents is known and can therefore be excluded in certain pathophysiological states and experimental (pharmacological) conditions with a reasonable reliability. Thus under well-defined conditions these 10% may just be considered as 'noise'.

The great advantage of our biopsy technique in human subjects compared to other techniques, such as isolated cells or animal experiments, is its close relation to the actual physiological or pathophysiological state (the 'in vivo' situation!) and its strict relation to the actual clinical problem. We have developed this technique because in our studies on anaphylactoid reactions to intravenous agents in man we have shown how doubtful results obtained from isolated cells can be (Fig. 9): the plasma substitute polygeline is undoubtedly a histamine releaser in man and dogs, but it is not only ineffective in isolated mast cell preparations, but even protects these cells against histamine release by several stimuli [48]. Dextran 70 is an excellent and classical histamine releaser on isolated cells, but even in lethal anaphylactoid reactions to dextran, no histamine release could be demonstrated by a highly sensitive in-vivo test in patients (for a detailed discussion of this problem see references [49–51]).

Thus in our opinion we need at least 2 strategies for elucidating the role of histamine in gastric secretion and peptic ulcer disease: studies on isolated tissues and tissue components *and* studies on models which are closely related to the in-vivo situation.

Summary

Some earlier and one recently developed concept on the interaction between histamine, gastrin and the vagus nerve in the regulation of gastric acid secretion are described.

This new concept was tested in a prospective controlled clinical trial in man measuring mucosal histamine stores and gastric acid secretion. There was support for the concept. The mast cell plays an important role in this concept. All the findings collected so far suggest that in human gastric mucosa atypical mast cells are histamine stores which release histamine and so stimulate the parietal cells to secrete hydrochloric acid.

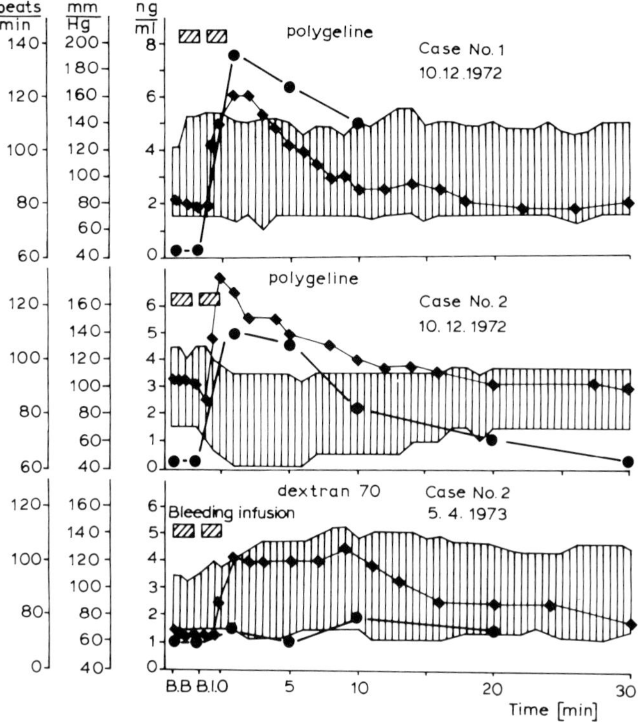

Fig. 9:   Two examples for completely contrasting results obtained from studies in vivo and from those on isolated mast cells. The figure shows plasma histamine concentration, heart rate and arterial pressure in 3 cases of anaphylactoid reactions to polygeline and dextran 70. Single values from each of the test subjects. ●———● = *plasma histamine concentration (ng/ml),* ||||| = *systolic and diastolic arterial pressure (mm Hg),* ◆———◆ = *heart rate (beats/min), B.B. = before bleeding, B.I. = before infusion. Reproduced with permission from [48].*

Acknowledgment

The authors are very grateful to Dr. Muriobayashi, A. Schmal, I. Stahlenberg and D. Weber for their excellent technical assistance in the experimental work which underlies this paper. Supervision of the English language by J. Parkin is highly appreciated.

References

1.   Babkin, B.P. (1950): Abnormal functioning of the gastric secretory mechanism as a possible factor in the pathogenesis of peptic ulcer. In: *Secretory Mechanisms of*

   the Digestive Glands, p. 547. Ed: P.B. Hoeber. Harper & Brothers, New York.

2. MacIntosh, F.C. (1938): Histamine as a normal stimulant of gastric secretion. *Q. J. Exp. Physiol. 28*, 87.

3. Emmelin, N. and Kahlson, G.S. (1944): Histamine as a physiological excitant of acid gastric secretion. *Acta Physiol. Scand. 8*, 289.

4. Code, C.F. (1956): Histamine and gastric secretion. In: *Ciba Foundation Symposium on Histamine*, p. 189. Eds: C.H. O'Connor and G.E.W. Wolstenholme. I. & A. Churchill, London.

5. Gregory, R.A. and Tracy, H.J. (1961): The preparation and properties of gastrin. *J. Physiol. (London) 156*, 523.

6. Grossman, M.I. (1966): After the conference: Review and Perspective. In: *Gastrin*, p. 325. Ed: M.I. Grossman. University of California Press Berkeley, Los Angeles.

7. Grossman, M.I. (1967): Some aspects of gastric secretion. *Gastroenterology 52*, 882.

8. Grossman, M.I. (1967): Neural and hormonal stimulation of gastric secretion of acid. In: *Handbook of Physiology*, Bd. 2, Chapter 47, p. 835. American Society of Physiology.

9. Code, C.F. (1965): Histamine and gastric secretion: A later look, 1955–1965. *Fed. Proc. 24*, 1311.

10. Lorenz, W. and Pfleger, K. (1968): Stoffwechsel und physiologische Funktion von Histamin im Magen. *Klin. Wochenschr. 46*, 57.

11. Johnson, L.R. (1971): Control of gastric secretion: no room for histamine? *Gastroenterology 61*, 106.

12. Håkanson, R. (1970): New aspects of the formation and function of histamine, 5-hydroxytryptamine and dopamine in gastic mucosa. *Acta Physiol. Scand. Suppl. 340*, 7.

13. Waton, N.G. (1971): Histamine and the parietal cell. *Am. J. Dig. Dis. 16*, 921.

14. Black, J.W. (1973): Speculation about the nature of the antagonism between metiamide and pentagastrin. In: *International Symposium on Histamine H_2-Receptor Antagonists*, p. 219. Eds: C.J. Wood and M.A. Simkins. Deltakos (UK) Ltd., London.

15. Troidl, H., Lorenz, W., Barth, H. et al. (1973): Augmentation of pentagastrin stimulated gastric secretion in the Heidenhain pouch dog by amodiaquine: inhibition of histamine methyltransferase in vivo? *Agents Actions 3*, 157.

16. Grossman, M.I. and Konturek, S.J. (1973): Inhibition of acid secretion in dog by metiamide, a histamine antagonist acting on H_2-receptors. In: *International Symposium on Histamine H_2-Receptor Antagonists*, p. 297. Eds: C.J. Wood and M.A. Simkins. Deltakos (UK) Ltd., London.

17. Lorenz, W., Barth, H. and Werle, E. (1970): Histamine and histamine methyltransferase in the gastric mucosa of man, pig, dog and cow. *Naunyn-Schmied. Arch. Pharmacol. 267*, 421.

18. Fielding, L.P., Curwain, B.P., Russell, R.C.G. and Bloom, S. (1975): Evidence for separate actions of an adrenergic β_2 stimulant and an histamine H_2-blocker on the oxyntic and gastrin cells. *Br. J. Surg. 62*, 157.

19. Lorenz, W., Barth, H., Kusche, J. et al. (1977): A critical view concerning metabolism and physiological function of histamine in the gastric mucosa. *Mat. Med. Pol. 9*, 155.

20. Bunce, K.T. and Parsons, M.E. (1977): The effect of hexamethonium on gastric acid secretion in the conscious rat. *Agents Actions 7,* 507.

21. Håkanson, R. and Liedberg, G. (1971): Evidence against histamine as final chemostimulator of gastric acid secretion. *Am. J. Physiol. 221,* 641.

22. Black, J.W., Duncan, W.A.M., Durant, C.J. et al. (1972): Definition and antagonism of histamine H_2-receptors. *Nature 236,* 385.

23. Kahlson, G. and Rosengren, E. (1971): *Biogenesis and Physiology of Histamine.* Eds: H. Davson, A.D.M. Greenfield, R. Whittam and G.S. Brindley. Edward Arnold Ltd., London.

24. Holton, P. (1973): *Pharmacology of Gastrointestinal Motility and Secretion,* Vol. I. Ed: G. Peters. Pergamon Press Ltd., Oxford.

25. Lorenz, W., Troidl, H., Barth, H. et al. (1975): Stimulus-secretion coupling in the human and canine stomach: role of histamine. In: *Stimulus Secretion Coupling in the Gastrointestinal Tract,* p. 177. Eds: R.M. Case and H. Goebell. MTP Press Ltd., Lancaster.

26. Schippert, B., Kovar, K.-A. and Sewing, K.-F. (1979): Determination of histamine and its metabolic products in the pig gastric mucosa. *Pharmacology 19,* 86.

27. Barth, H., Crombach, M., Schunack, W. and Lorenz, W. (1978): Gastric histamine methyltransferase has a less high acceptor substrate specificity. *Fed. Proc. 37,* 392.

28. Barth, H., Crombach, M., Schunack, W. and Lorenz, W. (1980): Evidence for a less high acceptor substrate specificity of gastric histamine methyltransferase: methylation of imidazole compounds. *Biochem. Pharmacol. 29,* 1399.

29. Lorenz, W., Troidl, H., Barth, H. and Rohde, H. (1978): Histamine, gastric secretion and peptic ulcer disease: An attempt to define special sources of error and problems in clinical-biochemical trials. In: *Cimetidine. Proceedings of an International Symposium on Histamine H_2-Receptor Antagonists,* p. 6. Ed: W. Creutzfeldt. Excerpta Medica, Amsterdam-Oxford.

30. Rohde, H., Lorenz, W., Troidl, H. and Weber, D. (1980): Histamine and peptic ulcer: influence of sample-taking on the precision and accuracy of fluorometric histamine assay in biopsies of human gastric mucosa. *Agents Actions 10,* 175.

31. Troidl, H., Lorenz, W., Rohde, H. et al. (1976): Histamine and peptic ulcer: a prospective study of mucosal histamine concentration in duodenal ulcer patients and in control subjects suffering from various gastrointestinal diseases. *Klin. Wochenschr. 54,* 947.

32. Troidl, H., Rohde, H., Lorenz, W. et al. (1978): Effect of selective gastric vagotomy on histamine concentration in gastric mucosa of patients with duodenal ulcer. *Br. J. Surg. 65,* 10.

33. Barth, H., Troidl, H., Lorenz, W. et al. (1977): Histamine and peptic ulcer disease: Histamine methyltransferase activity in gastric mucosa of control subjects and duodenal ulcer patients before and after surgical treatment. *Agents Actions 7,* 75.

34. Selye, H. (1965): *The Mast Cells.* Butterworths & Co., London.

35. Räsänen, T. (1958): Tissue eosinophils and mast cells in the human stomach wall in normal and pathological conditions. *Acta Pathol. Microbiol. Scand. Suppl. 129,* 11.

36. Norris, H.T., Zamcheck, N. and Gottlieb, L.S. (1963): The presence and

distribution of mast cells in the human gastrointestinal tract at autopsy. *Gastroenterology 44*, 448.

37. Håkanson, R., Lilja, B. and Owman, C. (1969): Cellular localization of histamine and monoamines in the gastric mucosa of man. *Histochemie 18*, 74.

38. Håkanson, R., Owman, C., Sjöberg, N.-O. and Sporrong, B. (1970): Amine mechanisms in enterochromaffin and enterochromaffin-like cells of gastric mucosa in various mammals. *Histochemie 21*, 189.

39. Steer, H.W. (1976): Mast cells of the human stomach. *J. Anat. 121*, 385.

40. Mohri, K., Reimann, H.-J., Lorenz, W. et al. (1978): Histamine content and mast cells in human gastric and duodenal mucosa. *Agents Actions 8*, 372.

41. Enerbäck, L. and Lundin, M. (1974): Ultrastructure of mucosal mast cells in normal and compound 48/80-treated rats. *Cell Tissue Res. 150*, 95.

42. Lorenz, W., Schauer, A., Hertland, St. et al. (1969): Biochemical and histo-chemical studies on the distribution of histamine in the digestive tract of man, dog, and other mammals. *Naunyn-Schmied. Arch. Pharmacol. 265*, 81.

43. Aures, D., Håkanson, R., Owman, C. and Sporrong, B. (1968): Cellular stores of histamine and monoamines in the dog stomach. *Life Sci. 7*, 1147.

44. Soll, A.H., Beaven, M.A. and Lewin, K. (1978): Identification and enrichment of histamine containing cells from canine gastric mucosa. *Clin. Res. 26*, 326A.

45. Soll, A.H., Lewin, K. and Beaven, M.A. (1979): Isolation of histamine-containing cells from canine fundic mucosa. *Gastroenterology 77*, 1283.

46. Troidl, H., Lorenz, W., Rohde, H. et al. (1975): Histamine content in human gastric mucosa: Its relation to pentagastrin-stimulated acid secretion and to selective gastric vagotomy with drainage. *Agents Actions 5*, 427.

47. Smith, A.N. (1961): Histamine and gastric secretion. *J. R. Coll. Surg. Edinburgh 6*, 276.

48. Lorenz, W., Doenicke, A., Messmer, K. et al. (1976): Histamine release in human subjects by modified gelatin (Haemaccel®) and dextran: An explanation for anaphylactoid reactions observed under clinical conditions? *Br. J. Anaesth. 48*, 151.

49. Keller, R. (1969): A study of the mastocytolytic effects of polyactions in the presence of certain plasma substitutes. *Bibl. Haematol. (Basel) 33*, 126.

50. Lorenz, W. (1975): Histamine release in man. *Agents Actions 5*, 402.

51. Lorenz, W. and Doenicke, A. (1978): Histamine release in clinical conditions. *M. Sinai J. Med. (N.Y.) 45*, 357.

52. Lorenz, W., Doenicke, A., Schöning, B. and Neugebauer, E. (1980): The role of histamine in adverse reactions to intravenous agents. In: *Monographs in Anaesthesiology*. Ed: A. Thomson. Elsevier Biomedical Press, North Holland (in press).

53. Saunders, J.H., Man, W.K. and Spencer, J. (1980): The effect of cimetidine and pentagastric stimulation on the histamine concentration in the gastric mucosa of patients with peptic ulcer. *Gut 21*, A452.

Neural regulation of gastric acid secretion

L. Olbe
Department of Surgery II, Sahlgren Hospital, Göteborg, Sweden

The contribution of neural mechanisms in the regulation of gastric acid secretion is far from clear, and consequently their importance in the pathogenesis of ulcer disease is uncertain. Some aspects of this problem will be discussed.

Vagal activation of acid secretion

Vagal activation of gastric acid secretion no doubt plays a decisive role as a stimulatory mechanism in man. Sham feeding, meaning that a meal is chewed and swallowed without reaching the stomach, is the classical method of demonstrating physiological activation of the vagal phase of gastric acid secretion. The simplest means of carrying out sham feeding in man is to have the subject chew and spit a meal, and to collect the gastric secretory output via a nasogastric tube. This method was used in 1951 by Noring [1], and resulted in a clear-cut acid response, although far from the maximal secretory capacity. Since sham feeding in dogs with an esophageal fistula has produced an acid sham feeding response equivalent to the maximal secretory capacity [2, 3], it could be argued that sham feeding in man using the 'chew-and-spit' technique might induce a submaximal vagal activation, due to the disturbing presence of a nasogastric tube during eating, and to the fact that swallowing of the meal is excluded. A more adequate sham feeding technique was therefore developed [4], allowing the meal to be eaten and swallowed without reaching the stomach and without the presence of a nasogastric tube. The method implied the presence of a gastrostomy through which a tube could be pushed up into the esophagus to deliver the meal to the exterior, and through which another tube could be introduced for collection of gastric secretion. This method can therefore only be used in patients undergoing surgery, such as closure of a perforated ulcer, antrectomy or vagotomy. As an additional measure a plastic sling was often placed around the esophagus, between the vagi and the esophageal musculature. The sling was exteriorized through a drainage tube in order to tighten the esophagus around the tube during the sham feeding, minimizing the leakage of food to the stomach. Over a period of several years this method has been applied in 85 operations on 78 carefully selected patients. Only 2 complications attributable to the preparations for the sham feeding procedure occurred – a splenic lesion necessitating splenectomy, and a subcutaneous abscess at the site of the gastrostomy [5]. Adequate sham feeding resulted in a peak acid response of about 55% of the maximal acid response to pentagastrin, independent of appetite, type of food served and whether the sham feeding period was 15 or 30 minutes [4]. The individual peak acid responses ranged between the extremes of 18% and 99% of the maximal acid response to pentagastrin, but showed good intraindividual reproducibility [4]. The acid response to sham feeding was not further increased by creating optimal conditions for vagal release of gastrin from the antrum, i.e. by neutralizing the gastric contents [6]. Whether these data can be interpreted as meaning that vagal activation under physiological conditions in man only evokes a submaximal stimulation of acid secretion, or involves both stimulatory and inhibitory mechanisms, is open to question.

Modified sham feeding by the 'chew-and-spit' technique produced an acid response equivalent to that induced by adequate sham feeding [7]. The simple procedure of modified sham feeding by the 'chew-and-spit' technique therefore seems to correctly reflect the vagal activation of gastric acid secretion under physiological conditions in man.

Vagal activation of acid secretion can also be induced pharmacologically, for instance by insulin hypoglycemia. Vagal activation using insulin hypoglycemia is the test most commonly used for postoperative checking of the completeness of vagotomy. In such a test, an insulin dose of 0.2 IU/kg body weight has usually been injected, since this dose of insulin has produced the highest acid response in subjects with an intact vagal innervation of the stomach [8, 9]. The acid response to insulin is dose-dependent, and the insulin hypoglycemia moreover evokes several stimulatory and inhibitory mechanisms, some of which are clearly extravagal (for references see [5]). The acid responses to insulin hypoglycemia and sham feeding are therefore not quite comparable, although the acid response to insulin in a dose of 0.1 IU/kg body weight most closely corresponds to the acid response to sham feeding in subjects with an intact vagal innervation of the stomach [7].

Vagal release of gastrin

Sham feeding in the dog produces a marked vagal release of gastrin from the antrum [10,11]. This vagally released gastrin seems to be of great significance for the vagal activation of gastric acid secretion in the dog, since the acid response to sham feeding in Pavlov pouch dogs is minimized by denervation or resection of the antrum and duodenal bulb [12, 13], and since the minimal acid response to sham feeding in antrum-denervated dogs is potentiated by subthreshold doses of exogenous gastrin [12].

In man, a just detectable vagal release of gastrin seems to exist. Sham feeding has evoked a significant increase in serum gastrin concentration of about 10 pg/ml in both healthy subjects and duodenal ulcer patients [14, 15], confirming previous results in duodenal ulcer patients [16], although this weak effect was not detectable in several studies [16–19]. A single study reported that sham feeding in duodenal ulcer patients evoked a substantial increase in plasma gastrin concentrations that was abolished by antrectomy [20]. A vagal release of gastrin in man is supported by the finding that sham feeding in healthy subjects and duodenal ulcer patients significantly increased the serum gastrin concentrations after pretreatment with anticholinergics [14, 21, 22]. The results suggest a noncholinergic vagal release of gastrin which is normally suppressed by a cholinergic mechanism. A cholinergic inhibition of gastrin release induced by bombesin has in fact been demonstrated [23]. Evidence collected to date thus favors a vagal release of gastrin in man, although the released gastrin is radioimmunologically just detectable in peripheral venous blood. The small vagal release of gastrin in man may be due to a concomitant cholinergic inhibitory effect on the gastrin cells, but is not due to an acid inhibition of gastrin release. Plasma gastrin concentrations did not significantly increase after sham feeding and neutralization of the antral milieu by a continuous gastric perfusion of the stomach with an alkaline buffer in duodenal ulcer patients [19].

The question which then remains is whether vagal release of gastrin in man, yielding an increase in serum gastrin of the order of 5–10 pg/ml, makes a significant contribution to the vagal activation of gastric acid secretion. There is no evidence that vagal activation by sham feeding changes the relationship between the serum concentrations of the various established gastrins that differ slightly in their acid-stimulatory efficiency. Sham feeding did not significantly change the plasma concentration of the heptadecapeptide gastrin (G-17), a potent acid stimulant among the endogenous gastrins [19]. It is, however, possible that current techniques for the radioimmunoassay of serum gastrins do not completely reflect the total gastrins. A gastrin of low molecular weight (G-4) has recently been found in the antral mucosa [24], and reasonable serum concentrations of this small peptide cannot be detected by present antisera.

Limited data clearly indicate that an antral factor contributes to the vagal activation of gastric acid secretion in man, but it is less certain whether this antral factor is composed only of vagally released gastrin. Acidification of the antral lumen to pH 1 reduced the gastric acid response to sham feeding in duodenal ulcer patients by almost 50% [6]. It is unknown whether this substantial reduction was solely due to abolition of vagal release of gastrin.

Electrical vagal stimulation in the cat has evoked release of both gastrin and somatostatin into the antral lumen, with release of only somatostatin during antral acidification [25]. The results were interpreted as indicating that antral acidification facilitated vagal release of somatostatin, which inhibited the gastrin release by a paracrine effect. During antral acidification a vagal release of somatostatin obviously may occur, and somatostatin − if transported to the fundus − is capable of exerting an inhibitory effect directly on the acid-secreting glands. Furthermore, another inhibitory mechanism that does not seem to involve somatostatin or inhibition of gastrin release can be elicited from the human antrum [26]. As a result, the possibility that the substantial reduction of the gastric acid response to sham feeding by antral acidification in duodenal ulcer patients is due to more factors than abolition of vagally released gastrin cannot be excluded.

The effect of antrectomy on the acid response to sham feeding in duodenal ulcer patients also suggests that an antral stimulatory factor − probably vagally released gastrin − contributes to some extent to the vagal activation of gastric acid secretion in man. The acid responses to sham feeding before and after antrectomy cannot, however, be directly compared, since antrectomy in man markedly reduces the capacity of the fundic glands to secrete acid, i.e. the maximal acid response to pentagastrin. This effect seems to be due, at least in part, to withdrawal of a 'trophic' effect of gastrin [27]. The relation between the acid sham feeding response and the maximal acid response to pentagastrin was, however, reduced by antrectomy from about 55% to about 35% [28]. A reduced but still substantial acid response to sham feeding in duodenal ulcer patients thus remained after resection of the antrum and duodenal bulb, implying that vagal release of gastrin from this region may contribute to, but is not essential for, vagal activation of gastric acid secretion in man.

Intravenous infusion of pentagastrin did not potentiate, and had only an additive effect on, the acid response to sham feeding in antrectomized duodenal ulcer patients [29], who in this respect seem to differ quite markedly from antrum-denervated Pavlov pouch dogs [12]. The results suggest that vagally released gastrin in man contributes to the vagal activation of gastric acid secretion as an additive stimulatory effect, without augmenting or potentiating the nervous excitatory effect on the acid secreting glands. In fact, it has been estimated from the acid secretory response to intravenous infusion of gastrin in man that an increase of serum gastrin concentration of the order of 5–10 pg/ml probably results in an increased acid output [30].

Effect of vagotomy

Vagal denervation of the acid-secreting mucosa by proximal gastric vagotomy in duodenal ulcer patients abolishes the acid response to sham feeding in the majority of patients [15, 22, 31, 32]. Since the antrum is intentionally left innervated by this operation, the small amount of vagally released gastrin seems incapable of evoking an acid response in the vagally denervated fundic mucosa. This result may, to some extent, be due to a concomitant vagal release of a chemically unidentified substance – the vagogastrone – that is characterized by inhibiting gastrin-stimulated acid secretion only in vagally denervated mucosa. The vagogastrone mechanism seems to exist in man, although it is less efficient than in the dog [33]. An acid response to sham feeding after proximal gastric vagotomy probably means an incomplete vagotomy. There is no method available by which the completeness of vagotomy can be proven. The insulin hypoglycemia that is often used to check the completeness of vagotomy has the disadvantage of evoking extravagal stimulatory as well as inhibitory mechanisms that influence the acid secretion. In fact, discrepancies have been found between the acid responses to sham feeding and insulin in patients that have been subjected to proximal gastric vagotomy [34]. These discrepancies – an acid response to sham feeding without an acid response to insulin, and vice versa – are probably explained by the extravagal influences of insulin hypoglycemia on acid secretion, in other words by falsely negative and positive insulin tests [35]. A falsely-negative insulin test was changed to a positive test by using an insulin dose of 0.1 IU/kg body weight, while a falsely-positive insulin test was changed to a negative one by pretreatment with an adrenergic blocker [35]. At present, sham feeding therefore seems to be a safe, and the most reliable, test for completeness of vagotomy, and could be recommended as a clinical test.

Vagal neurotransmission at the acid-secreting glands

It has previously been assumed that the nervous excitation of acid secretion by vagal activation is exerted via a cholinergic transmission, an assumption based partly on the fact that a large dose of atropine has completely abolished the acid response to sham feeding in the dog [10]. A large dose of atropine will, however, allow significant amounts of atropine to penetrate into the central nervous system, where it may interrupt a cholinergic transmission and thus eliminate a reflex response totally independent of the peripheral mechanism of transmission. In fact, a low dose of an anticholinergic with minimal cerebral action inhibited the acid response to sham feeding in man by about 65%, but did not abolish the acid response, and this result continued to be obtained with increasing doses of the anticholinergic [22]. The data indicate that the vagal neurotransmission at the acid-secreting glands is only partially cholinergic, at least in man. The nature of the missing hypothetical neurotransmitter is unknown. It may be relevant to emphasize that cimetidine almost eliminates the acid response to sham feeding in man [36], and that gastrin has been found in the vagal nerves [37]. One may speculate that gastrin or some other peptide may act as a peripheral co-transmitter in the vagal nerve.

Vagal hyperactivity in duodenal ulcer patients?

It has been claimed that hypersecretion of gastric acid in duodenal ulcer patients may be due to vagal hyperactivity [38]. There is no method available for direct determination of the vagal tone. The basal serum concentrations of pancreatic polypeptide may, however, serve as an indirect and rough measure of vagal tone. The pancreatic polypeptide is predominantly released by vagal activation which probably involves a pure cholinergic peripheral neuro-transmission. In each subject, the basal gastric acid secretion and the basal serum concentrations of pancreatic polypeptide oscillate synchronously [39], indicating that both secretions are under the influence of the basal vagal tone. The basal plasma concentrations of pancreatic polypeptide were low in young healthy subjects, and were high in some of the older healthy subjects. In duodenal ulcer patients of an age comparable to the older healthy subjects, the frequency of high basal plasma concentrations of pancreatic polypeptide was about the same as in the healthy subjects [39], arguing against the hypothesis that vagal hyperactivity is a common characteristic of duodenal ulcer patients. However, in a few patients sham feeding induced a very poor pancreatic polypeptide response, in spite of a simultaneous substantial gastric acid response and, furthermore, adequate sham feeding produced a significantly higher pancreatic polypeptide response than modified sham feeding in the same group of patients [40], indicating that the acid-secreting glands are more sensitive to vagal excitation than the pancreatic polypeptide-secreting cells. It is therefore questionable whether the basal plasma concentration of the pancreatic polypeptide is a completely reliable indicator of such a low-grade vagal activation as the vagal tone.

Fundic distension

Distension of the fundus generates a substantial gastric acid secretion in both healthy subjects and duodenal ulcer patients [41]. Separate graded distension of the fundus was produced by a balloon successively inflated to volumes of 150, 300 and 600 ml. The graded distension evoked an increasing acid secretion, and the balloon volume of 600 ml resulted in an acid response of the same magnitude as that evoked by sham feeding, i.e. about 50% of the maximal acid response to pentagastrin. Larger balloon volumes tended to induce epigastric fullness and nausea, with a subsequent decrease in acid secretion. A slight but statistically insignificant increase of plasma gastrin concentration occurred during fundic distension [42]. These experiments were performed both without and with neutralization of the gastric contents in order to optimize the conditions for release of gastrin from the antrum. The results were again in accordance with those obtained after sham feeding in man, and suggest that fundic distension in man evokes gastric acid secretion mainly by a neural reflex activation.

Proximal gastric vagotomy markedly reduced, but did not abolish, the acid response to fundic distension in duodenal ulcer patients [43]. In patients subjected to a complete proximal gastric vagotomy — as judged by the insulin test — the acid response to the largest balloon volume was about 20% of the maximal acid response to pentagastrin. The remaining acid response to fundic distension after a complete proximal gastric vagotomy strongly suggests that the activation is partly conveyed via short intramural reflex pathways. A vagotomy thus eliminates the vagal activation of acid secretion but it does not abolish neural reflex activation of the acid-secreting glands. The less efficient stimulation of acid secretion by fundic distension after complete vagotomy compared to the effect in the intact stomach indicates that a long vagovagal reflex also participates in the stimulation of acid secretion. This statement is supported by the finding that the acid response to fundic distension in patients with an incomplete vagotomy amounted to about 50% of the maximal acid response to pentagastrin. Atropine injected intravenously in a dose of 1 mg inhibited the acid response to fundic distension by 80% [43], while cimetidine completely abolished the response [36]. These drugs thus seem to have a similar inhibitory effect on acid secretion stimulated by fundic distension and that stimulated by sham feeding.

Antral distension

The effect of separate antral distension differs in some important respects from the effect of fundic distension in man. Distension of the antrum with a balloon inflated to 50, 100 and 150 ml stimulates gastric acid secretion in peptic ulcer patients, while it suppresses the basal acid secretion in healthy subjects [44]. The stimulation of acid secretion by antral distension in duodenal ulcer patients is probably a neural reflex activation, since the antral distension did not significantly increase the plasma gastrin concentration in peripheral venous blood [45] or portal blood [26]. During submaximal stimulation of gastric acid secretion by pentagastrin, antrum distension constantly inhibits the secretion by about 20% in healthy subjects, while it has no effect in duodenal ulcer patients [26, 46]. The results suggest that antral distension evokes both an inhibitory and a stimulatory mechanism in man. The inhibitory mechanism seems to be defective in duodenal ulcer patients, and its unravelment may therefore have pathophysiological interest. The nature of the inhibitory mechanism is unknown, although the prompt appearance and disappearance of the inhibition may hint at a reflex inhibition.

Inhibition by fat

Another inhibitory mechanism in man which surprisingly seems to involve a neural component is the inhibition of gastric acid secretion by fat administration into the duodenum. According to the classical view, fat inhibition of acid secretion is mediated by a humoral mechanism, the 'enterogastrone'. Some evidence has, however, been presented that vagotomy may impair the fat inhibition of acid secretion [47, 48]. In a recent study, the effect of graded volumes of intraduodenally-administered oleic acid on pentagastrin-stimulated gastric acid secretion showed that 20 ml of oleic acid evoked maximal inhibition in healthy subjects. The inhibitory effect of this volume of oleic acid was therefore studied in duodenal ulcer patients before and after proximal gastric vagotomy [49]. Before the vagotomy, the oleic acid evoked a significant inhibition that was abolished by the vagotomy. Obviously, the vagal nerves play a definite role in the duodenal fat inhibition of gastric acid secretion in man. Whether this vagal involvement implies a reflex inhibition or a hormone particularly active in the vagally innervated stomach is open to question.

Summary

Neural mechanisms seem to play an important part in the regulation of gastric acid secretion in man, and participate in both stimulatory and inhibitory actions. On the stimulatory side, a neural reflex activation of gastric acid secretion via the vagi is involved both in the cephalic phase of acid secretion and in the acid response to gastric distension. This direct vagal stimulation of the acid-secreting glands seems to be only partially a cholinergic transmitter mechanism. There is no evidence for vagal hyperactivity in duodenal ulcer patients. Gastric distension also activates a short intramural reflex pathway in stimulating gastric acid secretion. Furthermore, vagal activation seems to elicit a noncholinergic release of gastrin from the antrum that is markedly suppressed by a simultaneous cholinergic inhibitory mechanism. Present evidence supports the view that vagally released gastrin from the antrum has only an additive and no potentiating effect on the nervous excitation of the acid-secreting glands in man.

Inhibitory neural mechanisms are possibly involved in the cholinergic inhibition of gastrin release and in the inhibitory effect of antral distension, which is defective in duodenal ulcer patients. A vagal component is involved in the inhibition of gastric secretion evoked by intraduodenal fat in man.

References

1. Noring, O. (1951): Studies on the cephalic phase of gastric secretion in normal subjects and ulcer patients. *Gastroenterology 18*, 413.
2. Preshaw, R.M. and Webster, D.R. (1967): A comparison of sham feeding and teasing as stimuli for gastric acid secretion in the dog. *Q. J. Exp. Physiol. 52*, 37.
3. Preshaw, R.M. (1970): Gastric acid output after sham feeding and during release or infusion of gastrin. *Am. J. Physiol. 219*, 1409.
4. Knutson, U. and Olbe, L. (1973): Gastric acid response to sham feeding in the duodenal ulcer patients. *Scand. J. Gastroenterol. 8*, 513.
5. Stenquist, B. (1979): Studies on vagal activation of gastric acid secretion in man. *Acta Physiol. Scand. Sup. 465.*
6. Knutson, U., Bergegårdh, S. and Olbe, L. (1974): The effect of intragastric pH variations on the gastric acid response to sham feeding in duodenal ulcer patients. *Scand. J. Gastroenterol. 9*, 357.
7. Stenquist, B., Knuston, U. and Olbe, L. (1978): Gastric acid response to adequate and modified sham feeding and to insulin hypoglycemia in duodenal ulcer patients. *Scand. J. Gastroenterol. 13*, 357.
8. Baron, J.H., Cowley, D.J., Gutierrez, L.V. et al. (1972): Dose response of gastric acid to insulin in patients with duodenal ulcer. *Gastroenterology 62*, 203.
9. Kronborg, O. (1971): Dose dependence of insulin-activated gastric acid secretion in patients with duodenal ulcer before and after vagotomy. *Scand. J. Gastroenterol. 6*, 33.
10. Nilsson, G., Simon, J., Yalow, R.S. and Berson, S.A. (1972): Plasma gastrin and gastric acid responses to sham feeding and feeding in dogs. *Gastroenterology 63*, 51.
11. Tepperman, B.L., Walsh, J.H. and Preshaw, R.M. (1972): Effect of antral denervation on gastrin release by sham feeding and insulin hypoglycemia in dogs. *Gastroenterology 63*, 973.

12. Olbe, L. (1964): Potentiation of sham feeding response in Pavlov pouch dogs by subthreshold amounts of gastrin with and without acidification of denervated antrum. *Acta Physiol. Scand. 61*, 244.
13. Olbe, L. (1964): Effect of resection of gastrin releasing regions on acid response to sham feeding and insulin hypoglycemia in Pavlov pouch dogs. *Acta Physiol. Scand. 62*, 169.
14. Feldman, M., Richardson, C.T., Taylor, I.L. and Walsh, J.H. (1979): Effect of atropine on vagal release of gastrin and pancreatic polypeptide. *J. Clin. Invest. 63*, 294.
15. Feldman, M., Dickerman, R.M., McClelland, R.N. et al. (1979): Effect of selective proximal vagotomy on food-stimulated gastric acid secretion and gastrin release in patients with duodenal ulcer. *Gastroenterology 76,* 926.
16. Mayer, G., Arnold, R., Feurle, G. et al. (1974): Influence of feeding and sham feeding upon serum gastrin and gastric acid secretion in control subjects and duodenal ulcer patients. *Scand. J. Gastroenterol. 9*, 703.
17. Mignon, M., Galmiche, J.P., Accary, J.P. and Bonfils, S. (1974): Serum gastrin, gastric acid and pepsin responses to sham feeding in man. *Gastroenterology 66*, 856.
18. Konturek, S.J., Kwiecien, N., Obtulowicz, W. et al. (1979): Cephalic phase of gastric secretion in healthy subjects and duodenal ulcer patients: role of vagal innervation. *Gut 20*, 875.
19. Stenquist, B., Nilsson, G., Rehfeld, J.F. and Olbe, L. (1979): Plasma gastrin concentrations following sham feeding in duodenal ulcer patients. *Scand. J. Gastroenterol. 14*, 305.
20. Knutson, U., Olbe, L. and Ganguli, P.C. (1974): Gastric acid and plasma gastrin responses to sham feeding in duodenal ulcer patients before and after resection of antrum and duodenal bulb. *Scand. J. Gastroenterol. 9*, 351.
21. Feldman, M., Richardson, C.T., Taylor, I.L. and Walsh, J.H. (1978): Neural regulation of gastrin and pancreatic polypeptide release in man. *Clin. Res. 26*, 497A.
22. Stenquist, B., Rehfeld, J.F. and Olbe, L. (1979): The effect of proximal gastric vagotomy and anticholinergics on the acid and gastrin responses to sham feeding in duodenal ulcer patients. *Gut 20*, 1020.
23. Taylor, I.L., Walsh, J.H., Carter, D. et al. (1979): Effects of atropine and bethanechol on bombesin-stimulated release of pancreatic polypeptide and gastrin in dog. *Gastroenterology 77*, 714.
24. Rehfeld, J.F. and Larsson, L.-I. (1979): The predominant molecular form of gastrin and cholecystokinin in the gut is a small peptide corresponding to their COOH-terminal tetrapeptide amide. *Acta Physiol. Scand. 105*, 117.
25. Uvnäs-Wallensten, K., Efendic, S. and Luft, R. (1977): Vagal release of somatostatin into the antral lumen of cats. *Acta Physiol. Scand. 99*, 126.
26. Schöön, I.-M., Lundqvist, G., Rehfeld, J.F. and Olbe, L. (1980): A study of the effect of antral distension on gastric acid secretion in man. *Digestion.* (Accepted for publication).
27. Bergegårdh, S. and Olbe, L. (1976): The effect of long-term postoperative pentagastrin infusion on the maximal acid responses to pentagastrin in patients subjected to antrectomy. *Scand. J. Gastroenterol. 11*, 347.
28. Knutson, U. and Olbe, L. (1974): Gastric acid response to sham feeding before

and after resection of antrum and duodenal bulb in duodenal ulcer patients. *Scand. J. Gastroenterol. 9*, 191.

29. Knutson, U. and Olbe, L. (1974): The effect of exogenous gastrin on the acid sham feeding response in antrum-bulb resected duodenal ulcer patients. *Scand. J. Gastroenterol. 9*, 231.

30. Feldman, M., Walsh, J.H., Wong, H.C. and Richardson, C.T. (1978): Role of gastrin heptadecapeptide in the acid secretory response to amino acids in man. *J. Clin. Invest. 61*, 308.

31. Knutson, U. and Olbe, L. (1973): The gastric acid response to sham feeding in duodenal ulcer patients after proximal selective vagotomy. *Scand. J. Gastroenterol. Sup. 20*, 16.

32. Richardson, C.T. and Feldman, M. (1978): Sham feeding: a safe test for vagotomy. *Gastroenterology 74*, 1084.

33. Stenquist, B., Knutson, U. and Olbe, L. (1978): The vagogastrone mechanism in man. *Scand. J. Gastroenterol. 13*, 895.

34. Olbe, L. and Stenquist, B. (1979): Vergleich der Säuresekretion nach Scheinfütterung und Insulinstimulation nach proximaler gastrischer Vagotomie. In: *Selektive proximale Vagotomie − aktuelle Probleme*, p. 103. Eds: H. Pichlmaier and T. Junginger. Georg Thieme Verlag, Stuttgart.

35. Stenquist, B., Rehnberg, O. and Olbe, L. (1980): Sham feeding versus insulin as a test for completeness of vagotomy (abstract). *Hepato-Gastroenterol. Sup. XI*, International Congress of Gastroenterology, 138.

36. Schöön, I.-M. and Olbe, L. (1978): Inhibitory effect of cimetidine on gastric acid secretion vagally activated by physiological means in duodenal ulcer patients. *Gut 19*, 27.

37. Uvnäs-Wallensten, K., Rehfeld, J.F., Larsson, L.-I. and Uvnäs, B. (1977): Heptadecapeptide gastrin in the vagal nerve. *Proc. Nat. Acad. Sci. U.S.A. 74*, 5707.

38. Dragstedt, L.R. (1969): Peptic ulcer. An abnormality in gastric secretion. *Am. J. Surg. 117*, 143.

39. Schwartz, T.W., Stenquist, B., Olbe, L. and Stadil, F. (1979): Synchronous oscillations in the basal secretion of pancreatic-polypeptide and gastric acid. Depression by cholinergic blockade of pancreatic-polypeptide concentrations in plasma. *Gastroenterology 76*, 14.

40. Schwartz, T.W., Stenquist, B. and Olbe, L. (1979): Cephalic phase of pancreatic-polypeptide secretion studied by sham feeding in man. *Scand. J. Gastroenterol. 14*, 313.

41. Grötzinger, U., Bergegårdh, S. and Olbe, L. (1977): The effect of fundic distension on gastric acid secretion in man. *Gut 18*, 105.

42. Grötzinger, U., Rehfeld, J.F. and Olbe, L. (1977): Is there an oxyntopyloric reflex for release of gastrin in man? *Gastroenterology 73*, 753.

43. Grötzinger, U., Bergegårdh, S. and Olbe, L. (1977): The effect of atropine and proximal gastric vagotomy on the acid response to fundic distension in man. *Gut 18*, 303.

44. Bergegårdh, S. and Olbe, L. (1975): Gastric acid response to antrum distension in man. *Scand. J. Gastroenterol. 10*, 171.

45. Bergegårdh, S., Nilsson, G. and Olbe, L. (1976): The effect of antral distension on acid secretion and plasma gastrin in duodenal ulcer patients. *Scand. J. Gastroenterol. 11*, 475.

46. Schöön, I.-M., Bergegårdh, S., Grötzinger, U. and Olbe, L. (1978): Evidence for a defective inhibition of pentagastrin-stimulated gastric acid secretion by antral distension in the duodenal ulcer patients. *Gastroenterology 75*, 363.
47. Sircus, W. (1958): Studies on the mechanisms in the duodenum inhibiting gastric secretion. *Q. J. Exp. Physiol. 43*, 114.
48. Johnston, D. and Duthie, H.L. (1969): Effect of fat in the duodenum on gastric acid secretion before and after vagotomy in man. *Scand. J. Gastroenterol. 4*, 561.
49. Kihl, B. and Olbe, L. (1980): Fat inhibition of gastric acid secretion in duodenal ulcer patients before and after proximal gastric vagotomy. *Gut* (Accepted for publication).

Hormones and their role in ulcer disease

R. Arnold, H. Koop and W. Creutzfeldt
Division of Gastroenterology and Metabolism, Department of Medicine, University of Göttingen, Federal Republic of Germany

That peptic ulceration cannot be reduced to a single pathogenetic factor is unchallenged. Every newly arising ulcer results from an imbalance between aggressive and defensive factors. The defensive factors protect the mucosa against the aggressive potency of acid, pepsin and bile acids. Their effectiveness mainly depends upon the integrity of the so-called mucosal barrier, a superior principle which includes adequate mucosal blood flow, regeneration of the surface epithelium and production of a high quality mucus. Little is known about the physiological regulation of the mucosal barrier. However, a few observations in patients with Zollinger-Ellison syndrome and marked gastric acid hypersecretion who never get a peptic ulcer emphasize the importance of a well-functioning mucosal barrier. Due to our lack of awareness of defensive factor regulation, our concept of the pathogenesis and therapy of peptic ulceration rests unduly on the aggressive factors. This is even true regarding the role of humoral influences in ulcer disease. Most reports deal with their role in the regulation of acid or pepsin secretion and inactivation, whereas data on the regulation of the defensive factors by gastrointestinal hormones are scarce.

The significance of gastrointestinal hormones in the pathogenesis of peptic ulcers results from their mode of action:
— They modulate acid and pepsin secretion.
— They are partially responsible for neutralization of gastric acid and pepsin in the proximal duodenum.
— They influence motor activity of the gastrointestinal tract and, thus, contribute to an increased acid and pepsin transport into the duodenal bulb or to an increased reflux of alkaline duodenal content into the stomach.
— They influence mucosal blood flow and, by this, could affect epithelial regeneration.

Endocrine factors involved in the control of gastric acid secretion and their possible role in the pathogenesis of gastric acid hypersecretion are summarized in Table I. In discussing the significance of humoral factors in peptic ulcer disease one should not forget, however, that the pathogenesis of peptic ulcer may, in the majority of ulcer patients, never be explained by acid and pepsin alone.

Increased stimulation of parietal cells by gastrin

Autonomous gastrin hypersecretion

The Zollinger-Ellison syndrome is the classic example of a gastrointestinal endocrinopathy [1–3]. Parietal cell hyperplasia and gastric acid hypersecretion derive from the uncontrolled hormone release by a gastrin-producing tumor. Gastrinomas are mostly situated in the pancreas or duodenum. Gastrin concentrations and serum gastrin levels of 15 gastrinoma patients are

Table I: Possible role of gastrointestinal hormones in gastric acid hypersecretion.

Increased stimulation of parietal cells by gastrin
Autonomous gastrin hypersecretion
    Gastrinoma
Increased G-cell stimulation
    G-cell hyperfunction with and without G-cell hyperplasia
    Stomach outlet obstruction
    Disturbed gastric acid – gastrin feedback
    Elevated neural tone?
Defective inhibition of gastrin release
    Excluded antrum
    Short bowel syndrome
    Somatostatin deficiency?

Defective inhibition of parietal cell function
Endocrine factors
    Defective secretion of secretin
          gastric inhibitory polypeptide
          enterogastrone
Paracrine factors
    Somatostatin deficiency
Neurocrine factors
    Vasoactive intestinal polypeptide (VIP) deficiency

Defective neutralization of acid in the duodenal bulb
Pancreatic bicarbonate deficiency (secretin, VIP)
Rapid stomach emptying (motilin)

depicted in Figure 1 and compared to serum gastrin levels and antral gastrin concentrations of duodenal ulcer patients and controls. Four patients had duodenal gastrinomas and are characterized by an asterisk. In contrast to the markedly elevated circulating serum gastrin levels, tumor gastrin concentrations were surprisingly low and surpassed in only 5 patients antral gastrin concentration of controls and duodenal ulcer patients. There was no correlation between the tumor gastrin concentration and the peripheral serum gastrin concentration. Considering the size of the antral mucosa in controls and duodenal ulcer patients which contains 1–3% G-cells it can be concluded that a gastrinoma which rarely weighs more than one gram contains less gastrin than the antrum. Therefore, the serum gastrin levels in gastrinoma

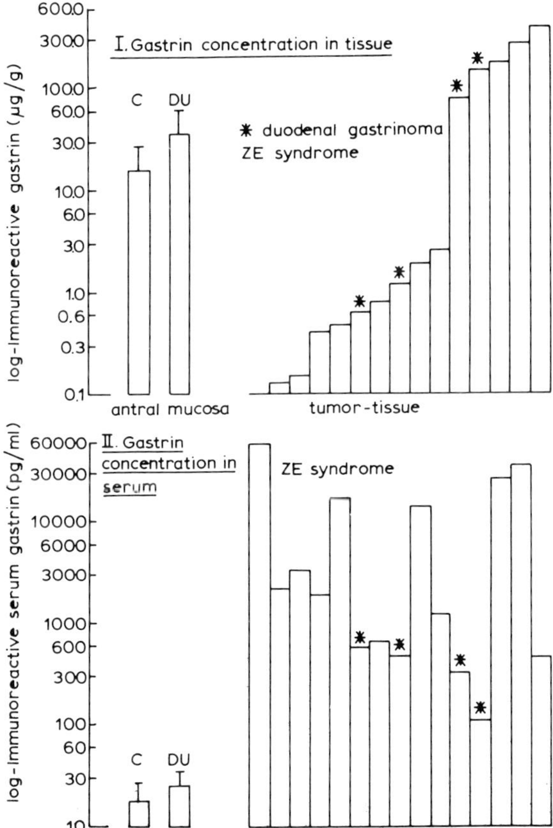

Fig. 1: Immunoreactive gastrin concentrations in serum and tumor extracts of 15 gastrinoma patients and in the antral mucosa of controls (C) and duodenal ulcer patients (DU).

patients demonstrate that hypergastrinemia results from a reduced storage capacity of the gastrinoma.

Increased G-cell stimulation

Antral G-cell hyperfunction   Another example for an increased stimulation of parietal cells by gastrin is represented by antral G-cell hyperfunction which may occur with and without G-cell hyperplasia [4–10].

Table II summarizes the data of 4 patients with intractable peptic ulcer disease, slightly or markedly elevated gastric acid secretion and moderately increased serum gastrin levels. All patients were male and had no previous gastric surgery. Antral G-cell density was in these patients significantly elevated if compared to that of normogastrinemic patients with duodenal ulcer, gastric ulcer or gastrinomas (Figs. 2 and 3). In 2 patients serum gastrin levels decreased to undetectable values after antrectomy. Patients Su and Fr improved during long-term treatment with cimetidine.

Recently, Lamers et al. reported a patient with gastric acid hypersecretion and hypergastrinemia without antral G-cell hyperplasia in which Billroth II antrectomy led to a normalization of serum gastrin within half an hour [9]. In this patient ingestion of a standard meal induced an early and steep increase in serum gastrin concentrations which was different from the postprandial gastrin response of gastrinoma patients which in Lamers' series showed only a distinct increase. The gastrin response to secretin was very weak in this patient.

The gastrin response of patients with antral G-cell hyperplasia to secretin differs as well from that reported in the majority of gastrinoma patients [7,

Table II: Findings in 4 patients with antral G-cell hyperfunction and antral G-cell hyperplasia.

Patient	Sex	Age (years)	BAO (mMol/hr)	MAO (mMol/hr)	Serum gastrin (pg/ml)	Antral G-cell density (cells/area*)
Du	m	17	16.1	37.6	105	94
Ha	m	27	10.3	44.0	269	100
Su	m	39	5.0	24.6	224	120
Fr	m	21	6.5	31.7	370	94
Upper limit in controls:					60	80

BAO = basal acid output, MAO = maximal acid output.
* size of area − 0.35 × 0.23 mm.

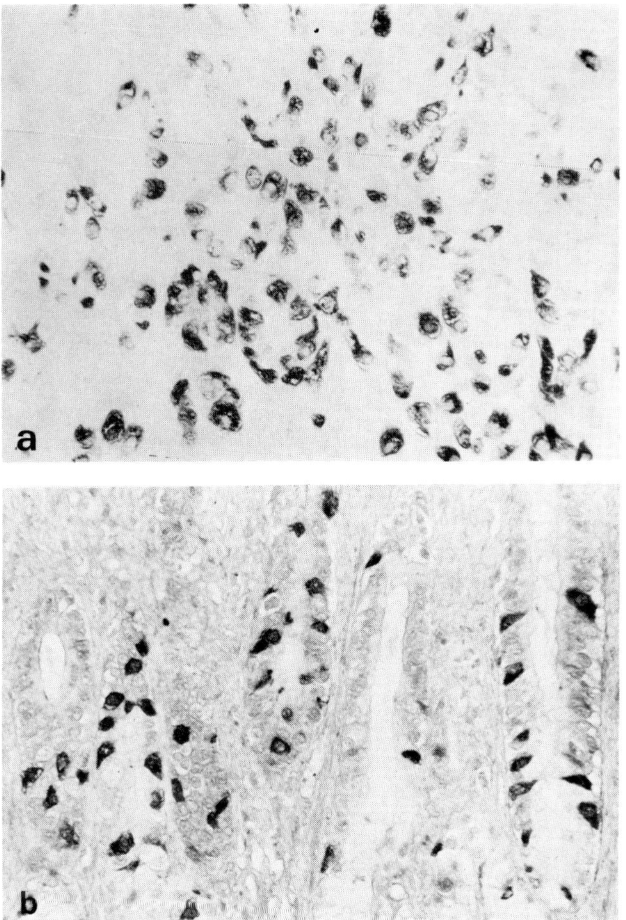

Fig. 2: a. Distribution of antral G-cells in a hypergastrinemic duodenal ulcer patient with gastric acid hypersecretion and G-cell hyperplasia. b. Distribution of antral G-cells in a normogastrinemic duodenal ulcer patient. Bouin fixation, paraffin embedding, PAP-technique. Magnification: 400×.

10]. Whereas in most gastrinoma patients secretin elicited a gastrin increase of more than 100% above basal values [2, 3, 11, 12], Russel et al. [7] and we have found in patients with G-cell hyperfunction due to antral G-cell hyperplasia either a small initial gastrin increase amounting to less than 50% which was followed by a significant decrease below the basal values or an immediate decrease of serum gastrin after secretin ingestion. Figure 4 illustrates the effect of intravenous secretin on the gastrin response of a gastrinoma patient, a patient with an excluded antrum at the duodenal stump after Billroth II resection and 13 duodenal ulcer patients. Note that the basal

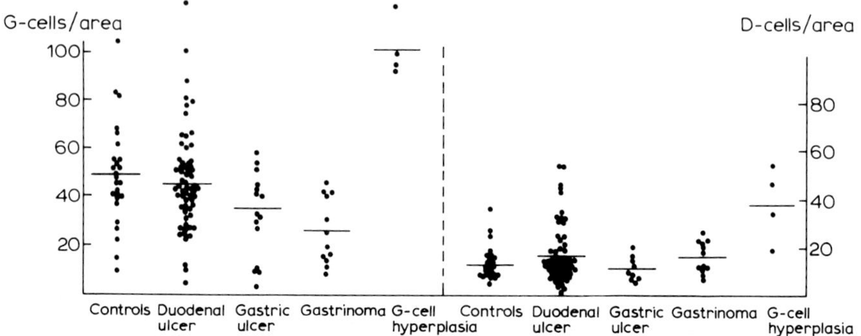

Fig. 3:   *G- and D-cells per area in pyloric biopsy specimens in controls, in duodenal ulcer patients, gastric ulcer patients, gastrinoma patients and in patients with G-cell hyperfunction (hypergastrinemia, gastric and hypersecretion and G-cell hyperplasia).*

gastrin levels in the hypergastrinemic subjects are almost identical. Therefore, a negative or a weak gastrin response to secretin but a strong gastrin increase in response to a test meal may be helpful criteria in the differential diagnosis of hypergastrinemic states of antral and gastrinoma origin. However, it should be considered that even in proven gastrinoma patients significant serum gastrin increases after a test meal [3], and weak gastrin responses to

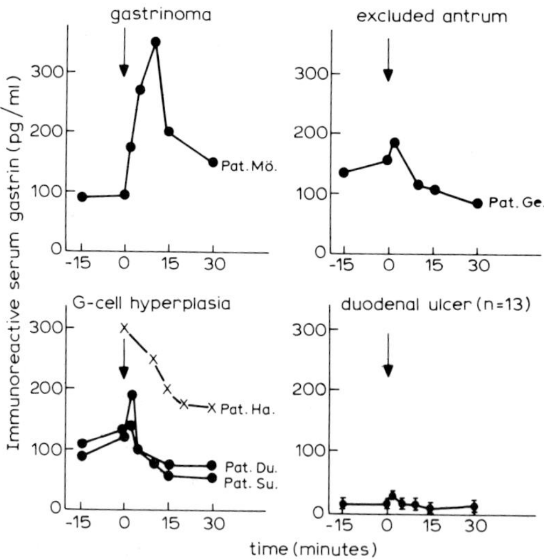

Fig. 4:   *Effect of intravenous injection of 75 KU secretin on serum gastrin in one patients with gastrinoma, one patient with excluded antrum, 3 patients with antral G-cell hyperplasia and 13 duodenal ulcer patients.*

secretin had been observed [3], indicating that both tests do at present not allow a definite conclusion as to the source of hypergastrinemia.

Whether antral G-cell hyperfunction represents a separate entity which does not underly the feedback inhibition by acid, thus appearing similarly autonomous as gastrinoma cells, or whether it is merely one extreme variant of the functional G-cell hyperactivity found in the majority of duodenal ulcer patients (see below) has to be established.

Stimulation by distension, catecholamines, calcium   By eliciting hypergastrinemia, endogenous or exogenous stimulation of antral G-cells could result in increased gastric acid secretion and thus contribute to the occurrence of peptic ulcers. For example, long-term treatment with glucocorticoids [13], injection of noradrenaline [14–16] or calcium [17] have been shown to increase serum gastrin. It was claimed that the increased incidence of peptic ulcer in patients with hyperparathyroidism results from direct stimulation of parietal cells by calcium which is amplified by the calcium-mediated increased G-cell stimulation [18, 19]. However, hypercalcemia from hyperparathyroidism or of other origin has been described to be associated with hypergastrinemia only in patients with gastrinoma or with achlorhydria [20]. In contrast, patients with hyperparathyroidism without a co-existing gastrinoma have not been shown to have increased serum gastrin, acid hypersecretion or a higher incidence rate of duodenal ulcer.

Since in healthy volunteers, stomach distention elicited a weak gastrin increase only [21], while gastric acid secretion increased independently of serum gastrin at low and high pressure, the increased gastric acid secretion of ulcer patients with stomach outlet obstruction was claimed to be the direct consequence of the stimulated parietal cell function by distention. However, in patients with stomach outlet obstruction basal and postprandial serum gastrin levels are elevated and acid response to exogenous tetragastrin exaggerated [22]. From these findings it was concluded that according to the original concept of Dragstedt [23] gastric acid hypersecretion in patients with stomach outlet obstruction may at least to some extent result from increased antral G-cell stimulation in response to antral stasis.

Disturbed gastric acid feedback   Antral gastrin release is inhibited by low pH and stimulated by neutral pH. The elevated serum gastrin levels in patients with pernicious anemia or after vagotomy are explained by a reduced or absent gastric acid secretion. Recently, Walsh et al. demonstrated that compared to controls duodenal ulcer patients released more gastrin and secreted more acid if the stomach was stimulated by an amino acid-cornstarch meal of different pH [24]. They could show that the degree of gastrin inhibition at low pH was significantly less in ulcer patients than in healthy volunteers [24]. By these findings a defect in the autoregulation of gastrin release and gastric acid secretion at low pH in ulcer patients was suggested, which as its consequence resulted in an increased functional G-cell activity.

Indeed, duodenal ulcer patients release more gastrin in response to a test meal than healthy controls as has been confirmed by several groups [25, 26]. Similarly, exaggerated gastrin responses were described during insulin hypoglycemia [27] and calcium infusion, whereas the reports on gastrin release during 'physiological' vagal stimulation (sham feeding) are controversial [25, 28, 29]. In contrast to previous findings we are at present unable to demonstrate, in recently-investigated ulcer patients using the same method of sham feeding and the identical radioimmunoassay system, a significant increase in serum gastrin as described earlier [25].

Taylor et al. could demonstrate by 2 different radioimmunoassay systems specific for G-17 and G-34 that duodenal and gastric ulcer patients release significantly more G-34 in response to a test meal than healthy subjects, whereas no differences in the increments in serum gastrin G-17 could be found between controls and ulcer patients [30]. The interpretation of this finding is difficult since the opposite was found by others [31].

In contrast to the elevated postprandial gastrin levels reports on basal serum gastrin in duodenal ulcer patients are controversial. Higher, lower and not significantly altered basal serum gastrin levels have been reported [25, 32, 33]. By comparing the serum gastrin levels of 233 duodenal ulcer patients with those of 124 unselected controls from a local insurance company we found significantly lower basal values in duodenal ulcer and gastric ulcer disease. However, these differences disappeared if duodenal ulcer patients were compared to age-matched controls with known gastric acid secretion (Fig. 5). The extremely high serum gastrin levels in some of the control groups with unknown acid secretion may derive from a clinically inapparent hypo- or achlorhydria. Therefore, the question of whether or not basal serum gastrin contributes to basal acid secretion in duodenal ulcer patients cannot be answered.

The exaggerated gastrin response of duodenal ulcer patients to food cannot be related to an increased antral and duodenal G-cell mass which could be confirmed by different groups ([34–39]; Table III; Fig. 3). It should, however, be stressed that one group showed a significant increase in the antral G-cell volume (not the number) of duodenal ulcer patients [36].

Antral gastrin concentration was reported to be slightly elevated by one group [34] but was found unchanged [40] or even lower [37] in other studies

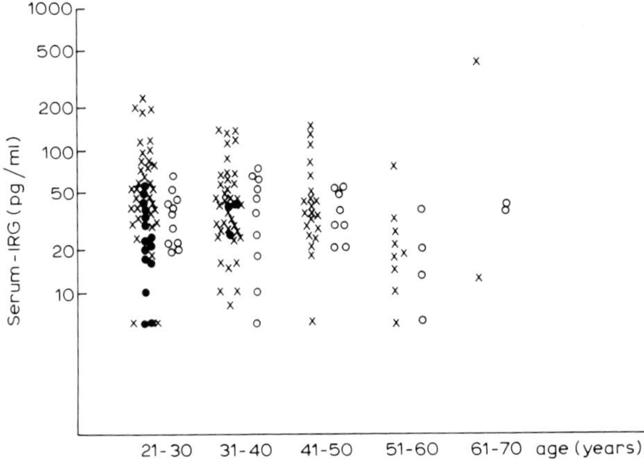

Fig. 5: Fasting serum gastrin levels in age-matched controls and duodenal ulcer patients. ● = controls with normal acid secretion, × = controls with unknown acid secretion, ○ = duodenal ulcer patients.

compared to the antral gastrin concentration of controls. Therefore, the data available at present concerning antral gastrin concentration do nothing to contribute to the understanding of the mechanism by which ulcer patients release more gastrin than healthy controls.

Ultrastructurally, the secretory granules of antral G-cells in duodenal ulcer patients contain significantly more electron-lucent 'empty' granules than G-cell granules of healthy subjects in which G-cells display a broad scale of varying electron density [34]. The results of these studies have shown that the

Table III: Antral G-cells in duodenal ulcer patients.

Study	Year	Controls	Duodenal ulcer patients
Creutzfeldt et al. [34]	1976	38.7 ± 3.4/area	41.2 ± 2.6/area
Royston et al. [35]	1978	6.5 – 13.6/mm strip	3.1 – 25.7/mm strip
Oberholzer et al. [36]	1978	207.4 ± 19.8/cm^3 epithelium	81.4 ± 12.4/cm^3 epithelium
		1221.1 μ^3 (volume)	2654.6 μ^3 (volume)*
Barbara et al. [37]	1978	23.5 ± 9.8/area	15.9 ± 12.3/area*
Piris and Whitehead [38]	1979	86 – 470/unit	43 – 643/unit
Arnold et al. [39]	1980	49.2 ± 4.2/area	46.7 ± 2.5/area

* Significantly different versus controls.

G-cells have a significantly higher functional activity in duodenal ulcer disease.

A defective inhibition of antral G-cell function by hormones that inhibit gastrin release could be an attractive hypothesis to explain the exaggerated postprandial gastrin release of duodenal ulcer patients. A potent inhibitor of both gastric acid secretion and gastrin release is somatostatin which is situated in close vicinity to antral G-cells and to fundic parietal cells. A significant somatostatin release into the veins draining the stomach and into the gastric lumen could be demonstrated by several authors supporting the suggestion that somatostatin acts physiologically as a modulator of gastrin and gastric acid secretion [39].

We investigated the number of D-cells in different states of peptic ulcer disease and did not find significant differences in the number of antral D-cells between controls and duodenal and gastric ulcer patients (see Fig. 3). However, findings on the somatostatin concentration in antral and fundic mucosa samples of duodenal ulcer patients are controversial: a significantly lower somatostatin concentration in the antral mucosa of duodenal and gastric ulcer patients [41] and no difference from that in controls [42] were reported. In contrast, no difference in fundic somatostatin concentration could be found in ulcer patients. From this it may be concluded that a defective inhibition of gastrin release cannot be due to a lack of somatostatin-producing D-cells, while a functional defect of D-cells cannot be ruled out.

It has been speculated that the defective autoregulation of gastrin release and gastric acid secretion at low pH shown in ulcer patients could explain the higher functional activity state of antral G-cells. Alternatively a higher neural tone may alter the activity of antral G-cells and could as well be responsible for the increased parietal cell mass and the increased sensitivity of parietal cells to gastrin.

Recently it was proposed that basal pancreatic polypeptide (PP) levels may serve as an indicator of the abdominal vagal tone. Schwartz et al. demonstrated that spontaneous fluctuations in acid secretion of duodenal ulcer patients are paralleled by simultaneous fluctuations in plasma PP levels suggesting that plasma PP may serve as an indicator of the abdominal vagal tone [43].

We investigated basal PP levels in duodenal ulcer patients compared to age-matched controls and found significantly higher basal PP levels in age-matched duodenal ulcer patients (Fig. 6). In addition, serum PP of duodenal ulcer patients responded significantly stronger to modified sham feeding than controls. However, in individual subjects we were unable to confirm a congruent behavior of acid secretion and PP levels both in the basal period

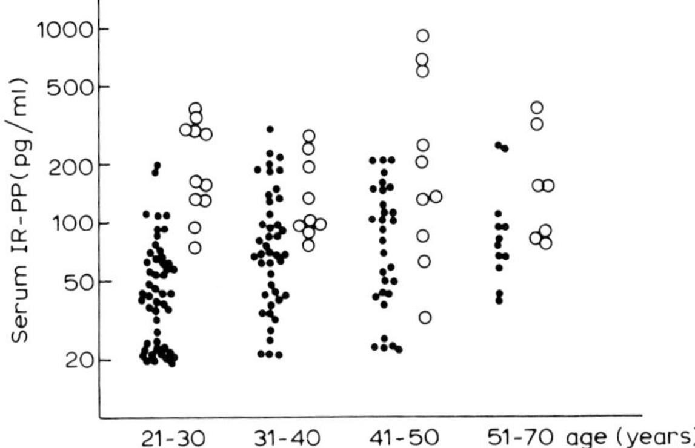

Fig. 6: Basal serum pancreatic polypeptide levels in controls and duodenal ulcer patients. ● = controls, ○ = duodenal ulcer patients.

and during vagal stimulation (see Fig. 7). In addition, there was a significantly negative correlation of acid output and integrated PP secretion during one hour sham feeding [44].

Further studies have, therefore, to be performed in order to elucidate the validity of PP measurements as a parameter of the vagal tone.

Interesting results are available concerning the registration of sympathetic nervous activity in duodenal ulcer patients. Plasma noradrenaline, when measured by a precise and sensitive assay, serves as a reliable index of the sympathetic tone [45]. Earlier it was shown that epinephrine stimulates the secretion of gastrin in man and to a higher extent in duodenal ulcer patients [46] and that it is at least partially responsible for the rise in serum gastrin during insulin hypoglycemia [16].

Overnight fasting and mean supine plasma noradrenaline were found to be significantly elevated in duodenal ulcer patients compared to controls. However, there was no correlation between plasma noradrenaline and serum gastrin in ulcer patients [45]. Therefore plasma noradrenaline is unlikely to be directly responsible for the abnormality in gastrin secretion. Although the significance of increased noradrenaline levels in duodenal ulcer patients has to be established these findings suggest that adrenergic mechanisms could be involved in the faulty control of gastrin release in duodenal ulcer patients.

Defective inhibition of gastrin release

Excluded antrum   G-cells of an excluded antrum at the duodenal stump after Billroth II resection release excess gastrin because they are not inhibited by

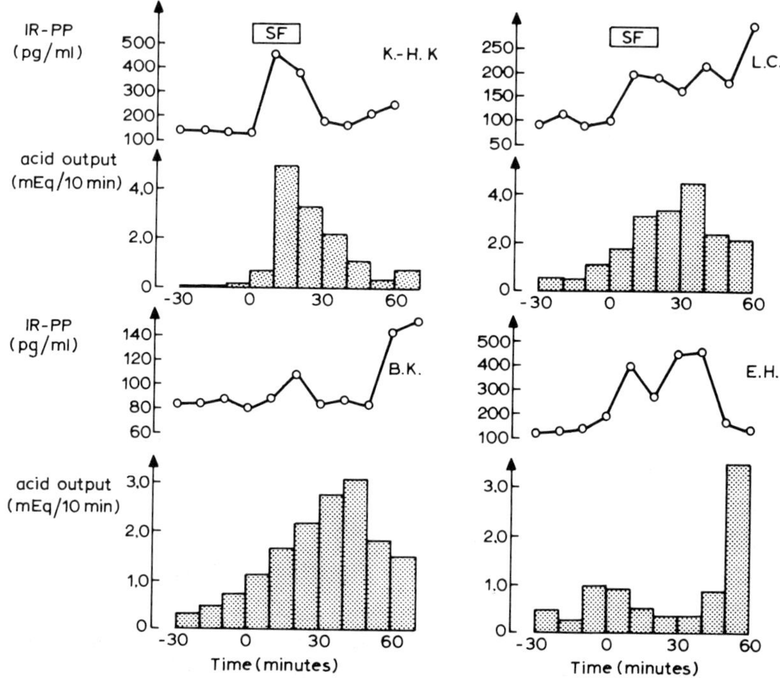

Fig. 7:   Serum pancreatic polypeptide levels and gastric acid secretion in 4 duodenal ulcer patients before and in response to 20 minutes sham feeding (spit-and-chew technique).

gastric acid. They increase in number as antral G-cells in pernicious anemia or after vagotomy. The unrestrained gastrin release results in acid hypersecretion and, by that, in relapsing ulcer disease that is indistinguishable from Zollinger-Ellison syndrome. Gastrin response from the excluded antrum to secretin is weak as shown by Figure 4 [46].

Short bowel syndrome   The small intestine, as the kidney, is a major catabolism site of gastrointestinal hormones. Extensive small-bowel resection is, therefore, occasionally followed by gastric acid hypersecretion and an increased incidence of peptic ulcers [47]. Since basal and postprandial serum gastrin levels are elevated in the majority of patients after small-bowel resection [48], it was suggested that gastrin participates in evoking gastric acid hypersecretion in these states.

Defective inhibition of parietal cell function

When exogenously administered, several hormones inhibit gastric acid secretion. These are secretin, GIP, VIP, somatostatin, neurotensin and other candidate enterogastrones as well as pancreatic glucagon and calcitonin. The physiological significance of these findings which are achieved by the application of pharmacological doses of hormones is unsettled. Whether diminished release of these peptides contributes to the gastric acid hypersecretion in duodenal ulcer disease cannot be answered at present.

Endocrine factors

Contradictory results had been reported on basal and stimulated secretin levels in duodenal ulcer patients: lower and elevated basal and postprandial hormone concentrations were observed [49–52]. However, by improving the radioimmunoassay technique, reports on elevated secretin levels in duodenal ulcer patients [52] and on very high levels in Zollinger-Ellison syndrome [51] seem to reflect the real conditions. Thus the present data do not support the suggestion that a defect in secretin secretion or a resistance to the biological effects of secretin contributes to the increased acid secretion and to the increased acidity of the duodenal bulb in duodenal ulcer patients.

GIP-hyposecretion could also be ruled out as a pathogenetically-significant factor in ulcer disease. It could be demonstrated that basal and food- or glucose-stimulated GIP levels are even elevated in duodenal ulcer patients, presumably due to a more rapid rate of gastric emptying in these patients [53–55]. In addition to these findings it has been shown that, in man at least, GIP is a very poor inhibitor of gastric acid secretion [56]. Exogenously-administered GIP in doses that elevated serum GIP concentrations to levels comparable to those achieved during food uptake failed to inhibit pentagastrin- and food-stimulated gastric acid secretion.

Paracrine and neurocrine factors

Nothing is known about circulating somatostatin levels in peptic ulcer disease. Since somatostatin is postulated to be a peptide that is released in a paracrine, not in an endocrine way [57], measurements of peripheral somatostatin may fail to answer the question whether somatostatin release is faulty in ulcer patients. The same holds true for VIP which in the gastrointestinal tract is exclusively present in nerve fibers and acts as a neurotransmitter. It could be shown that these peptides reach the portal vein after acidification of the duodenum [58], but its physiological and pathophysiological significance for the control of pancreatic exocrine secretion and of gastric acid secretion are unsettled.

Other gastrointestinal peptides

There are several hormones and hormone candidates in the gastrointestinal tract which could theoretically contribute to the known abnormalities in peptic ulcer disease. As far as the increased gastric emptying rates in duodenal ulcer disease and the delayed gastric emptying known for gastric ulcer patients result from disturbed hormone secretion, and by that contribute to the development of peptic ulcers in the duodenal bulb or in the stomach, has not been ascertained. Motilin which in pharmacological doses increases gastric emptying could be a candidate [59]. The same holds true for endorphins and substance P which could modulate both secretory and motor function as well as mucosal blood flow of the gastrointestinal tract [60, 61].

Summary

A significant pathogenetic role of gastrointestinal hormones in ulcer disease could be ascertained for gastrin in patients with gastrinoma and for patients with hypergastrinemia and acid hypersecretion due to antral G-cell hyperfunction. In duodenal ulcer patients the exaggerated postprandial gastrin response which is predominantly due to an increased secretion of G-34 and the significantly lower degree of gastrin inhibition at low pH is reflected by the increased functional activity of antral G-cells at the ultrastructural level. This increased functional activity of antral G-cells could be the consequence of a defective autoregulation of gastrin release and gastric acid secretion at low pH and of an elevated neural (vagal and/or sympathetic) tone. There is no evidence for a faulty release of secretin and gastric inhibitory polypeptide in duodenal ulcer disease. There is at present no information available to decide the role of hormones in the pathogenesis of peptic ulcer which are postulated to be released in a paracrine or neurocrine way.

References

1. Ellison, E.H. and Wilson, D. (1964): The Zollinger-Ellison syndrome: reappraisal and evaluation of 260 registered cases. *Ann. Surg. 160*, 512.
2. Isenberg, J.I., Walsh, J.H. and Grossman, M.I. (1973): Zollinger-Ellison syndrome. *Gastroenterology 65*, 140.
3. Creutzfeldt, W., Arnold, R., Creutzfeldt, C. and Track, N.S. (1975): Patho-

morphologic, biochemical, and diagnostic aspects of gastrinomas (Zollinger-Ellison syndrome). *Hum. Pathol. 6*, 47.

4. Cowley, D.J., Dymock, I.W., Boyes, B.E. et al. (1973): Zollinger-Ellison syndrome type I: clinical and pathological correlations in a case. *Gut 14*, 25.

5. Dimango, E.P. and Go, V.L.W. (1974): Malabsorption secondary to antral gastrin-cell hyperplasia. *Mayo Clin. Proc. 49*, 727.

6. Ganguli, P.C., Polak, J.M., Pearse, A.G.E. et al. (1974): Antral-gastrin-cell hyperplasia in peptic-ulcer disease. *Lancet I*, 583.

7. Russel, R.C.G., Bloom, S.R., Davies, W.A. et al. (1975): Hypergastrinemia in a peptic ulcer patient with antral gastrin cell hyperplasia. *Br. Med. J. 4*, 441.

8. Straus, E. and Yalow, R.S. (1975): Differential diagnosis of hypergastrinemia. In: *Gastrointestinal Hormones*, pp. 99–113. Ed: J.C. Thompson. University of Texas Press, Austin.

9. Lamers, C.B.H., Ruland, C.M., Joosten, H.J.M. et al (1978): Hypergastrinemia of antral origin in duodenal ulcer. *Am. J. Dig. Dis. 23*, 998.

10. Creutzfeldt, W. and Arnold, R. (1979): Endocrinology of duodenal ulcer. *World J. Surg. 3*, 605.

11. Arnold, R., Fuchs, K., Siewert, R. et al. (1974): Zur Morphologie, Klinik, Diagnostik und Therapie des Zollinger-Ellison-Syndroms. *Dtsch. Med. Wochenschr. 99.* 607.

12. Stage, J.G., Stadil, F., Rehfeld, J.F. et al. (1978): Secretin and the Zollinger-Ellison syndrome: reliability of secretin tests and pathogenetic role of secretin. *Scand. J. Gastroenterol. 13*, 501.

13. Seino, S., Seino, Y., Matsukura, S. et al. (1978): Effect of glucocorticoids on gastrin secretion in man. *Gut 19*, 10.

14. Hayes, J.R., Ardill, J., Kennedy, T.L. et al. (1972): Stimulation of gastrin release by catecholamines. *Lancet I*, 819.

15. Stadil, F. and Rehfeld, J.F. (1973): Release of gastrin by epinephrine in man. *Gastroenterology 65*, 210.

16. Brandsborg, O., Brandsborg, M. and Christensen, N.J. (1975): Plasma adrenaline and serum gastrin studies in insulin-induced hypoglycemia and after adrenaline infusions. *Gastroenterology 68*, 455.

17. Becker, H.D., Reeder, D.D. and Thompson, J.C. (1974): Der Einfluß des Calciums auf den Serumgastrinspiegel und die Magensekretion beim Menschen. *Klin. Wochenschr. 52*, 433.

18. McGuigan, J.E., Colwell, J.A. and Franklin, J. (1974): Effect of parathyroidectomy on hypercalcemic hypersecretory peptic ulcer disease. *Gastroenterology 66*, 269.

19. Christiansen, J. (1974): Primary hyperparathyroidism and peptic ulcer disease. *Scand. J. Gastroenterol. 9*, 111.

20. Lamers, C.B.H. and van Tongeren, J.H.M. (1977): Serum gastrin response to acute and chronic hypercalcaemia in man: studies on the value of calcium-stimulated serum gastrin levels in the diagnosis of Zollinger-Ellison syndrome. *Eur. J. Clin. Invest. 7*, 315.

21. Soares, E.C., Zaterka, S. and Walsh, J. (1977): Acid secretion and serum gastrin at graded intragastric pressures in man. *Gastroenterology 72*, 676.

22. Tani, M. and Shimazu, H. (1977): Meat-stimulated gastrin release and acid secretion in patients with pyloric stenosis. *Gastroenterology 73*, 207.

23.   Dragstedt, L.R. (1956): A concept of the etiology of gastric and duodenal ulcers. *Gastroenterology 30*, 208.
24.   Walsh, J.H., Richardson, C.T. and Fordtran, J.S. (1975): pH dependence of acid secretion and gastrin release in normal and ulcer subjects. *J. Clin. Invest. 55*, 462.
25.   Mayer, G., Arnold, R., Feurle, G. et al. (1974): Influence of feeding and sham feeding upon serum gastrin and gastric acid secretion in control subjects and duodenal ulcer patients. *Scand. J. Gastroenterol. 9*, 703.
26.   Brandsborg, O., Brandsborg, M., Løvareen, N.A. and Christensen, N.J. (1978): Increased plasma noradrenaline and serum gastrin in patients with duodenal ulcer. *Eur. J. Clin. Invest. 8*, 11.
27.   Stadil, F. (1974): Gastrin and insulin hypoglycaemia. A review of studies in gastrin determination and hypoglycaemic release of gastrin in man. *Scand. J. Gastroenterol. 9, Suppl. 23*, 1.
28.   Konturek, S.J., Kwiecień, N., Obtułowicz, W. et al. (1979): Cephalic phase of gastric secretion in healthy subjects and duodenal ulcer patients: role of vagal innervation. *Gut 20*, 875.
29.   Stenquist, B., Nilson, G., Rehfeld, J.F. and Olbe, C. (1979): Plasma gastrin concentrations following sham feeding in duodenal ulcer patients. *Scand. J. Gastroenterol. 14*, 305.
30.   Taylor, I.L., Dockray, G.J., Calam, J. and Walker, R.J. (1979): Big and little gastrin responses to food in normal and ulcer subjects. *Gut 20*, 957.
31.   Stadil, F., Rehfeld, J.F., Christiansen, L.A. and Malmström, J. (1975): Patterns of gastrin components in serum during feeding in normal subjects and duodenal ulcer patients. *Scand. J. Gastroenterol. 10*, 863.
32.   Trudeau, W.L. and McGuigan, J.E. (1970): Serum gastrin levels in patients with peptic ulcer disease. *Gastroenterology 59*, 6.
33.   Walsh, J.H. (1979): Pathogenetic role of gastrins. In: *Gastrins and the Vagus*, pp. 181–198. Ed: J. Rehfeld. Academic Press, New York.
34.   Creutzfeldt, W., Arnold, R., Creutzfeldt, C. and Track, N.S. (1976): Mucosal gastrin concentration, molecular forms of gastrin, number and ultrastructure of G-cells in patients with duodenal ulcer. *Gut 17*, 745.
35.   Royston, C.M.S., Polak, J., Bloom, S.R. et al. (1978): G-cell population of the gastric antrum, plasma gastrin, and gastric acid secretion in patients with and without duodenal ulcer. *Gut 19*, 689.
36.   Oberholzer, M., Heitz, U., Kasper, M. et al. (1978): Immunhistochemie und Morphometrie der Magenantrumschleimhaut beim Gesunden und bei Patienten mit Ulcus duodeni. *Verh. Dtsch. Ges. Pathol. 62*, 398.
37.   Barbara, L., Biasco, G., Saleva, M. et al. (1978): Antral G-cells and mucosal gastrin concentration in normal subjects and in patients with diodenal ulcer. *Adv. Exp. Med. Biol. 106*, 97.
38.   Piris, J. and Whitehead, R. (1979): Gastrin cells and fasting gastrin levels in duodenal ulcer patients: a quantitative study based on multiple biopsy specimens. *J. Clin. Pathol. 32*, 171.
39.   Arnold, R. and Lankisch, P.G. (1980): Somatostatin and the gastrointestinal tract. *Clin. Gastroenterol. 9*, 733.
40.   Malmström, J. and Stadil, F. (1975): Measurement of immunoreactive gastrin in gastric mucosa. *Scand. J. Gastroenterol. 10*, 433.
41.   Chayvialle, J.A.P., Descos, F., Bernard, C. et al. (1978): Somatostatin in mucosa

of stomach and duodenum in gastrointestinal disease. *Gastroenterology 75*, 13.

42. McIntosh, C., Arnold, R., Bothe, E. et al. (1978): Gastrointestinal somatostatin: extraction and radioimmunoassay in different species. *Gut 19*, 655.

43. Schwartz, T.W., Stenquist, O., Olbe, L. and Stadil, F. (1979): Synchronous oscillations in the basal secretion of pancreatic-polypeptide and gastric acid. *Gastroenterology 76*, 14.

44. Koop, H., Arnold, R., Becker, H.D. et al. (1980): Vagale pancreatic-polypeptide (PP)-Freisetzung bei der Ulkus-Krankheit – ein Indikator für den Vagotonus? *Verh. Dtsch. Ges. Inn. Med. 86* (In press).

45. Brandsborg, O., Christensen, N.J., Løvgreen, N.A. et al. (1978): Increased sensitivity of gastrin release to adrenaline in duodenal ulcer. *Gut 19*, 202.

46. Korman, M.G., Scott, D.F., Hansky, J. and Wilson, H. (1972): Hypergastrinaemia due to an excluded gastric antrum: a proposed method for differentiation from Zollinger-Ellison syndrome. *Aust. N. Z. J. Med. 3*, 266.

47. Osborne, M.P., Sizer, J. and Frederick, P.L. (1967): Massive bowel resection and gastric hypersecretion. *Am. J. Surg. 114*, 393.

48. Straus, E., Gerson, C.D. and Yalow, R.S. (1974): Hypersecretion of gastrin associated with short bowel syndrome. *Gastroenterology 66*, 175.

49. Isenberg, J.I., Cano, R. and Bloom, S.R. (1977): Effect of graded amounts of acid instilled into the duodenum on pancreatic bicarbonate secretion and plasma secretion in duodenal ulcer patients and normal subjects. *Gastroenterology 72*, 6.

50. Bloom, S.R. and Ward, A.S. (1975): Failure of secretin release in patients with duodenal ulcer. *Br. Med. J. I*, 126.

51. Straus, E. and Yalow, R.S. (1977): Hypersecretinemia associated with marked basal hyperchlorhydria in man and dog. *Gastroenterology 72*, 992.

52. Chey, W.Y., Lee, Y.H., Hendricks, J.G. et al. (1978): Plasma secretin concentrations in fasting and postprandial state in man. *Am. J. Dig. Dis. 23*, 981.

53. Arnold, R., Creutzfeldt, W., Ebert, R. et al. (1978): Serum gastric inhibitory polypeptide (GIP) in duodenal ulcer disease: relationship to glucose tolerance, insulin, and gastrin release. *Scand. J. Gastroenterol. 13*, 41.

54. Cataland, S., O'Dorisio, T.M., Brooks, R. and Mekhjian, H.S. (1977): Stimulation of gastric inhibitory polypeptide in normal and duodenal ulcer patients. *Gastroenterology 73*, 19.

55. Lauritsen, K.B. and Moody, A.J. (1978): The response of gastric inhibitory polypeptide (GIP) and insulin to glucose in duodenal ulcer patients. *Diabetologia 14*, 149.

56. Arnold, R., Ebert, R., Creutzfeldt, W. et al. (1978): Inhibition of gastric acid secretion by gastric inhibitory polypeptide (GIP) in man. *Scand. J. Gastroenterol. 13, Suppl. 49*, 11.

57. Creutzfeldt, W. (1976): Effects of gastrointestinal hormones – physiological or pharmacological? In: *Stimulus-Secretion Coupling in the Gastrointestinal Tract*, pp. 415–428. Eds: R.M. Case and H. Goebell. MTP Press Ltd, Lancaster.

58. Schusdziarra, V., Harris, V., Conlon, J.M. et al. (1978): Pancreatic and gastric somatostatin release in response to intragastric and intraduodenal nutrients and HCl in the dog. *J. Clin. Invest. 62*, 509.

59. Christofides, N.D., Modlin, I.M., Fitzpatrick, M.L. and Bloom, S.R. (1979): Effect of motilin on the rate of gastric emptying and gut hormone release during a test breakfast. *Gastroenterology 76*, 903.

60. Liljedahl, S.O., Mattson, O. and Pernow, B. (1958): The effect of substance P on intestinal motility in man. *Scand. J. Clin. Lab. Invest. 10*, 16.
61. Konturek, S.J. (1978): Endogenous opiates and the digestive system. *Scand. J. Gastroenterol. 13*, 257.

Discussion

Parietal cell function

Several issues were raised by discussants of the previous papers. An important one is whether isolated cell systems reflect the behavior of normal intact mucosa with regard to parietal cell function. At the present time, it seems reasonable to assume that it does, but this is an open-ended question. Within the parietal cell, the likely source of hydrogen ion is water which is split into protons and hydroxyl ion. Transmucosal sodium flux from blood to lumen appears to follow a paracellular not a transcellular route. The $H^+:K^+$ exchange ATPase is located in the wall of the canaliculi during active acid secretion but the precise location of the enzyme in resting parietal cells is not known. The enzyme is probably unresponsive to somatostatin or prostaglandins.

Parietal cell receptors

Dealing with possible interactions between H_1-receptor antagonists and H_2-receptor antagonists, it should be noted that imidazole compounds can affect histamine-forming and histamine-metabolizing enzymes. Methyltransferase has been found to be strongly associated not only with parietal cells but with a number of other cells as well. It is possible that histamine undergoes some metabolic transformation prior to receptor binding but this needs further investigation.

It was noted that impromidine provides about 50% of the stimulation of adenylate cyclase activity observed with histamine and about 50% of the acid response as well. To explain these findings, Lewin proposes a model in which histamine receptors can provide a dual response: stimulatory and inhibitory. A single molecule, such as impromidine, may incorporate agonist and antagonist moieties, bind simultaneously to both sites of the receptor and thus provide half of the total possible response.

Work on partially purified parietal cell preparations obtained from dog mucosa (Soll and Grossman; pages 164–175) suggests the existence of 3 separate parietal cell receptors: to histamine, to acetylcholine and to gastrin. Gland preparations from rabbit mucosa (Sachs et al.; pages 139–146) failed to detect a gastrin receptor. This could be due to species difference or to technical factors that will need clarification in the future. Whereas it is conceivable that small amounts of histamine in the impure (70%) parietal cell preparation could be responsible for the small stimulating effect caused by gastrin, this possibility seems unlikely since the response to gastrin, although small, was not slowed by the H_2-receptor antagonists. This appears to be true also in humans in whom gastrin-stimulated secretion cannot be completely abolished with cimetidine. Some residual secretion remains, about the same order as observed in isolated parietal cells.

Histamine

Histamine release from human gastric mucosa in response to pentagastrin has been demonstrated by comparing the levels of histamine in plasma and gastric secretion during stimulation. Some evidence for this has also been obtained in the dog. Spencer, Saunders and Mann have looked at mucosal histamine in subjects with duodenal ulcer and in normal control subjects. Although there is much overlap, histamine levels were lower in ulcer patients but not significantly so. Values in ulcer subjects were significantly lower than in other ulcer subjects under treatment with cimetidine. Therefore, cimetidine raises mucosal histamine. These authors have also looked at mucosal histamine before and after pentagastrin infusion (as part of an acid secretion test) in man. There was a fall in 10 of 11 subjects after pentagastrin and, in the other subject no change was seen. The difference between the 2 sets of values was highly significant. Thus, in man, gastric secretion in response to pentagastrin is accompanied by a fall in mucosal histamine.

Neural regulation

Sham feeding tests may be a simpler, safer, and more reliable indicator of completeness of vagotomy than insulin tests. However, sham feeding tests first need to be standardized and applied to larger populations of postsurgical cases. Also, patients need to be followed for relatively long periods of time to determine whether recurrences can be predicted by responses to the test. The response of pancreatic polypeptide as index of completeness of truncal vagotomy has recently been questioned (see paper by Arnold et al. pages 207–224, and [1]).

There appear to be both inhibitory and stimulatory effects on acid secretion and on gastrin release. Sham feeding, for instance, has been shown to inhibit the acid secretion of a Heidenhain pouch being stimulated by pentagastrin.

This and other work suggests that there is vagal release of a hormonal agent, probably extragastric, which is suppressing secretion in the denervated pouch. This agent has not been identified. With regard to gastrin release, it appears that the vagal inhibitory component involves a cholinergic mechanism since gastrin release can be augmented by giving an anticholinergic. There is also some evidence that it may act in the fundus rather than in the antrum itself since vagal denervation of the fundus may augment antral gastrin production. Thus, the inhibitory effect of the vagus may involve, at least in part, a pathway other than directly to the antrum.

Hormones

The relationship of hormones to peptic ulcer remains controversial. The endocrine system of the gut has special features that make it difficult to study its physiology and pathophysiology, particularly in man. First, we have not been able yet to map out the entire spectrum of hormones and biologically active peptides released into the blood (the endocrine form of secretion). Secondly, there exists a paracrine system where these substances are released locally and exert their actions locally. Paracrine secretion cannot be reliably quantified at this time. Thirdly, important interactions among hormones and hormones and nerves do exist, further complicating interpretation of observed phenomena involving simple measurement of hormones and peptides by radioimmunoassay. The 'peptidergic' system, released locally by nerve ends, is as yet poorly explored. We are left with simple observation of hormone release and open-ended interpretations.

The relationship between antral G-cell number, acid secretion, and serum gastrin response to food in duodenal ulcer patients remains obscure. Lam and Sircus have described 2 groups of duodenal ulcer patients: those with high acid secretion and normal gastrin release and those with low or normal acid secretion and high gastrin release [2]. These differences may represent part of a spectrum or may reflect heterogeneity in ulcer disease. This needs to be investigated further. For every 4 G-cells in the antrum there is one D cell, that is, a somatostatin-secreting cell. It is known that these D cells have long processes which reach the G cells making it likely that their effects are exerted locally. It is not surprising, under the circumstances, that contradictory results have been obtained with somatostatin concentrations in gastric mucosa. Some groups have found that duodenal ulcer patients have reduced somatostatin concentrations in gastric mucosa and others have found the opposite. Regional differences between antrum and fundus somatostatin concentrations have been described but again these findings are difficult to interpret and need further study.

References

1. Taylor, I.L., Gulsrud, P.O., Chew, P. and Meyer, J.H. (1980): Effect of vagotomy on the pancreatic polypeptide (PP) response to gastric distention. (Abstract). *Gastroenterology 78*, 1276.
2. Lam, S.K. and Sircus, W. (1975): Studies in duodenal ulcer, the clinical evidence for the existence of two populations. *Q. J. Med. 44*, 369.

Regulation of gastric secretory functions: a critical overview

R.A. Levine
State University of New York, Upstate Medical Center, Syracuse, New York, U.S.A.

This introductory chapter emphasizes a look into the future as well as a review or update of past research accomplishments. The rapid developments in technology to study gastric secretory physiology will certainly advance our understanding of its theories. Most of the observations reported in this scientific session are consistent with, but do not establish the hypothesis that acid secretion is generated by certain metabolic requirements such as adenosine triphosphate (ATP); that adenosine 3′,5′-phosphate (cyclic AMP; cAMP) plays a key second messenger role; that the secretagogue histamine is the most likely common pathway for acid secretion; that separate receptors exist on the parietal cell for histamine, gastrin and acetylcholine; and that potentiating interactions exist between these agents and effects of these interactions may explain the apparent nonspecificity of inhibitors of acid secretion in vivo [1].

I will not attempt to review the excellent papers in this chapter but rather emphasize certain areas where future research or cautious reservations are worthwhile. Particular attention will be given to the mechanisms for secretagogue action at the cellular level. Acid secretion is influenced by the key transmitters acetylcholine, histamine and gastrin acting through their respective neurocrine, paracrine and endocrine pathways to the parietal cell. Specific parietal cell receptors to these transmitters probably exist and potentiating interactions between secretagogues probably occur at the parietal cell itself. This interdependence between histamine and other secretagogues is emphasized in the paper by Soll and Grossman. Dr. Lewin's paper presents new techniques for in-vivo and in-vitro approaches to parietal cell receptors. I agree that cAMP probably plays a second messenger role in acid secretion, but would disagree that cholinergic receptors have not yet been documented in the parietal cell. Unpublished work by M.H. Parsons has shown that there are acetylcholine receptors in the rat stomach and this kind of data is supported in canine stomach by the work of Soll. As Dr. Lewin points out, the regulation of gastrin may be partly enhanced by the number of gastrin receptors present. Thus, gastrin may play a role in this regulatory process as suggested by Takeuchi et al. [2]. The paper by Olbe emphasizes the importance of the vagus input into acid secretion.

One area not sufficiently emphasized in this section is the important modulating role of endogenous prostaglandins on gastric acid secretion as opposed to other candidate hormones. Like prostaglandins and histamine, somatostatin may also have an important paracrine role, however, nothing is known yet about its true physiologic function. The paper by Arnold et al. reviews the hormonal influences in acid secretion. At the present time it still remains controversial whether or not tissue gastrin concentrations can be correlated with serum gastrin levels in most patient groups.

Isolated cell models

There has been a major discrepancy between biochemical and functional responses in vivo and in vitro. Much of the past confusion relating to the possible regulatory role of cAMP in acid secretion rests with experiments performed in intact mucosa. Prior studies from our own laboratory in intact canine antral and fundic mucosa failed to implicate cAMP or cyclic guanylic acid (cGMP) as mediators of stimulated canine gastric acid secretion [3]. Similarly, infusion of PGE_2 alone or in combination with indometacin, the prostaglandin synthetase inhibitor, also failed to result in generation of cAMP in gastric canine mucosa [4]. In contrast, in our laboratory using the isolated rabbit fundic gland [5] and in Dr. Soll's laboratory using the isolated canine parietal cell preparation [6, 7], histamine and prostaglandin have both been shown to stimulate cAMP production. The explanation for the disparity between studies in intact mucosa and parietal cell preparations is unclear. It is unlikely that the secretagogues or PGE_2 utilized in our intact animal studies failed to accumulate intracellularly because physiological responses to the infused agents were demonstrated in these canine preparations [3, 4]. Furthermore, in contrast to the situation in intact mucosa, phosphodiesterase inhibition does exaggerate the biochemical and secretory responses induced by histamine in both isolated rabbit glands and in isolated parietal cells [5, 6–8].

With advances in techniques for cell separation, the biochemical basis for gastric secretion has become clearer. Isolated mammalian gastric mucosa is a weak secretor even in the presence of secretagogues. Nevertheless, the isolated rabbit gland preparation is actually a functional stomach where parameters of parietal cell activity can be evaluated. Isolated glands contain 2 cell types, predominantly parietal and peptic cells in equal proportions. Since acid secretion can be evoked in a number of ways, an isolated system can be used to trace down possible sequential stimulation or multireceptor interactions on the parietal cell. Unfortunately, only the direct effect of secretagogues can be detected in an isolated cell system. Indirect actions via release of other compounds or modulators would not be evident due to dilution.

Both gastric glands and gastric cells can be prepared, oxygenated, and maintained in a highly viable state. The glands appear to be somewhat less fragile and represent a more intact system. Parietal cell stimulation can be monitored by changes in oxygen consumption, alterations in parietal cell morphology and acid formation as measured by an indirect method using the weak base aminopyrine (AP). Thus the isolated gland or cell preparation had advantages over intact mucosa despite some loss of cellular polarity with enzyme treatment and cell dispersion. Problems involving cell separation and limitations of isolated cell models are apparent. Differences in isolated systems or in species utilized are becoming evident as more investigators use isolated gastric glands or other more enriched cell preparations.

It is possible that there is destruction of gastrin receptors during the preparation of isolated model systems which accounts for the failure of gastrin to elicit biochemical responses. It is clear that histamine involvement is present in the gastrin response and histamine may serve as a moderator of or activator of the gastrin response, although the concentration must be very small. The role of prostaglandins as modulator of histamine's response has been explored in the studies by Kohen et al. [5] and Soll and coworkers [7] and is discussed below.

Dr. Lewin raises the problem of discrepancy in reaction to secretagogues based upon technical difficulty with attempts to preserve intact receptors in vitro. It is clear that some functional and biochemical responses in the isolated gland preparation of Berglindh [9, 10] is at variance with studies in the isolated canine parietal cell preparation of Soll [8]. For example, the cAMP and AP responses to carbachol are muted in the isolated gland preparation [11] and exaggerated in the isolated parietal cell preparation [8]. In contrast, histamine stimulation of cAMP is more prominent in isolated rabbit glands than in isolated dog parietal cells. Certainly the effects of enzyme treatment, possible calcium removal, morphologic damage to intracellular communications and altered cell polarity may all account for differences between intact mucosal responses to secretagogues and the results seen in isolated systems. On balance, however, there are more similarities than differences in terms of parietal cell response to secretory stimulants and inhibitors. Results from cell separation studies will continue to complement those observed with intact preparations.

Parietal cell receptors and the role of histamine

The role of histamine and other agents has been clarified by the analytical use of the receptor-specific agonists and antagonists that are now available. The paper by Lorenz et al. reviews the importance of histamine and its role in acid secretion. Their interpretation that gastrin may directly release histamine from the mast cell is speculative and has not been supported by direct evidence at the present time.

The hypothesis that the parietal cell has specific receptors for each of the classical 3 stimulants, histamine, gastrin and acetylcholine, and that antagonists act in a predictable, specific fashion seems to be supported by work in isolated cell systems. Histamine appears to be the only secretagogue capable of stimulating and maintaining acid secretion, while cholinergic agents and possibly gastrin are regulatory devices which determine the magnitude of the histamine response. It is apparent that a background concentration of histamine greatly potentiates the actions of both acetylcholine and gastrin. It is assumed that histamine is constantly released by intact gastric mucosa and it may be likely that an inhibitory action of cimetidine on such stimulants as gastrin and acetylcholine can be accounted for by removing the potentiating action of this histamine background, as postulated by Soll and Grossman in their paper. In the isolated parietal cell, even after enzyme treatment, classical muscarinic and H_2 receptors are functionally intact. There appears to be an interaction between histamine and cholinergic stimulations beyond the H_2-receptor site. It is also apparent that dibutyryl cAMP and cAMP act distal to the H_2 receptor.

If we postulate that there are gastrin, acetylcholine and histamine receptors on the parietal cell, as emphasized by Soll and Grossman (the 3-receptor hypothesis), another question that remains to be answered is the exact localization of the acid secretory process in intact tissue. Studies by DiBona et al. have documented that histamine stimulation results in the development of intracellular spaces within the parietal cells compatible with an expanded canaliculus and proven by special staining techniques for the cellular site of gastric secretion [12]. In stimulated glandular parietal cells, red fluorescent areas coincided with the secretory canaliculi and were dependent on the presence of acid as evident from the effects of the gastric acid inhibitor potassium thiocyanate. Glands were made permeable to solutes by dielectric breakdown of cell membranes. Following electric shocking, the glands lost their ability to accumulate AP and showed no red dye fluorescence. Addition of ATP and potassium rapidly restored AP accumulation and red fluorescence, even in the presence of mitochondrial inhibitors like cyanide, azide or amobarbital.

Little is known about the factors that regulate the synthesis, storage and release of histamine or how it is delivered in the parietal cell. We also do not know how histamine interacts with other stimuli at the parietal cell to produce potentiated responses. Histamine's importance as a modulator of gastrin responses in acid secretion is clear since gastrin needs the presence of histamine to elicit its secretory action. Histamine plays a central role for activation of the parietal cell, without which no acid secretion would take place. Once histamine is activated, acetylcholine and gastrin serve as regulatory devices for the secretion rate. Perhaps gastrin and acetylcholine are involved in regulation of the magnitude of histamine release, but there is no definite relationship.

Phosphodiesterase inhibition

Phosphodiesterase inhibitors in isolated glands and in dog parietal cells normalize the influence of secretagogues, partly by a response in the cAMP pathway.

The potentiation of a hormone by a phosphodiesterase inhibitor is an important criterion to indicate that the hormone acts via adenylate cyclase activation [13]. In studies in isolated systems, the ability of the phosphodiesterase inhibitor isobutylmethyl-xanthine (IMX) to enhance both cAMP production and AP accumulation to histamine and carbachol has been examined. Histamine in the presence of phosphodiesterase inhibitors has a more pronounced effect than when solely presented to a parietal cell system [8]. In our laboratory, histamine-induced cAMP and AP accumulation were both markedly potentiated by IMX while carbachol's effect appeared additive to the effects of IMX. Although gastrin does not stimulate acid in certain species, in the presence of phosphodiesterase inhibition by IMX, a strong and dose-dependent potentiation of the IMX response is seen [6, 8]. Another of the criteria established to implicate cAMP as a mediator of a hormone is that the hormone's action can be mimicked by the application of exogenous cAMP. Berglindh et al. showed that exogenous dibutyryl cAMP stimulated oxygen consumption in the isolated rabbit gastric gland [10]. On the basis of our results [5] and previous work in the rabbit and canine models [6, 8, 11], cAMP fulfills all of the criteria necessary to implicate it as a biochemical mediator of histamine. The actual level of cAMP may not be as important as the turnover of the cyclic nucleotide. The role of cGMP appears to be minimal in acid secretion based on data in our laboratory.

Relationship between prostaglandins and cAMP

Prostaglandins have been shown to inhibit gastric acid secretion in the presence of histamine, but not alone. In certain species they also elevate fundic mucosal cAMP [14, 15]. In intact gastric mucosa, prostaglandins generally fail to stimulate cAMP but in isolated rabbit glands and in isolated canine parietal cells, prostaglandins stimulate the cyclic nucleotide [5, 6]. The disparity between stimulation of fundic cAMP by both prostaglandins and histamine and their opposite effects on acid secretion can be explained by actions on different cell populations within the gastric mucosa. Thus prostaglandins may have the ability to preferentially stimulate cAMP in nonparietal cells. In vivo, prostaglandins have been shown to increase mucus production [16] and bicarbonate secretion [17], stimulate a gastric mucosal sodium pump [17] and alter gastric blood flow [18]. Such actions by prostaglandins are unrelated to their known antisecretory mechanism and are believed to depend on nonparietal cell effects.

Recent studies in vitro have emphasized the inverse relationship between prostaglandin stimulation of cAMP production and parietal cell concentration [6, 19, 20]. Our results in isolated rabbit glands [5] are consistent with the hypothesis that histamine and prostaglandins stimulate cAMP in parietal and nonparietal cells, respectively. These findings therefore support the work in isolated parietal cells cited by Soll and Grossman. PGE_2 at concentrations above 1 μM stimulated cAMP production. However, such stimulation was negatively correlated with the parietal cell content of the fractions indicating a minor stimulation by prostaglandins on parietal cell adenylate cyclase [7]. In our studies in isolated rabbit glands, prostaglandins stimulated cAMP concentrations in a dose-dependent manner but failed to affect acid secretion as measured by AP accumulation [5]. The basal AP accumulation ratio remained unchanged with PGE_2 despite a significant stimulation of cAMP over a dose range of 1 μM to 1 mM. The lack of a detectable increase in AP accumulation even at high concentrations of PGE_2 is evidence against PGE_2-induced cAMP generation in parietal cells.

In enriched canine parietal cells or in rabbit fundic glands, prostaglandins have been documented to inhibit the histamine H_2-receptor-mediated elevation of cAMP. Soll [7], Major and Scholes [19], and Sonnenberg et al. [20] showed that E-type prostaglandins preferentially increased cAMP in nonparietal as compared to parietal cells. PGE_2 has also been shown to specifically inhibit histamine-stimulated AP accumulation over a wide dose range and at lower concentrations below 1 μM inhibit histamine-stimulated cAMP concentration [5, 7]. Such effects are probably related to prostaglandin inhibition of parietal cell function. Prostaglandins did not inhibit gastrin responses in isolated cell systems, as studied by Soll, unless histamine was also present in combination. There is also no inhibition of dibutyryl cAMP stimulation of gastrin responses in the presence of prostaglandins.

Our studies in rabbit glands complement the findings in isolated canine parietal cells whereby histamine stimulation of biochemical and secretory responses is inhibited by prostaglandins. However, in our studies this observation was carried out in the absence of phosphodiesterase inhibition. It is conceivable that the background enrichment with IMX in isolated canine parietal cells [7] could have added another indeterminable factor to interpret the specific inhibition by prostaglandins of histamine-stimulated AP and cAMP production. In rabbit glands, IMX increased both cAMP and cGMP, and together with histamine, IMX enhanced the AP output and cAMP accumulation. PGE$_2$ can block IMX-stimulated AP accumulation and possibly other aspects of parietal cell function [5]. It is possible that IMX may have effects independent of phosphodiesterase inhibition. If, in fact, IMX stimulation of AP uptake represents potentiation of histamine release or utilization, then the interactions with histamine may be more important than the potentiation by IMX with other secretagogues.

In canine parietal cells, the addition of histamine, in the presence of IMX, potentiates the interactions of PGE$_2$ with carbachol and gastrin [7]. PGE$_2$ at a concentration of $10^{-6}M$ was observed by Soll not to inhibit histamine-stimulated AP accumulation by larger concentrations of histamine between 10^{-4} and $10^{-5}M$ in isolated rabbit parietal cells. On the other hand, in isolated rabbit glands [5], PGE$_2$ inhibition of histamine-stimulated AP was not overcome by high concentrations of histamine (10^{-3}, 10^{-4} and $10^{-5}M$). Thus, there are apparent differences between the responses found in isolated parietal cells and isolated fundic glands, as previously noted for gastrin, carbachol and histamine.

Prostaglandins have been found in the gastric mucosa in relatively large amounts and prostacyclin (PGI$_2$) and PGE$_2$ are the most abundant prostaglandins present in the gastric mucosa [21, 22]. Extraction of prostaglandin-like material from gastric mucosa show concentrations 2-fold higher in the gastric antrum than in the corpus [21]. Similarly, prostaglandins have been shown to stimulate adenylate cyclase from gastric antral mucosa to a significantly greater extent than the analogous preparations from fundus [23]. The localization of a prostaglandin-responsive adenylate cyclase mainly in antral tissue suggests that the smaller cAMP response seen in the fundus induced by PGE_2 is less well correlated with parietal cell function. Furthermore, maximal stimulation by prostaglandins is additive to maximal stimulation by histamine in fundic tissue [5, 7, 15, 23]. This would suggest that the fundic mucosa contains different cyclase systems for prostaglandins and for histamine. It remains unknown whether prostaglandins exert their antisecretory and cytoprotective effects solely or partly by acting on the membrane-bound adenylate cyclase–cAMP system. This is a key area for future study.

In summary, prostaglandins alone do not alter parietal cell function but rather modulate interactions with histamine and possibly other secretagogues. There is a remarkable similarity between the inhibitory action of PGE_2 on secretagogue stimulation of biochemical and secretory responses in isolated rabbit glands and the ability of prostaglandins to modulate cAMP-mediated hormonal effects in tissues other than the stomach, including adipose, corpora luteal, parathyroid and hepatic tissues [24]. Our findings in isolated rabbit gastric gland are particularly similar to our findings in isolated perfused rat liver [24]. PGE_2 inhibited glucagon-mediated gluconeogenesis and concomitantly inhibited cAMP content, while PGE_2 alone failed to induce gluconeogenesis or stimulate hepatic cAMP concentrations. It thus appears likely that PGE_2, like a number of polypeptides, modulates hormone or drug-induced physiological actions at the cellular level by affecting cAMP concentration or tissue susceptibility to the nucleotide.

The prostaglandin receptor

There is little information on the prostaglandin receptors in acid function. The characteristics of the adenylate cyclase-linked prostaglandin receptor have been evaluated by specific sensitivity to blockade in parietal cells. Recent evidence for functional prostaglandin receptors has been found in porcine fundic mucosa [25]. At the present time we do not understand the physiological significance of the activation of adenylate cyclase and cAMP by prostaglandins. This is an extremely important area which should be explored in the future. If one can demonstrate correlation between the binding of prostaglandins and the activation of adenylate cyclase in the parietal cell, then it would appear that activation of cAMP upon interaction with structure specific receptors is the basis of at least part of the physiological effects of certain prostaglandins in the stomach. It is possible that multiple classes of cyclase-linked PGE receptors may exist in the stomach.

Role of calcium

Calcium appears critical for the acetylcholine-induced acid response. Cholinergic action seems to be related to enhanced calcium influx or efflux possibly localized at the parietal cell. The calcium influx step may be related to cAMP dependence, but more investigation is needed on this point. Histamine action appears to be linked to the generation of cAMP and is unrelated to calcium presence. cAMP-induced secretion is not affected by a calcium-free medium nor is calcium necessary to affect the response to gastrin, as discussed by Soll and Grossman. Further studies on the calcium interdependence to gastrin's involvement will be required in several model systems in order to exclude a role of extracellular calcium on the action of gastrin.

Role of ATP in acid secretion

The paper by Sachs and colleagues emphasizes the importance of ATP as a generating energy source for hydrogen ion secretion. The interactions involved at the membrane require further study.

With the additional use of new probes such as AP and the fluorescent acridine orange, there is accumulating evidence that exogenous ATP can drive acid formation in the secretory canaliculi of the parietal cell [26]. The isolated gastric glands are a particularly good model for studying the substrate-level energy dependence of gastric secretion. There are a variety of agents which S.J. Hersey has reported at the 64th annual meeting of the American Physiological Society (1980) that show restoration of histamine responsiveness in the isolated gastric gland. These agents include pyruvate, lactate, acetate, butyrate, all of which are effective in restoring histamine responsiveness. Although the level of ATP is critical for the response, the action of the parietal cell does not seem to be totally dependent on the maintenance of ATP levels.

Future perspective

The biochemical and morphologic changes, the ion requirements and the membrane adaptations which occur in isolated cell systems provide optimal cellular models for studying acid formation. Hopefully, future technological developments will further advance our knowledge of the complete spectrum of reactions leading to acid secretion.

References

1. Soll, A.H. and Grossman, M.I. (1978): Cellular mechanisms in acid secretion. *Ann. Rev. Med. 29*, 495.
2. Takeuchi, K., Speir, G.R. and Johnson, L.R. (1980): Mucosal gastrin receptor. III. Regulation by gastrin. *Am. J. Physiol. 238 (Gastrointest. Liver Physiol. 1)*, G135.
3. Levine, R.A., Schwartzel, E.H. Jr., Bachman, S. and Talev, J.N. (1978): Effects of secretagogues and theophylline on canine gastric mucosal cyclic nucleotides. *J. Lab. Clin. Med. 92*, 813.
4. Levine, R.A., Schwartzel, E.H. Jr., Randall, P.A. and Bachman, S. (1979): Failure of prostaglandins E_1 and E_2 to alter canine gastric mucosal cyclic nucleotides. *Prostaglandins 18*, 63.
5. Kohen, K.R., Schwartzel, E.H. Jr. and Levine, R.A. (1980): Interactions of prostaglandin E_2 (PGE_2) and histamine (H) on cyclic AMP (cAMP) and acid production in isolated gastric glands. *Gastroenterology 78*, 1197.
6. Wollin, A., Soll, A.H. and Samloff, I.M. (1979): Actions of histamine, secretin, and PGE_2 on cyclic AMP production by isolated canine fundic cells. *Am. J. Physiol. 237*, E437.
7. Soll, A.H. (1980): Specific inhibition by prostaglandins E_2 and I_2 of histamine-stimulated ^{14}C-aminopyrine accumulation and cyclic AMP generation by isolated canine parietal cells. *J. Clin. Invest. 65*, 1222.
8. Soll, A.H. and Wollin, A. (1979): Histamine and cyclic AMP in isolated canine parietal cells. *Am. J. Physiol. 237*, E444.
9. Berglindh, T. and Obrink, K.J. (1976): A method of preparing isolated glands from the rabbit gastric mucosa. *Acta Physiol. Scand. 96*, 150.
10. Berglindh, T., Helander, H.F. and Obrink, K.J. (1976): Effects of secretagogues on oxygen consumption, aminopyrine accumulation and morphology in isolated gastric glands. *Acta Physiol. Scand. 97*, 401.
11. Chew, C.S., Hersey, S.J., Sachs, G. and Berglindh, T. (1980): Histamine responsiveness of isolated gastric glands. *Am. J. Physiol. 238 (Gastrointest. Liver Physiol. 1)*, G312.
12. Dibona, D.R., Ito, S., Berglindh, T. and Sachs, G. (1979): Cellular site of gastric acid secretion. *Proc. Natl. Acad. Sci. U.S.A. 76*, 6689.
13. Robison, G.A., Butcher, R.W. and Sutherland, E.W. (1971): Experimental approaches used in the study of hormones which stimulate adenyl cyclase. In: *Cyclic AMP*, pp. 36–47. Academic Press, New York–London.
14. Thompson, J.W. and Jacobson, E.D. (1977): Comparison of the effects of secretory stimulants and inhibitors on gastric mucosal adenyl cyclases of various species. *Proc. Soc. Exp. Biol. Med. 154*, 377.
15. Wollin, A., Code, C.F. and Dousa, T.P. (1976): Interaction of prostaglandins and histamine with enzymes of cyclic AMP metabolism from guinea pig gastric mucosa. *J. Clin. Invest. 57*, 1548.
16. Chaudhury, T.K. and Jacobson, E.D. (1978): Prostaglandin cytoprotection of gastric mucosa. *Gastroenterology 74*, 59.
17. Garner, A., Flenstrom, G. and Heylings, J.R. (1979): Effects of anti-inflammatory agents and prostaglandins on acid and bicarbonate secretions in the amphibian-isolated gastric mucosa. *Gastroenterology 77*, 451.

18. Main, I.H.M. and Whittle, B.J.R. (1974): Prostaglandins and gastrointestinal function and disease. In: *Prostaglandin Synthetase Inhibitors*, pp. 363–372. Raven Press, New York.
19. Major, J.S. and Scholes, P. (1978): The localization of a histamine H_2-receptor adenylate cyclase system in canine parietal cells and its inhibition by prostaglandins. *Agents Actions 8*, 324.
20. Sonnenberg, A., Hunziker, W., Koelz, H.R. et al. (1978): Stimulation of endogenous cyclic AMP (cAMP) in isolated gastric cells by histamine and prostaglandin. *Acta Physiol. Scand. Spec. Suppl.,* 307.
21. Bennett, A., Stamford, I.F. and Stockley, H.L. (1977): Estimation and characterization of prostaglandins in the human gastrointestinal tract. *Br. J. Pharmacol. 61*, 579.
22. Moncada, S., Salmon, J.A., Vane, J.R. and Whittle, B.T.R. (1977): Formation of prostacyclin (PGI_2) and its product, 6-Oxo-$PGF_{1\alpha}$, by the gastric mucosa of several species. *J. Physiol. (London) 275*, 4.
23. Dozois, R.R., Kim, J.K. and Dousa, T.P. (1978): Interaction of prostaglandins with canine gastric mucosal adenylate cyclase-cyclic AMP system. *Am. J. Physiol. 235*, E546.
24. Levine, R.A. and Schwartzel, E.H. Jr. (1980): Prostaglandin E_2 inhibition of glucagon-induced hepatic gluconeogenesis and cyclic adenosine $3',5'$-monophosphate accumulation. *Biochem. Pharm. 29*, 681.
25. Tepperman, B.L. and Soper, B.D. (1980): Evidence for a specific prostaglandin E (PGE) binding site in porcine fundic mucosa. *Gastroenterology 78*, 1276.
26. Berglindh, T. and Sachs, G. (1980): The site and energy source of mammalian gastric acid. *Gastroenterology 78*, 1140.

Chapter IV: Pathophysiology and diagnosis of ulcer disease

Gastric secretion in ulcer disease

J.I. Isenberg
Department of Medicine, University of California at San Diego, San Diego, California, U.S.A

As recently reviewed by Baron, Prout, in the 1820's, was the first to demonstrate that gastric juice contained hydrochloric acid [1]. Two German investigators, Tiedemann and Gmelin, unaware of Prout's observations, independently reported that gastric juice contained hydrochloric acid [2]. However, it was not until the 1870's, when von Leube developed the gastric tube for collecting gastric juice, that the practice of measuring gastric secretion developed [3]. Although this procedure is now well developed gastric secretory measurements are not able to provide all the answers to the riddles of peptic ulceration.

The purpose of this article is to review gastric acid secretion abnormalities in patients with peptic ulcer. It must be emphasized, however, that a number of well-designed studies carried out to examine the precise pathophysiologic abnormality in ulcer patients versus healthy subjects have yielded widely divergent results. The explanation for these differences is unclear. In some of the pre-endoscopic studies, one might question the accuracy of ulcer diagnosis. However, even in recent studies where ulcer diagnosis was endoscopically confirmed, divergent results sometimes still prevail. The most likely explanation for this discrepancy is that peptic ulcer, both duodenal and gastric, is the net result of the interaction of a number of genetic, environmental, pathophysiologic, psychological and other factors. The relative importance of each of these variables is not fully understood. If acid pepsin secretion were the sole cause of ulcer disease, one would expect that all gastrinoma (Zollinger-Ellison Syndrome) patients with massive amounts of gastric acid and pepsin secretion would develop ulcer. This is not the case. There are gastronoma patients with marked gastric acid hypersecretion but without evidence of ulcer [4]. Although efforts have been largely directed towards the 'aggressive' factors in the pathogenesis of both duodenal and gastic ulcer, those factors which maintain the integrity of the gastrointestinal mucosa may be considerably more important in ulcer pathogenesis.

Duodenal ulcer

Increased secretory capacity

In 1952, Cox reported that the number of parietal cells in the stomachs of duodenal ulcer patients was approximately 2-fold greater than that in healthy subjects (Fig. 1; [5]). The overlap between the duodenal ulcer patients and the normal subjects was large; approximately two-thirds of the ulcer patients fell within the normal range. This important study requires validation.

The role of genetic factors in the pathogenesis of duodenal ulcer is gradually being unravelled. Immediate relatives of ulcer patients have about a 2-fold greater likelihood of developing ulcers than the general population [6]. Rotter et al. have recently demonstrated that hyperpepsinogenemia I, closely correlated with maximal acid output, is inherited as a single autosomal dominant gene [7]. It would be important to know if the parietal cell number is also inherited.

Duodenal ulcer patients, as a group, tend to release greater amounts of gastrin when compared with normal subjects in response to meal [8].

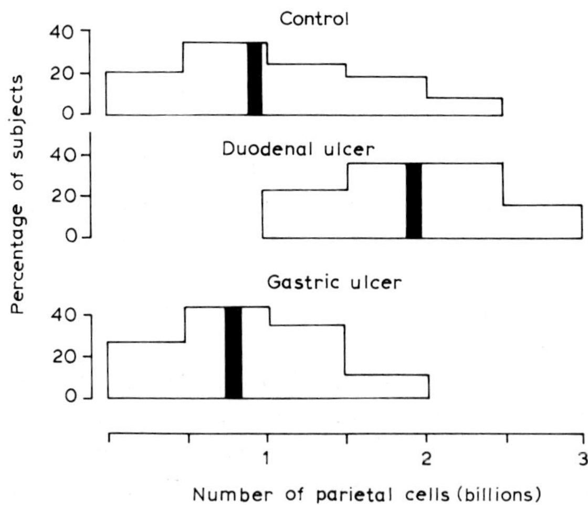

Fig. 1:   Number of parietal cells in normal stomachs versus stomachs of patients with duodenal or gastric ulcer. Adapted with permission from Cox, A.J. (1952): Stomach size and its relation to chronic peptic ulcer. Arch. Pathol. 54, 407. Copyright 1952, American Medical Association.

However, in some studies gastrin release was similar in both groups [9]. One wonders whether or not the genetic predisposition to duodenal ulcer results in a greater postprandial gastrin release which in turn produces an increased parietal cell number. In order to address this important question, longitudinal studies are needed in subjects before they develop ulcer disease.

Increased 'drive' to secrete acid

As a group, duodenal ulcer patients have a greater 'drive' to secrete acid when contrasted with nonulcer subjects [10]. This is reflected as a greater basal, or resting, gastric acid secretion. The ratio of basal acid secretion in duodenal ulcer patients compared to normal subjects ranges from 2–3 to 1, while in other series, it was as low as 1 to 1. The explanation for the differences between series is not clear, but probably reflects differences between population groups. If it is assumed that the basal secretory rate in duodenal ulcer patients is often greater than normal, the explanation for this difference is still unknown. It may be entirely due to the increased parietal cell number in the average duodenal ulcer patient or may be due to other imbalances in neural or humoral control of gastric secretion.

There are no perfect methods which permit measurement of vagal activity, or 'tone', in man. Therefore, the precise role of vagal activity in either resting or stimulated gastric acid secretion in duodenal ulcer patients and normal man is not known.

Increased sensitivity to gastrin and its analogues

Most studies indicate that patients with duodenal ulcer are more sensitive – i.e., require significantly lower doses of exogenous pentagastrin or gastrin to produce one-half maximal gastric acid output; therefore, the dose response curve is shifted to the left (Fig. 2; [11]). Recent studies by Lam et al. demonstrated that gastric acid secretion in response to graded doses of intragastric peptone resulted in a positive correlation ($r = 0.9$; $p = <0.001$) between gastrin release and acid secretion [12]. More importantly, duodenal ulcer patients were significantly more sensitive to their endogenous gastrin than nonulcer patients (Fig. 3). For example, the mean ($\pm$ SE) D_{50} for endogenous gastrin in the duodenal ulcer patients was 29.9 ± 2.7 and in the normal subjects was 40.0 ± 1.9 mmol; $p < 0.05$. These observations indicate that the parietal cells in duodenal ulcer patients are more responsive to both exogenous gastrin and pentagastrin, and endogenously-released gastrin. The cellular explanation for these differences is unknown.

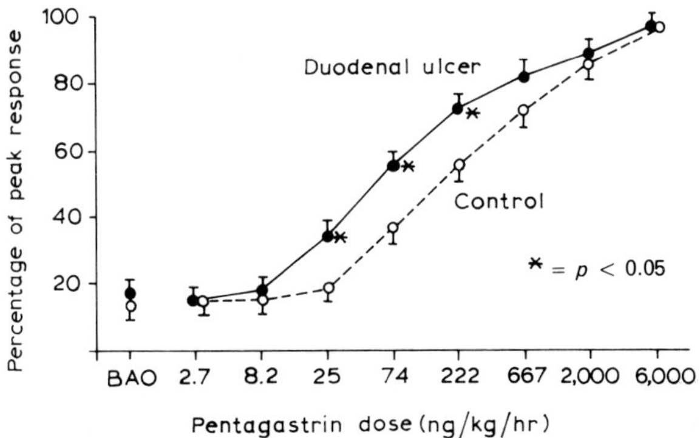

Fig. 2:   Dose-response curve to graded doses of pentagastrin in duodenal ulcer and normal subjects. The dose required for one-half maximal response (D₅₀), is significantly lower in duodenal ulcer patients. Reproduced with permission from [11].

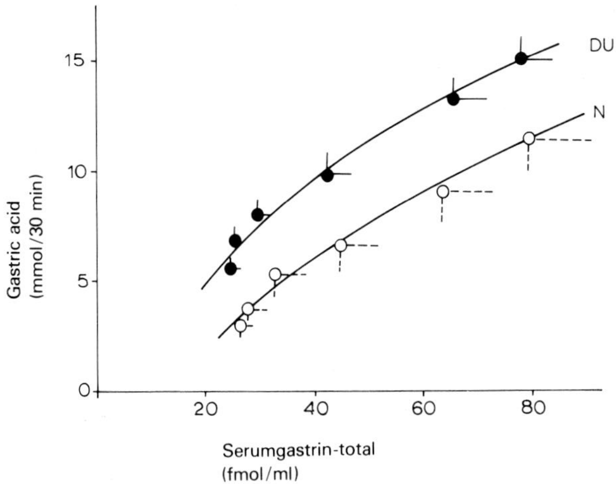

Fig. 3:   Comparison of the relationship between mean serum G17 and mean gastric acid output after graded peptone meals in duodenal ulcer (DU) and normal (N) subjects. The horizontal and vertical bars represent one standard error of the mean. For each incremental change in serum gastrin, gastric acid secretion was greater in duodenal ulcer patients compared to normal subjects. Reproduced with permission from [12].

Decreased inhibition of acid secretion by acidified meals

Walsh et al. reported that gastric acid secretion as well as gastrin release were almost completely abolished in normal subjects after instillation and intragastric titration of an acidified amino acid and corn starch meal at pH 2.5 [13]. However, in duodenal ulcer patients, neither gastric acid secretion nor gastrin release in response to the acidified meal was abolished (Fig. 4). Lam et al., using a technique of measuring gastric acid secretion which permits the meal to seek its natural pH, also observed that gastric acid secretion was greater after acidified meals in duodenal ulcer versus normal subjects [14]. For example, in normal subjects mean gastric acid secretion following 500 ml of 10% peptone at pH 1.5 was 0.5 mEq/2 hr, while in duodenal ulcer patients it was 6.9 mEq/2 hr ($p<0.05$). These results suggest that: there seems to be a defect in the acid-induced inhibition of gastric acid secretion in many duodenal ulcer patients; and there is greater gastrin release at intragastric acid pH's in duodenal ulcer patients compared with nonulcer subjects.

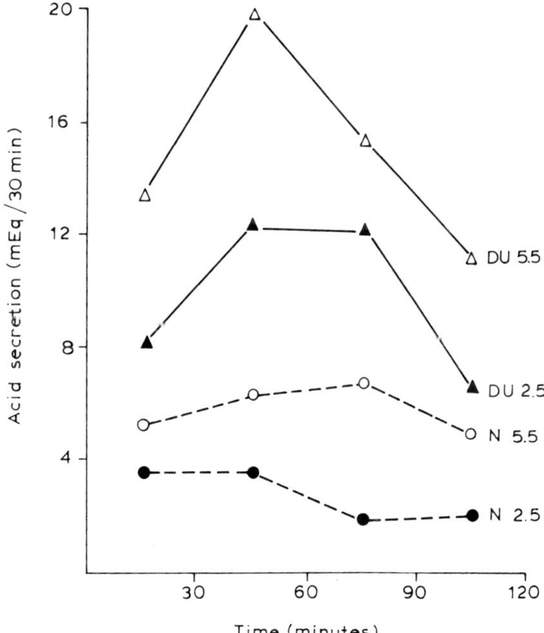

Fig. 4: Gastric acid secretion expressed as a percentage of the peak response to histamine in serum gastrin after amino acid plus cornstarch meals at either pH 5.5 or 2.5 in 6 duodenal ulcer patients and 6 normal subjects. Reproduced with permission from [13].

248   *J.I. Isenberg*

Rapid gastric emptying, duodenal acid load, and duodenal pH

In 1920, Hurst [15] and in 1944, Shay [16] reported that gastric emptying of liquid meals was more rapid in duodenal ulcer patients than in normal subjects. However, as with each pathophysiologic abnormality, these observations are counterbalanced by studies which have failed to observe differences in emptying [17]. The bulk of evidence to date, however, indicates that the emptying, particularly of liquids, is more rapid in duodenal ulcer patients than in normals. Also, there are preliminary data which suggest that duodenal acidification slows the basal electrical activity of the normal stomach while acidification failed to produce this effect in patients with duodenal ulcer [18]. This would suggest that there is some impairment of the inhibition of emptying by acid. It appears that duodenal ulcer patients have more rapid emptying of liquids and/or solids than normals but other ulcer patients do not.

Studies by Malagelada et al. [9] and Cano et al. [19] have reported an increase in duodenal acid load in response to meals in duodenal ulcer patients when contrasted to normal controls (Fig. 5). Lam and colleagues recently compared the gastric acid secretion, duodenal acid load and gastric emptying in response to 3 liquid meals at pH's 7, 3, and 1.5 [14]. Gastric acid secretion, duodenal acid load and gastric emptying were significantly greater in the duodenal ulcer patients than in normal subjects.

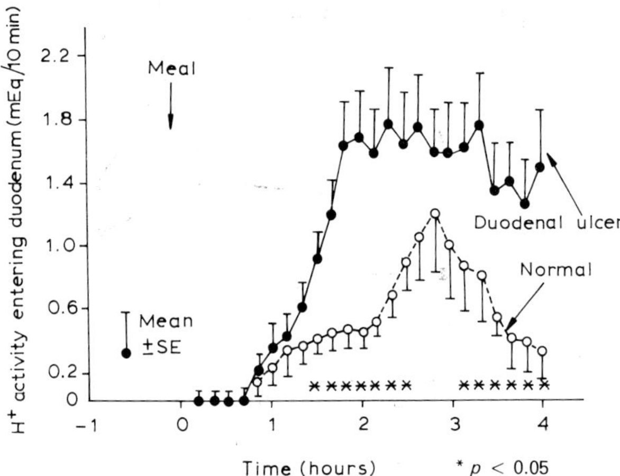

*Fig. 5: Duodenal hydrogen ion load after meals in 12 patients with duodenal ulcer and in 8 healthy volunteers. *=significant difference at each 10-minute interval. Reproduced with permission from [9].*

A number of studies have measured the duodenal pH in duodenal ulcer and normal subjects. As with gastric emptying studies, the methods have varied; some have used pH electrodes while others aspirated duodenal contents. Each method has its own inherent problems. Rune reviewed the literature on duodenal pH in ulcer and normal subjects, and summarized that duodenal bulbar pH tends to be lower in duodenal ulcer patients than in normal subjects, both fasting and after feeding [20]. In fasting subjects the pH of the second portion of the duodenum is comparable in duodenal ulcer and normal subjects. However, after a meal the pH in the postbulbar duodenum, the second portion, tends to be lower in duodenal ulcer patients than in normal subjects. As with each of the other pathophysiologic parameters, additional studies are needed to determine the prevalence and importance of an abnormally low duodenal pH in relation to other pathophysiologic abnormalities and in relation to the clinical course of duodenal ulcer (e.g., do patients with lower duodenal pH's have more ulcer recurrences, a more aggressive course of ulcer disease, etc.).

Duodenal inhibitor factors

One of the potential explanations for the increased gastric acid secretion in duodenal ulcer patients could be impaired release of either neural or humoral inhibitors of acid secretion. The only inhibitory hormone which has been thoroughly examined is secretin. Most of the evidence suggests that serum secretin either basal, postprandial, or following duodenal acidification is at least as great in duodenal ulcer patients as in normals (Fig. 6; [21]). Therefore, there is no evidence of a defect in the release of secretin in duodenal ulcer patients. In fact, serum secretin is elevated in patients with gastric acid hypersecretion and those with Zollinger-Ellison syndrome. Also, there is no evidence of impaired inhibition of gastric acid or pepsin secretion by fat in patients with duodenal ulcer, compared to normal subjects. Of potential physiologic importance (see Fig. 7), compared to a protein plus carbohydrate meal, a protein plus fat meal significantly inhibited gastrin release in normal subjects but not in a small group of duodenal ulcer patients [22]. This observation deserves further study.

Duodenal disposal of acid

A contributing factor to the apparent lower duodenal pH in patients with duodenal ulcer could be attributed to abnormal removal of acid either by neutralization or absorption from the proximal duodenum. As summarized

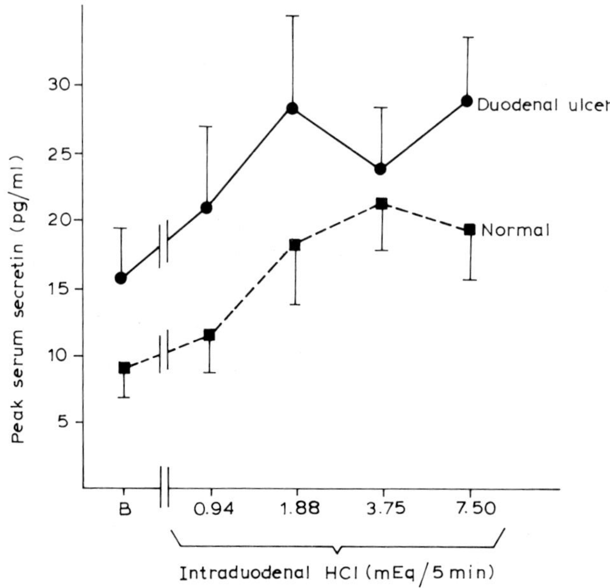

Fig. 6:   Mean peak plasma secretin before (B) and after instillation of graded amounts of hydrochloric acid into the duodenum in duodenal ulcer and in normal subjects. Reproduced with permission from [21].

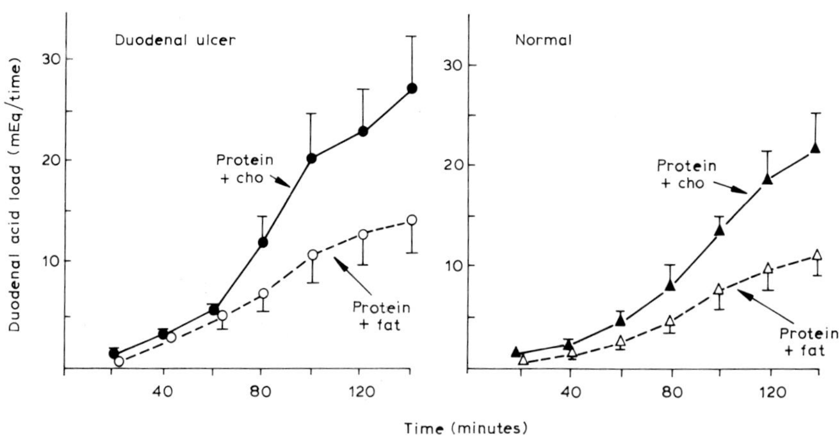

Fig. 7:   Gastric acid secretion in response to a protein plus carbohydrate (cho) meal versus a protein plus fat meal in 10 duodenal ulcer and 10 normal subjects. Reproduced with permission from [22].

by Wormsley, patients with duodenal ulcer secrete as much or more bicarbonate in response to exogenous secretin [23]. There are conflicting data, however, regarding the effect of duodenal acidification and its effect on pancreatic bicarbonate secretion. Studies in our laboratory suggested that graded amounts of acid resulted in greater amounts of bicarbonate secretion in patients with duodenal ulcer than normal subjects (Fig. 8; [21]). Also, although the dose of exogenous secretin required for one-half maximal response was reportedly greater in duodenal ulcer patients than normals, the maximal response in duodenal ulcer patients to exogenous secretin is at least as great as in normal subjects [24]. As I interpret these data, they suggest that there is no obvious defect in duodenal or jejunal disposal of acid in duodenal ulcer patients.

Gastric ulcer

The mucosal functional abnormalities in patients with gastric ulcer are discussed by others (see papers by Domschke – pp. 57–71, Robert – pp.

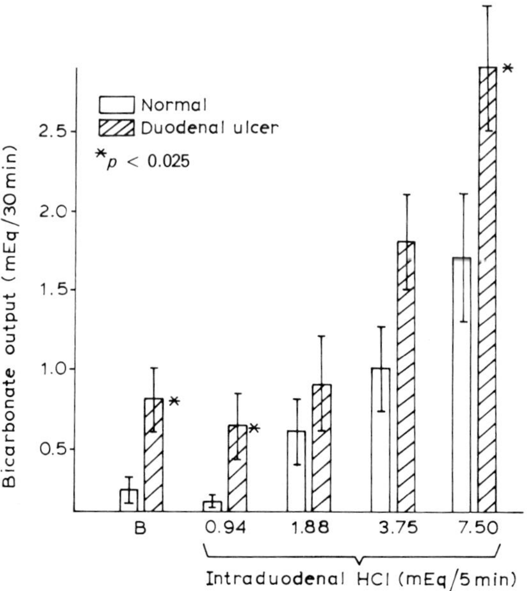

Fig. 8: Mean bicarbonate output before (B) and after instillation of graded doses of hydrochloric acid into the duodenum of duodenal ulcer patients versus normal subjects. The results represent the mean of 9 normal subjects and 9 duodenal ulcer patients. Reproduced with permission from [21].

72–77, Waldron-Edward – pp. 87–100, and Guth – pp. 101–109). However, gastric ulcer patients as a group secrete 'normal' or slightly less than 'normal' amounts of acid at rest in response to betazole, pentagastrin, etc. [25]. Patients with gastric ulcer involving the body of the stomach tend to secrete lower amounts of acid than normal subjects. The explanations for the decreased acid secretion include: gastritis, duodenal gastric reflux, and possibly back-diffusion of acid, etc. Patients with gastric ulcers near the gastroduodenal junction, or pyloric channel ulcers, secrete acid at rates that are comparable to duodenal ulcer patients.

Although most gastric ulcer patients secrete acid in response to pentagastrin, etc., there have been a few bona fide patients with benign gastric ulcer and histamine- or pentagastrin-fast achlorhydria [26]. The pathologic factors which are operative in these patients are not understood. However, Schwarz's dictum should not dictate clinical judgment in this unusual group of gastric ulcer patients.

Summary and the future

Gastric acid secretion has been exhaustively studied in patients with both gastric and duodenal ulcer. There are a number of pathophysiologic defects present in the 'average' duodenal ulcer patient; i.e. 1. an increased capacity to secrete acid; 2. an increased sensitivity to stimulants of acid secretion; 3. an increased drive to secrete; 4. a decreased inhibition of gastric acid secretion in the presence of intragastric acid; 5. an increased emptying of liquids; and finally 6. an increased duodenal acid load.

Studies are badly needed at a tissue and cellular level to explore the possible mechanisms which produce these abnormalities. Studies are also needed to correlate the presence of one abnormality with another in specific patients with duodenal ulcer, and more importantly to correlate these pathophysiologic abnormalities with the course of duodenal ulcer. Finally, it seems necessary at this time, 160 years since the discovery of gastric hydrochloric acid, to shift the emphasis from studies of the 'aggressive' factors to careful examination of the various abnormalities of 'defensive' factors.

References

1.   Baron, J.H. (1979): The discovery of gastric acid. *Gastroenterology 76*, 1056.
2.   Tiedemann, F. and Gmelin, L. (1826): *Die Verdauung nach Versuchen*. K. Groos, Heidelberg.

3. von Leube, W.O. (1871): *Sitz Phys Med. Soc. Erlangen* 106.

4. Isenberg, J.I., Walsh, J.H. and Grossman, M.I. (1973): The Zollinger-Ellison Syndrome. *Gastroenterology 65*, 140.

5. Cox, A.J. (1952): Stomach size and its relation to chronic peptic ulcer. *Arch. Pathol. 54*, 407.

6. Grossman, M.I. (1979): *Peptic ulcer pathogenesis and pathophysiology. 15th ed. of Textbook of Medicine,* pp. 1502–1567. Eds: P.B. Beeson and W. McDermott. W.B. Company, Philadelphia.

7. Rotter, J.I., Petersen, G., Samloff, M. et al. (1979): Genetic heterogeneity of hyperpepsinogenemic I and normopepsinogenemic I duodenal ulcer disease. *Ann. Intern. Med. 91*, 372.

8. McGuigan, J.E. and Trudeau, W.L. (1973): Differences in rates of gastrin release in normal persons and patients with duodenal ulcer disease. *N. Engl. J. Med. 288*, 64.

9. Malagelada, J.R., Longstreth, G.F., Deering, T.B. et al (1977): Gastric secretion and emptying after ordinary meals in duodenal ulcer. *Gastroenterology 73*, 989.

10. Baron, J.H. (1963): Studies of basal and peak acid output with an augmented histamine test. *Gut 4*, 136.

11. Isenberg, J.I., Grossman, M.I., Maxwell, V. and Walsh, J.H. (1975): Increased sensitivity to stimulation of acid secretion by pentagastrin in duodenal ulcer. *J. Clin. Invest. 55*, 330.

12. Lam, S.K., Isenberg, J.I., Grossman, M.I. et al. (1980): Gastric acid secretion is abnormally sensitive to endogenous gastrin released after peptone test meals in duodenal ulcer patients. *J. Clin. Invest. 65*, 555.

13. Walsh, J.H., Richardson, C.T. and Fordtran, J.S. (1975): pH dependence of acid secretion and gastrin release in normal and ulcer subjects. *J. Clin. Invest. 55*, 462.

14. Lam, S.K., Isenberg, J.I., Hogan, D. et al. (1979): Effect of neutral and acid meals on gastric acid secretion (GAS), duodenal acid load (DAL), and gastric emptying (GE) in duodenal ulcer (DU) and normals (N). (abstract). *Gastroenterology 76*, 1178.

15. Hurst, A.F. (1920): New views on the pathology, diagnosis and treatment of gastric and duodenal ulcer. *Br. Med. J. 1*, 559.

16. Shay, H. (1944): The pathologic physiology of gastric and duodenal ulcer. *Bull. N.Y. Acad. Med. 20*, 264.

17. Bromster, D. (1969): Gastric emptying rate in gastric and duodenal ulceration. *Scand. J. Gastroenterol. 4*, 193.

18. Coutourier, D., Roze, C., Sainz, R. et al. (1974): Activité électrique de l'estomac en réponse à la stimulation acide duodénale: résultats chez des sujets normaux et au cours de l'ulcère duodénal en évolution. *Biol. Gastroentérol. (Paris) 7*, 91.

19. Cano, R. and Isenberg, J.I. (1975): Demonstration of increased duodenal acid load in duodenal ulcer patients. *Clin. Res. 23*, 97A.

20. Rune, S.J. (1973): pH in the human duodenum. *Digestion 8*, 261.

21. Isenberg, J.I., Cano, R. and Bloom, S.R. (1977): Effect of graded amounts of acid instilled into the duodenum on pancreatic bicarbonate secretion and plasma secretin in duodenal ulcer patients and normal subjects. *Gastroenterology 72*, 6.

22. Gross, R.A., Isenberg, J.I., Hogan, D. et al. (1978): The effect of fat on meal-stimulated duodenal acid load, duodenal pepsin load, and serum gastrin in duodenal ulcer and normal subjects. *Gastroenterology 75*, 357.

23. Worsmley, K.G. (1974): The pathophysiology of duodenal ulceration. *Gut 15*, 59.
24. Berstad, A., Roland, M., Petersen, H. et al. (1974): The pancreatic exocrine secretion in duodenal ulcer patients before and after selective proximal vagotomy of the stomach. *Scand. J. Gastroenterol. 9*, 431.
25. Fiddian-Green, R.G., Marks, I.N., Bank, S. et al. (1976): Maximum acid output and position of peptic ulcers. *Lancet II*, 1370.
26. Korn, E.R. and Foroozan, P. (1974): Pyloric channel ulcer with betazole-fast-achlorhydria. *Gastroenterology 67*, 1248.

Gastric motor function in ulcer disease*

J.-R. Malagelada and **J.-R. Larach**
Gastroenterology Unit, Mayo Clinic and Mayo Foundation, Rochester, Minnesota, U.S.A.

Introduction

A search of the medical literature for information on motor abnormalities in ulcer disease (gastric and duodenal ulcers) reveals a large number of studies extending over several decades. However, much of these data need to be looked at in light of new concepts about the etiology of ulcer disease. Evidence has accumulated that duodenal ulcer disease, as we recognize it clinically, represents a mixture of disorders with different etiologies but a common pathologic expression, a concept described as genetic heterogeneity [1]. For gastric ulcer, specific etiologic factors have been recognized in some cases (such as drug ingestion) [2], and gastric ulcer has been subdivided into types exhibiting characteristic features. Johnson, for instance, recognizes 3 types of gastric ulcer [3, 4]. Type 1 occur proximal to the incisura of the stomach, usually along the lesser curvature, and their pathogenesis is poorly understood. Type 2 are associated with duodenal ulcer and may be sharing common pathogenetic factors; and type 3 are located in the antral area, and they are often associated with ingestion of acetylsalicylic acid or other known ulcerogenic drugs. Therefore, etiologic heterogeneity in gastric ulcer disease is likely to exist and genetic heterogeneity is also a possibility.

The pathophysiologic implications of heterogeneity are considerable. Because of their cost and technical complexity, many pathophysiologic studies have involved relatively small populations of patients with ulcer disease. Data from patients with different genetic background, secretory data, and even clinical presentations are analyzed together. From these studies, a multiplicity

* This work was supported in part by Research Grant AM 26428 from the National Institutes of Health, Bethesda, Maryland.
** Dr. Malagelada is the recipient of Research Career Development Award AM 00330 from the National Institutes of Health.

of defects, sometimes contradictory, has been revealed. It is possible that some confusing results are due to failure to recognize patient heterogeneity when designing the experiments. The information reviewed here needs to be evaluated with an understanding of these limitations.

Nevertheless, the information obtained from investigations on unselected groups should not be readily dismissed. A useful cohesive pathophysiologic pattern has emerged from these studies, and unselectivity may have allowed identification of defects common to many types of duodenal or gastric ulcers. It is quite possible that pathophysiologic abnormalities link etiologically heterogeneous disorders in the same way that common clinical expressions do.

Gastric motor abnormalities in duodenal ulcer

Motor and secretory functions in the fasting and postprandial states

Gastric secretion and gastric emptying are 2 functions that cannot be considered independently from each other. However, their interrelationships are different in 2 separate states: fasting and the postprandial period. During fasting, which extends physiologically during nocturnal rest and early morning, gastric secretion appears to be determined by 2 physiologic processes. One, the so-called circadian rhythm, determines changes over a long period and is responsible for gastric secretion peaking around midnight and then declining steadily until the early hours of the morning. The mechanisms regulating this circadian rhythm are unknown. The other process, operating simultaneously, is the so-called interdigestive motor-secretory cycles [5]. These cycles develop in healthy man approximately every 1–2 hours and consist of intense motor activity (designated as phase III) beginning in the upper gut and progressing distally to the terminal ileum. Recently, these cycles were shown to have a secretory counterpart. Gastric, pancreatic, and biliary secretions increase in close temporal association with bursts of motor activity [6, 7].

DeFilippi and Valenzuela have recently examined the pattern of interdigestive motor complexes in patients with duodenal ulcer and found that cycles occur at a normal frequency [8]. However, preliminary data suggest that increases in duodenal pH associated with each complex (due to bicarbonate secretion) are lower in ulcer patients than in healthy individuals. If these results are confirmed, they would indeed be of great significance in our understanding of the role of duodenal acidification in the pathogenesis of duodenal ulcer.

Despite the variations caused by both the circadian rhythm and the interdigestive motor-secretory complexes, gastric secretion and emptying interrelationships over a long period (for instance, during the night) are essentially in a steady state. Thus, the volume of gastric juice secreted equals the amount emptied, and intragastric volume remains constant. Estimates of the fasting intragastric volume in healthy man vary between 10 and 30 ml, and the amount of gastric juice secreted and emptied is about 1 ml/min, respectively. These are obviously approximations, since gastric secretory rates in normal persons are known to be extremely variable. If we accept that, as a group, patients with duodenal ulcer secrete more gastric water, acid and pepsin than normals, the implication is that in the fasting state the duodenal loads of these substances would be correspondingly greater.

Ingestion of a meal abruptly disrupts steady-state kinetics between gastric secretion and emptying because of several factors that, unlike what happens during fasting, lead to a rise in intragastric volume. First, the meal itself constitutes a considerable volume that the stomach must accommodate by exerting its 'reservoir' capacity through the mechanism called 'receptive relaxation'. Second, gastric secretion surges rapidly because of the stimulatory effect of the meal. Peak gastric secretion after a meal is at least 2–3 times higher than the highest rate observed during fasting. The third factor that disturbs the steady state is the stimulation of several inhibitory mechanisms of gastric emptying located in the duodenum that respond to pH, osmolality, and so forth.

Because of the nonsteady-state conditions between gastric emptying and secretion operating postprandially, duodenal acid load (a key variable in duodenal ulcer pathophysiology) cannot be predicted simply by measuring gastric secretory rates, whether the measurement is made during fasting, during stimulation by secretagogues, or even after ingestion of food. Therefore, methods allowing simultaneous measurement of gastric secretion and gastric emptying are required to elucidate the determinants of conditions prevailing in the duodenal bulb after meals.

In recent years, we have developed and refined a method that enables us to measure simultaneously gastric secretion and emptying after ingestion of a solid and liquid meal [9, 10]. The duodenal acid and volume load can thus be calculated. Our data show that after ingestion of the meal, gastric secretion increases sharply and reaches a peak by the end of the first hour. Peak acid secretory rate is similar in duodenal ulcer patients and healthy persons. However, patients with duodenal ulcer have an abnormally prolonged gastric secretory response to food, with acid secretion returning to baseline rate more slowly than in healthy persons. Since patients with duodenal ulcer, as a group, have higher 'maximal' secretory response to histamine or pentagastrin, it comes as a surprise to find that their postprandial secretory 'peak' is normal. Nevertheless, we have also found that peak acid outputs after pentagastrin correlate poorly with outputs after a meal [10]. Gross et al. also found that an increased peak gastric secretory response to food is not a constant feature in patients with duodenal ulcer, although their patients, unlike ours, did not have a higher than normal response after pentagastrin [11]. The observations, however, are in contrast with those of Fordtran and Walsh, who noted a higher peak acid output in response to meals in duodenal ulcer disease and noted a good correlation between acid responses to food and to histamine [12]. The difference in results might be due to the fact that these authors measure gastric secretion by a method that requires maintaining the gastric pH at 5.5, whereas our method and that used by Gross et al. [11] allow physiologic fluctuation of pH. A higher secretory response might have been obtained by Fordtran and Walsh because inhibitory mechanisms triggered by luminal acidification were not allowed to come into play.

Furthermore, our studies suggest an abnormality in regulatory mechanisms controlling the duodenal acid load. In patients with duodenal ulcer, who had an abnormally prolonged secretory response to the meal, the gastric reservoir function was not fully utilized to retain in the stomach the higher quantity of acid secreted during the late postprandial period [10]. Instead, acid was delivered in proportion to its secretion, that is, faster than in normal persons, so that duodenal acid load was increased. Since, according to Fordtran and Walsh, buffer is also emptied faster in duodenal ulcer [12], the extra duodenal acid load that occurs during the second and third hours would be composed of dissociated hydrogen ions to a greater extent than in healthy persons and would magnify the lower action of gastric acid on duodenal bulb pH. These data suggest that duodenal feedback mechanisms, which should slow gastric secretion in response to an increased duodenal acid load, are impaired in duodenal ulcer disease. However, proving that duodenal acid-sensitive mechanisms are deficient has not been an easy task, and the results of different investigations, as we discussed earlier, have often been conflicting.

Studies of gastric emptying in duodenal ulcer

Gastric emptying in patients with duodenal ulcer has been evaluated by many investigators. It would seem useful to reexamine the results reported to date in the medical literature (Table I).

In 1957, Hunt studied the influence of hydrochloric acid on gastric secretion and emptying in 16 patients with duodenal ulcer and 27 volunteers who served as controls [13]. He used his method of serial aspiration with a

Table I: Gastric emptying in duodenal ulcer.

Study	Year	No. of patients	Ulcer active	Meal		Method of measurement (marker)	Gastric secretory rate measured	Gastric emptying rate
				Physical characteristics	Description			
Hunt [13]	1957	16	?	Liquid	750 ml of 10% glucose	Serial aspiration	Yes	Normal
Buckler [14]	1967	193	?	Semisolid	Mashed potatoes, 150 g	Serial aspiration	No	Normal
George [15]	1968	20	?	Liquid	750 ml of water	Serial marker dilution (phenol red)	No	Normal
Griffith et al. [16]	1968	27	?	Solid	Bread, butter, porridge, milk, water; total volume 550 ml	Gamma camera (^{51}Cr)	No	Accelerated
Cobb et al. [17]	1971	12	Probably active	Liquid	750 ml of water	Serial marker dilution (phenol red)	No	Normal
Wormsley [18]	1972	14	Probably active	Liquid	Normal saline, 500 ml	Serial marker dilution (^{57}Co)	No	Accelerated
Fordtran and Walsh [12]	1973	7	Probably active	Solid	Steak, bread, butter, water; total volume, 500 ml	Disappearance of meal buffer	Yes	Accelerated
Stubbs and Hunt [19]	1975	250*	?	?	—	—	No	Accelerated
Howlett et al. [20]	1976	27	?	Solid	Meat, peas, mashed potatoes; weight, 250 g	Gamma camera (^{113m}In-DTPA)	No	Accelerated**
Malagelada et al. [10]	1977	12	Active	Solid	Steak, bread, butter, ice cream, water; total volume 400 ml	Perfusion and sampling; double marker (PEG/^{14}C-PEG)	Yes	Accelerated
Miyaoka et al. [21]	1977	16	Active	Liquid	750 ml of water	Serial marker dilution	No	Normal
Faxén et al. [22]	1978	15	?	Liquid	750 ml of 10% glucose	Serial marker dilution	No	Accelerated
Hinder and Morris [23]	1978	16	Active	Liquid	Milk	Serial marker dilution	No	Accelerated
Harasawa et al. [24]	1979	65	Active	Semisolid	200 ml of pastry (Okunos-A)	Plasma acetaminophen concentration	No	Accelerated
Lam et al. [25]	1979	8	?	Liquid	500 ml of 10% peptone	Serial marker dilution	No	Accelerated

*Collected from the literature.
**In one subgroup of duodenal ulcer patients.

meal consisting of 750 ml of water containing 100 g of glucose and 20 mEq of hydrochloric acid per liter. Hunt found gastric emptying to be similar in duodenal ulcer patients and healthy controls. However, he interpreted these results to mean that patients with duodenal ulcer were overreactive in their response to the meal, because the amount of acid emptied would be 'normal' for duodenal ulcer patients, who tend to be hypersecretors. Later, Stubbs and Hunt studied the relationship between energy of food and gastric emptying in patients with duodenal ulcer by gathering data from the medical literature about the volume and energy density of meals whose emptying had been quantified by a variety of methods [19]. They concluded that duodenal ulcer patients have abnormally rapid gastric emptying, especially for meals of high energy density. Buckler used a radiologic method to assess gastric emptying in 93 duodenal ulcer patients [14]. His meal of mashed potatoes and starch was semisolid. He found the overall pattern of emptying similar to that in the normal population. Emptying times tended to be longer in patients with marked hypersecretion.

Griffith et al. studied gastric emptying in 19 healthy controls and 27 duodenal ulcer patients. They used a 550 ml meal labeled with ^{51}Cr [16]. Emptying was measured by external monitoring with a gamma camera of the disappearance of the isotope from the stomach at half-hourly intervals. They found that the mean half-life of the isotope in the stomach in duodenal ulcer patients was significantly lower than the mean for the controls and thus concluded that gastric emptying in patients with duodenal ulcer was abnormally rapid.

Howlett et al. investigated gastric emptying in patients with duodenal ulcer by using a small (250 ml) semisolid meal of mashed potatoes tagged with ^{113m}DTPA [20]. The disappearance of the isotope from the gastric area was quantified by an external gamma camera. Twenty-six normal persons and 27 patients with duodenal ulcer were studied. These authors did not detect any statistically significant difference in mean gastric emptying of the isotope between duodenal ulcer and control groups. However, a closer look at their distribution appeared to reveal 2 groups of duodenal ulcer patients. One group had initially faster emptying.

Miyaoka et al. examined the dynamic aspects of gastric emptying of a liquid meal in patients with peptic ulcer, taking into account the different evolutionary stages of ulcer disease [21]. They studied 16 duodenal ulcer patients and 7 healthy controls with a serial dilution method and found no differences in gastric emptying between healthy persons and duodenal ulcer patients, although the emptying time in 5 of 7 duodenal ulcer patients showed a tendency to shorten as the ulcers healed. Faxén et al. also examined gastric emptying of a liquid meal in 18 healthy controls and 15 patients with duodenal ulcer disease [22]. They measured the emptying of the meal by the serial dilution test. Since this method primarily gives information on changes in the total volume of gastric contents (meal plus secretions), they compared the regression line for the postprandial decline in gastric volume in health and in duodenal ulcer. Duodenal ulcer patients had faster initial emptying (in the first 20 minutes) and shorter total emptying time than normal persons.

Fordtran and Walsh evaluated gastric emptying in 6 normal subjects and 7 patients with chronic duodenal ulcer disease by measuring the disappearance of buffer from the stomach after a hamburger meal [12]. They found that by 2 hours after eating the meal, the ulcer subjects had less than half as much buffer in the stomach as the controls. Although several factors besides gastric emptying influence the amount of buffer present in the stomach, the results suggest rapid gastric emptying of protein ingested in solid form.

Cobb et al. measured the gastric emptying of liquid meals in 12 patients with duodenal ulcer and 9 patients with diseases presumed to be unrelated to the stomach [17]. The 'meal' consisted of 750 ml of distilled water containing phenol red as a marker. Emptying was measured by the serial dilution method, with estimations repeated at 10-minute intervals during the first half hour and less frequently afterward. These authors could not demonstrate any difference in the emptying rate of the meal in patients with duodenal ulcer and in those with normal gastrointestinal tract.

Hinder and Morris performed a comparative study of the gastric emptying pattern in 19 normal subjects and in 16 patients with active duodenal ulcer [23]. They used a milk meal of 10 ml/kg of body weight incorporating 125 radioactive iodinated human serum albumin as a marker; the emptying from the stomach was quantified by serial dilution. The standard milk meal emptied faster in duodenal ulcer patients than in healthy persons. In addition, patients with duodenal ulcer appeared to have a greater intragastric volume, which the authors speculated could be due to either increased amounts of secretion or reflux. There was a trend for gastric emptying correlating with intragastric volume.

Harasawa et al. evaluated gastric emptying by a noninvasive method based on determining blood concentrations of paracetamol, a rapidly absorbable substance, incorporated into a test meal [24]. They found that duodenal ulcer patients had higher blood levels of paracetamol than normal controls, a result suggesting that their gastric emptying was also more rapid. They also found significantly more rapid emptying in duodenal ulcer patients with hypersecretion than in those with normal secretion or hyposecretion.

Studies on the effect of acidification of gastric or duodenal contents on gastric emptying in duodenal ulcer (Table II)

Johnston and Duthie have demonstrated the inhibitory effect of duodenal acidification on gastric secretion stimulated by gastrin in healthy individuals [27]. In an elegant series of studies, Wormsley examined the effect of duodenal acidification on gastric secretion and gastric emptying in patients with duodenal ulcer [28]. He demonstrated that infusion of acid into the duodenum produced a marked decrease in the gastric secretory response to pentagastrin in normal subjects as well as in patients with duodenal ulcer. However, the reduction in acid secretion during acidification was followed by an apparent 'rebound' increase in secretion, so that there was little or no net change in secretory rate when the entire test was considered. In a later study, Wormsley examined the effect of duodenal acidification on gastric emptying of normal saline or acidified saline [18]. The response observed in the duodenal ulcer group was not uniform. A subgroup of 6 patients had a reversal of the normal pattern, with an increase in the rate of gastric emptying during acidification. Another 5 patients had accentuation of the normal slowing of gastric emptying by acid in the duodenum.

Lam et al. measured gastric emptying in 8 duodenal ulcer patients and 7 healthy controls by a marker dilution method after ingestion of isosmotic liquid peptone meals that had been adjusted to pH 7, 3, and 1.5, respectively [25]. They found that the time to empty half of the test meal was significantly less in ulcer patients than in normal subjects after the meals at pH 3 and 1.5 but not after the meals adjusted at pH 7. However, both the total volume of gastric contents passing through the pylorus and the percentage of gastric contents emptied per unit of time (fractional gastric emptying) were significantly higher in ulcer patients than in normal subjects after all meals. Acidification of the meals from pH 7 to 3 decreased gastric emptying in normal controls but not in ulcer patients; this result suggests that the ability to slow gastric emptying in response to an increased duodenal acid load is impaired in duodenal ulcer patients.

In our laboratory, we tested the hypothesis that patients with duodenal ulcer have impaired duodenal acid feedback inhibition of gastric emptying [26]. The studies involved instilling acid into the duodenum and observing its effects on gastric emptying of a saline instillate. Saline was used to circumvent the problems of multiple mechanisms being stimulated by more complex meals. Acid output after saline instillation was similar in the group of patients with duodenal ulcer and in healthy controls; thus, differences could not be attributed to hypersecretion in the ulcer group. Saline left the stomach faster

Table II: Effect of duodenal acidification on gastric emptying in duodenal ulcer.

Study	Year	Number of ulcer patients	Ulcer active	Meal	Method of duodenal acidification	Secretion	Gastric emptying	
							Without acidification	With acidification
Hunt [13]	1957	16	?	750 ml of 10% glucose	HCl, 20 mEq/l, added to the meal	No change	Normal	Delayed, same as in normals
Wormsley [18]	1972	12	Active	500 ml of normal saline	Duodenal perfusion of: HCl, 50 mM; NaCl, 105 mM } 240 ml	Decreased; more in normals than in DU patients	Accelerated	Variable response
Lam et al. [25]	1979	8	?	Liquid isotonic peptone solution	Meal adjusted to pH 7, 3, 1.5	Decreased; more in normals than in DU patients	Accelerated	Delayed, but less than in normals
Coleman and Malagelada [26]	1979	6	Active	400 ml of normal saline	Duodenal perfusion of HCl, 0.1 N, 12 mEq/hr	Decreased; same in normals and in DU patients	Accelerated	No change; remained accelerated in DU patients

in duodenal ulcer patients than in healthy controls, a result in agreement with those of most studies, which have found rapid gastric emptying of simple crystalloid solutions and meals of varying composition in these patients. Acidification of the duodenum by instillation of isotonic hydrochloric acid greatly reduced gastric secretion in patients with duodenal ulcer and, to a similar extent, in healthy controls. However, it had no effect on gastric emptying of saline, emptying remaining significantly faster in duodenal ulcer patients during duodenal acidification. These results suggest that the main inhibitory feedback to increased duodenal acid load works by turning off gastric secretion in preference to slowing gastric emptying, although both mechanisms may come into play if the duodenal acid load is greatly increased. This feedback response to an increased duodenal acid load was normal in duodenal ulcer patients, although even under the inhibitory effect of duodenal acidification on gastric secretion, gastric emptying remained faster in the ulcer group. We have interpreted these results as indicating that patients with duodenal ulcer have abnormally rapid gastric emptying of fluid and acid, and that this abnormality is not simply due to the failure of acid-sensitive inhibitory mechanisms in the duodenum, since it occurs within a wide range of duodenal acid loads. This conclusion agrees with the work of Lam et al. who found increased gastric emptying in duodenal ulcer patients after liquid meals adjusted at pH's between 7 and 1.5 [29].

If it is not exclusively impaired duodenal feedback, what then is the cause of rapid gastric emptying in duodenal ulcer? We may need to turn to considerations of gastric and duodenal motility, but, unfortunately, little work has been done to date in measuring electrical and pressure patterns at the gastroduodenal junction in ulcer patients. DeFilippi and Valenzuela recently reported that normal interdigestive duodenal motor complexes are present in duodenal ulcer patients but that they are associated with a smaller increase in bulb pH than in healthy persons [30]. Whether this finding indicates a motility disorder or a weaker secretory counterpart of the migrating motor complex is not known. As Johnson pointed out, duodenal acid load and alkaline secretion are not the only 2 factors determining duodenal bulb pH [31]. Coordination in the arrival of alkaline and acid solutions to the area and their mixing may be crucial. Yet little is known about human duodenal motility and its fine control, either in health or in disease.

At present, no hypothesis can be developed to accommodate the results obtained by all investigators on the pathophysiology of gastric emptying in patients with duodenal ulcer. However, a plausible scheme can be presented as follows: in duodenal ulcer patients, gastric emptying is abnormally rapid because of some unspecified alteration of gastric or duodenal motility. After a meal, rapid gastric emptying and a higher secretory response (particularly after the first postprandial hour) cause an abnormally higher duodenal acid load. Inhibitory mechanisms are operative but insufficient to reduce duodenal acid load to normal levels (which would require a proportionally greater than normal inhibition of gastric secretion and emptying). The increased duodenal acid load is not matched by an appropriate increase in alkaline secretion (or its delivery to the duodenal bulb); thus, pH in the proximal duodenum decreases, and susceptibility of the duodenal mucosa to injury increases.

This hypothetical model does not take into account heterogeneity in duodenal ulcer, which could mean, in this context, that not all patients in the group need to have the same abnormality. Nevertheless, the concurrence of many reports involving together a large number of ulcer patients suggests that rapid gastric emptying, if not a constant feature, certainly is a prevalent physiopathologic feature of duodenal ulcer disease.

Gastric motor abnormalities in gastric ulcer

Types of gastric ulcer and their relationship to ulcer pathogenesis

As we alluded to earlier, type-1 gastric ulcers, those occurring proximally to the incisura, are those whose pathogenesis is less well understood [3, 4]. Type 2, associated with duodenal ulcer, and type 3, antral and often related to analgesic drug ingestion, probably involve different pathogenetic mechanisms. Whereas some pathophysiologic studies have included patients from all 3 groups, there has been a progressive tendency to study each of these groups separately, and more commonly type 1. In light of current knowledge the distinction of 3 separate groups of gastric ulcers is sound.

Gastric emptying in gastric ulcer

The number of studies examining gastric emptying in gastric ulcer has not been as numerous as with duodenal ulcer (Table III). George measured the emptying of water by his dye dilution technique and found delayed emptying [15]. Emery and Monroe, using a radiologic method, also found delayed emptying of liquid barium in gastric ulcer [34]. Griffith et al., employing a γ-labelled semisolid meal and external scanning, also found delayed emptying, although in this study it is not certain what proportion of the radiolabel remained attached to nutrients in the stomach [16]. More recently Morguelan et al. reexamined gastric emptying in patients with gastric ulcer employing a stable solid marker ^{99m}Tc-labelled chicken liver incorporated into a meal of

Table III: Gastric emptying in type-1 gastric ulcer.

Study	Meal	Method	Gastric emptying
George (1968) [15]	Water	Dye dilution	Delayed
Griffith et al. (1968) [16]	Semisolid	γ-label	Normal
Morguelan et al. (1978) [32]	Solid	γ-label	Delayed
Miller et al. (1980) [33]	Solid and liquid	Triple marker dilution	Delayed (solids) Normal (liquid)

beef stew [32]. They quantified gastric emptying by external radioscintiscanning and found gastric emptying of solids to be delayed. Studies carried out in our laboratory on patients with type-1 gastric ulcer revealed slower gastric emptying of solids and normal gastric emptying of liquids after ingestion of a mixed solid and liquid meal [33]. Therefore, there is general agreement among previous studies on the finding of gastric stasis of solids with either normal or delayed emptying of liquids in patients with gastric ulcer. Some of these studies have suggested that abnormalities of gastric emptying in patients with gastric ulcer may be reserved after healing of the ulcer [35]. Thus, the question arises whether the abnormalities described are primary or secondary. However, earlier results may have been influenced by inclusion of patients with antral ulcers [35], and ulceration in this area could have interfered physically with antral function. Also, the question might be unanswerable because causes may be intermittent. Further, whether the abnormalities described are cause or effect, they are probably important in either case. The dysfunctions of the stomach described could be implicated either in the pathogenesis of the original ulcer or in the progression or lack of healing of an already developed lesion.

The finding in our study that gastric emptying of solids was slow and that absolute emptying of liquids was normal [33] is suggestive of dysfunction of the antrum since current physiologic concepts assign to this portion of the stomach a role primarily concerned with the emptying of solids, whereas the fundus is thought to influence the emptying of liquids [36]. However, interactions between both mechanisms probably exist [37]. The antrum probably has several complex functions – forward propulsion of solids, grinding and dispersion of solids, and solid-liquid discrimination [38] – permitting independent emptying of nutrients in these 2 different physical states. Indeed, recent experimental studies have shown that only very fine meal particles are permitted to pass into the duodenum [39], whereas the larger ones are retropulsed [36]. Our study provides good evidence of normal solid-liquid discrimination in patients with type-1 gastric ulcer since, as in healthy controls, these patients emptied very little solids early in the postprandial period when liquid emptying was maximal [33]. Therefore, our data are consistent with antral dysfunction (failure to grind, disperse, and propel solids) but a normal 'filtering' mechanism, allowing liquids to be emptied preferentially.

Indeed, morphometric study of the antropyloric region in patients with gastric ulcer has revealed irregular areas of thickening and muscle hypertrophy [40]. However, direct evidence of antral hypomotility is limited to a short observation (120 minutes) of fasting motor activity [35]. These observations were not synchronized with phases of the interdigestive motor cycle [41]. Further, there are large differences in fasting and postprandial motility. At least in health, solid meals induce pronounced early postprandial antral hyperactivity [42]. Metoclopramide, a drug which is known to stimulate gastric contractions and accelerate gastric emptying, was able, in our study [33], to normalize gastric emptying of solids. The fact that metoclopramide accelerated gastric emptying of solids in our study further suggests a predominant effect on an abnormal antrum. Although previous clinical trials with this drug have produced equivocal results, this could have been due to inclusion of a heterogeneous patient group or a variable action of the drug during chronic administration [43, 44]. Further clinical studies with metoclopramide or similar pharmacologic agents seem warranted.

Duodenogastric reflux in gastric ulcer

Increased reflux of bile acids into the stomach has been documented in patients with gastric ulcer during fasting and after liquid meals [45–48]. Our study also suggested increased reflux of bile acids after a solid and liquid meal [33]. The timing of the increased reflux, early after ingestion of the solid meal, coincides with the normal peak in antral motor activity [49]. This raises the further possibility that antral dysfunction could be responsible for alterations in both solid emptying and duodenogastric reflux. It also seems possible that pyloric dysfunction plays a role as suggested by the studies of Fisher's group [50, 51]. As is true for gastric emptying abnormalities, it is somewhat uncertain whether increased duodenogastric reflux is a preexisting defect in patients with gastric ulcer or whether it completely disappears when the ulcer heals.

Interactions among gastric secretion, gastric emptying, and duodenogastric reflux in gastric ulcer

Patients with type-1 gastric ulcer tend to have less acid in their stomach than do normals [3, 52–57]. However, it is debatable whether this actually represents hyposecretion, increased backdiffusion of hydrogen ions across the mucosal barrier [58], or neutralization by refluxed duodenal contents [59, 60]. Our own studies [33], in carefully selected patients with type-1 gastric ulcer, revealed fasting and postprandial hypersecretion of acid, pepsin, and water. Decrease in postprandial acid recovery in the gastric lumen of patients with gastric ulcer was similar to the decreases in recovery of pepsin and water. Assuming normal secretory ratios for these 3 components of gastric juice in gastric ulcer, for which limited evidence exists [61], these data suggest that diminished secretory response to the meal mainly reflects reduced glandular secretion (of acid, water, and pepsin) rather than the backdiffusion of hydrogen ions. The latter would be expected to affect net acid output more than that of water or the pepsin molecule, which cannot backdiffuse.

Therefore, 3 abnormalities of postprandial gastric function have been identified in these patients with type-1 gastric ulcer: slowed gastric emptying of solids; gastric hyposecretion; and increased bile acid concentration in gastric contents. Substantial interactions may occur among these 3 abnormalities. An important consequence of the hyposecretion of gastric juice observed in patients with gastric ulcer is to increase concentrations of bile acid in the gastric contents, thus magnifying the effect produced by increased duodenogastric reflux. This has not been previously appreciated, since earlier studies measured only concentrations of bile acids without quantification of intragastric volume [45]. It could also be speculated that the combination of delayed emptying of solids, hyposecretion, and bile acid reflux permits prolonged exposure of the gastric mucosa to high concentrations of potential irritants in food or drug particles and high concentrations of bile acids or other refluxed substances, all having potentially damaging effects. Gastric hyposecretion could also aggravate gastric stasis of solids. Meyer (personal communication) has recently shown in the dog that gastric acid-pepsin concentrations play a role in accelerating trituration and liquefaction of digestible solids in the stomach. Reduced secretion in gastric ulcer could magnify a motor failure in the antrum and delay or impair trituration of solid particles to a size which would allow them to avoid discrimination by the antropyloric region. Through such a process gastric stasis could be aggravated.

Conclusion

Abnormalities in motor and secretory function have been described in gastric ulcer and there is reasonable agreement among different studies as to the occurrence of such abnormalities in groups of gastric ulcer patients. It is also possible, as we have attempted in this review, to ascribe a theoretical pathogenetic role to these abnormalities and interactions which occur among them.

However, it seems appropriate to reiterate here what we have stated at the beginning. Groups of patients studied tend to be small; patients with different clinical features and ulcer types may be lumped together; and further, new concepts about genetic heterogeneity in ulcer disease raise doubts about the interpretation of the abnormalities described. Therefore, the significance of what is presently known about gastric emptying in ulcer disease cannot be fully ascertained and the need for continuing work in this area of ulcer research is more compelling than ever.

References

1. Rotter, J.I. and Rimoin, D.L. (1977): Clinical trends and topics. Peptic ulcer disease – a heterogeneous group of disorders? *Gastroenterology 73*, 604.
2. Cameron, A.J. (1975): Aspirin and gastric ulcer. *Mayo Clin. Proc. 50*, 565.
3. Johnson, H.D. (1965): Gastric ulcer: classification, blood group characteristics, secretion patterns and pathogenesis. *Ann. Surg. 162*, 996.
4. Johnson, H.D. (1957): The classification and principles of treatment of gastric ulcers. *Lancet II*, 518.
5. Code, C.F. and Marlett, J. (1975): The interdigestive myo-electric complex of the stomach and small bowel of dogs. *J. Physiol. (London) 246*, 289.
6. Keane, F.B., DiMagno, E.P., Dozois, R.R. and Go, V.L.W. (1979): Relations of canine interdigestive pancreatic and biliary secretions to duodenal motor activity (Abstract). *Gastroenterology 76*, 1167.
7. Vantrappen, G., Peeters, T.L. and Janssen, S.J. (1979): The interdigestive complexes of man have both secretory and motor components (Abstract). *Gastroenterology 76*, 1264.
8. DeFilippi, C. and Valenzuela, J. (1980): Acid in duodenum and propagation of the interdigestive mortility complex (IDMC) (Abstract). *Gastroenterology. 78*, 1154.
9. Malagelada, J.-R., Longstreth, G.F., Summerskill, W.H.J. and Go, V.L.W. (1976): Measurement of gastric functions during digestion of ordinary solid meals in man. *Gastroenterology 70*, 203.
10. Malagelada, J.-R., Longstreth, G.F., Deering, T.B. et al. (1977): Gastric secretion and emptying after ordinary meals in duodenal ulcer. *Gastroenterology 73*, 989.
11. Gross, R.A., Isenberg, J.I., Hogan, D. and Samloff, I.M. (1978): Effect of fat on meal-stimulated duodenal acid load, duodenal pepsin load, and serum gastrin in

duodenal ulcer and normal subjects. *Gastroenterology 75*, 357.

12. Fordtran, J.S. and Walsh, J.H. (1973): Gastric acid secretion rate and buffer content of the stomach after eating: results in normal subjects and in patients with duodenal ulcer. *J. Clin. Invest. 52*, 645.

13. Hunt, J.N. (1957): Influence of hydrochloric acid on gastric secretion and emptying in patients with duodenal ulcer. *Br. Med. J. 1*, 681.

14. Buckler, K.G. (1967): Effects of gastric surgery upon gastric emptying in cases of peptic ulceration. *Gut 8*, 137.

15. George, J.D. (1968): New clinical method for measuring the rate of gastric emptying; the double sampling test meal. *Gut 9*, 237.

16. Griffith, G.H., Owen, G.M., Campbell, H. and Shields, R. (1968): Gastric emptying in health and in gastroduodenal disease. *Gastroenterology 54*, 1.

17. Cobb, J.S., Bank, S., Marks, I.N. and Louw, J.H. (1971): Gastric emptying after vagotomy and pyloroplasty. *Am. J. Dig. Dis. 16*, 207.

18. Wormsley, K.G. (1972): Response to duodenal acidification in man. IV. Effect on gastric emptying. *Scand. J. Gastroenterol. 7*, 631.

19. Stubbs, D.F. and Hunt, J.N. (1975): A relation between the energy of food and gastric emptying in men with duodenal ulcer. *Gut 16*, 693.

20. Howlett, P.J., Sheiner, H.J., Barber, D.C. et al. (1976): Gastric emptying in control subjects and patients with duodenal ulcer before and after vagotomy. *Gut 17*, 542.

21. Miyaoka, T., Misaki, F., Sasaki, Z. et al. (1977): Dynamic aspects of gastric emptying in patients with peptic ulcer according to ulcer stages. *Digestion 16*, 10.

22. Faxén, A., Kewenter, J. and Kock, N.G. (1978): Gastric emptying of a liquid meal in health and duodenal ulcer disease. *Scand. J. Gastroenterol. 13*, 735.

23. Hinder, R.A. and Morris M.W. (1978): A comparative study of the gastric emptying pattern in normal subjects and in patients with duodenal ulceration, truncal vagotomy or proximal gastric vagotomy. *S. Afr. J. Surg. 16*, 55.

24. Harasawa, S., Tani, N., Suzuki, S. et al. (1979): Gastric emptying in normal subjects and patients with peptic ulcer. *Gastroenterol. Jpn. 14*, 1.

25. Lam, S.K., Isenberg, J.I., Hogan, D. et al. (1979): Effect of neutral and acid meals on gastric acid secretion (GAS), duodenal acid load (DAL), and gastric emptying (GE) in duodenal ulcer (DU) and normals (N) (Abstract). *Gastroenterology 76*, 1178.

26. Coleman, S.L. and Malagelada, J.-R. (1979): Effect of duodenal acidification on gastric secretion and emptying in duodenal ulcer (DU) (Abstract). *Clin. Res. 27*, 264A.

27. Johnston, D. and Duthie, H.L. (1965): Inhibition of gastric secretion in the human stomach: effect of acid in the duodenum. *Lancet II*, 1032.

28. Wormsley, K.G. (1970): Response to duodenal acidification in man. II. Effects on the gastric secretory response to pentagastrin. *Scand. J. Gastroenterol. 5*, 207.

29. Lam, S.K., Isenberg, J.I., Lane, W. et al. (1979): Gastric acid secretion (GAS) is more sensitive to endogenous gastrin in duodenal ulcer (DU) than in normals (N) (Abstract). *Gastroenterology 76*, 1178.

30. DeFilippi, C. and Valenzuela, J. (1980): Acid in the duodenum and propagation of the interdigestive motility complex (Abstract). *Gastroenterology 78*, 1154.

31. Johnson, A.G. (1979): Peptic ulcer and the pylorus. *Lancet I*, 710.

32. Morguelan, B., Ippoliti, A. and Sturdevant, R. (1978): Gastric emptying in

patients with gastric ulcer (GU) (Abstract). *Gastroenterology 74*, 1070.

33. Miller, L.J., Malagelada, J.-R., Longstreth, G.F. and Go, V.L.W. (1980): Dysfunctions of the stomach with gastric ulceration. *Dig. Dis. Sci.* (In press).

34. Emery, E.S. Jr. and Monroe, R.T. (1931): Peptic ulcer: the diagnostic value of the roentgen ray before and after treatment. *Am. J. Roentgenol. 25*, 51.

35. Garrett, J.M., Summerskill, W.H.J. and Code, C.F. (1966): Antral motility in patients with gastric ulcer. *Am. J. Dig. Dis. 11*, 780.

36. Dozois, R.R., Kelly, K.A. and Code, C.F. (1971): Effect of distal antrectomy on gastric emptying of liquids and solids. *Gastroenterology 61*, 675.

37. Meyer, J.H., Strunz, U., Carter, D. and Kauffman, G. (1978): The distal stomach may regulate fluid outflow at constant pressure (Abstract). *Gastroenterology 74*, 1067.

38. Malagelada, J.-R. (1977): Quantification of gastric solid-liquid discrimination during digestion of ordinary meals. *Gastroenterology 72*, 1264.

39. Meyer, J.H., Shadchehr, A., Cohen, M.B. and Mandiola, S. (1978): Effect of ulcer operations on size of food particles passed from the canine stomach (Abstract). *Gastroenterology 74*, 1067.

40. Liebermann-Meffert, D. and Allgöwer, M. (1977): The morphology of the antrum and pylorus in gastric ulcer disease. *Prog. Surg. 15*, 109.

41. Szurszewski, J.H. (1969): A migrating electric complex of the canine small intestine. *Am. J. Physiol. 217*, 1757.

42. Rees, W.D.W., Go, V.L.W. and Malagelada, J.-R. (1978): The antroduodenal motor response to solid-liquid and homogenized meals in man (Abstract). *Gastroenterology 74*, 1083.

43. Gutz, H.J. (1973): Metoclopramide in treatment of gastroenterologic disorders. *Medicamentum 14*, 201.

44. Hoskins, E.O.L. (1973): Metoclopramide in benign gastric ulceration. *Postgrad. Med. J. 4*, Sup. 49, 95.

45. Rhodes, J., Barnardo, D.E., Phillips, S.F. et al. (1969): Increased reflux of bile into the stomach in patients with gastric ulcer. *Gastroenterology 57*, 241.

46. Capper, W.M., Airth, G.R. and Kilby, J.O. (1966): A test for pyloric regurgitation. *Lancet II*, 621.

47. Flint, F.J. and Grech, P. (1970): Pyloric regurgitation and gastric ulcer. *Gut 11*, 735.

48. Cocking, J.B. and Grech, P. (1973): Pyloric reflux and the healing of gastric ulcers. *Gut 14*, 555.

49. Rees, W.D.W., Go, V.L.W. and Malagelada, J.-R. (1978): The antroduodenal motor response to solid-liquid and homogenized meals in man (Abstract). *Gastroenterology 74*, 1083.

50. Fisher, R.S. and Cohen, S. (1973): Pyloric-sphincter dysfunction in patients with gastric ulcer. *N. Engl. J. Med. 288*, 273.

51. Fisher, R.S. and Boden, G. (1975): Reversibility of pyloric sphincter dysfunction in gastric ulcer. *Gastroenterology 69*, 591.

52. Marks, I.N. and Shay, H. (1959): Observations on the pathogenesis of gastric ulcer. *Lancet I*, 1107.

53. Ball, P.A.J. (1961): The secretory background to gastric ulcer. *Lancet I*, 1363.

54. Baron, J.H. (1963): An assessment of the augmented histamine test in the diagnosis of peptic ulcer: correlations between gastric secretion, age and sex of patients, and site and nature of the ulcer. *Gut 4*, 243.

55. Wormsley, K.G. and Grossman, M.I. (1965): Maximal histalog test in control subjects and patients with peptic ulcer. *Gut 6,* 427.
56. Aukee, S. (1972): Gastritis and acid secretion in patients with gastric ulcers and duodenal ulcers. *Scand. J. Gastroenterol. 7,* 567.
57. Dahlgren, S. and Nordgren, B. (1973): Gastric acid secretion in patients with gastric ulcer and gastric cancer investigated during continuous intravenous infusion of histamine. *Acta Chir. Scand. 139,* 529.
58. Davenport, H.W. (1965). Is the apparent hyposecretion of acid by patients with gastric ulcer a consequence of a broken barrier to diffusion of hydrogen ions into the gastric mucosa? *Gut 6,* 513.
59. James, A.H. and Pickering, G.W. (1949): The role of gastric acidity in the pathogenesis of peptic ulcer. *Clin. Sci. 8,* 181.
60. Watkinson, G. (1951): A study of the changes in pH of gastric contents in peptic ulcer using the twenty-four hour test meal. *Gastroenterology 18,* 377.
61. Makhlouf, G.M., McManus, J.P.A. and Card, W.I. (1967): Comparative effects of gastrin II and histamine on pepsin secretion in man. *Gastroenterology 52,* 787.

Current views on symptomatology of ulcer disease

W. L. Peterson
Departments of Internal Medicine, Dallas Veterans Administration Medical Center and Southwestern Medical School, Dallas, Texas, U.S.A.

An important goal in the treatment of peptic ulcer disease is relief of the patient's symptoms. In discussing the topic of ulcer symptoms, 3 questions will be addressed. First, are the 'classic' symptoms of peptic ulcer reliable? Second, is the pain of peptic ulcer produced by gastric acid? Third, do ulcer symptoms correlate with the presence of an ulcer crater?

The pain of uncomplicated peptic ulcer is visceral [1]. As such, it is dull, poorly localized, and, because of bilateral sensory afferent nerves, midline. Descriptions of visceral pain include such terms as boring, aching, gnawing, hunger-like and burning. Only with ulcer penetration or perforation does the pain become parietal (e.g., sharp and localized). The 'classic' symptoms of peptic ulcer are listed in Table I. Recent studies have demonstrated that this description of ulcer symptoms is neither reliably sensitive nor specific for peptic ulcer [2, 3].

Earlam examined 100 patients with radiographically documented duodenal ulcer. While ulcer pain was epigastric, frequently nocturnal, episodic, and often relieved with antacids, there was no relationship to meals in over half the patients. Indeed, many patients noted worsening of the pain with food. Furthermore, almost half noted pain upon awakening in the morning and

Table I: Classic symptoms of duodenal (DU) and gastric ulcer (GU).

DU and GU:	— Epigastric pain occurring 1–3 hours after meals — Pain not present before breakfast — Night pain frequent — Pain relieved by food or antacid
DU:	— Pain occurs with frequent exacerbations and remissions (episodic 'clusters') — Appetite enhanced
GU:	— Appetite decreased

only 20% had enhanced appetite [2]. Because endoscopic confirmation was not required for this study, the correlation of these symptoms with active duodenal ulceration is unknown.

Horrocks and De Dombal studied 360 patients with dyspepsia and tabulated symptoms of patients ultimately found to have duodenal ulcer, gastric ulcer, or 'functional' disease. Their results are displayed in Table II. These findings generally agree with those of Earlam and, in particular, dispel the notions that there is a prominent relation of ulcer pain to ingestion of food and that patients with duodenal ulcer eat more often to 'feed their ulcer'. The fact that less than 40% of patients with peptic ulcer in this study experienced relief of pain with antacids may be a reflection of the severity of the disease, since most patients ultimately underwent surgery for their symptoms. Although patients classified as 'functional' had either negative laparotomy, negative endoscopy findings, or no recurrence of symptoms after 1–2 years, follow-up was not long enough to fully exclude a diagnosis of peptic ulcer disease. In summary, keeping in mind the limitations of these studies, it appears that 'classic' symptoms do not ensure the diagnosis of peptic ulcer nor do their absence in any way exclude the diagnosis.

The presence of a duodenal or gastric ulcer has long been considered an acid-related phenomenon. As such, it has been assumed that ulcer symptoms are also produced by gastric acid. Palmer [4] and Bonney and Pickering [5] noted in pooly-controlled studies that ulcer pain could be relieved by aspiration of gastric contents and initiated by reinfusion of gastric contents. However, pain did not occur if gastric juice was neutralized before reinfusion.

Table II: Incidence of symptoms in functional disease, duodenal ulcer and gastric ulcer.

Symptoms	Functional (N = 50)	Duodenal ulcer (N = 80)	Gastric ulcer (N = 50)
Epigastric pain	50%	86%	66%
>3 years of symptoms	35%	70%	30%
'Clusters' of pain	35%	56%	16%
Night pain	32%	70%	32%
Effect of food:			
none	65%	50%	55%
relief	4%	20%	2%
Relief with antacids	26%	39%	36%
Weight loss	32%	44%	61%

Reproduced with permission of the Editor from Horrocks, J.C. and De Dombal, F.T. (1978): Clinical presentation of patients with dyspepsia. *Gut 19*, 19.

Bonney and Pickering found a pH threshold for pain of 1.5 to 2.5 in patients with duodenal ulcer and 2.2 to 3.0 in patients with gastric ulcer. More recent observations, carried out under more rigorous scientific conditions, suggest that this simplistic explanation is not entirely correct. Isenberg's group has reported a carefully controlled, preliminary study in which solutions of varying pH were blindly infused into the stomach of controls and patients with endoscopically-documented duodenal ulcer [6]. Their results are shown in Table III. It is clear that gastroduodenal acidification failed to consistently reproduce pain in this small number of patients with duodenal ulcer. It is possible, of course, that other components of gastric juice, such as pepsin, must be present for acid to reproduce ulcer pain.

Another approach to the study of ulcer pain is to determine if pharamacologic reduction of gastric acidity relieves ulcer pain. Reduction of gastric acidity may favorably influence ulcer pain in 2 ways. First, a dose of antacid may abort an individual episode of ulcer pain (immediate relief). Second, a continued regimen of ulcer medications may shorten the period of time needed for a patient to become free of pain episodes (long-term relief).

The ability of single doses of a potent liquid antacid to relieve individual episodes of pain has been compared to a similar appearing and tasting placebo in patients with duodenal ulcer [7]. There was no significant difference between antacid and placebo in time to onset, degree, or duration of pain relief. Antacid resulted in 75% pain relief in 60% of patients after antacid and in 50% after placebo. Contrasting results were found in another study when either an antacid (30 ml of aluminium magnesium hydroxide) or saline was instilled blindly via a nasogastric tube into duodenal ulcer patients at the time of pain [8]. Antacid produced complete pain relief in 95% of instillations while saline relieved pain only 43% of the time. Analysis of these 2 studies suggests that while antacid relieves pain in a large proportion of patients, a

Table III: Proportion of subjects studied who experienced ulcer pain with several infused solutions.

	Infused solution	Duodenal ulcer	Control
Study 1	0.1 M Citrate pH1	1/5	0/5
	0.1 M Citrate pH3	0/5	0/5
	0.1 M Citrate pH7	0/5	0/5
Study 2	0.15 M HCl pH1	3/6	0/5
	0.1 M Citrate pH7	1/6	0/5

Reproduced with permission from [6].

white, creamy placebo swallowed by the patient will work just as well. The patient's expectation of pain relief with such a liquid produces a remarkable placebo effect.

A number of controlled trials have assessed the ability of a wide variety of drug regimens to promote long-term ulcer symptom relief. This discussion will use as examples those trials using antacid or cimetidine as means of reducing gastric acidity. The results of 3 well-controlled trials of antacids in outpatients with peptic ulcer have been reported [9–11]. One study demonstrated significantly better relief of gastric ulcer symptoms with antacid than with placebo (although only 8 patients were included in each group) but no significant benefit in patients with duodenal ulcer [9]. Similar results were obtained in 2 studies of duodenal ulcer, even when large doses of antacid were used [10, 11]. The results from one of these studies are depicted in Figure 1. There was no significant difference in reduction of ulcer symptoms, as measured by an unbiased interviewer, between patients taking antacid or a similar appearing and tasting placebo. Again, this may not be a reflection of poor results with antacid but of impressive results with placebo.

More trials evaluating pain relief have been performed with cimetidine than

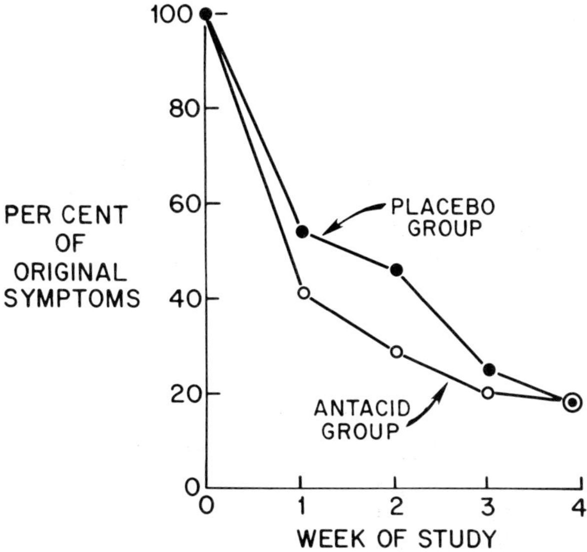

Fig. 1: Per cent of original symptoms remaining at each week of a 4-week comparison of antacids and placebo in duodenal ulcer. Reproduced with permission from Peterson, W., Sturdevant, R.A.L., Frankl, H.D. et al. (1977): Healing of duodenal ulcer with an antacid regimen. New Engl. J. Med. 297, 341.

with antacids. Studies of gastric ulcer conducted outside the United States show trends toward superior relief of pain with cimetidine when compared to placebo [12–14], although results from only one reached statistical significance [14]. The only 'placebo'-controlled trial performed in the United States demonstrated only a slight trend toward better results with cimetidine [15]. This trial, however, is clouded by the fact that placebo-treated patients consumed moderate amounts of supplemental antacids.

In duodenal ulcer the results are clearer. Each non-United States trial, summarized by Winship [16], demonstrated better pain relief with cimetidine than with placebo. Results from one of these are shown in Figure 2 [17]. A discouraging note was sounded by the large cooperative trial conducted in the United States [18]. In this study, symptom relief with cimetidine, while excellent, was superior to placebo only at week one of a 6-week trial. In contradistinction to non-United States trials, however, placebo-treated patients in the United States were allowed supplemental liquid antacid. Although a regimen of large-dose antacid prompts duodenal ulcer pain relief as well as a regimen of cimetidine [19], it remains unclear whether patients in

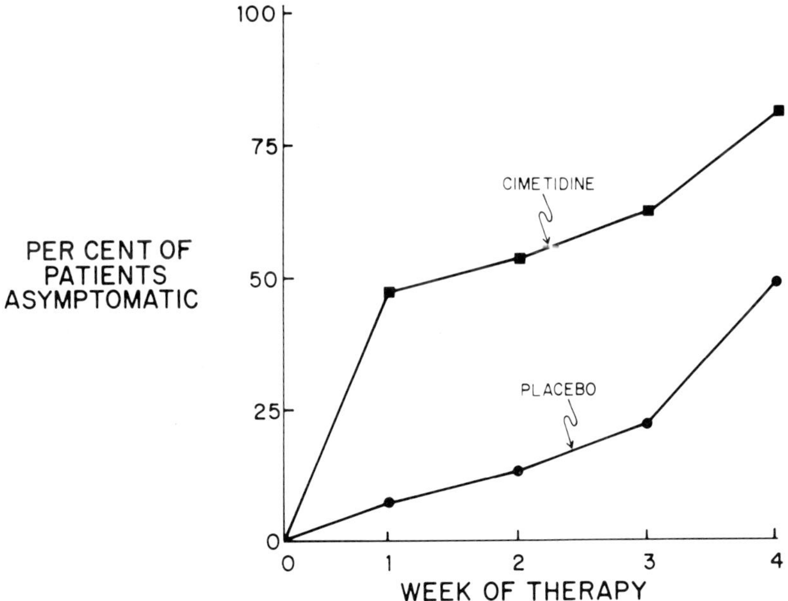

Fig. 2: Per cent of patients who were asymptomatic at each week of a 4-week comparison of cimetidine and placebo in duodenal ulcer. Reproduced with permission from [17].

the United States cimetidine trial taking placebo experienced pain relief comparable to patients taking cimetidine because of antacid or because of the placebo effect of the white, creamy liquid.

Based on the forgoing data, it is this author's opinion that, once mucosa is damaged, the most likely physiologic stimulus for ulcer pain is gastric secretion but perhaps not solely hydrochloric acid. As such, neutralization or reduction of gastric secretion promotes pain relief. Just as important, however, from the point of view of a patient's subjective response to these stimuli, is the psychological aspect. Appropriately suggestible patients may respond to a placebo as well as to an agent that either neutralizes or reduces gastric secretion. Just how gastric secretion prompts pain remains unclear, although some investigators believe disordered gastroduodenal motility may play a role [20, 21].

The increasing use of fiberoptic endoscopy in controlled clinical trails of ulcer pharmacotherapy has allowed correlation of ulcer symptoms with morphologic mucosal abnormalities. In one large placebo-controlled trial of antacids in duodenal ulcer there was poor correlation between ulcer symptoms and ulcer healing [10]. However, because most patients taking liquid placebo do very well symptomatically, it is important to look to trials where placebo patients do not respond as well. The results of one such trial, the large United Kingdom placebo-controlled trial of cimetidine, are shown in Table IV [22]. Once again, ulcer healing is neither necessary for, nor guarantees relief of ulcer symptoms. Results in gastric ulcer are similar [13]. Clearly, the presence or absence of an endoscopically-documented ulcer crater does not correlate well with ulcer symptoms.

Neither do symptoms correlate well with an endoscopic diagnosis of duodenitis. In one trial comparing antacids and cimetidine in duodenal ulcer, it was found that ulcer symptoms after 4 weeks of therapy occurred in 50% of patients with either an active ulcer or duodenitis but in only 5% of patients

Table IV: Ulcer healing versus symptomatic response after 4 weeks of therapy.

Status of ulcer	Symptomatic	Asymptomatic
Healed	40/101	61/101
	(40%)	(60%)
Not healed	47/78	31/78
	(60%)	(40%)

Reproduced with permission of the Editor from Bardhan, K.D., Saul, D.M., Edwards, J.L. et al. (1979): Comparison of two doses of cimetidine and placebo in the treatment of duodenal ulcer: a multicentre trial. *Gut 20*, 68.

with a normal bulb [19]. On the other hand, another study found no difference in symptom relief between patients with duodenitis and those with a normal bulb [10].

The preceding discussion leads one to question 'What is peptic ulcer disease?' Ulcer symptoms occur in patients without documented ulcer craters and can be relieved without healing of an ulcer crater. Although 40% of patients with nonulcer dyspepsia (or 'pseudo-ulcer') reportedly will ultimately develop a peptic ulcer, these data are not based on endoscopic confirmation [23]. Further, there is no good evidence that duodenitis, either histologic or endoscopic, is a 'pre-ulcer' lesion. Spiro has speculated that ulcer disease is a spectrum of abnormalities, which he calls Moynihan's Disease [24]. While duodenitis and a visible ulcer crater may be one part of the spectrum, there are other aspects which have yet to be characterized histologically or functionally. These may be present in patients with ulcer-like dyspepsia and normal appearing mucosa. What is needed is a study of large numbers of unselected patients with dyspepsia, using endoscopy as the 'gold-standard' of active ulceration and long-term follow-up as the 'gold-standard' of peptic ulcer disease.

In summary it can be said that: many of the classic symptoms of peptic ulcer are unreliable; ulcer pain is most likely caused by gastric secretions; reduction or neutralization of gastric secretion promotes ulcer-pain relief, often despite nonhealing of the ulcer crater; and the placebo effect often promotes pain relief as well as active medications.

How does all of this affect patient management? When someone comes to a physician with ulcer-like symptoms, the prime goal is to relieve these symptoms, regardless of the mucosal appearance. Evidence suggests this can be accomplished as well with placebo as with active medication, at least in the United States. However, patients should be treated with an active drug such as antacid or cimetidine for 3 reasons. First, placebo is not marketed. Second, there are ethical concerns involved in administering placebo to the unsuspecting patient. Third, antacids and cimetidine promote ulcer healing to a greater degree than placebo. Although the consequences of an unhealed, asymptomatic ulcer are not known, it appears rational to heal the ulcer, especially since antacids and cimetidine are known to be safe.

References

1. Way, L.W. (1978): Abdominal pain and the acute abdomen. In: *Gastrointestinal Disease*, 2nd ed., Vol I, Chapter 20, p. 394. Eds: M. Sleisenger and J. Fordtran. W.H. Saunders, Philadelphia.

2. Earlam, R. (1976): A computerized questionaire analysis of duodenal ulcer symptoms. *Gastroenterology 71*, 314.
3. Horrocks, J.C. and De Dombal, F.T. (1978): Clinical presentation of patients with dyspepsia. *Gut 19*, 19.
4. Palmer, W. (1927): The 'acid test' in gastric and duodenal ulcer. *J. Am. Med. Assoc. 88*, 1778.
5. Bonney, G.L.W. and Pickering, G.W. (1946): Observations on the mechanism of pain in ulcer of the stomach and duodenum. I. The nature of the stimulus. *Clin. Sci. 6*, 63.
6. Harrison, A., Hagie, L., Schapira, M. and Isenberg, J.I. (1979): Gastroduodenal acidification failed to induce pain consistently in patients with active symptomatic duodenal ulcer. (Abstract). *Gastroenterology 76*, 1152.
7. Sturdevant, R.A.L., Isenberg, J.I., Secrist, D. and Ansfield, J. (1977): Antacid and placebo produced similar pain relief in duodenal ulcer patients. *Gastroenterology 72*, 1.
8. Lorber, S.H., Stelzer, F.A. and Mayer, E.M. (1978): Effect of antacid and placebo on pain of duodenal ulcer. (Abstract). *Gastroenterology 74*, 1058.
9. Hollander, D. and Harlan, J. (1973): Antacids vs placebos in peptic ulcer therapy. A controlled double-blind investigation. *J. Am. Med. Assoc. 226*, 1181.
10. Peterson, W., Sturdevant, R.A.L., Frankl, H.D. et al. (1977): Healing of duodenal ulcer with an antacid regimen. *New. Engl. J. Med. 297*, 341.
11. Lam, S.K., Lam, K.C., Lai, C.L. et al. (1979): Treatment of duodenal ulcer with antacid and sulpiride. *Gastroenterology 76*, 315.
12. Bader, J.P., Morin, T., Benier, J.J. et al. (1977): Treatment of gastric ulcer by cimetidine. In: *Cimetidine: Proceedings of the 2nd International Symposium on Histamine H₂-Receptor Antagonists,* p. 287. Eds: W.L. Burland and M.A. Simkins. Excerpta Medica, Amsterdam.
13. Frost, F., Rahbek, I., Rune, S.J. et al. (1977): Cimetidine in patients with gastric ulcer: a multicentre controlled trial. *Br. Med. J. 2*, 795.
14. Ciclictira, P.J., Macbell, R.J., Forthing, M.J. et al. (1977): A controlled trial of cimetidine in the treatment of gastric ulcer. In: *Cimetidine: Proceedings of the 2nd International Symposium on Histamine H₂-Receptor Antagonists,* p. 283. Eds: W.L. Burland and M.A. Simkins. Excerpta Medica, Amsterdam.
15. Dyck, W.P., Belsito, A., Fleshler, B. et al. (1978): Cimetidine and placebo in the treatment of benign gastric ulcer. A multicenter double blind study. *Gastroenterology 74*, 410.
16. Winship, D.H. (1978): Cimetidine in the treatment of duodenal ulcer. Review and commentary. *Gastroenterology 74*, 402.
17. Bardhan, K.D. (1978): Cimetidine in duodenal ulceration. In: *Cimetidine: The Westminster Hospital Symposium,* p. 31. Eds: C. Wastell and P. Lance. Churchill Livingstone, Edinburgh.
18. Binder, H. J., Cocco, A. and Crossley, R.J. (1978): Cimetidine in the treatment of duodenal ulcer. A multicenter double blind study. *Gastroenterology 74*, 380.
19. Ippoliti, A.F., Sturdevant, R.A.L., Isenberg, J.I. et al. (1978): Cimetidine versus intensive antacid therapy for duodenal ulcer. A multicenter trial. *Gastroenterology 74*, 393.
20. Bolton, C. (1928): Interpretation of gastric symptoms. *Lancet I*, 1159.
21. Ruffin, J.M., Baylin, G.J. and Legerton, C.W. (1953): Mechanism of pain in peptic ulcer. *Gastroenterology 23*, 252.

22. Bardhan, K.D., Saul, D.M., Edwards, J.L. et al. (1979): Comparison of two doses of cimetidine and placebo in the treatment of duodenal ulcer: a multicentre trial. *Gut 20*, 68.
23. Krag, E. (1965): Pseudo-ulcer and true peptic ulcer. A clinical, radiographic, and statistical follow-up study. *Acta Med. Scand. 178*, 713.
24. Spiro, H.M. (1974): Moynihan's Disease? The diagnosis of duodenal ulcer. *New Engl. J. Med. 291*, 367.

Endoscopy in the diagnosis of duodenal ulcer*

M. Classen, H. Dancygier and H.F. Fuchs
Departments of Gastroenterology and Diagnostic Radiology I, Johann Wolfgang Goethe University, Frankfurt/Main, Federal Republic of Germany

Introduction

As a result of the introduction of fiber-glass endoscopes, the combined examination of esophagus, stomach and duodenum in a single procedure has been made possible. The advantages of this procedure for diagnostic and therapeutic purposes are obvious. As a consequence, upper gastrointestinal endoscopy has been fully integrated into the practice of gastroenterology over the last few years. Even now, however, there is still a need for a discussion of the role of endoscopy in the diagnosis of duodenal ulcer (DU), and of its relevance in clinical trials.

Role of endoscopy in the diagnosis of DU

There is general acceptance that radiological methods are less sensitive than endoscopy in detecting overt ulceration, especially when the duodenal cap is deformed.

In previously reported studies, if the results of routine barium meals were taken into consideration, about 25–35% of DU's were not seen radiologically [1, 2]. Ten per cent of the radiologically diagnosed ulcers were not found on endoscopy [3]. These retrospective studies did not, however, completely exhaust the efficacy of the 2 methods. A prospective study was therefore carried out.

X-ray studies and endoscopy of the duodenum were carried out by examiners having personal experience of several thousand procedures. The clinical information collected for each patient was identical, and the information was collected by a neutral colleague and not given to the partner

*This work was supported by E. Merck, Darmstadt.

examiner. The endoscopist used direct and lateral viewing endoscopes, and the radiologist applied hypotonic duodenography if this was felt to be necessary. One hundred patients with dyspeptic complaints were studied.

In 74 patients, endoscopy and X-ray gave the same results. In 4 patients the DU was diagnosed only by endoscopy, while in 5 patients a radiologically diagnosed ulcer was not confirmed endoscopically. Minor discrepancies were found in the remaining 17 patients.

The 4 X-ray-negative DUs comprised less than 10% of the total 42 DUs diagnosed by both methods. There is no proof as to whether the 5 ulcers not seen by the endoscopist were in fact present or not. The absolute value of endoscopy cannot, therefore, be precisely assessed, since there is no objective criterion against which judgments can be made. However, this study confirmed our assumption that endoscopy is a sensitive tool in the diagnosis of DU.

Need for histological examination of DU

Malignant ulceration in the duodenal bulb is extremely rare. Only 3 cases (0.2%) were diagnosed by Ottenjann in his series of 15,000 consecutive endoscopic examinations of the duodenum [4]. Ulcerative lesions in Crohn's disease of the duodenum seem to be becoming more common, so that the general opinion that it is not necessary to biopsy DUs may be revised in the future. It is not unlikely that DUs which do not respond to conventional peptic ulcer therapy are in fact Crohn's ulcers, and should be biopsied.

Endoscopy in DU trials

Endoscopic studies and controlled clinical trials for the assessment of therapeutic agents have shown no correlation between the so-called ulcer symptoms and the existence, size or location of DUs [5]. In addition, data collected during follow-up of patients with healed DUs in trials of maintenance therapy also indicate a discrepancy between endoscopically confirmed recurrence of the ulcer and symptomatic relapse [6]. Radiological examination is also insufficiently sensitive to demonstrate partial or complete healing of the duodenal ulceration [7].

Endoscopic estimations of ulcer size and changes in size were hindered by variations in apparent object size with image distance. Sonnenberg et al. have recently demonstrated that endoscopic estimations of the ulcer size with forceps or graduated probe as reference lengths are unreliable. These authors advise complete healing of the ulcer as the criterion to be used in ulcer trials [8].

New electronic systems for the assessment of ulcer size

H. Dancygier and other members of the Department of Gastroenterology at the J.W. Goethe University, Frankfurt/Main, have adapted a computer-assisted semi-automatic device for stereological analyses for use in endoscopy. The basic elements are an electronic planimeter with an evaluation tablet coupled with an electronic calculator, the latter being attached to a TV monitor. The measurement of various geometric parameters, namely areas, perimeters and maximal diameters, is performed by tracing the structure with a marking stylo. The area analysis can be carried out either on a photograph or directly on a TV monitor.

The principle of measurement is as follows: the current impulses emitted from the tablet sides induce magnetostrictive pulses in the magnetic steel wires running beneath the tablet surface in the X and Y directions. If the magnetostrictive pulses pass the receiver coil incorporated in the drawing pen, the running time (which is proportional to the displacement) will be electronically measured. Therefore, the coordinates of the image point touched will be obtained in mm. The integrated microprocessor with floppy disk drives processes the measured coordinate values. The accuracy of the measuring device is to within 0.1 mm for the coordinates, $<1\%$ for the area, and $<1\%$ for the length (according to information supplied by the producer).

The endoscopic picture obtained, using a Siemens TV camera, from the endoscope and transmitted to a TV monitor can be stored on video tape. The ulcerated area can be measured directly on the TV monitor by means of an electronic overlay marker. The path of the marker remains visible on the screen, so that the surrounded lesion is exactly labeled. From the relation of a known and endoscopically introduced reference area to the ulcerated test area, the latter can be calculated by the computer. It is important that the reference area lies in the plane of the ulcer. The optical distortions for the 2 areas are then almost identical, and an evaluation is possible. Differences in image distance and angles of viewing can then be neglected. Multiple measurements with different distances, different angles of vision and different reference areas revealed an error of $4.2 \pm 0.5\%$.

The inter-observer variation resulting from 5 measurements of an endoscopic picture of a DU by 6 different examiners (5 working with the device for the first time) was $2.9 \pm 1.2\%$.

Our experience with this new system is preliminary, but its advantages are clear. With electronic planimetry, measurements of ulcerated areas obtained in clinical trials allow judgments of alterations in ulcer sizes to be made. A re-evaluation of previous findings is possible because they are taped. Electronic planimetry seems to be rapid and accurate enough for the clinical assessment of ulcer healing [9].

Principles of DU trials

Patients admitted into clinical trials are those with peptic ulceration well-established by endoscopy. It has to be borne in mind, however, that they belong to a highly selected group, due to protocol requirements, the reasons for referral to the hospital or center, their degree of compliance, and possibly the stage in the ulcer's natural history [6].

Endoscopies should be performed by an experienced examiner who has no knowledge of the treatment in use. Modern direct and lateral viewing endoscopes should be used. In previous studies, it was found that 13–25% of duodenal pathology was demonstrable only with a lateral viewer [3, 10].

Upper gastrointestinal endoscopy can be performed without premedication on an outpatient basis. Duodenal ileus may be advisable for measurements of ulcerated areas (10 mg of scopolamine butyl bromide, 1 mg of glucagon). Planimetry of the ulcer on a photograph or on a TV monitor seems to be the best discriminating tool currently available in ulcer treatment.

Summary

Endoscopy is a sensitive method for the diagnosis of duodenal ulcer (DU). Histological examination for the diagnosis of bulbar malignancies is not necessary. In DU trials, endoscopy should be used for assessment of complete healing. Endoscopic planimetry of ulcerated areas should permit judgement on the dynamics of ulcer healing.

References

1. Jenny, S., Frühmorgen, P., Bäurle, H. et al. (1971): Endoskopisch-radiologische Diagnostik (Ulkus, Narbe). *Dtsch. Med. Wochenschr. 97*, 118.
2. Belber, J.P. (1971): Endoscopic comparison of the duodenal bulb: A comparison with endoscopy. *Gastroenterology 61*, 55.
3. Salmon, P.R. (1973): Endoscopic observations on the healing of duodenal ulcer. In: *Das Peptische Ulkus*, pp. 79–84. Eds: L. Demling, K. Moser and W. Rösch. Schattauer, Stuttgart-New York.
4. Ottenjann, R. (1979): Ösophagogastroduodenoskopie. In: *Gastroenterologische Endoskopie Lehrbuch und Atlas*, pp. 3–69. Eds: R. Ottenjann and M. Classen. Enke, Stuttgart.
5. Frühmorgen, P., Jenny, S., Classen, M. et al. (1972): Anamnese bei Ulkus und Narben im Bulbus duodeni. *Dtsch. Med. Wochenschr. 97*, 188.

6. Misiewicz, J.J. (1978): Peptic ulceration and its correlation with symptoms. In: *Endoscopy. Clinics in Gastroenterology*, Vol. 7, No. 3. Ed: K. Schiller. W.H. Saunders, London-Philadelphia-Toronto.
7. Kawai, K., Ida, K., Misaki, F. et al. (1971): Comparative study for duodenal ulcer by radiology and endoscopy. *Endoscopy 1*, 118.
8. Sonnenberg, A., Giger, M., Kern, L. et al. (1979): How reliable is determination of ulcer size by endoscopy? *Br. Med. J. 2,* 1322.
9. Langman, M.J.S. (1978): Treatment trials and their design. In: *Endoscopy. Clinics in Gastroenterology*, Vol. 7, No. 3. Ed: K. Schiller, W.H. Saunders, London-Philadelphia-Toronto.
10. Classen, M. (1973): Endoscopy in benign peptic ulcer. In: *Peptic Ulceration. Clinics in Gastroenterology*, Vol. 2, No. 2. Ed: W. Sircus. W.H. Saunders, London-Philadelphia-Toronto.

Endoscopy in the diagnosis of gastric ulcer

K. Ewe
I Medizinische Klinik und Poliklinik Johannes Gutenberg Universität, Mainz, Federal Republic of Germany

The role of endoscopy is not confined to the macroscopic diagnosis of gastric ulcer (GU) where it competes with radiology, but includes other equally important facets, namely guided biopsy and cytology. The role of directed biopsy, the problems of endoscopy as compared to radiology, problems arising in estimating the size and healing of GU, and the differentiation of benign and malignant ulcers will therefore be discussed in this paper.

GU is traditionally defined anatomically and not functionally, with the pylorus being taken as the border for the duodenal bulb and the duodenal ulcer (DU), although the prepyloric ulcer and the ulcus ad pylorum also share the characteristics of a DU. The generally accepted classification of Johnson et al. divides GU into 3 major groups [1]. In the first, the ulcer is located at the angulus or above; this group accounts for 57% of cases, and the acid output is usually low. In the second the ulcer is located in the same area as in the first group, but there is in addition a DU or the scar of a DU; this group accounts for 21% of the cases, and the acid output is usually high. The third type is the prepyloric ulcer, which as a rule is confined to a distance within one inch (2.5 cm) from the pylorus; the acid output is normal or high.

Endoscopic biopsies have revealed different histological changes for the 3 types of ulcers, from serial biopsies from different parts of the stomach. The most common site of GU is the border of the antrum and the acid-forming fundus of the stomach [2, 3]. It has been shown by Stadelmann et al. that the higher the ulcer is located, the higher is the rate of chronic atrophic gastritis and the lower the rate of normal mucosa and/or superficial gastritis, with corresponding changes in gastric acid production (Fig. 1; [4]).

Comparison of endoscopy and radiology

To diagnose ulcerative lesions in the stomach, 2 methods may be employed:

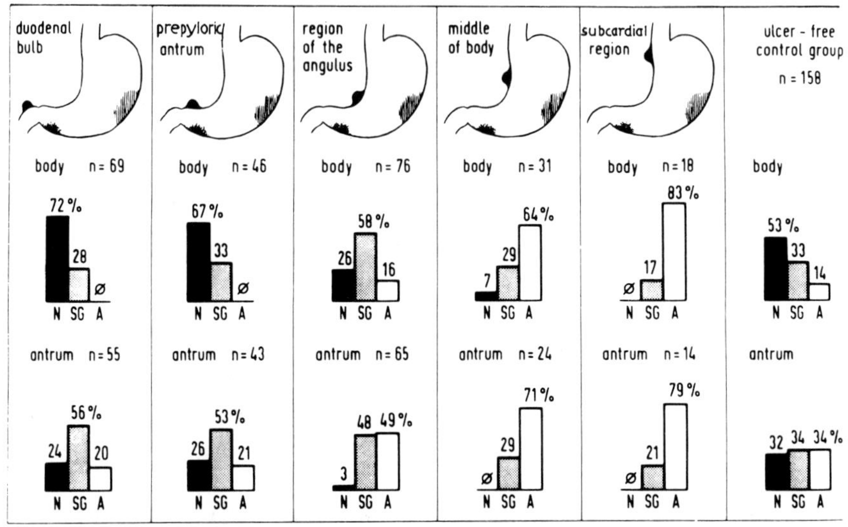

Fig. 1:   Correlation of mucosal histology obtained at gastroscopy and location of ulcer: body and antrum gastritis depending on the site of the ulcer. Reproduced with permission from [4], and the Universitetsforlaget.

endoscopy and radiology. It is generally stated that endoscopy is superior to radiology in the diagnosis of GU. Figures from the literature give a failure rate of 25–50% for radiology [5–8], with pathological findings being overlooked in about two-thirds of these cases (false-negative), and about one-third not being verified by endoscopy (false-positive) [8, 9]. But these findings must be evaluated in greater detail, and it has been found to be very difficult to prove this point [10], for various reasons.

Firstly, there has been a lack of prospective trials. A comparative trial should be prospective, but this has rarely been the case in GU studies [8]. Most trials are retrospective, with all the adherent problems of this kind of examination.

A second reason has been the heterogeneity of comparative trials. Many comparative trials of radiology and endoscopy have included all types of gastric and duodenal pathology, with GU being just one among other lesions. Therefore, the numbers of cases are usually small, and a special study on the efficacy of either method in the detection of GU alone has not been carried out, except for the diagnosis of ulcerative lesions in early cancer [11, 12].

A third problem has been the selection of patients. In several studies, patients underwent gastric radiology because of dyspeptic complaints with negative results, and gastroscopy was then performed. Others exhibited doubtful findings on radiology and were sent for endoscopy to clarify the diagnosis [13].

A further problem has been the lack of a reference method. If 2 methods are to be compared, there should be a reference method which is absolutely reliable. In the present case, this would mean surgery or autopsy, but this kind of comparison has been done only exceptionally [14].

There is also a great variability in the examiners' experience. Gastroscopy with the modern fiberscopes is a new method compared to X-ray examination. Therefore, in most trials an experienced endoscopist initiated the study. For comparison, routine roentgenograms were obtained from the X-ray department, and had been performed by various radiologists with varying experience [8, 11, 15].

Another variable is the time interval between radiological and endoscopic examination, which should be short but can be as long as weeks or even up to one month in the different studies [6, 15, 16], and is not mentioned at all in many reports.

Finally, if 2 methods are to be compared, this should be done under optimal conditions. This is usually the case for the modern fiberscopes, but not for the X-ray examination. The vast majority of studies were still performed as standard barium meals and did not employ the currently generally advocated double contrast barium meal [8, 11, 17, 18].

An example illustrating the importance of some of these points is given in the study of Moule et al. [8]. In this prospective study of 149 patients, gastroscopic results were compared to those obtained from routine barium meal and from double contrast barium meal performed by a single, experienced radiologist. In the first comparison there was a disagreement between the 2 methods of 49%, the discrepancy being highest in differentiating GU from cancer, with radiology being erroneous in 46%. In the second comparison the disagreement was 16%. Among the controversial diagnoses, one case of GU was not seen by the radiologist but diagnosed at gastroscopy, and 2 were described at radiology but not seen by the endoscopist. The question as to who was right and who wrong could not be settled, as none of the patients were operated upon or autopsied.

All in all, it is evident from the present data that it is hardly possible to prove objectively the superiority of either method. It would appear from studies on early cancer [11, 19] that both methods are equally efficient in the primary diagnosis of an ulcerative gastric lesion, but as the definitive diagnosis of cancer in a GU can only be made histologically, radiology has to be supplemented by guided biopsy.

Estimation of ulcer size and endoscopic criteria of ulcer healing in therapeutic trials

Although it is usually possible to measure the diameter of an ulcer in at least one direction, this seems to be most unreliable for estimating the exact surface area, and hence quantifying ulcer healing [20, 21].

Apart from new methods, such as that described in the previous paper (see pages 282–286), it must be postulated that complete ulcer healing should be taken as the final criterion of success or failure in a therapeutic trial, and not the diminution of ulcer size. Complete healing is defined as the ulcer being completely covered by gastric epithelium. It should be kept in mind, however, that malignant ulcers may also heal, as is seen below.

Differentiation of benign and malignant GU

The generally employed classification of malignant GU is that of the Japanese Society for Gastrointestinal Endoscopy (Fig. 2). The depressed types are the most common ones, accounting for about 80% of all early cancers. Among these, type IIc is the most frequent [22].

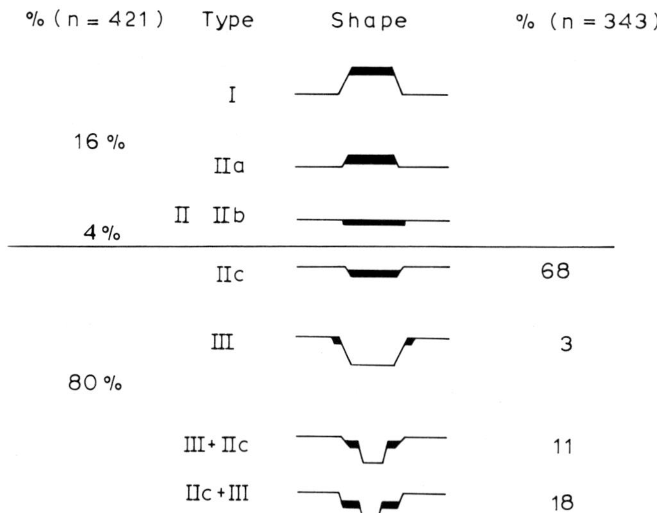

Fig. 2:   Classification of early gastric cancer and statistical distribution of various types. Reproduced with permission from [22].

Most malignant ulcers can be diagnosed macroscopically: the folds are rigid, there is narrowing at the tip, clubbing, fusion of folds and sudden break; the ulcer is irregularly shaped, and the ground is nodular. Sometimes, however, it is difficult or even impossible to differentiate between benign and malignant ulcer endoscopically, especially in type III early cancer. Therefore, endoscopic histology or cytology is of special importance. Most authors recommend taking 6–10 biopsies from the margin and the base, because the cancer may involve only parts of an ulcer (Fig. 3). In fact, it has been shown by Kasugai that the correct diagnosis can be made with 6–7 biopsies in nearly 100% of cases, but in only 75% if 3 biopsies are taken [23]. Other reasons for false-negative results may be that biopsy particles are small and the cancer may be missed if serial sections are not performed. Finally, it is sometimes impossible to biopsy all areas for technical reasons, or there may be cancer at one area of the wall only, or the ground may be covered by necrotic tissue. All this explains why there are a certain number of false-negative results. In a survey by Rösch, it was found to range from 2–46% (see Table), the higher values mostly dating back to the late sixties or early seventies [24]. With modern endoscopes, the percentage of false-negative results will be 10% or less.

Biopsy may be supplemented by guided brush cytology or by jet cytology. It is generally accepted that cytology adds to the accuracy of differentiating benign from malignant ulcer [24, 25]. However, because of the high diagnostic yield of guided biopsy, some authors have abandoned cytology [26]. Moreover, there are a certain number of false-positive results, in 1.8% of cases (n = 7,091), for cytology, which is only exceptional in the case of biopsy. Therefore, it seems reasonable to perform supplementary cytology if adequate biopsy is difficult for technical reasons or the diagnosis is in doubt.

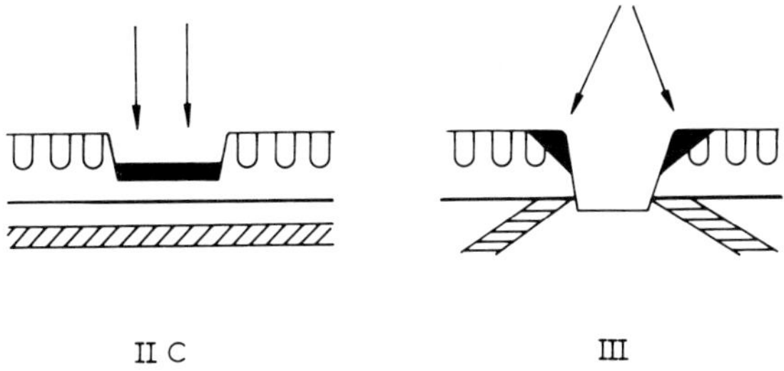

Fig. 3:   Sites of biopsies for diagnosis or exclusion of malignancy.

Table: Positive biopsy in early gastric cancer.

Author	Number of cases	Percentage positive
Okuda	232	98
Kasugai	126	96
Kobayashi	153	96
Shirakabe	63	95
Fukuchi	74	94
Yamakawa	55	93
Kawai	54	93
Yoshkatsu	115	92
Heinkel	37	92
Elster	78	91
Büttner	27	89
Stadelmann	16	88
Seifert	26	83
Sato	41	83
Figus	37	81
Fuchigami	66	79
Wiendl	24	64
Miller	1,099	54

Reproduced with permission from [24].

Healing of malignant ulcer

Endoscopy plays an important role in determining the healing of benign and malignant ulcers. It has been shown that malignant ulcers may heal completely, and the crater is epithelialized [26]. Sakita et al. observed significant healing in 51 out of 72 malignant GU, that is in 71% (Fig. 4; [27]). The authors summarized their interpretation of this phenomenon in the life cycle of malignant ulcer (Fig. 5). The malignant ulcer may begin as an ulceration in an area of mucosal cancer, or as malignant degeneration of the margin of the benign ulcer. An ulcer Type III (A) develops, which heals when benign tissue grows in from the margin (B). Next, the scar is again invaded by cancer or a fresh ulceration occurs, completing the life cycle of malignant ulcer. The growth of malignant tumors in the stomach is slow and, theoretically, this cycle could repeat itself several times.

As a consequence of these observations, it is recommended that biopsies should also be taken from healing ulcers and the scar [19]. Conditions for obtaining a positive biopsy may even be better when taking a biopsy from a scar than from the acute ulcer, because of the better correlation of cancer (black) with benign ulcer (Fig. 6).

Healing tendency of ulcer in early gastric cancer		Number of cases O : Intramucosal cancer, ● : Cancerous invasion limited to submucosal layer.	Total
Remarkable		○○○○○○○○○○○○ ●●●●●●	18
Appreciable		○○○○○○○○○○○○○ ○○○○○○○○○○○○○ ●●●●●●●●●●	33
No change	Open ulcer → Open ulcer	○○○○○○○○○○○○○ ●●●●●●●●	21
	Scar → Scar	○○○○○○○○○○○○○○○○○○ ○○○○○○○○○○○○○○ ○○○○ ●●●●●●●●●●●●●●	50
			122

Fig. 4:   Healing in early gastric cancer. Reproduced with permission from [27].

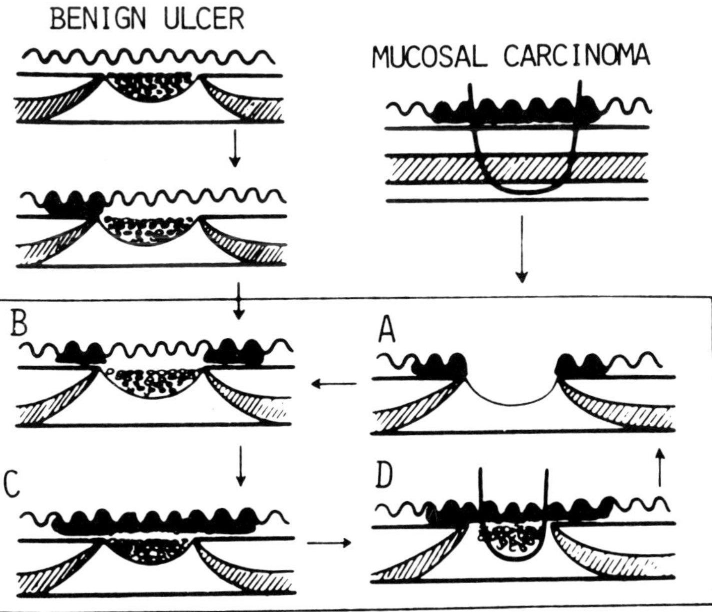

Fig. 5:   Life cycle of malignant ulcer. Reproduced with permission from [27].

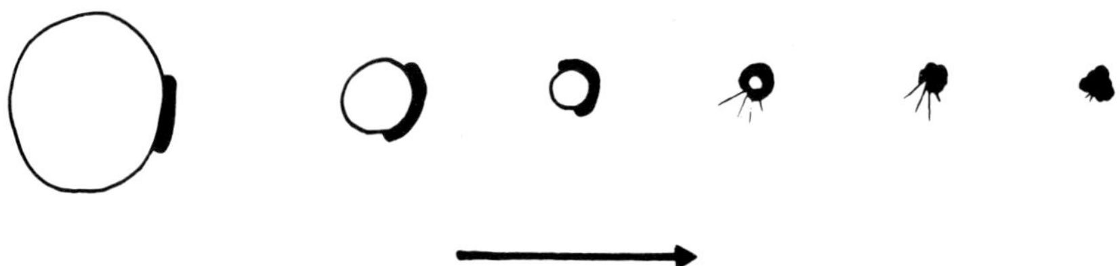

Fig. 6: *Relative increase of malignant area during ulcer healing. Reproduced with permission from [20].*

Summary

Superiority of endoscopy over barium meal with double contrast in the diagnosis of gastric ulcer (GU) cannot be proven because of a lack of comparable trials. Both methods seem to be similarly efficient in the primary diagnosis of an ulcerative gastric lesion. However, endoscopically guided biopsy has to supplement the macroscopic diagnosis in order to exclude cancer. Complete healing of GU only must be taken as proof of success in therapeutic trials, since estimations of diminution in ulcer size are unreliable. The most important role of endoscopy in regard to GU is in the differentiation of benign from malignant ulcer. Six to 10 biopsies from edge and base usually suffice to establish the correct diagnosis, with an accuracy of more than 90%. Malignant ulcers may diminish in size or even heal. Consequently, biopsies should be taken from healing ulcers and ulcer scars as well.

References

1. Johnson, H.D., Love, A.H.G., Rogers, N.C. and Wyatt, A.B. (1964): Gastric ulcer blood groups and acid secretion. *Gut 5*, 402.
2. Du Plessis, D.J. (1965): Pathogenesis of gastric ulceration. *Lancet I*, 974.
3. Oi, M., Yoshida, K. and Shugimura, S. (1959): The location of gastric ulcer. *Gastroenterology 36*, 45.
4. Stadelmann, O., Elster, K., Stolte, M. et al. (1971): The peptic gastric ulcer – histotopographic and functional investigations. *Scand. J. Gastroenterol. 6*, 613.
5. Cameron, A.J. and Ott, B.J. (1977): The value of gastroscopy in clinical diagnosis. A computer-assisted study. *Mayo Clin. Proc. 5*, 806.
6. Cotton, P.B. (1973): Fibreoptic endoscopy and the barium-meal results and implicatons. *Br. Med. J. 2*, 161.
7. Laufer, I., Mullens, J.E. and Hamilton, J. (1975): The diagnostic accuracy of barium studies of the stomach and duodenum – correlation with endoscopy. *Radiology 115*, 569.

8. Moule, B., Cochrane, K.M., Sokhi, G.S. et al. (1975): A comparative study of the diagnostic value of upper gastrointestinal endoscopy and radiography. *Gut 16*, 411.

9. Nelson, R.S., Urrea, L.B. and Lanza, F.L. (1976): Evaluation of gastric ulcerations. *Am. J. Dig. Dis. 21*, 389.

10. Ewe, K. and Farack, U. (1978): Magendiagnostik: Endoskopie statt Röntgen? *Med. Klin. 73*, 1409.

11. Mountford, R.A., Brown, P., Salmon, P.R. et al. (1980): Gastric cancer detection in gastric ulcer disease. *Gut 21, 9*.

12. Shirakabe, H., Nishizawa, M., Hayakawa, H. and Maruyama, M. (1973): Röntgenologisch-endoskopische Diagnostik des Magenfrühcarcinoms. *Leber Magen Darm 3*, 60.

13. Barnes, R.J., Gear, M.W.L., Nicol, A. and Dew, A.B. (1974): Study of dyspepsia in a general practice as assessed by endoscopy and radiology. *Br. Med. J. 4*, 214.

14. Jensen, S.K., Elsborg, L. and Andersen, D. (1976): The diagnostic value of endoscopy and X-ray examination in gastroduodenal disease. *Aktuel. Gastroenterol. 5*, 339.

15. Renner, M., Böttger, E., Adolphs, H.-P. and Manegold, B.-C. (1974): Vergleichende Untersuchung über die Diagnosemöglichkeiten der Radiologie und Endoskopie bei Erkrankungen des Magens und des Duodenums. *Fortschr. Röntgenstr. 121*, 744.

16. Rogers, I.M., Moule, B., Sokhi, G.S. et al. (1976): Endoscopy and routine and double contrast barium meal in diagnosis of gastric and duodenal disorders. *Lancet I*, 901.

17. Herlinger, H., Glanville, J.N. and Kreel, L. (1977): An evaluation of the double contrast barium meal against endoscopy. *Clin. Radiol. 28*, 307.

18. Treichel, H. and Oeser, H. (1975): Die Doppelkontrastmethode: Optimale Technik der röntgenologischen Magenuntersuchung. *Dtsch. Med. Wochenschr. 100*, 2226.

19. Ichikawa, H. (1973): Differential diagnosis between benign and malignant ulcers. *Clin. Gastroenterol. 2*, 329.

20. Classen, M., Dancygier, H. and Fuchs, H.F. (1980): Endoscopy in the diagnosis of duodenal ulcer: This publication, pp. 282–286.

21. Sonnenberg, A., Gieger, M., Kern, L. et al. (1979): How reliable is determination of ulcer size by endoscopy? *Br. Med. J. 2*, 1322.

22. Sakita, T. (1973): Endoscopy in the diagnosis of early ulcer cancer. *Clin. Gastroenterol. 2*, 345.

23. Kasugai, T. (1968): Gastric lavage cytology and biopsy for early gastric cancer under direct vision of the fiberscope. *Gastrointest. Endosc. 14*, 205.

24. Rösch, W. (1976): Diagnose und Prognose des Magenfrühkarzinoms. In: *Ergebnisse der Gastroenterologie*, pp. 128–136. Eds: U. Ritter and M. Classen. Karl Demeter Verlag, Gräfelfing.

25. Witte, S. (1978): *Magencytologie. Gastroenterolg. Kompendium 5*. G. Witzstrock Verlag, Baden-Baden.

26. Murakami, T., Yasui, A. and Takekawa, H. (1966): Non cancerous regenerated area at the center of ulcer-cancer. *Trans. Soc. Pathol. Jpn. 55*, 229.

27. Sakita, T., Oguro, Y., Takasu, S. et al. (1971): Observations on the healing of ulcerations in early gastric cancer. *Gastroenterology 60*, 835.

Discussion

Pathophysiology

The first 2 papers included in this Chapter have dealt with aspects of the pathophysiological disturbances found in some patients with peptic ulcers, especially with the point that only some, and usually the minority, of patients with peptic ulcers have these functional abnormalities. Most patients with ulcers respond to test situations like 'control' individuals, but that is perhaps because the tests are too crude and nonspecific and also because we do not know who has, or is going to have, an ulcer in an apparently normal population, so that 'control' does not mean 'nonulcer' for the purpose of population studies.

The other problem concerns the actual significance of the pathophysiological disturbances that have been found. Do they represent epiphenomena, like color of eyes, that may be used as convenient and perhaps even genetic labels but are of no etiological significance? Alternatively, are these disturbances of function primarily involved in the etiology of ulcer disease, or even secondarily in that they represent functional reactions which, in turn, aggravate the underlying ulcer? If the answer to either possibility in the latter question is affirmative, then clearly the pathophysiological abnormalities of function must be corrected by treatment.

There remains, theoretically, a third possibility − that the pathophysiological disturbances are in some manner a 'protective' reaction to the underlying mucosal ulceration. If the latter were the case, we should not try to correct the observed functional abnormalities but should concentrate more on healing the ulcers or correcting the primary abnormalities.

In summary, we must distinguish between pathophysiological disturbances of function and etiological bases of ulceration, since these 2 aspects of ulcer disease may not be synonymous.

Symptoms

The reliability of classic symptoms as indicators of ulcer disease and the value of endoscopy in diagnosing gastric and duodenal ulcer, and in following up their healing process during therapy were discussed. The difficulty in assessing ulcer symptoms as indicators of active ulcer disease is in part due to the lack of prospective data defining in large populations the predictive value of true ulcer symptoms and ulcer-like symptoms. The most reliable symptoms to discriminate duodenal ulcer disease from dyspepsia are night pain and a duration of pain greater than 3 years. Relief by food is a specific symptom for duodenal ulcer disease but is only present in 20% of the patients [1]. In contrast, relief of symptoms by antacids does not discriminate between the different forms of dyspepsias. Relief of symptoms by antacids has been documented in patients with peptic ulcer as well as in patients with gastric carcinoma or 'functional' dyspepsia [1]. Blum et al. analyzed the specificity and sensitivity in detecting ulcer disease in 876 hospitalized patients of different age groups with and without associated diseases [2]. Ulcer symptoms were present in 52% of patients with active duodenal ulcer below the age of 60, and in 27% of those above the age of 60. The respective figures for gastric ulcers were 26% for both age groups. In the presence of associated diseases, ulcer symptoms were noted even less frequently; even so, active ulcers were documented by upper endoscopy. It would seem therefore that the incidence of ulcer symptoms would depend on the absence of associated disease and on the age of patients. Furthermore, the presence of ulcer-like symptoms may even more frequently be associated with duodenal scarring than with an active ulcer [3]. The results of these studies indicate that the 'data base' for classifying ulcer disease on the basis of symptoms may well be insufficient.

It is tempting to speculate that some of the discrepancies reported about the effect of drugs on ulcer symptoms may be due to difficulties in discriminating between ulcer symptoms and dyspeptic symptoms of other causes based on the standard description of these diseases in textbooks. Future trials investigating the effect of the patients' symptoms should not only consider the fact that many so-called ulcer symptoms are not very reliable markers of ulcer disease but also make an attempt in determining the 'observer error' when classifying symptoms and relief of symptoms. The knowledge of the degree of concordance between ulcers and symptoms would be valuable in conducting epidemiological studies.

Diagnosis

In regard to the role of endoscopy there was general agreement that endoscopy is the procedure of choice in determining the presence and the healing of an ulcer. Even when double-contrast barium meal is used the potential accuracy of this method in detecting gastric or duodenal ulcers was shown to be 96% of that accorded to fiber endoscopy [4]. The assessments were done with both techniques by experienced specialists in their respective fields. Since there is marked intra- and interobserver variation in determining ulcer size by conventional methods, only complete ulcer healing should be assessed as the end point when drug efficacy is tested in clinical trials. The newly designed electronic planimeter (see paper by Classen et al., pages 282–286) will need further testing in a larger number of patients with gastric or duodenal ulcer. It was suggested that comparative measurements of ulcer size in patients immediately prior to surgery and in the excised gastric specimens should be undertaken to assess the accuracy of this method.

If endoscopy is accepted as the 'gold standard' for diagnosing peptic ulcers, certain criteria will need to be fulfilled in clinical trials. Endoscopy should be carried out by experienced examiners in a standardized fashion using instruments with prograde and side-viewing optics. The observer error should be assessed by 2-independent investigators, especially when changes like mucosal redness, etc. are recorded [5]. The presence of the ulcer and changes in the surrounding mucosa should be documented by photography and by biopsies taken from different parts of the lesion including the scar following a prospectively designed protocol to allow an independent review of the findings by different examiners in multicenter trials.

The relevance of duodenitis was briefly touched upon. There was general agreement that duodenitis may be diagnosed by endoscopic findings like edema with thickened mucosal folds, reddening of the mucosa, petechial hemorrhages, and erosions. These findings should be confirmed histologically. There is marked observer variation in the interpretation of subtle mucosal changes [5]. It is still controversial whether duodenitis can cause symptoms and the importance of excluding other causes of the patients' complaint does not need to be emphasized. From the data available it is unclear whether duodenitis is part of the spectrum of duodenal ulcer disease [6, 7]. Prospective long-term studies are required in patients with duodenitis and in patients being at risk for developing duodenal ulcer disease (patients with hyperpepsinogenemia I) to determine the natural history of this disease and its relationship to duodenal ulcer disease.

References

1. Horrocks, J.C. and de Dombal, F.T. (1978): Clinical presentation of patients with 'dyspepsia'. *Gut 19*, 19.
2. Hess, H., Würsch, T.G., Killer-Walser, R. et al (1980): How often does peptic ulcer produce 'typical' ulcer symptoms? *Hepato-Gastroenterol. 27*, 57.
3. Frühmorgen, P., Jenny, S., Classen, M. et al. (1972): Anamnese bei Ulkus und Narben im Bulbus duodeni. *Dtsch. Med. Wochenschr. 97*, 188.

4. Herlinger, H., Glanville, J.N. and Kreel, L. (1977): An evaluation of the double contrast barium meal (DCBM) against endoscopy. *Clin. Radiol. 28*, 307.
5. Holden, R.J. and Crean, G.P. (1977): Assessment of observer error in upper gastrointestinal endoscopy. *Gut 18*, 941.
6. Joffe, S.N., Lee, F.D. and Blumgart, L.H. (1978): Duodenitis. *Clin. Gastroenterol. 7*, 635.
7. Tweedle, D.E.F. and Ravenscroft, M.M. (1979): Duodenitis. *Gut 20*, 434.

Chapter V: Medical treatment of ulcer disease

Goals of medical therapy in ulcer disease

K.-H. Holtermüller
I. Medizinische Klinik und Poliklinik, Johannes Gutenberg-Universität, Mainz, Federal Republic of Germany

Introduction

The decision to treat any kind of disease has to take into account the following factors: the natural history of the disease to be treated; the influence of therapy on the course of the disease; and the risks and benefits of the therapy chosen. Knowledge of the natural history allows definition of specific therapeutic aims and prospective assessment of the efficacy of the treatment chosen.

Natural history of ulcer disease

It has been claimed that one in 5 Europeans is afflicted at some time in his life by ulcer disease. The incidence of gastric ulcer is reported to be 0.35/1,000 and for duodenal ulcer 2.85/1,000 [1]. Ulcer disease is characterized by a high rate of spontaneous remissions and a marked tendency to relapses. The half-life of ulcers (that is, the time which is necessary to achieve a 50% size reduction) has been reported to be 1.7 weeks for gastric ulcer and 1.9 weeks for duodenal ulcer in a prospective study to determine spontaneous healing [2]. The long-term course of ulcer disease has also been investigated in a few well-documented studies. Both gastric ulcer and duodenal ulcer are characterized by the high incidence of recurrence (Tables I and II) [3–8]. Due to failure of medical therapy, surgery was necessary in 16–39% of the patients in the past, but there are no data to support the theory that elective surgery is likely to reduce the mortality of duodenal ulcer disease by preventing future fatal complications. Rather, the mortality associated with operation is likely to be as great as the mortality from the disease itself. A recent study [9] analyzing ulcer-specific deaths and using an actuarial analysis of life expectancy showed that ulcer disease does influence survival. The 9-year cumulated risk

Table I: Natural history of gastric ulcer disease.

Study*	Number of patients			Recurrences (%)		Gastric surgery (%)	
	Total	Males	Females	Males	Females	Males	Females
Krause (25 years)	247	134	113	67.9	61.9	38.1	27.4
Fry (15 years)	53	28	25	68	74	18	20
Krag (17–27 years)	58	38	20	76	50	22**	
Littman (2 years)	638	638		42		11	

*   Figures in parentheses refer to length of follow-up observations.
** Males + females.

Table II: Natural history of duodenal ulcer disease.

Study*	Number of patients			Recurrences (%)		Gastric surgery (%)	
	Total	Males	Females	Males	Females	Males	Females
Krause (25 years)	349	258	91	88.7	83.5	57.4	53.8
Fry (15 years)	212	176	36	45	41	16	14
Krag (15–27 years)	251	190	61	74	57	39**	

*   Figures in parentheses refer to length of follow-up observations.
** Males + females.

of dying from peptic ulcer is 1.8%. This increase in deaths is small and was only present in the first 1 or 2 years after diagnosis. The life expectancy was not significantly different for men and women. No increase in deaths was found in patients who were under the age of 50 years at diagnosis [9].

Goals of therapy

The natural history of ulcer disease reviewed above forms the basis for the definition of therapeutic goals in ulcer disease.

Pain relief and the speeding of ulcer healing are the goals of therapy in ulcer exacerbation. This exacerbation, which is usually of short duration, will be referred to as 'ulcer activity', clinically recognized as an episode of gastric or duodenal ulcer with a characteristic pain pattern. It has to be realized that endoscopically-proven ulcer craters may occur without associated symptoms. Although the definition of 'ulcer activity', as given above, will not cover the entity of painless ulcer, it nevertheless may be useful in the decision-making process of daily clinical practice and might facilitate the evaluation of the therapeutic efficacy of drugs used in the treatment of patients with duodenal or gastric ulcer.

In contrast to ulcer activity 'ulcer disease' refers to repetitive cycles of ulcer recurrence with clinical symptoms, and a tendency to develop ulcer complications with increasing duration of the disease. Control of ulcer activity, with pain relief and the speeding of healing, is only one of the goals of therapy. The medical treatment of ulcer disease additionally requires the prevention of recurrences and complications, thereby influencing the natural course of the disease entity 'peptic ulcer' (Table III).

In the following sections, objective evaluation of the specific therapeutic aims will be discussed. Furthermore, criteria should be established for clinical studies in order to define the requirements for a therapy altering the natural history of ulcer disease.

Pain relief

Periodic epigastric pain, occurring with a regular food-related rhythm, and nocturnal pain are considered typical ulcer-like symptoms [10]. For patients below the age of 60 years with endoscopically proven duodenal or gastric ulcers, these symptoms were present in 52% and in 26%, respectively. For

Table III: Goals of ulcer therapy.

Relief of pain Speeding of ulcer healing	Influence on ulcer activity
Prevention of complications Prevention of ulcer recurrences	Influence on ulcer disease

patients over 60 years of age with endoscopically proven duodenal or gastric ulcer, typical symptoms were present in 27% and in 26%, respectively. The presence of associated diseases further decreased the incidence of ulcer-like symptoms [11]. From such results it can be concluded that the ulcer-like symp-

Table IV: Comparison of 'spontaneous' ulcer healing with healing under medical therapy (antacids, carbenoxolone, pirenzepine, colloidal bismuth).

Drug	Country	Number of patients	Percentage of ulcers healed after 4 weeks of therapy	
			Placebo	Barbipyrine
Antacid	U.S.A.	16	50	100
Antacid	U.S.A.	74	45	78
Antacid	Germany	45	73	100
Carbenoxolone	England	46	27	45
Carbenoxolone	England	34	22	69
Carbenoxolone	Germany	360	55	70
Pirenzepine	Germany	36	55	94
Colloidal bismuth	England	20	36	91

Table V: Comparison of 'spontaneous' ulcer healing with healing under medical therapy (anticholinergics, cimetidine).

Drug	Country	Number of patients	Percentage of ulcers healed after 4 weeks of therapy	
			Placebo	Barbipyrine
Anticholinergics	Australia	40	25	55
Anticholinergics	U.S.A.	30	57	81 (NS)*
Cimetidine	Germany/ Switzerland	78	58	79
Cimetidine	Germany	67	79	88 (NS)
Cimetidine	France	53	37	69
Cimetidine	England	89	29	63/76**
Cimetidine	Norway	42	60	85 (NS)
Cimetidine	Scotland	40	25	85
Cimetidine	Sweden	44	17	67*
Cimetidine	U.S.A.	178	47	56 (NS)

* Percentage healed after 3 weeks.
** 63% healing with cimetidine 1,000 mg/day; 76% healing with cimetidine 2,000 mg/day.
NS = not significant.

toms described above indicate ulcer disease with a high specificity (96%) but a low sensitivity (23%) [11].

Scientific evaluation of the symptom 'ulcer pain' and documentation of the relief of pain by a chosen treatment requires reproducibility of the method used to measure pain. The assumption implicit in clinical trials, as in many other kinds of research, is that the sample with which one is working can be defined well, and that the methods can be clearly described so that others may confirm the observations [12].

In order to evaluate a symptom like pain, objectively, it is necessary that more than one investigator classifies the pain as 'ulcer-like', and that the degree of concordance is defined. Furthermore, the severity of symptoms will need to be graded on a measuring scale and agreement as to the degree of pain may be evaluated in a similar way. This might be one way of determining whether the clinical method of assessing pain is a reproducible 'measuring device'.

An unpredictably large number of placebo responses not identifiable in advance, as well as the group refractory to treatment, combine to greatly reduce the sensitivity of the experiment. This sort of predicament is known as the type II, or Beta, error − a failure of an experiment to demonstrate a difference between treatments when such a difference does exist to a meaningful degree. Statistical evaluation of clinical trials requires that type-I error (risk of a false-positive result) and type-II error (risk of a false-negative result) can be calculated from the data. The absence of calculated or calculable type-II error in a randomized clinical trial may well make the study useless [12].

Furthermore, the evaluation of pain relief must also measure the impact of an individual physician's method of counseling on the patient's response to medical therapy of ulcer disease. Sarles et al. showed that, in the same ulcer population, different physicians can influence the patient's response to medical therapy to a different degree, as measured in days with pain after starting therapy [13]. These data further show that on the patient's part there is an expectation of pain relief while receiving medical therapy. This expectation, which is not directly related to the physician, will certainly modify the affective response of the patient.

Critical assessment of pain relief as a goal of therapy   An objective assessment of pain relief, if possible at all, requires determination of the observer error, measurement of the placebo effect of the physician, and evaluation of the affective response of the patient. Most clinical trials have not considered these factors and some conclusions drawn about the efficacy of drugs in regard to pain relief could be misleading. The patient with ulcer disease is primarily interested in a symptomatic improvement; the relief of pain is thus an important goal of ulcer therapy. Symptomatic improvement is not, however, necessarily paralleled by ulcer healing [14]. Any effective medical treatment of ulcer activity and ulcer disease has therefore to promote healing as well as to relieve ulcer symptoms if these symptoms are typical for ulcer activity.

Some studies have shown that pain relief can be achieved equally well by placebo or barbipyrine [15, 16]. Failure of antacids to produce either consistent marked relief of pain or significantly better relief than placebo indicates that factors other than acid neutralization are important in the acute relief of pain.

Healing of ulcers

Speeding of ulcer healing, prevention of complications and pain relief are the major goals in the treatment of ulcer diseases. A clearly defined end-point is necessary if studies are to be comparable.

We suggest that only complete endoscopic healing of a crater should be used. Since the healing rate of an ulcer depends also on the initial size of the ulcer, a sufficiently large number of patients must be included in clinical trials in order to come to meaningful conclusions. We do not recommend measurements of ulcer size, especially that of duodenal ulcer, since the accuracy and reproducibility of endoscopically assessed ulcer size has not been examined in the therapeutic trials published to date [12]. In a recent study determining the reproducibility of endoscopic measurements of the surface area of artificial ulcers in a rubber manikin, 80% of the measurements underestimated the true size of the ulcer: the mean ($\pm$ SD) underestimation was $-29 \pm 40\%$. The largest and the smallest estimate of the same ulcer by different endoscopists varied on average by a factor of 4.5 ± 3.8 [17]. In a group of artificial ulcers of identical size, the smallest estimate differed from the largest estimate by a mean factor of 2.3 ± 0.6, showing that the endoscopists not only understimated the ulcer size but were inconsistent in their estimations. These studies demonstrate that estimation of ulcer size by endoscopy is very inaccurate [17]. The results thus confirm our recommendation that in therapeutic ulcer trials it is advisable not to use changes in ulcer size as an index of the effect of anti-ulcer drugs, but instead to use only complete healing of the ulcer as criterion of drug efficacy [12]. This on its own may be difficult, because the macroscopical aspects of an ulcer site (persisting duodenitis, erosions) do not always allow an assessment of whether an ulcer is completely healed, but errors are less likely to occur than with a method which gives a false impression of scientific accuracy.

Recently published trials of ulcer therapy document differing placebo healing rates (Tables IV and V) [14, 18–35]. This placebo healing rate is not a true placebo healing rate, since ancillary treatments (antacids, bed rest, etc.) have not been standardized. Furthermore, the different responses could also be attributed to the known heterogeneity of ulcer disease [36]. A number of abnormalities have now been identified in many patients with duodenal ulcer, namely abnormalities of secretory response, gastrin response to a meal, and gastric emptying – all of which suggest heterogeneity. It is tempting to speculate that the therapeutic response of duodenal ulcer disease may be influenced by the heterogeneity of ulcer disease. However, the clinical trials differ in patient selection, patient characteristics, group size, follow-up period and ancillary treatment [37]. The standardization of these factors will make clinical trials more comparable and their results can then be applied to a general patient population. It would be naive, however, to believe that controlled trials will remove the disagreement among experts concerning therapy. In order for one treatment to be clearly superior to another, it is necessary that its expected utility be greater for alle possible patients.

Critical assessment of the promotion of ulcer healing as a goal of therapy The healing of ulcers and the speeding of this healing process are 2 of the goals of ulcer therapy. Since medical therapy only hastens ulcer healing, which means a more rapid closure of a mucosal defect, we have to assume that such a complication of ulcer disease as scarring will occur with unaltered frequency. An increase in healing rate will not prevent this complication, which can only be avoided by a cure of ulcer disease.

The risk of such complications as bleeding or perforation in a primarily un-complicated episode of ulcer activity is low. Expressing the risk of such com-plications as bleeding, perforation and obstruction in terms of patients at risk over a period of 2 years, the rate was 4% [7]. This incidence may be higher in untreated patients, since in the Veterans Administration Study [6, 7], patients with complications were excluded at entry, and possibly because the demon-stration of radiographic healing had been required for entry into the group at risk.

It is important to recognize that a short-term therapy of ulcer activity has so far not been proven to have an advantage for the patient, except for accelerat-ing the healing of the ulcer and providing a partial symptomatic relief.

Prevention of ulcer recurrences and complications

It is not known which factors are responsible for periodic recurrences of ulcer disease. Healing of ulcer activity is of little avail if recurrences and complications are not obviated by the treatment chosen. The major goal of medical therapy should be that of altering the long-term course of the disease.

The rate of ulcer recurrence has been reported to be between 42% and 88%. In more recent prospective studies, the recurrence rates for duodenal ulcer have been given as 80–83% [8, 38]. During a one-year observation of the results of placebo treatment in patients with ulcer disease of long duration, 33% had 2 recurrences per year. Selective proximal vagotomy was recommended to 50% of the placebo-treated patients because of repeated relapses or intractable symptoms during the relapse [38]. The presence of recurrence is indicated by ulcer symptoms in only about 75% [39].

The incidence of complications in terms of patients at risk has been reported to be between 4% and 11% per year, depending on the patient population studied [7, 38]. In long-term studies, the incidence of such complications as perforation was 5.6% and of bleeding 21% (gastric ulcer) and 25% (duodenal ulcer) over a follow-up period of 17–27 years [5]. Studies in outpatients report a complication rate over 15 years of 14% for bleeding and 6% for perforation [4]. In this regard it should be noted that 40% of the patients in whom bleeding developed during the observation period also had hematemesis or melena on first admission [5].

The intensity of ulcer disease should be analyzed by cumulative assessment or by separate assessment of each 5-year period. The intensity of the ulcer disease is greatest during the first few years after diagnosis and then decreases, but only after 15–20 years does it adjust to a more or less constant level [5].

If a meaningful statement about long-term results of therapy is to be made, a minimum of 5 years of observation is required. The possibility of preventing relapses and complications does not solely depend on the availability of effective drugs for ulcer therapy, but also on the side effects of the compounds used. This factor will also influence the decision as to whether surgical therapy, despite its risk, will be given preference over medical therapy.

The efficacy of medical ulcer therapy can be measured by its effectiveness to reduce the incidence of recurrences and complications. Because of the frequency of relapses it is easy to determine whether a treatment will fulfill this criterion. Furthermore, an effective medical treatment should lower mortality and decrease the rate of elective surgery. Since an increase in deaths from ulcer disease has only been documented in patients older than 50 years it will be very difficult to prove an influence of therapy on this factor. Effective therapy should, however, also reduce the rate of hospitalization.

Socioeconomic influence of therapy

A further important factor to be considered is the socioeconomic impact of ulcer disease. This economic impact has 3 components: the direct costs of the resources diverted to medical care of the disease; the indirect costs resulting from loss of individual productivity due to disability caused by the disease; and the indirect costs resulting from the loss of future productivity of individuals whose death is attributed to the disease. The estimated cost of peptic ulcer disease in 1963 in the U.S.A. was 1,005 million dollars, representing 12.8% of the total cost of digestive disease [40]. These costs of ulcer disease should be markedly decreased by an effective medical treatment. Such parameters as the number of patients off work, the total number of days off work, insurance expenses, etc., can be measured objectively and must be taken into consideration when the therapeutic goals are defined. Future studies should also document the socioeconomic impact of treatment as well as the influence of therapy on ulcer activity and ulcer disease.

Conclusions

The goals listed in Table VI should be influenced by an effective treatment of ulcer disease. The strict criteria established for randomized clinical trials [37] and the observation of the therapeutic goals will enable the drawing of conclusions which can be applied to future patients. Results of a well-designed study with clearly defined therapeutic goals will influence the decision-making process of physicians. Based on inductive inference of conclusions the physician will make decisions concerning the therapy to be chosen. This process can effectively change the therapeutic approach to a disease, as evidenced by the study of chronic active hepaptitis [41]. The cure of ulcer disease is the ultimate aim of surgical and medical therapy. Further

Table VI: Goals of ulcer therapy: parameters which should be influenced by effective treatment.

1.	To lower mortality
2.	To decrease the number of elective gastric operations
3.	To influence the duration of convalescence and of the time off work
4.	To decrease the need for hospitalization
5.	To lower the rate of recurrences and prevent relapses
6.	To speed ulcer healing
7.	To achieve pain relief
8.	To have no serious side effects in comparison to current medical therapy

investigations will be necessary to decide whether this aim can be achieved by some regimen of nonsurgical therapy.

Summary

The natural course of chronic ulcer disease is marked by cycles of remissions and exacerbations. In patients with peptic ulcer an acute exacerbation is defined as ulcer activity, presenting with pain and a mucosal lesion. The goals of therapy in ulcer activity are therefore alleviation of pain and healing of the ulcer. Ulcer disease is characterized by relapses and complications, and their prevention will alter the natural course of the disease. Ulcer disease, like any chronic disease, will generate costs by diverting resources to medical care of the disease and through loss of productivity due to disability. Any form of effective treatment must lower these costs. Thus, the efficacy of ulcer therapy should be evaluated by the following parameters: lowering mortality, decreasing the number of elective gastric operations, decreasing the incidence of relapses and complications, diminishing the need for hospitalization, shortening the time for convalescence, promoting ulcer healing and achieving pain relief.

References

1. Monson, R.R. and MacMahon, B. (1969): Peptic ulcer in Massachusetts physicians. *N. Engl. J. Med. 281*, 11.
2. Scheurer, U., Witzel, L., Halter, F. et al. (1977): Gastric and duodenal ulcer healing and placebo treatment. *Gastroenterology 72*, 838.
3. Krause, U. (1963): Long term results of medical and surgical treatment of peptic ulcer. *Acta Chir. Scand. (Sup.) 310*, 1.
4. Fry, J. (1964): Peptic ulcer: a profile. *Br. Med. J. 2*, 809.
5. Krag, E. (1966): Long term prognosis in medically treated peptic ulcer. *Acta Med. Scand. 180*, 657.
6. Littman, A. (1971): The Veterans Administration Cooperative Study on Gastric Ulcer. *Gastroenterology 61*, 567.
7. Hanscom, D.H. and Buchman, E. (1971): The follow-up period. *Gastroenterology 61*, 585.
8. Gudmand-Høyer, E., Birger-Jensen, K., Krag, E. et al. (1978): Prophylactic effect of cimetidine in duodenal ulcer disease. *Br. Med. J. 1*, 1095.
9. Bonnevie, O. (1978): Survival in peptic ulcer. *Gastroenterology 75*, 1055.
10. Earlam, R. (1976): A computerized questionnaire analysis of duodenal ulcer symptoms. *Gastroenterology 71*, 314.
11. Blum, A.L., Sonnenberg, A., Hess, H. et al. (1978): Ulcer like symptoms are specific but not sensitive signs of ulcer disease (Abstract). *Gastroenterology 74*, 1116.
12. Holtermüller, K.-H. (1978): Therapieziele beim peptischen Ulcus. In: *Ulcusthera-*

pie, 1st edition, Chapter 21, pp. 256–268. Eds: A.L. Blum and J.R. Siewert. Springer Verlag, Berlin-Heidelberg-New York.

13. Sarles, H., Camatte, R. and Sahel, J. (1977): A study of the variations in the response regarding duodenal ulcer when treated with placebo by different investigators. *Digestion 16*, 289.

14. Peterson, W.L., Sturdevant, R.A.L., Frankl, H.D. et al. (1977): Healing of duodenal ulcer with an antacid regimen. *N. Engl. J. Med. 297*, 341.

15. Sturdevant, R.A.L., Isenberg, J.I., Secrist, D. and Ansfield, D. (1977): Antacid and placebo produced similar pain relief in duodenal ulcer patients. *Gastroenterology 72*, 1.

16. Littman, A., Welch, R., Fruin, R.C. and Aronson, A.R. (1977): Controlled trials of aluminium hydroxide gels for peptic ulcer. *Gastroenterology 73*, 6.

17. Sonnenberg, A., Giger, M., Kern, L. et al. (1979): How reliable is determination of ulcer size by endoscopy? *Br. Med. J. 2*, 1322.

18. Hollander, D. and Harlan, J. (1973): Antacids vs placebo in peptic ulcer therapy. *J. Am. Med. Assoc., 226*, 1181.

19. Kunert, H. and Ottenjann, R. (1979): Effekt eines Mg-Al-hydroxid-haltigen Antazidums auf die Heilungsdauer von Ulcera duodeni – randomisierte Doppelblindstudie. *Z. Gastroenterol. 27*, 630.

20. Hampel, K.E., Billich, C., Dannenmeier, H.D. et al. (1972): Therapie des Ulcus ventriculi et Ulcus duodeni mit Carbenoxolon-Natrium (Doppelblindversuch). *Münch. Med. Wochenschr. 114*, 925.

21. Gheorghiu, Th., Frotz, H. and Dole, A. (1975): The therapeutic effect of carbenoxolone in duodenal ulcer. Preliminary analysis of a multi-centre double blind trial. In: *Fourth Symposium on carbenoxolone*, pp. 1–255. Eds: F. Avery Jones and D.V. Parke. Butterworth, London.

22. Doll, R., Hill, I.D. and Hutton, F.C. (1965): Treatment of gastric ulcer with carbenoxolone sodium and oestrogens. *Gut 6*, 19.

23. Davies, W.A. and Reed, P.I. (1977): Controlled trial of Duogastrone in duodenal ulcer. *Gut 18*, 78.

24. Ludwig, H. (1977): Behandlung von Ulcus ventriculi und Ulcus duodeni mit LS 519 – eine Doppelblindstudie. *Therapiewoche 27*, 1664.

25. Salmon, P.R., Brown, P., Williams, R. and Read, H.E. (1974): Evaluation of colloidal bismuth (DeNol) in the treatment of duodenal ulcer employing endoscopic selection and follow up. *Gut 15*, 189.

26. Baume, P.E., Hunt, J.H. and Piper, D.W. (1972): Glycopyronium bromide in the treatment of chronic gastric ulcer. *Gastroenterology 63*, 399.

27. Bowers, J., Forbes, J. and Freston, J. (1977): Effect of nighttime anisotropine methylbromide (AMB) on duodenal ulcer (DU) healing: a controlled trial. *Gastroenterology 62*, 6.

28. Peter, P., Kiene, K., Gonvers, J.J. et al. (1978): Cimetidin in der Behandlung des Ulcus duodeni. *Dtsch. Med. Wochenschr. 103*, 1163.

29. Malchow, H., Sewing, K.-Fr., Albinus, M. et al. (1978): Cimetidin in der stationären Behandlung des peptischen Ulkus. I. Wirkung auf die Heilung des Ulcus duodeni. *Dtsch. Med. Wochenschr. 103*, 149.

30. Gillespie, G., Gray, G.R., Smith, I.S. et al. (1977): Short term and maintenance treatment in severe duodenal ulceration. In: *Cimetidine. Proceedings of the Second International Symposium on Histamine H_2-Receptor Antagonists*, pp.

240–247. Eds: W.L. Burland and M.A. Simkins. Excerpta Medica, Amsterdam-Oxford.

31. Semb, L.S., Berstad, A., Myren, J. et al. (1977): A double blind multicenter comparative study of cimetidine and placebo in short term treatment of active duodenal ulceration. In: *Cimetidine. Proceedings of the Second International Symposium on Histamine H₂-Receptor Antagonists*, pp. 248–253. Eds: W.L. Burland and M.A. Simkins. Excerpta Medica, Amsterdam-Oxford.

32. Multicentre trial (1977): The effect of cimetidine on duodenal ulceration. In: *Cimetidine. Proceedings of the Second International Symposium on Histamine H₂-Receptor Antagonists*, pp. 260–271. Eds: W.L. Burland and M.A. Simkins. Excerpta Medica, Amsterdam-Oxford.

33. Multicentre trial (1977): Treatment of gastric ulcer by cimetidine. In: *Cimetidine. Proceedings of the Second International Symposium on Histamine H₂-Receptor Antagonists*, pp. 287–292. Eds: W.L. Burland and M.A. Simkins. Excerpta Medica, Amsterdam-Oxford.

34. Binder, H.J., Cocco, A., Crossley, R.J. et al. (1978): Cimetidine in the treatment of duodenal ulcer. A multicenter double blind study. *Gastroenterology 74*, 380.

35. Bodemar, G., Norlander, B. and Walan, A. (1977): Cimetidine in the treatment of active peptic ulcer disease. In: *Cimetidine. Proceedings of the Second International Symposium on Histamine H₂-Receptor Antagonists*, pp. 224–239. Eds: W.L. Burland and M.A. Simkins. Excerpta Medica, Amsterdam-Oxford.

36. Rotter, J.I., Peterson, G., Samloff, I.M. et al. (1979): Genetic heterogeneity of hyperpepsinogenemic I and normopepsinogenemic I duodenal ulcer disease. *Ann. Intern. Med. 91*, 372.

37. Christensen, E., Juhl, E. and Tygstrup, N. (1977): Treatment of duodenal ulcer. Randomized clinical trials of a decade (1964 to 1974). *Gastroenterology 73*, 1170.

38. Bodemar, G. and Walan, A. (1978): Maintenance treatment of recurrent peptic ulcer by cimetidine. *Lancet I*, 403.

39. Cargill, J.M., Peden, N., Saunders, J.H.B. and Wormsley, K.G. (1978): Very long-term treatment of peptic ulcer with cimetidine. *Lancet II*, 1113.

40. Blumenthal, I.S. (1968): Digestive disease as a national problem. III. Social cost of peptic ulcer. *Gastroenterology 54*, 86.

41. Soloway, R.D., Summerskill, W.H.J., Baggenstoss, A.H. et al. (1972): Clinical, biochemical and histological remission of severe chronic active liver disease: a controlled study of treatments and early prognosis. *Gastroenterology 63*, 820.

Pharmacologic requirements of the 'ideal' ulcer drug

K.-F. Sewing
Department of General Pharmacology, Medical College, Hannover, Federal Republic of Germany

When asked to create the ideal anti-ulcer drug, I immediately ceased my deliberations, prepared a joint, and started smoking Indian hemp, bearing in mind that the late Sir John Gaddum had written in his textbook on pharmacology in 1959: 'The man who has chewed, swallowed, or smoked hemp appears first dull, and then fatuous and excited before he finally goes to sleep, but he may be dreaming of gardens gay with houris or perhaps, if his mind works that way, of fantastic new chemical compounds bedecked with steroid rings and polypeptide chain.' I leave it to you to decide in which way my mind worked, but as a result of this adventure I can tell you that neither a new steroid ring, nor a polypeptide chain, nor even the ideal anti-ulcer structure emerged. The only offspring were new H_2-receptor antagonists with a potency 100 times higher than that of those known to date, and a new anticholinergic with specific actions on gastric cholinergic receptors. None of this really helps us.

It is therefore necessary to approach the problem from another angle. The medications available for gastric and duodenal ulcers are the same giving rise to the illusion that the pathophysiology of the 2 ulcer types is identical. We must therefore briefly review the pathogenesis of the 2 ulcer types.

Recent review articles on this subject regularly return to the following features which duodenal ulcer patients have in common: increased secretory capacity, increased susceptibility to secretory stimuli, defective acid inhibition, and increased gastric emptying. The overall result is an increased duodenal acid load.

The situation is different for gastric ulcers, for which the most discussed factors are: defective mucosal barrier, bile reflux, and various local factors such as impaired cell renewal, impaired mucus secretion, and reduced blood supply.

Things become even more complicated when we consider ulcerogenic drugs.

First, there is little reliable data on the incidence and character of gastro-intestinal ulceration related to various anti-inflammatory drugs, except for the fact that prostaglandins are involved. Even less is known about those processes caused by prostaglandin synthetase inhibition.

In summary, therefore, it seems that there is no common cause for peptic ulceration of the gastrointestinal tract. Consequently there cannot be a single anti-ulcer drug which will prevent or heal all the different types of peptic ulcer. It would therefore create a deep conflict for a professional drug developer, whose philosophy is directed towards drugs with a highly specific spectrum of action, were he to be asked to develop a chemical compound that stops acid secretion, promotes cell regeneration, improves membrane resistance to ulcerogenic noxae and emotionally stabilizes the ulcer-prone patient.

Let us accept for a while that there are drugs available that have been shown unequivocally to promote ulcer healing and to reduce the relapse rate when given over a long period of time. They have special pharmacodynamic and pharmacokinetic features, making them applicable for the purpose in question. However, I think they are all far from ideal. They have a major disadvantages.

Firstly, they affect only a few, or even only one, of the factors involved in ulcer pathogenesis. It is no secret that we have drugs which suppress acid secretion very effectively. But again it must be emphasized that gastric secretion is only one component causing and maintaining peptic ulceration. That is perhaps the reason why a certain proportion of ulcers is always resistant to treatment with antisecretory agents. These drugs can therefore be regarded as helpful, but they are not ideal.

Secondly, the effectiveness of some of the drugs has not been demonstrated. Lists of the most common drugs give numerous preparations said to be helpful in peptic ulcer disease. But a search of the literature to find support for the claim that these drugs, or just single components, are effective in ulcer disease fails. So again this is no ideal situation.

Thirdly, the drugs have inconvenient pharmacokinetic properties. Since it is very difficult to define the kind of pharmacokinetic properties required of anti-ulcer drugs, we cannot exactly specify complaints concerning the pharmacokinetic features of drugs currently available. We must return to this problem later.

Finally, the drugs have intolerable side effects. It is well-known that drugs that are effective also have unwanted side effects. In this much all anti-ulcer drugs are equal, but there are some which are associated with more severe and more frequent side effects than others. Again, this is not an ideal situation.

Given these conditions, in a search for the ideal drug we must focus our attention on at least 3 aspects.

First, we need more insight into the cellular machinery promoting ulcerogenesis, and our goal is eventually to influence these basic principles. One of the very early events in ulcer formation seems to be a functional damage of the mucosal cell membrane. If it were possible to stabilize the gastric mucosal cell membrane, and thereby to keep the interior milieu intact, this would be a great step forward.

Secondly, it is very important to minimize untoward effects of the currently known effective anti-ulcer drugs. I am aware of the fact that if we eliminate one side effect we will probably be faced with another, or may eliminate the therapeutic efficacy. Since side effects are very difficult to predict, one can only hope for an increase in drug safety.

Finally, a promising direction would seem to be an improvement of the pharmacokinetic properties of the known and effective anti-ulcer drugs, and the development of new drugs with adequate pharmacokinetic features. The pharmacokinetics of anti-ulcer drugs seems to be a field that should attract more attention. Since all the ulcerogenic factors are to be found together in a lesion of the gastric and/or duodenal mucosa, it seems reasonable that the drug in question should accumulate in the area of damage. With ulcer disease we have a great advantage in that we can easily obtain access to the area of damage by simple oral administration of the drug. However, I know of no anti-ulcer drug currently available that accumulates in the mucosa for an appreciable length of time. Such an accumulation can occur independent of absorption, which should be poor if not absent, since any absorption is likely to be associated with unwanted systemic effects. If we want no absorption, it is irrational to make speculations concerning biological half-lives in the conventional sense of the word. Therefore, we must postulate that the drug concentration in the mucosa be maintained at a high enough level to be effective. We can leave open the question as to how long, since that can be a matter of debate. If such a drug is not being absorbed, we also do not have to consider drug disposition and half-lives in renal or hepatic disease. Consideration must be given to the ways in which we can approach the problem in order to reach these goals. I think one of the most promising ways would be to study the affinity of potentially effective drugs for gastric and duodenal cells in relation to their affinity for other cells in the body.

I do not know whether such an approach as that described above will be sufficient for the development of an even half-ideal anti-ulcer drug, or whether such a drug will ever be obtained. But when considering such a topic it must be possible to make speculations in any direction. This was, I am sure, just one such direction.

Histamine H₂-receptor antagonists in short- and long-term treatment of duodenal ulcer

J.J. Misiewicz
Department of Gastroenterology, Central Middlesex Hospital, London, England

Recent developments in the therapeutic modalities available for the practical management of duodenal ulcer are likely to affect substantially the management of this common condition, even if doubt remains whether the eventual outcome of the disease will be significantly influenced, or whether the natural history of duodenal ulcer might be in any way altered. The factors that have contributed to the progress of medical therapy in this area are of considerable interest, not only to the practicing clinician, but also to those committees or organizations that seek to direct medical research along the most fruitful pathways. These has been an intensive study of gastric acid secretion and the mechanisms that control it, and an information explosion in the field of gastrointestinal polypeptide hormones and other biogenic substances (e.g. prostaglandins).

The preceeding papers in this symposium demonstrate the wealth of new data that has accumulated in these areas. Despite these considerable advances in gastric and duodenal physiology, the cause of duodenal ulcer remains unknown. One can postulate that this is so because there may not be a single cause for the majority of duodenal ulcers, the etiology of the disease being multifactorial. Moreover, ulcers in different individuals, or in different geographical areas, or in different ethnic groups may have different causes, with one or other factor predominating in the etiology. Ignorance of precise mechanism of causation need not preclude effective medical therapy however, and examples of this can at present be readily found in medical therapeutics. Advances, such as they are, in the medical treatment of duodenal ulcer have come about not through a major breakthrough in the understanding of causes, but through the introduction of new drugs (carbenoxolone sodium, cimetidine), because of technological advances allowing measurement of ulcer healing to be vastly more accurate (fiberoptic endoscopy), and lastly through a critical reappraisal of older remedies using the new techniques and a stringently critical approach to the evaluation of treatment in properly controlled, double-blind clinical trials.

Although valid data have been collected in this way, they must be interpreted in the knowledge that relatively small numbers of patients have been intensively studied and that they are a highly selected population that satisfied the entry criteria of the various trial protocols. Results of trials on patients referred to specialist centers may or may not be relevant to those seen by the primary care physician, or those in another country. This contention is supported by the occasional discordant results of short-term clinical trials of cimetidine in the treatment of duodenal ulcer, by the varying placebo healing rates in different trials and similar phenomena. Whether the factors that operate to produce these differences are environmental, dietary, or genetic, or whether they relate to the selection of patients, or their consumption of tobacco or alcohol, or to the degree of compliance, remains to be determined.

General considerations

Evaluation of therapy must be based on accurate definition and diagnosis of the lesion studied. Acute erosive ulcers must be clearly differentiated from chronic, recurrent duodenal ulcers. Juxtapyloric ulcers (pyloric canal ulcers) are thought to behave like duodenal ulcers. This may be useful in formulating a therapeutic strategy for the individual patient, but patients with juxtapyloric ulcers should perhaps be studied separately, until more is known about the clinical characteristics of such ulcers. In general, only trials in which the results have been assessed with fiberoptic endoscopy are acceptable and the end-point should be the complete healing of the ulcer. This is partly because endoscopic assessments of changes in ulcer diameter tend to be unreliable, but also because an incompletely healed ulcer is a doubtful benefit of medication. It need hardly be mentioned that the endoscopist should not be aware of the nature of the treatment and ideally should not be involved in the clinical supervision of the patient in the trial.

Results of short-term treatment (up to 12 weeks) must be clearly distinguished from maintenance therapy (6 months, or longer), intended to prevent relapses. The relapse should be precisely defined, because recent studies have shown that the incidence of asymptomatic relapses of duodenal ulcer on maintenance therapy with either placebo or cimetidine lies between 10 and 38% [1], while the correlation between ulcer healing and symptomatic improvement is poor [2].

Short-term treatment

The main recent interest in this area has been the results of endoscopically-controlled trials using cimetidine, antacids, anticholinergics, carbenoxolone and prostaglandins. Newer histamine H_2-receptor antagonists, such as raniti-dine, are more potent [3] and possibly longer acting than cimetidine, but their clinical efficacy has not been evaluated at the time of writing. Cimetidine is at present the most extensively studied drug for the short-term management of duodenal ulcer and the one with specific and well-characterized pharma-cological actions [4]. The therapeutic effects of H_2-receptor blockade stem from the marked inhibition of acid output, amounting to a 60% diminution of meal-stimulated gastric secretion [5]. In most trials cimetidine heals a significantly higher percentage of duodenal ulcers than placebo, both groups of patients receiving ad lib supplies of antacid (Table I; [6–18]). In a small number of studies, cimetidine has not been shown to be better than either placebo, or intensive antacid therapy (Table II; [19–24]).

Table I: Percentage healing of duodenal ulcer on cimetidine or placebo. Results of double-blind trials showing a significant advantage of cimetidine over placebo. (Not a complete list of available trials).

Study	Number of patients	Daily dose of cimetidine (g)	Time (weeks)	Percentage healing	
				Cime-tidine	Placebo
Albano et al. [6]	157	1	4	72	34
Bank et al. [7]	38	1.2–1.6	6	84	42
Multicentre trial [8]	180	1	4	61	28
		2		70	
Blackwood et al. [9]	23	1.6	6	82	25
Bodemar and Walan [10]	44	0.8	6	80	36
		1.2		93	
Cremer et al. [11]	32	1	6	73	42
Dobrilla et al. [12]	34	1	4	80	40
Gray et al. [13]	40	1	4	85	20
Hetzel et al. [14]	85	1.2	6	84	38
Lambert et al. [15]	140	1	4	76	59
Moshal et al. [16]	55	0.8	6	74	42
		1.2		65	
Northfield and Blackwood [17]	74	1.6	6	62	19
			12	88	27
Manousos et al. [18]	22	1	4	76	44

Table II: Percentage healing of duodenal ulcer on cimetidine, placebo or high dose antacid (1,000 mMol· day^{-1}) showing no significant difference between the treatment groups.

Study	Number of patients	Daily dose of cimetidine (g) (g)	Time (weeks)	Percentage healing	
				Cime-tidine	Placebo
Binder et al. [19]	217	1.2	2 (IP)	56	37 (P)
			2	56	30 (P)
			4	57	48 (P)
Villalobos et al. [20]	45	1	4	96	77 (P)
Malchow et al. [21]	77	1.2	4 (IP)	88	79 (P)
Semb et al. [22]	40	1.2	4	85	60 (P)
Ippoliti et al. [23]	94	0.8	4	59	–
		1.2		64	–
		–		–	52 (A)
Peter et al. [24]	78	1	4	79	58 (P)

IP = inpatients, P = placebo, A = antacid.

Maintenance treatment

Cimetidine remains the drug of choice in the maintenance therapy for duodenal ulcer, there being no satisfactory data available for the other compounds shown to be effective in the short-term management of duodenal ulceration. An analysis of ongoing maintenance trials in the United Kingdom, European countries and South Africa (Table III; [24]) shows a highly significant advantage of cimetidine 400 mg at night or 400 mg twice daily, over placebo. Overall the smaller dose appears to be as effective as the larger one, although theoretically it might be advantageous to give more drug to patients with hypersecretion of acid. After 6 months' maintenance therapy approximately 85% of duodenal ulcer patients on cimetidine 400 or 800 mg daily will be in remission, compared with only 40% of those on placebo. At 12 months the number of patients analyzed at the time of writing is too small to permit meaningful interpretation. On the data at present available the annual recurrence rate of duodenal ulcer while on long-term treatment with 400 or 800 mg daily can be calculated to be approximately 23%, but it is 100% on placebo in less than 12 months. In one study, however, of 42 patients with duodenal ulcer treated with either cimetidine 800 mg daily, or placebo only, 16% relapsed during one year's treatment with the drug, while 78% of the control group relapsed [26].

Table III: Analysis of ongoing maintenance trials of cimetidine versus placebo in duodenal ulcer for 12 months.

Reference	Number of patients at entry	Daily dose of cimetidine (g)	Reulceration	
			Symptomatic	Asymptomatic
			% (no. examined)	% (no. examined)
Burland et al. [25]	179	0.4	13.4 (24)	5.3 (75)
	184	0.8	13.0 (24)	9.3 (75)
	333	Placebo	47.4 (158)	30.0 (73)

In another trial, analyzed on the basis of symptomatic recurrence only, the relapse rate after one year's treatment was 12% on cimetidine 400 mg nightly and 80% on placebo [27]. As the number of patients followed up in controlled trials for one year is still relatively small, conclusions regarding the relapse rate during long-term treatment with cimetidine must be tentative.

Discussion

The clinician has now a choice of therapeutic agents active in promoting the healing of duodenal ulcer in the short-term. Each of the available drugs will significantly increase the percentage of ulcers healed, but each has advantages and disadvantages and the weight of evidence supporting the assessment of therapeutic efficacy is not evenly matched throughout the range of the compounds.

Treatment with cimetidine in the dose range of 1–2 g daily for 4–6 weeks will result in the healing of almost 80% of duodenal ulcers. Prompt and marked relief of symptoms will be experienced by most patients and after the first few days supplementary antacid therapy will be unnecessary. The patient can be encouraged to eat a normal diet, taking care to space the meals evenly throughout the day. On the basis of the published data, similar rates of duodenal ulcer healing can be expected from therapy with carbenoxolone sodium administered in the 'positioned-release' capsule, or from antacids. The symptomatic relief from carbenoxolone sodium, however, appears to be slower and less marked than with cimetidine. Although no formal comparisons have been made, patients on carbenoxolone probably need more antacids. Moreover, medication has to be continued for 6 weeks or longer, in order to achieve results comparable to cimetidine and there is an appreciable incidence of side-effects. Antacids used in large quantities as the sole treatment for duodenal ulcer are inconvenient to take, especially for the patient who remains at work. They also may produce troublesome unwanted effects.

Although the great majority of clinical trials show an advantage of cimetidine over placebo in the short-term treatment of duodenal ulcer, there are several where the differences from control groups have not been significant (see Table II). The reasons why some studies do not show a significant advantage for cimetidine are not immediately apparent. Selection of patients and racial and environmental differences must all play an important part. Epidemiological studies show very clearly that the clinical characteristics of duodenal ulcer can vary with geographical location, as evidenced, for example, by the marked differences in the rates of perforated ulcer between England and Scotland. The interval between the onset of relapse and the initial endoscopy may also affect the results, and waiting time for endoscopic assessment varies widely from country to country.

The placebo healing rate is highly variable in the reported studies (see Tables I and II). The factors discussed above can all affect the placebo healing rate, which can also be influenced by the amount of antacid consumed by the patients in the control groups. One study has shown that high-dose antacids are an effective therapy for duodenal ulcer [28] and although this needs to be confirmed in a larger number of patients, it seems reasonable to suggest that substantial consumption of base by patients in control groups might blur the differences between cimetidine and placebo.

Safety is another aspect of treatment that may influence the choice of a drug for the short-term treatment of duodenal ulcer. Short-term treatment with cimetidine is a remarkably safe procedure. In the United Kingdom the number of untoward effects associated with administration of the drug reported to the Committee for Safety of Medicines, the manufacturers, or published in the medical press, totals but a fraction of one per cent of the patients treated and none have been serious. Detailed analysis of patients in short-term trials shows that 17% of patients on cimetidine reported untoward effects, but 19% of patients receiving a placebo did so as well. Diarrhea, tiredness, dizziness, drowsiness, or rash occurred with a slightly higher frequency in cimetidine-treated patients. Comparison of cimetidine- with placebo-treated groups showed no significant hematological abnormalities, while raised levels of plasma creatinine and hepatic enzymes occurred only slightly more frequently in the patients receiving the drug. Occasional cases of gynecomastia or of galactorrhea have been reported, mainly in association with gastrinomas [29]. Other evidence of antiandrogenic action has been published [30], but reports of erectile impotence, or of decreased sperm count must await further evaluation before the risk can be accurately assessed [31, 32]. Chronic oral administration of cimetidine does not affect the release of prolactin or other anterior pituitary hormones [33], but has some effect on glucose metabolism, increasing sensitivity to insulin [34]. Interactions with anticoagulants (warfarin) and with benzodiazepines (diazepam) have been reported and must be borne in mind [35, 36]. Another clinically important unwanted effect is mental confusion which occurs sporadically in elderly or ill patients with other metabolic abnormalities [37]. However, impaired hepatic or renal function does not preclude therapy with cimetidine, although the dose has to be smaller in the presence of the latter. Cimetidine therapy increases the bacterial population of the upper alimentary tract [38]: whether this may have clinical consequences in terms of colonization of the gut, or in terms of production of potentially carcinogenic nitrosamines or nitrosamides, is at present unknown.

Whichever drug is chosen to treat the duodenal ulcer patient in the short term, there will remain a residuum of 20–30% of ulcers which will be resistant to therapy. Why this should be so is unclear. The usual clinical factors of previous ulcer history, age, sex, etc., do not appear to provide the answer. One study suggested that nonhealers have a higher acid output [13], but this has not been borne out by a more detailed examination of pentagastrin- and insulin-stimulated gastric secretion and basal gastrin levels by others [39]. Patient compliance has not been extensively studied (a neglected area in most clinical trials, whatever the specialty!), but then it is unlikely that the same percentage of patients fail to take medication in so many studies. There is a great need for controlled investigations using combined therapy with anti-secretory (e.g. cimetidine), together with mucosal-protective (e.g. carbenoxo-lone), or other drugs, to see whether the percentage healing rate can be increased.

After the ulcer has healed, the crux of medical long-term management of duodenal ulcer is the prevention of relapses. Cimetidine is the drug of choice, there being no evidence to suggest that the other compounds discussed in the following chapters affect the relapse rate. Review of safety data culled from patients in clinical trials of long-term cimetidine therapy does not indicate any reason to limit the dose, or duration of treatment, or to restrict the type of ulcer patients to be treated [29].

As acidification of the antrum is the main mechanism of suppression of the release of gastrin, there is a theoretical possibility that prolonged ad-ministration of cimetidine may lead to hypergastrinemia, with consequent hyperplasia of the parietal cell mass and, upon cessation of cimetidine therapy, rebound hypersecretion of acid and reulceration. This has not so far been borne out by human studies lasting up to 12 months. Although acid output is inhibited, the mean intragastric pH is raised only slightly during treatment with cimetidine, because anacidity is not achieved in the majority of patients [40]. Despite that, the release of gastrin in response to food is increased by cimetidine [41, 42]. Administration of cimetidine in very high doses to rats (equivalent to over 70 $g \cdot day^{-1}$ in a 75-kg man) leads to a significant increase in parietal cells counts after 1 or 2 years; this increase is also seen at lower doses, equivalent to 11.25 $g \cdot day^{-1}$ on the human scale. On the other hand, patients with duodenal ulcer on cimetidine 1.6 $g \cdot day^{-1}$ for prolonged periods have unchanged pre- and post-treatment maximally histamine-stimulated acid secretion, although the integrated gastrin response to a meal is increased [43]. Fasting gastrin, pentagastrin- and insulin-stimulated acid secretion were unchanged after long-term maintenance therapy for duodenal ulcer in another study [39]. Investigation of gastric function before and after treatment with cimetidine at 1–2 $g \cdot day^{-1}$ for 4–8 weeks followed by 1.2 $g \cdot day^{-1}$ for 6 months showed that fasting serum gastrin concentrations were raised during and 5 days after stopping treatment. The integrated gastrin response to food was significantly raised during treatment but normal after it, and there were no significant changes in basal, or in the pentagastrin-stimulated maximal acid output after therapy was stopped [44]. These studies taken together indicate that although hypergastrinemia does occur during treatment with cimetidine, it is insufficient to produce parietal cell hyperplasia and therefore hypersecretion of acid does not take place. It should be borne in mind that these conclusions are valid only within the limits of the dosage and duration of the experiments on which thcy are based.

Studies of relapses of duodenal ulcer after one year of cimetidine therapy do not show any increase in the rate at which relapses occur. Indeed, the incidence of relapse of duodenal ulcers appears remarkably unaffected by prolonged blockade of histamine H₂-receptors [27].

Financial considerations apart, it would seem that cimetidine is the most convenient drug for the short-term treatment of duodenal ulcer, and the only compound shown to diminish the probability of the ulcer recurring in the long term. The pharmacological properties and specificity of action are clearly defined for cimetidine, while the mode of action of other drugs, apart from antacids, remains somewhat conjectural. Other drugs may be cheaper, but the calculation of treatment costs is not easy, as time taken off work and loss of productivity have to be taken into account. This is especially so in long-term treatment with cimetidine, as was clearly shown in one report [26]. If the ulcer does not heal after 4 weeks' cimetidine at $1-2 \text{ g} \cdot \text{day}^{-1}$, it is worth persevering for a further 2–3 weeks, as some ulcers appear to heal only after a more prolonged therapy. Accurate diagnosis, preferably endoscopic, is mandatory at the start of management of the patient suspected of having an ulcer. Endoscopy-negative dyspepsia, in the absence of frank duodenitis, does not respond to cimetidine [45]. In clinical practice it is doubtful whether repeat endoscopy is strictly necessary after treatment. All the same, it has to be admitted that correlation of ulcer healing with symptomatic remission is less than perfect and the incidence of nonhealed, or relapsed, but symptom-free ulcers, appreciable [1, 25]. The management of the asymptomatic ulcer will be the subject of lively debate at gastroenterological meetings for years to come.

Cimetidine does not cure duodenal ulcers, which can be expected to recur. Not every patient requires continuous maintenance treatment, however. Those with well-defined relapses and remissions can be treated by on-demand regimes, as soon as symptoms reappear. Purists might object, but there is no a priori reason why a patient with an ulcer should not have a supply of cimetidine at home and begin treatment as soon as the pain comes back. If there is no response within a week, a doctor should be consulted. Those with more continuous symptoms need continuous therapy; for how long, it is difficult to say at present. Maintenance treatment is obviously indicated for those who are unsuitable for surgery for any reason. In the uncomplicated case, the decision between medical therapy or surgery must be made by the patient, with informed guidance from the doctor. Some patients, for example those living or working in remote areas, where the risk of perforation or hemorrhage from the ulcer is substantial, should be advised to have surgery. We do not yet know how the availability of H_2-histamine receptor antagonists will affect the incidence of surgery in duodenal ulcer. This partly because it is, as yet, too early to collect data, partly because developments in surgical techniques confuse the picture and partly because the ulcer diathesis itself may be evolving new clinical attributes.

References

1. Bardhan, K.D. (1979): Cimetidine in duodenal ulceration. In: *Cimetidine: The Westminster Hospital Symposium*, Chapter 3, p. 31. Eds: C. Wastell and P. Lance. Churchill Livingstone, Edinburgh-Harlow.
2. Misiewicz, J.J. (1978): Peptic ulceration and its correlation with symptoms. In: *Clinics in Gastroenterology. Endoscopy*, Vol. 7, No. 3, Chapter 2, p. 571. Ed: K.F.R. Schiller. W.B. Saunders Company Ltd., London-Philadelphia-Toronto.

3. Walt, R.P., Male, P.-J., Rawlings, J. et al. (1979): 24-Hour intragastric acidity in duodenal ulcer patients on a new twice-daily H_2-receptor antagonist. *Gut 20*, A904.

4. Burland, W.L. and Simkins, M.A. (Editors) (1977): *Cimetidine. Proceedings of the Second International Symposium on Histamine H_2-Receptor Antagonists.* Excerpta Medica, Amsterdam-Oxford.

5. Pounder, R.E., Williams, J.G., Russell, R.C.G. et al. (1976): Inhibition of food-stimulated gastric acid secretion by cimetidine. *Gut 17*, 161.

6. Albano, O., Barbara, M., Miglioli, M. et al. (1978): Trattamento a breve termine con cimetidina nell'ulcera duodenale. Risultati di una ricerca policentrica controllata. In: *Cimetidine: Farmacologia e clinia*, p. 149. Eds: P. Luchelli. Smith, Kline and French, Milano.

7. Bank, S., Barbezat, G.O., Novis, B.H. et al. (1976): Histamine H_2-receptor antagonists in the treatment of duodenal ulcers. *S. Afr. Med. J. 50*, 1981.

8. A multicentre trial (1979): *Gut 20*, 68.

9. Blackwood, W.S., Maudgal, D.P., Pickard, R.G. et al. (1976): Cimetidine in duodenal ulcer, controlled trial. *Lancet II*, 174.

10. Bodemar, G. and Walan, A. (1976): Cimetidine in the treatment of active duodenal and prepyloric ulcers. *Lancet II*, 161.

11. Cremer, M., Derumier, J., Deltenre, M. and Toussaint, J. (1978): Etude en double avangle de l'effet de la cimetidine dans l'ulcere duodenal et dans l'ulcere gastrique. In: *Proceedings of the 6th World Congress on Gastroenterology* (Abstract), p. 19.

12. Dobrilla, G., Valentini, M., Filippini, M. et al. (1978): Therapie mit Cimetidin bein ulkus duodeni. *Munch. Med. Wochenschr. 120*, 839.

13. Gray, G.R., McKenzie, I., Smith, I.S. et al. (1977): Oral cimetidine in severe duodenal ulceration. *Lancet I*, 4.

14. Hetzel, D.J., Taggart, G.J., Hansky, J. et al. (1977): Cimetidine in the treatment of duodenal ulcer. *Med. J. Aust. 1*, 317.

15. Lambert, R., Bader, J.P., Bernier, J.J. et al. (1977): Treatment of gastric and duodenal ulcers with cimetidine. *Gastroenterol. Clin. Biol. 1*, 855.

16. Moshal, M.G., Spitaels, J.M. and Bhoola, R. (1977): Treatment of duodenal ulcers with cimetidine. *S. Afr. J. Med. 52*, 760.

17. Northfield, T.C. and Blackwood, W.S. (1977): Controlled clinical trial of cimetidine for duodenal ulcer. *Gut 20*, 272.

18. Manousos, O.N., Zografos, A., Nicolaou, A. et al. (1978): A double-blind study of cimetidine in patients with duodenal or gastric ulcer in Greece. *J. Int. Med. Res. 6*, 381.

19. Binder, H.J., Cocco, A., Crossley, R.J. et al. (1978): Cimetidine in the treatment of duodenal ulcer. *Gastroenterology 74*, 380.

20. Villalobos, J.J., Elizondo, J., Guevara, L. and Centeno, F. (1978): Cimetidine in the treatment of duodenal ulcer: double-blind study. *J. Int. Med. Res. 6*, 351.

21. Malchow, H., Sewing, K.F., Albinus, M. et al. (1978): In-patient treatment of peptic ulcer with cimetidine. 1. Effect on the healing of duodenal ulcer. *Dtsch. Med. Wochenschr. 103*, 149.

22. Semb, L.S., Berstad, A., Myren, J. et al. (1977): A double-blind multicentre comparative study of cimetidine and placebo in short-term treatment of active duodenal ulceration. In: *Cimetidine. Proceedings of the Second International*

Symposium on Histamine H_2-Receptor Antagonists, pp. 248–253. Eds: W.L. Burland and M.A. Simkins. Excerpta Medica, Amsterdam-Oxford.
23. Ippoliti, A.F., Sturdevant, R.A.L., Isenberg, J.I. et al. (1978): Cimetidine versus intensive antacid therapy for duodenal ulcer. A multicenter trial. *Gastroenterology 74*, 393.
24. Peter, P., Kiene, K., Gonvers, J.J. et al. (1978): *Dtsch. Med. Wochenschr. 103*, 1163.
25. Burland, W.L., Hawkins, B.W., Horton, R.J. and Beresford, J. (1978): The longer-term treatment of duodenal ulcer with cimetidine. In: *Cimetidine: The Westminster Hospital Symposium*, Chapter 5, p. 66. Eds: C. Wastell and P. Lance. Churchill Livingstone, Edinburgh-Harlow.
26. Bodemar, G. and Walan, A. (1978): Maintenance treatment of recurrent peptic ulcer by cimetidine. *Lancet I*, 403.
27. Gudman-Høyer, E., Birger Jensen, K., Krag, E. et al. (1978): Prophylactic effect of cimetidine in duodenal ulcer disease. *Br. Med. J. 1*, 1095.
28. Peterson, W.L., Sturdevant, R.A.L., Frankl, H.D. et al. (1977): Healing of duodenal ulcer with an antacid regimen. *N. Engl. J. Med. 297*, 341.
29. Burland, W.L. (1978): Evidence for the safety of cimetidine in the treatment of peptic ulcer disease. In: *Cimetidine. Proceedings of an International Symposium on Histamine H_2-Receptor Antagonists*, p. 238–255. Ed: W. Creutzfeldt. Excerpta Medica, Amsterdam-Oxford.
30. Winters, S.J., Banks, J.L. and Loriauk, D.L. (1979): Cimetidine is an anti-androgen in the rat. *Gastroenterology 76*, 504.
31. Peden, N.R., Cargill, J.M., Browning, M.C.K. et al. (1979): Male sexual dysfunction during treatment with cimetidine. *Br. Med. J. 1*, 659.
32. Van Thiel, D.H., Gavaler, J.S., Smith, W.I. and Paul, G. (1979): Hypothalamic, pituitary-gonadal dysfunction in men using cimetidine. *N. Engl. J. Med. 300*, 1012.
33. Delitala, G., Stubbs, W.A., Wass, J.A.H. et al. (1978): Hypothalamic-pituitary effects of cimetidine. *Lancet II*, 1054.
34. Stubbs, W.A., Delitala, G., Besser, G.M. et al. (1979): Blood glucose regulation in man: a role for histamine receptors. (Abstract.) In: *10th Congress of International Diabetes Federation*, Vienna. 582F:225.
35. Serlin, M.J., Mossman, S., Sibeon, R.G. et al. (1979): Cimetidine: interaction with oral anticoagulants in man. *Lancet II*, 317.
36. Klotz, V. and Reimann, I. (1980): Delayed clearance of diazepam due to cimetidine. *N. Engl. J. Med. 302*, 1012.
37. Schentag, J.J., Calleri, G., Cerra, F.B. et al. (1979): Pharmacokinetic and clinical studies in patients with cimetidine-associated mental confusion. *Lancet I*, 177.
38. Ruddell, W.S.J., Axon, A.T.R., Findlay, J.M. et al. (1980): Effect of cimetidine on the gastric bacterial flora. *Lancet I*, 672.
39. Venables, C.W., Stephen, J.G., Blair, E.L. et al. (1978): Cimetidine in the treatment of duodenal ulceration and the relationship of this therapy to surgical management. In: *Cimetidine: The Westminster Hospital Symposium*, Chapter 2, p. 13. Eds: C. Wastell and P. Lance. Churchill Livingstone, Edinburgh-Harlow.
40. Pounder, R.E., Hunt, R.H., Vincent, S.H. et al. (1977): 24-Hour intragastric acidity and nocturnal acid secretion in patients with duodenal ulcer during oral administration of cimetidine and atropine. *Gut 18*, 85.

41. Heading, R.C., Logan, R.F.A., McLoughlin, G.P. et al. (1977): Effect of cimetidine on gastric emptying. In: *Cimetidine. Proceedings of the Second International Symposium on Histamine H₂-Receptor Antagonists*, p. 145–152. Eds: W.L. Burland and M.A. Simkins. Excerpta Medica, Amsterdam-Oxford.

42. Longstreth, G.F., Malagelada, J.R. and Go, V.L.W. (1977): Postprandial gastric, pancreatic and biliary response to histamine H₂-receptor antagonists in active duodenal ulcer. *Gastroenterology 72*, 9.

43. Spence, R.W., Celestin, L.R., McCormick, D.A. and Owens, C.J. (1977): The effect of 3 months' treatment with cimetidine on basal and 'oxo'-stimulated serum gastrin. In: *Cimetidine. Proceedings of the Second International Symposium on Histamine H₂-Receptor Antagonists*, pp. 163–174. Eds: W.L. Burland and M.A. Simkins. Excerpta Medica, Amsterdam-Oxford.

44. Forrest, J.A.H., Fettes, M., McLoughlin, G. and Heading, A.C. (1978): The effect of long-term cimetidine on gastric acid secretion, serum gastrin and gastric emptying. In: *Cimetidine: The Westminster Hospital Symposium*, Chapter 4, p. 57. Eds: C. Wastell and P. Lance. Churchill Livingstone, Edinburgh-Harlow.

45. La Brooy, S., Lovell, D. and Misiewicz, J.J. (1978): The treatment of non-ulcer dyspepsia. In: *Cimetidine: The Westminster Hospital Symposium*, Chapter 2, p. 131. Eds: C. Wastell and P. Lance. Churchill Livingstone, Edinburgh-Harlow.

Histamine H$_2$-receptor antagonists in short- and long-term treatment of gastric ulcer

W. Dölle

I Department of Internal Medicine, University Medical Clinic, Tübingen, Federal Republic of Germany

Much less data are available on the subject of gastric ulcer than on duodenal ulcer, due to the difference in incidence of the 2 types of peptic ulcer.

The following can, however, be said of the natural course of gastric ulcer [14]: recurrence of peptic ulcer is common; in 70% of patients with gastric ulcer, clinical symptoms of recurrence occur within the first 10 years; an average of 22% of patients with gastric ulcer undergo operation due to failure of conservative therapy; in 11% of patients with peptic ulcer, the ulcer is the direct cause of death; and there may be a dissociation between ulcer symptoms and the presence of an ulcer.

Table I shows the variation of recurrence to be between 42 and 76% in various studies. Between 11 and 38% of patients needed operation. The mortality, including the operative mortality, varied from 0–8.9% [11].

Table II gives the results of short-term treatment with cimetidine. Seven studies compare cimetidine with placebo, and 3 with other treatments such as

Table I: Natural course of gastric ulcer disease [11].

Study*		No. of patients			Recurrences (%)		Operations (%)		Mortality (%)	
		Total	M	F	M	F	M	F	M	F
Krause	(25 years)	247	134	113	67.9	61.9	38.1	27.4	3.7	8.9
Fry	(15 years)	53	28	25	68.0	74.0	18.0	20.0	0	0
Krag	(17–27 years)	58	38	20	76.0	50.0	22.0**		8**	
Littman	(2 years)	638	638		42.0		11.0		0	

* Figures in parentheses refer to length of follow-up observations.
** Males (M) + females (F).

colloidal bismuth [1], a bismuth preparation, carbenoxolone and antacid.

In only 2 of 6 studies did cimetidine treatment result in a significantly greater healing than placebo after 4 weeks or 6 weeks. These studies were carried out in France and Denmark. In 2 studies in the U.S.A. and in one study each in Australia and the United Kingdom, however, no effect of cimetidine on the healing rate could be shown. Our own study in the Federal

Table II: Results of short-term treatment with cimetidine.

Study	No. of patients	Dose	Duration of treat- ment	Rate of healing	Significance
Ciclitira et al. 1979, United Kingdom	35 25	1,000 mg Placebo	4 weeks	66% 52%	NS
Bader et al. 1977, France	26 27	1,000 mg Placebo	4 weeks	69% 37%	$p < 0.02$ (χ^2-test)
Frost et al. 1978, Denmark	23 22	1,000 mg Placebo	6 weeks	78% 27%	$p < 0.005$
Dyck et al. 1978, U.S.A.	30 29	1,200 mg Placebo	6 weeks	60% 41%	NS
Englert et al. 1978, U.S.A.	68 62	1,200 mg Placebo	6 weeks	59% 61%	NS
Landecker et al. 1978, Australia	25 23	1,200 mg Placebo	5 weeks	64% 57%	NS
Sewing et al. 1978, Federal Republic of Germany**	20 16	1,200 mg Placebo	4 weeks	65% 50%	NS
Tanner et al. 1979, Australia	27 57	1,200 mg Colloidal bismuth	6 weeks	63% 66%	NS
Hunt et al. 1977, United Kingdom	12 12	800 mg Carben- oxolone	4 weeks	83% 30%	$p < 0.03$ (Fischer's exact test)
La Brooy et al. 1979, United Kingdom	27 27	800 mg Carben- oxolone	6 weeks	78% 52%	NS

* In- and outpatients.
** Inpatients.
NS = not significant.

Republic of Germany was performed only on hospitalized patients whereas, with the exception of Englert's study on both in- and outpatients, all other investigations were performed on outpatients. Cimetidine does not seem to be more effective than colloidal bismuth, carbenoxolone or antacid. Only in Hunt's study was a significantly better result achieved with cimetidine than with carbenoxolone. Tables III and IV give the healing rates.

It would appear that a significant effect of cimetidine can be achieved only if the healing rate on placebo is remarkably low. In the 2 studies with a significant effect of cimetidine the healing rate on placebo was 27% and 37%, respectively, whereas in the remaining 5 studies, with one exception, the healing rates on placebo were at least 50%.

The varying healing rates for peptic ulcer in different parts of the world have been pointed out before. Scheurer [21] showed that 83.3% of gastric ulcers were healed on placebo after 6 weeks. The average healing rate after 4 weeks is about 50% in Europe, with the exception of the United Kingdom, where it is about 20–30% [11].

Let us turn now to long-term treatment: information on 4 studies is given in Table V [2, 17–19, 25]. Cimetidine in a dose of 800 mg/day was compared with placebo administered over a period of 11 or 12 months. In all studies, a

Table III: Short-term treatment of gastric ulcer by cimetidine or placebo: studies showing no significant differences between results of the 2 treatments (5 studies).

	Percentage healed		
	4 weeks	5 weeks	6 weeks
Cimetidine	66 65	64	60 59
Placebo	52 50	57	41 61*

*Antacid.

Table IV: Short-term treatment of gastric ulcer by cimetidine or placebo: studies with significant difference between results of the 2 treatments (2 studies).

	Percentage healed	
	4 weeks	6 weeks
Cimetidine	69	78
Placebo	37	27

Table V: Long-term treatment with cimetidine.

Study	No. of patients	Dose	Duration of treatment	Rate of re- currence	Signifi- cance
Bodemar et al.,	32	800 mg	12 months	18.8%	
1978	36	Placebo		83.3%	
Machell et al.,	6	800 mg	11 months	16.7%	$p<0.002$
1978	11	Placebo		81.8%	
Mekel, 1978	26	800 mg	12 months	19.2%	
	14	Placebo		100.0%	
Wulff and Rune,	10	800 mg	12 months	0%	$p<0.025$
1978	9	Placebo		55.6%	

remarkable lowering of the recurrence rate was achieved with cimetidine. Thus, cimetidine is effective in the long-term treatment of gastric ulcer over at least 12 months.

La Brooy et al. [15] showed that the incidence of rebleeding in patients with severe hemorrhage due to gastric ulcer was reduced in those treated with cimetidine, although not significantly so. Hoare et al. [10] showed no significant effect on the bleeding from duodenal ulcers, but only 2 of 14 patients with gastric ulcer showed renewed bleeding on cimetidine, compared with 10 of 19 patients on placebo. The authors therefore concluded that 'Cimetidine may help to prevent hemorrhage from gastric ulcer. There is, of course, the need for more investigations on the effect of cimetidine in bleeding gastric ulcer'. It would seem, however, that treatment of a bleeding gastric ulcer with cimetidine is justified for the present.

With respect to the use of cimetidine in the treatment of gastric ulcer, the following can thus be said.

Cimetidine has 3 advantages: firstly, it is possible to achieve an increase in the healing rate, especially in outpatients, thereby eliminating the need for hospital admission [22]; this applies to outpatients in regions with low healing rates on placebo. Secondly, complete healing of the initial ulcer produces a prolonged remission. This effect is not, however, related to the kind of treatment [20]. Finally, cimetidine may help to prevent hemorrhage from a gastric ulcer. The disadvantages of cimetidine are that it will at least temporarily control the dyspepsia of gastric cancer, a malignant ulcer may appear to heal on cimetidine, and cimetidine has possible side effects.

At the present time, the general opinion seems to be not to treat an uncomplicated first gastric ulcer with cimetidine. Prolonged dyspepsia and/or pain not responding to antacids and/or lack of diminution of the ulcer are indications for cimetidine. Recurrence of gastric ulcer, suggesting long-term treatment, needs therapy of the ulcer episode with cimetidine.

Summary

In only 2 of 7 studies did cimetidine result in a significantly greater healing rate than placebo after 4 or 6 weeks of treatment. It would appear that a significant effect of cimetidine can be achieved only if the healing rate on placebo is remarkably low. Cimetidine is effective in the long-term treatment of gastric ulcer, and may help to prevent hemorrhage from gastric ulcer. The general opinion at the present time seems to be not to treat an uncomplicated first gastric ulcer with cimetidine. Prolonged symptoms and/or lack of response to antacids are indications for cimetidine. Recurrence of gastric ulcer suggesting long-term treatment needs therapy of the ulcer episode with cimetidine.

References

1. Bader, J.P., Morin, E., Bernier, J.J. et al. (1977): Treatment of gastric ulcer by cimetidine: a multicenter trial. In: *Cimetidine. Proceedings of the Second International Symposium on Histamine H_2-Receptor Antagonists*, pp. 287–292. Eds: W.L. Burland and M.A. Simkins. Excerpta Medica, Amsterdam-Oxford.
2. Bodemar, G. and Walan, A. (1978): Maintenance treatment of recurrent peptic ulcer by cimetidine. *Lancet I*, 402.
3. Bonnevie, D. (1977): Causes of death in duodenal and gastric ulcer. *Gastroenterology 73*, 1000.
4. Ciclitira, P.J., Machell, R.J., Farthing, M.J. et al. (1977): A controlled trial of cimetidine in the treatment of gastric ulcer. In: *Cimetidine. Proceedings of the Second International Symposium on Histamine H_2-Receptor Antagonists*, pp. 283–286. Eds: W.L. Burland and M.A. Simkins. Excerpta Medica, Amsterdam-Oxford.
5. Ciclitira, P.J., Machell, R.J., Farthing, M.J. et al. (1979): Double-blind controlled trial of cimetidine in the healing of gastric ulcer. *Gut 20*, 730.
6. Dyck, W.P., Belsito, A., Fleshler, B. et al. (1978): Cimetidine and placebo in the treatment of benign gastric ulcer. *Gastroenterology 74*, 410.
7. Englert, E. Jr., Freston, J.W., Graham, D.Y. et al. (1978): Cimetidine, antacid and hospitalization in the treatment of benign gastric ulcer. *Gastroenterology 74*, 416.
8. Freston, J.W. (1978): Cimetidine in the treatment of gastric ulcer. *Gastroenterology 74*, 426.
9. Frost, F., Rahbek, I., Rune, S.J. et al. (1977): Cimetidine in patients with gastric ulcer; a multicentre controlled trial. *Br. Med. J. II*, 795.
10. Hoare, A.M., Bradhy, G.V.H., Hawkins, C.F., et al. (1979): Cimetidine in bleeding peptic ulcer. *Lancet II*, 671.
11. Holtermüller, K.H. (1978): Natürlicher Verlauf der Ulcuskrankheit. In: *Ulcus-

Therapie, 6, pp. 63–70. Eds: A.L. Blum and J.R. Siewert. Springer, Berlin-Heidelberg-New York.

12. Holtermüller, K.H. (1978): Therapieziele beim peptischen Ulcus. In: *Ulcus-Therapie*, pp. 256–268. Eds: A.L. Blum and J.R. Siewert. Springer, Berlin-Heidelberg-New York.

13. Hunt, R.H., Vincent, S.H., Milton-Thompson, G.J. et al. (1977): Cimetidine in the treatment of gastric ulcer. In: *Cimetidine. Proceedings of the Second International Symposium on Histamine H₂-Receptor Antagonists*, p. 293. Eds: W.L. Burland and M.A. Simkins. Excerpta Medica, Amsterdam-Oxford.

14. Krag, E. (1963): Long-term prognosis in medically treated peptic ulcer. *Acta Med. Scand, 180*, 657.

15. La Brooy, S.J., Misiewicz, J.J., Edwards, J. et al. (1979): Controlled trial of cimetidine in upper gastrointestinal haemorrhage. *Gut 20*, 892.

16. Landecker, K.D., Crawford, J., Hunt, J.H. et al. (1979): Cimetidine and gastric ulcer healing. *Med. J. Aust. 2*, 43.

17. Machell, R.J., Ciclitira, P.J., Farthing, M.J.G. et al. (1979): Cimetidine in the prevention of gastric ulcer relapse. *Postgrad. Med. J. 55*, 393.

18. Mekel, R.C.P.M. (1978): Long-term treatment with cimetidine. *S. Afr. Med. J. 54*, 1089.

19. Piper, D.W., Shinners, J., Greig, M. et al. (1978): Effect of ulcer healing on the prognosis of chronic gastric ulcer. *Gut 19*, 419.

20. Piper, D.W. (1979): Treatment of peptic ulcer in the cimetidine era. *Med. J. Aust. 1*, 446.

21. Scheurer, V., Halter, F., Keller, H.M. et al. (1977): Gastric and duodenal ulcer healing and placebo treatment. *Gastroenterology 72*, 838.

22. Sewing, K.-F., Malchow, H., Albinus, M. et al. (1978): Cimetidin in der stationären Behandlung des peptischen Ulcus. II. Doppelblindstudie bei Ulcus ventriculi. *Dtsch.Med.Wochenschr. 103*, 152.

23. Tanner, A.R., Cowlisham, J.L., Cowen, A.E. and Ward, M. (1979): Efficacy of cimetidine and tri-potassium di-citrato bismuthate (De-Nol) in chronic gastric ulceration. *Med. J. Aust. 1*, 1.

24. Wulff, H.R. and Rune, S.J. (1978): A comparison of studies on the treatment of gastric ulceration with cimetidine. In: *Cimetidine*, pp. 281–288. Eds: C. Wastell and P. Lance. Churchill Livingstone, Edinburgh-London-New York.

Comparison of the acid inhibitory effects of ranitidine and cimetidine

S.J. Konturek, W. Obtułowicz, N. Kwiecień, E. Sito and J. Oleksy
Institute of Physiology and District Hospital, Kraków, Poland

Since the discovery by Black and his colleagues of a new class of drugs that specifically block the action of histamine on gastric secretion [1], a number of clinical studies have shown that these agents are superior to placebo in relieving ulcer pain, in decreasing antacid requirement and in expediting ulcer healing [2]. At present, cimetidine is the only widely accepted representative of this type of agent that blocks histamine H_2-receptors and this action is thought to be due to the imidazole ring present in its structure [3].

Recently, a new H_2-receptor blocker, ranitidine has been synthesized which does not contain an imidazole ring but which inhibits gastric acid secretion and is more potent than cimetidine [4, 5]. This study was undertaken to compare the effects of ranitidine and cimetidine given intravenously on pentagastrin- or histamine-induced gastric secretion and to determine the action of ranitidine and cimetidine on the cephalic and gastrointestinal phases of gastric secretion and on pancreatic secretion in duodenal ulcer patients.

Method

The studies were performed on patients with well established chronic duodenal ulcer disease and a mean age of 22 years (range 19–24 years), and mean weight of 68 kg (range 62–72). All these patients were in clinical remission when their study period began and they were divided into 3 groups, each consisting of 6–8 subjects. The patients received no anticholinergics or any other antisecretory drug for at least 5 days before the secretory studies were begun.

In all tests performed on group-I and group-III patients, a double lumen Dreiling tube was inserted early in the morning for secretory studies as described previously [6].

Gastric secretory studies

The comparison of intravenous administration of ranitidine and cimetidine on pentagastrin- and histamine-induced gastric secretion was studied in 6 subjects (group I). Throughout each study 154 mM of NaCl was infused in an arm vein at 80 ml/hr by peristaltic pump. Two 15-minute collections of gastric juice were first obtained to determine basal gastric secretion and then pentagastrin (2 μg/kg/hr) or histamine (40 μg/kg/hr) was infused at a constant dose throughout the study. After 60 minutes' infusion, when the secretory rate reached a peak, ranitidine or cimetidine was added to the infusion in graded doses, each dose being infused for a 60-minute period. Gastric juice was collected continuously throughout the study and divided in 15-minute aliquots. The volume of each sample was recorded and acid and pepsin outputs were determined as described previously [6].

The effects of ranitidine or cimetidine on the cephalic and gastroduodenal phases of gastric secretion were studied in 8 subjects (group II). Cephalic phase stimulation was induced by chewing and expectorating an appetizing meal consisting of 250 g of beefsteak, 150 g of French fried potatoes and 250 ml of water. This sham-feeding procedure was performed over a 30-minute period. All meals were prepared in a separate building so that the subjects could not see or smell the food until the time for the sham feeding. Each subject was trained, in a preliminary study, not to swallow food during sham feeding. During all tests gastric aspirates were carefully checked for swallowed food particles and none were found.

Pancreatic secretory studies

The effects of ranitidine on pancreatic secretion were examined in 8 subjects (group III). One 15-minute basal sample was collected first and then secretin, 1 clinical unit/kg/hr and cholecystokinin-pancreozymin, 1 Crick Harper, Raper unit/kg/hr were infused intravenously at a constant dose for 13 15-minute periods. After the initial 5 periods of secretin plus cholecystokinin-pancreozymin infusion, ranitidine was added to the infusate in a dose of 0.5 mg/kg/hr which was found in this study to cause over 90% inhibition of maximal pentagastrin-induced gastric acid secretion. The infusion of ranitidine or cimetidine was started 45 minutes before the start of sham feeding and continued during and following this procedure. Ranitidine was given in a dose of 0.5 mg/kg/hr whereas cimetidine was in a dose of 2.0 mg/kg/hr.

In the gastrointestinal phase tests a modification of the intragastric titration technique was applied [6]. The test meal used for intragastric titration consisted of a 10% aqueous solution of a liver concentrate powder and was allowed to flow continuously into the stomach from a reservoir barostat. Acid output was measured by intragastric titration with the end pH point of 5.5. Ranitidine or cimetidine was added to intravenous infusion after a 45-minute period of intragastric titration, when acid output reached a well sustained plateau, which continued for 60 minutes. The doses of these H_2-blockers were similar to those in the sham-feeding tests. For a comparison of the secretory responses to cephalic or gastrointestinal phases, each subject was tested with pentagastrin given in a constant dose of 2 μg/kg/hr for a 90-minute period to achieve the maximal acid output.

In pancreatic secretory tests secretin plus cholecystokinin-pancreozymin without ranitidine was given for the duration of the secretory test. Gastric and duodenal aspirates were collected continuously in 15-minute samples. Gastric aspirates were rejected and duodenal samples were measured regarding volume flow, bicarbonate and protein output as described previously [7]. In all tests during the cephalic and gastroduodenal phases of gastric secretion, venous blood samples were obtained from a peripheral vein for measurement of serum gastrin level. In tests during cephalic phase, blood samples were taken at 30 and 15 minutes before the start of H_2-blocker infusion, 15 minutes before the beginning of sham feeding, and then at 15, 30, 45, 60, 90 and 120 minutes following the procedure. In tests during the gastrointestinal phase, blood samples were withdrawn 30 and 15 minutes before, and every 30 minutes during the test meal. Serum gastrin was measured by radioimmuno-assay [8]. Antibody to gastrin was used at a final dilution 1:100,000. With this antibody all major molecular forms of gastrin were measured on a nearly equimolar basis. All determinations were made in duplicate. The within-assay variation was 9% and interassay variation was 16%. The immunoassay system was sufficiently sensitive to detect 5 pg/ml of serum gastrin.

Results are expressed as the mean $\pm$ SEM. Student's t-test was used to determine the significance of difference between the means with significances giving a p value of less than 0.05 being considered significant.

Results

Comparison of ranitidine and cimetidine in the inhibition of pentagastrin- and histamine-induced gastric secretion

The effect of graded doses of ranitidine or cimetidine infused against a constant background dose of pentagastrin (2 μg/kg/hr) or histamine (40

μg/kg/hr) producing the highest observed acid response is presented in Figures 1 and 2. Increasing the H_2-blocker dose resulted in a corresponding increase in the inhibition of gastric acid secretion. The dose required for 50% inhibition of maximal response (ID_{50}) to pentagastrin equalled about 0.12 mg/kg/hr of ranitidine and 1.04 mg/kg/hr of cimetidine. The ID_{50} for histamine stimulation was about 0.15 mg/kg/hr of ranitidine and 1.30 mg/kg/hr of cimetidine. Thus, the inhibitory potency of ranitidine was about 8 times greater than that of cimetidine. The administration of 0.5 mg/kg/hr of ranitidine or 3.0 mg/kg/hr of cimetidine caused almost complete inhibition of acid response to pentagastrin or histamine.

Pepsin outputs in tests with pentagastrin plus an H_2-blocker paralleled acid outputs. With increasing H_2-blocker doses the pepsin output fell dose-dependently and this decrease was almost entirely due to a reduction in the volume flow of gastric juice without significant change in pepsin concentration.

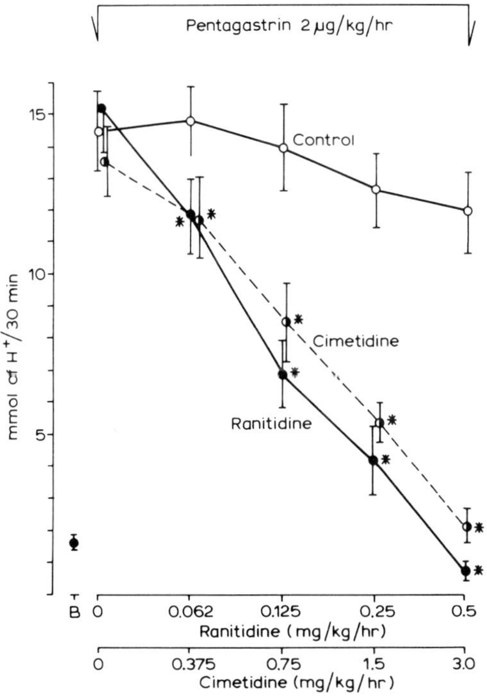

Fig. 1:   Effect of graded doses of ranitidine or cimetidine on pentagastrin-induced gastric acid secretion in duodenal ulcer patients. Mean $\pm$ SEM of 6 tests in 6 patients. Asterisks indicate significant decrease below control value.

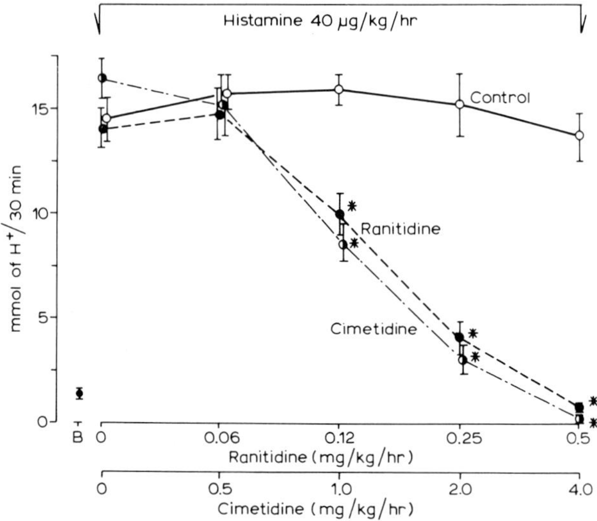

Fig. 2:   Effect of graded doses of ranitidine or cimetidine on histamine-induced gastric acid secretion in duodenal ulcer patients. Mean ± SEM of 6 tests in 6 patients. Asterisks indicate significant decrease below control value.

Effects of ranitidine or cimetidine on cephalic phase or gastrointestinal phase of gastric secretion and serum gastrin level

In control tests with sham feeding, the mean peak acid output (PAO) amounted to about 66% of the pentagastrin maximum. Ranitidine in a dose of 0.5 mg/kg/hr strongly reduced basal acid output (BAO) and almost completely prevented the increase in acid secretion in response to sham feeding. Cimetidine in a dose of 2 mg/kg/hr also reduced BAO and decreased, by about 70%, the response to sham feeding (Fig. 3). An increase in acid secretion in response to sham feeding was accompanied by a rise in pepsin secretion due to an increase in both volume of gastric juice and pepsin concentration. Ranitidine almost completely abolished pepsin response to sham feeding, whereas cimetidine reduced this response to about 50% of control value.

No significant changes in serum gastrin levels were observed during or after sham feeding and neither ranitidine nor cimetidine significantly affected these levels.

Gastric acid response to a LE meal introduced into the stomach to evoke the gastrointestinal phase of secretion was as high as that to pentagastrin and

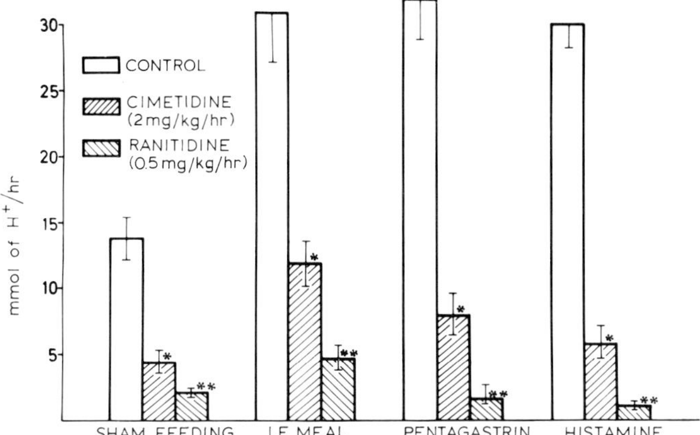

Fig. 3:   Effect of ranitidine (0.5 mg/kg/hr) and cimetidine (2.0 mg/kg/hr) on sham feeding and gastric LE meal-induced gastric acid secretion in duodenal ulcer patients. Mean ± SEM of 8 tests in 8 patients. For comparison, the degree of inhibition of pentagastrin- and histamine-induced acid secretion by the same doses of ranitidine or cimetidine are presented. Single asterisk indicates significant decrease below the control value; 2 asterisks indicate significant decrease below the value obtained with cimetidine.

remained relatively well sustained throughout the control experiment (Fig. 3). It was accompanied by an increase in serum gastrin level from a basal value of about 40 pg/ml to 100 pg/ml. Ranitidine given in a dose of 0.5 mg/kg/hr resulted in an immediate and almost complete inhibition of acid response, which remained suppressed even after the withdrawal of ranitidine infusion.

Cimetidine (2 mg/kg/hr) also dramatically inhibited postprandial acid secretion, which fell to about 75% of control values at the end of cimetidine infusion but then showed a tendency to increase when the H₂-blocker was withdrawn. Neither ranitidine nor cimetidine significantly influenced the postprandial elevation of serum gastrin level.

Effect of ranitidine on secretin and cholecystokinin-pancreozymin-stimulated pancreatic secretion

The rate of secretion of volume flow, bicarbonate and protein outputs in response to secretin plus cholecystokinin-pancreozymin alone (control) given in a constant dose reached a peak at the end of the first hour of infusion and was followed by a relatively well-sustained plateau (Figs. 4 and 5). In tests with ranitidine, pancreatic volume flow, bicarbonate and protein output was

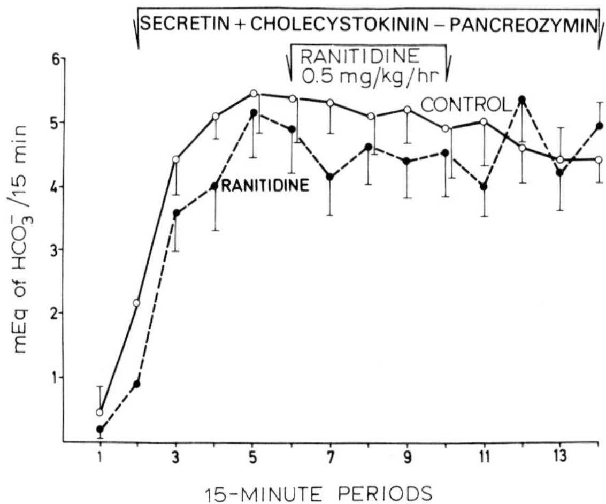

Fig. 4: Effect of ranitidine on pancreatic bicarbonate response to secretin plus cholecystokinin-pancreozymin. Mean ± SEM of 8 tests in 8 duodenal ulcer patients.

not significantly different from those with pancreatic secretagogues alone.

No symptoms or side effects were recorded with intravenous administration of any dose of ranitidine or cimetidine.

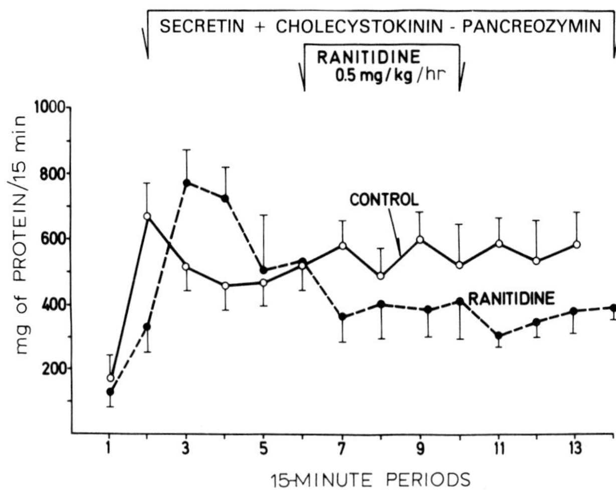

Fig. 5: Protein output in tests mentioned in Figure 4.

Discussion

Previous studies on the structure-function relationship of conventional H_2-receptor antagonists such as metiamide and cimetidine suggested that the imidazole ring is a necessary feature of these agents in order to recognize and bind specifically with the histamine H_2-receptor site for competitive antagonism [3]. The present study shows that ranitidine, which does not contain the imidazole ring but is a substituted amino-alkyl furan, is a potent inhibitor of basal and stimulated gastric secretion (Fig. 6).

Ranitidine given intravenously to duodenal ulcer patients appears to produce a dose-dependent inhibition of pentagastrin- or histamine-induced gastric acid secretion, being about 8 times more potent than cimetidine in this respect. This finding is in good agreement with a recent report from Domschke et al., who found that ranitidine infused intravenously to healthy volunteers is several times more effective than cimetidine in inhibiting pentagastrin-induced acid secretion [4]. Our studies extend this observation by studying the effects of ranitidine on sham feeding- and real feeding-induced gastric secretion and serum gastrin levels.

Our observation that ranitidine is capable of completely abolishing the sham feeding-induced acid and pepsin secretion provides strong evidence for the important role of histamine and H_2-receptors in cholinergic activation of the oxyntic cells. Since blockade of cholinergic receptors by atropine only partially inhibited sham feeding-induced gastric secretion in duodenal ulcer

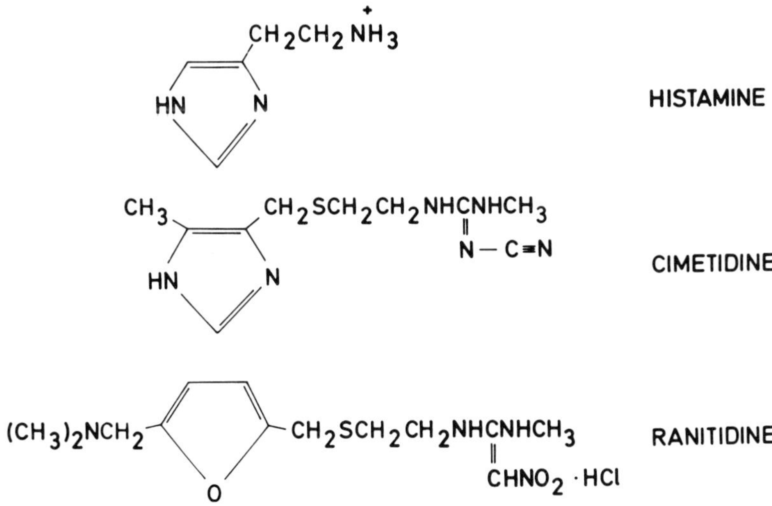

Fig. 6: The structures of histamine and 2 H₂-blockers, ranitidine and cimetidine.

patients [9], it may be concluded that H_2-receptors are more important than cholinergic receptors in the cholinergic activation of the oxyntic cells.

Gastric and intestinal phases of secretion are mediated by gastrin-cholinergic nerves and other ill-defined stimulants of gastric and intestinal origin. The principal mechanism of this secretion is by release of gastrin, which probably is due to direct excitation of the gastrin-producing cells, gastric distention and antral neutralization. Like the cephalic phase, the gastrointestinal phase of gastric secretion evoked by the introduction of the LE meal into the stomach was almost entirely suppressed by ranitidine without affecting serum gastrin response to this meal. This can be interpreted simply that H_2-receptors are not involved in postprandial gastrin release and this remains in agreement with previous findings in this respect [10]. The fact that both ranitidine and cimetidine can abolish postprandial gastric acid response indicates that histamine and H_2-receptors mediate also the stimulation of the oxyntic cells in the gastrointestinal phase. The question of whether histamine is the 'final common mediator' or 'general sensitizer' of the oxyntic cells to other stimuli involved in the postprandial secretion remains to be answered, but the studies on the isolated oxyntic cells support the latter function of this biogenic amine.

In addition to higher efficacy and potency in the inhibition of gastric secretion, ranitidine seems to be free of the various side effects attributed to cimetidine [11–13]. For these reasons ranitidine may prove more suitable for peptic ulcer therapy, particularly when prolonged treatment is required. The pathophysiological processes underlying duodenal ulceration are not fully explained but there are some indications that one of them may be an inadequate neutralization of an excessive gastric juice entering the duodenal bulb [14]. It seems obvious that agents which decrease the amount of acid and pepsin secretion entering the duodenum may increase the effectiveness of duodenal defense mechanisms and speed the healing rate of peptic ulceration. In view of the powerful inhibitory effects of ranitidine on gastric secretion it was pertinent to examine its action on pancreatic secretion, which provides most of the alkali for neutralizing gastric acid in the duodenum. The dose of ranitidine used in this study was found to cause about over 90% inhibition of pentagastrin-stimulated gastric secretion but did not effect significantly exogenously-stimulated pancreatic secretion. Specifically, the administration of ranitidine was not associated with significant changes in pancreatic volume flow, bicarbonate or protein output. The absence of any effect on pancreatic secretion indicates that histamine and H_2-receptors are not involved in mediating the action of secretin and cholecystokinin-pancreozymin on the pancreas. The action of ranitidine on pancreatic secretion in man has not been studied, but metiamide was reported to have no effect on pancreatic secretion in man [15].

Summary

The effects of ranitidine, a new H_2-receptor antagonist that does not contain an imidazole ring, and those of cimetidine on pentagastrin-, histamine-, the cephalic phase- and gastroduodenal phase-stimulated gastric acid secretion, and serum gastrin responses in duodenal ulcer patients have been determined. Compared with cimetidine, ranitidine was found to be about 8 times more potent an inhibitor of gastric acid secretion without affecting serum gastrin levels. Ranitidine, given in a dose inhibiting gastric acid secretion by over 90%, did not affect pancreatic secretion induced by secretin plus cholecystokinin-pancreozymin in duodenal ulcer patients. The availability of ranitidine, a more powerful inhibitor of gastric secretion, provides the opportunity for alternative treatment for peptic ulcer and related diseases.

References

1. Black, J.W., Duncan, W.A.M., Durant, G.J. et al. (1972): Definition and antagonism of histamine H_2-receptors. *Nature 236*, 385.
2. Binder, H.J., Cocco, A., Crossley, R.J. et al. (1978): Cimetidine in the treatment of duodenal ulcer. A multicenter double blind study. *Gastroenterology 74*, 380.
3. Brimblecombe, R.W., Duncan, W.A.M., Durant, G.J. et al. (1978): Characterization of development of cimetidine as a histamine H_2-receptor antagonist. *Gastroenterology 78*, 339.
4. Domschke, W., Lux, G. and Domschke, S. (1979): Gastric inhibitory action of H_2-antagonists ranitidine and cimetidine. *Lancet I*, 320.
5. Peden, M.R., Saunders, J.H.B. and Wormsley, K.G. (1979): Inhibition of pentagastrin-stimulated and nocturnal gastric secretion by ranitidine. *Lancet I*, 690.
6. Konturek, S.J., Biernat, J., Kwiecień, N. and Oleksy, J. (1975): Effect of glucagon on meal-induced gastric secretion in man. *Gastroenterology 68*, 448.
7. Konturek, S.J., Kwiecień, N., Swierczek, J. and Oleksy, J. (1979): Effect of methylated PGE_2 analogs given orally on pancreatic response to secretin in man. *Am. J. Dig. Dis. 22*, 16.
8. Yalow, R.S. and Berson, S.A. (1970): Radioimmunoassay of gastrin. *Gastroenterology 58*, 1.
9. Konturek, S.J., Kwiecień, N., Obtułowicz, W. et al. (1979): Comparison of the cephalic phase of gastric secretion in healthy subjects and duodenal ulcer patients. Role of vagal innervation. *Gut 20*, 875.
10. Konturek, S.J., Tasler, J., Obtułowicz, W. and Rehfeld, J.E. (1974): Effect of metiamide, a histamine H_2-receptor antagonist, on mucosal blood flow and serum gastrin level. *Gastroenterology 66*, 982.
11. Dell Fave, O.F., Tamburrano, G. and De Magistris, L. (1977): Gynecomastia with cimetidine. *Lancet I*, 1319.

12. Akaidon, P.G. and Karim, S.M.M. (1979): Male sexual dysfunction during treatment with cimetidine. *Br. Med. J. 1*, 17872.
13. McMillen, M.A., Ambis, D. and Siegel, J.H. (1978): Cimetidine and mental confusion. *N. Engl. J. Med. 298*, 284.
14. Wormsley, K.G. (1974): The pathophysiology of duodenal ulceration. *Gut 15*, 59.
15. Thjodleifsson, B. and Wormsley, K.G. (1975): Effect of metiamide on the response to secretin and cholecystokinin in man. *Gut 5*, 33.

Medical therapy of ulcer disease after gastric resection*

K.-H. Holtermüller, H. Weis, P. Herzog, M. Rothmund and J. Gröninger
I. Medizinische Klinik and Poliklinik, and Chirurgische Klinik, Johannes Gutenberg-Universität, Mainz, Federal Republic of Germany

Recurrent peptic ulceration has been reported after all types of operations performed for duodenal ulcer, except total gastrectomy. In general, operations which effect a greater reduction in acid secretion are followed by a lower incidence of recurrence than those which reduce gastric secretion to a lesser extent. Recurrence rates over a 5-year observation period differ from 3.7% (after subtotal gastrectomy alone) to 0.7% (if vagotomy and antrectomy are performed) [1].

Once the diagnosis of jejunal ulcer is established, operative treatment is in general advised to the patients [2]. The rationale behind such a recommendation is the belief that if medical management failed to control the initial ulceration, additional medical therapy will not control recurrent ulceration. Traditional medical management of recurrent ulcers is complicated by a redevelopment of ulcers in 42.1%; in contrast, surgery is followed by a second recurrence in only 14.3%; [3]. Since the development of recurrent ulcer following surgery is believed to reflect an inadequacy of the initial procedure, surgery is advised despite the fact that the mortality is about 4% and reoperation is successful in only about 70% of the cases.

It has been previously shown that H_2-receptor antagonists as well as antacids are beneficial in the treatment of duodenal ulcer [4–8]. The present study was designed to assess in a randomized trial the efficacy of the H_2-receptor antagonist cimetidine or of a magnesium aluminium hydroxide gel in the treatment of patients with jejunal ulcerations following gastric resection. Furthermore, whether the prophylactic use of cimetidine or antacid would prevent ulcer recurrences was studied.

* Part of this work was presented at the 34th meeting of the Deutsche Gesellschaft für Verdauungs- und Stoffwechselkrankheiten 1979. Supported by a grant from the Deutsche Forschungsgemeinschaft (Ho 349/6).

Patients and methods

Eighteen patients with jejunal ulcerations following gastric resection with Billroth II (B II) anastomosis were studied. The ulcer was confirmed by endoscopy within 3 days of entering the trial. Only patients with ulcers greater than 7 mm in diameter were admitted to the trial. Patients older than 65 years, and those with a marked impairment of renal function (serum creatinine greater than 2 mg/100 ml) and retained antrum or gastrinoma (Zollinger-Ellison syndrome) were excluded.

In the first phase (Phase I) of the trial, the influence of the 2 drugs on ulcer activity was evaluated. In the second phase (Phase II) an assessment was made of whether the 2 treatments were effective in preventing ulcer relapse.

All patients with jejunal ulcers were hospitalized (Phase I) for a 4-week period, during the acute attack of ulcer activity. The patients receiving bed rest were randomly allocated to cimetidine, 200 mg 3 times a day after meals and 400 mg at bed time, or a liquid magnesium aluminium antacid (Maaloxan® , 564 mEq/day), in a dose of 30 ml one and 3 hours after each meal and at bed time (7 doses/day).

A standard gastric analysis using pentagastrin, 6 μg/kg, was performed prior to the study if possible and in all patients following the study. Patients were asked to record such symptoms as epigastric pain, night pain and vomiting. All patients were seen during daily ward rounds by one of the attending physicians and were asked for details of symptoms and side effects. Before the study, and then at weekly intervals, routine hematological and biochemical studies and urine analysis were performed.

After 4 weeks of treatment, the endoscopy was repeated and ulcers were recorded as healed or unhealed. Ulcer healing was defined as disappearance of a crater and absence of, erosions. Patients in whom the ulcer did not heal within 4 weeks were classified as treatment failures.

Patients whose ulcer had not healed during antacid regimen received cimetidine for 4 weeks as outpatients. Patients whose ulcer had not healed during a 4-week course of cimetidine were advised to continue therapy for 3 more weeks as outpatients. If endoscopy still showed a persisting ulcer after 7 weeks in either of the 2 treatment groups, the patients were referred to surgery.

After completion of the trial, all patients whose ulcer had healed within 4 weeks entered the prophylactic outpatient trial (Phase II of the study), receiving either 400 mg of cimetidine twice daily or 7 doses of the magnesium aluminium antacid. Over a period of one year, repeated endoscopies were performed at 4-month intervals and on the occurrence of symptoms suggestive of an ulcer relapse. The hematologic and biochemical studies were repeated at

2-month intervals, and the symptoms and side-effect records were checked by the physician at these office visits. Compliance was evaluated by counting tablets, recording the number of antacid bottles used, and by assessing the number of bowel movemens. For statistical comparison Fisher's exact test was used.

Results

Patient characteristics

Patients characteristics are given in Table I. There were no significant differences between the 2 treatment groups with regard to age, sex, duration of disease, recent upper gastrointestinal bleeding, serum gastrin levels, and gastric acid secretion. All patients had had previous gastric resection without vagotomy for duodenal ulcer. In one patient, the B II resection was carried out because of gastric and duodenal ulcer. The average interval between previous gastric surgery and recurrent symptoms was 1.8 years. The majority of patients had had 2–3 operations related to their ulcer disease. One patient had a total of 7 abdominal operations, of which 3 were related to the ulcer disease. The duration of ulcer disease was comparable in the 2 groups and extended to 7.7 ± 2.4 years in the cimetidine group and 8.2 ± 2.6 years in the antacid group (Table I).

Table I: Patient characteristics.

	Cimetidine	Antacid
Mean age (years)	42 ± 7.4	40 ± 5.6
Males/females	8/1	9/10
Mean duration of disease (years)	7.7 ± 2.4	8.2 ± 2.6
Mean time elapsed since last gastric surgery (years)	1.9 ± 0.8	1.8 ± 0.6
Number of previous gastric operations	1 – 3	1 – 3
Patients with upper gastrointestinal bleeding on admission	4	2
Location of the ulcer		
Proximal loop	2	0
Distal loop	7	9
Mean peak acid output (mEq/hour)	11.2 ± 4.3	12.6 ± 5.6
Mean serum gastrin (pg/ml)	44 ± 8	47 ± 9

Mean values are expressed as mean ± SEM.

Symptoms, signs and ulcer localization

Pain was reported by all patients admitted to the study. The pain was localized in the upper part of the abdomen, being more frequently localized on the left than on the right side. Pain radiated into the back in 4 patients.

In 6 patients, the initial manifestation of recurrent ulcer was a history of gastrointestinal bleeding with melena. On physical examination, abdominal tenderness was the most frequent finding. The laboratory data were unrewarding except for anemia in patients who had previously experienced bleeding.

The site of the jejunal ulcer was the distal loop of the jejunum in 17 patients. In one patient the ulcer was localized in the proximal loop. In addition, in 5 patients gastric ulcers near the anastomosis were seen at the initial endoscopy. The healing of these anastomotic ulcers was recorded, but did not influence the decision concerning the efficacy of treatments applied, which was based solely on the healing of jejunal ulcerations.

Results of treatment

In the cimetidine group, ulcers healed within the 4 weeks of hospitalization in 8 of 9 patients treated. In contrast, only 3 out of 9 patients had completely healed ulcers while taking antacids. This difference was statistically significantly different at the 2.5% level.

Analysis of the duration of disease, ulcer size and gastric secretion revealed no difference between patients whose ulcers were healed and patients whose ulcers did not heal. Furthermore, there was no significant difference in the largest diameter of the ulcers measured during initial endoscopy. It should be noted that in patients treated with antacids only there was a decrease in ulcer size, but complete healing was only achieved in 3 patients (Table II).

Symptoms were analyzed as days and nights with ulcer pain. The symptoms in the week before the trial did not differ significantly between the 2 treatment groups. Symptoms improved markedly within both groups during the first few days of hospitalization. Cimetidine seemed to be more effective in relieving pain during the first 2 days, but this impression could not be statistically confirmed because of a wide variation in partial relief and decreased frequency of symptoms. During the short-term trial, no side effects were seen except for an increased stool frequency in patients during antacid therapy. The stools were soft and occasionally watery.

In the cimetidine group one patient had an ulcer which was not healed within 4 weeks. During continuous treatment with cimetidine complete

Table II: Ulcers healed after 4 weeks of therapy and number of relapses during maintenance therapy. (Figures in parentheses refer to total numbers of patients studied.)

	Cimetidine	Antacid
Ulcer healing in 4 weeks	8 (9)	3 (9)
Percentage healed	88	33*
Relapse within 1 year	0 (6)	2 (5)

* $p < 0.025$.

healing was seen after a total of 7 weeks of treatment. Six patients in the antacid group had ulcers that did not heal; they were treated with cimetidine, 1 g/day, for 4 weeks as outpatients. During that time 4 patients showed complete ulcer healing. The 2 patients whose ulcer had not healed and who were symptomatic as outpatients were advised to have surgery but refused. Both patients were lost to follow-up.

Recurrences

After completion of the trial, all patients whose ulcer had healed within 4 weeks were rerandomized for the prophylactic study (Phase II). Eleven patients were available for further study. Six received cimetidine and 5 received the antacid.

Two patients in the antacid group showed a symptomatic relapse after 3 and 5 months, respectively. Both were treated with a full dose of cimetidine for 4 weeks, and their ulcers healed. In the patients treated with cimetidine, no asymptomatic or symptomatic relapse occurred.

During long-term treatment with the H_2-receptor antagonist, a transient and moderate rise of SGPT serum glutamic pyruvic transaminase was seen in one patient. There were no changes in serum testosterone levels.

During the long-term study there was a significant difference between the 2 groups in the days off work. In the antacid group, 64 days of work were lost, in contrast to the cimetidine group, where no day off work was noted because of recurrent ulcer ($p < 0.01$).

After completion of the long-term trial all patients were advised to continue to take cimetidine in a dose of 400 mg at bedtime. The patients were cared for by their home physicians, who were asked to refer the patients for follow-up if symptoms compatible with recurrent ulcer were present.

Discussion

The present study was designed to test the efficacy of cimetidine and an antacid in promoting ulcer healing in hospitalized patients with jejunal ulcerations following gastric surgery. Furthermore following complete ulcer healing an assessment was made of whether the 2 treatment regimens were effective in preventing ulcer relapse.

Cimetidine promoted ulcer healing in patients with recurrent jejunal ulcerations after B II gastrectomy. The H_2-receptor antagonist was significantly more efficient than an antacid with a buffering capacity of 80 mEq/dose.

In the present study, we chose to treat patients with jejunal ulcers as inpatients, since more than 50% of these patients present with upper gastrointestinal bleeding, according to data in the literature [2]. In our own series, one third of the patients were admitted to the hospital because of bleeding from the jejunal ulceration. In hospitalized patients we found a healing rate of 88% within 4 weeks, which is the same as has been found in patients with duodenal ulcer during hospitalization and cimetidine treatment [9].

The assessment of ulcer pain was difficult since the symptoms disappeared within the first week; similar observations were made by others [9]. There was no significant difference between cimetidine and antacid with regard to the relief of ulcer pain.

Antacids have recently been shown to heal duodenal ulcers in hospitalized patients in the dosage used in this study [8]. However, in jejunal ulceration following B II gastrectomy antacids were much less effective. This is most likely due to a decreased utilization due to gastric emptying in operated patients [10].

Our results are in accordance with the data reported by Delle Fave et al. [11], who documented the healing of postgastrectomy ulcers with a dosage of 1.6 g of cimetidine over 8 weeks in 9 of 10 patients. In 2 randomized double-blind studies including patients with anastomotic ulcers following B I or B II gastrectomy, the effect of medical therapy on ulcer healing was assessed [12, 13]. The healing rate in outpatients after one month of cimetidine treatment was 67%, and this increased to 86% after 2 months [12]. In the second study, the healing rate was 85% (6 of 7 patients) during a 4-week treatment period, and increased to 100% after 8 weeks. The healing rates in the control groups of the 2 studies were 11% and 12.5% respectively [12, 13].

Furthermore, Hoare et al. [14] observed healing of ulcers that recurred after operation in 19 of 20 patients after 8 weeks of cimetidine in a dose of 1 g day. Saunders et al. [15] reported healing in 10 of 13 patients with recurrent and stomal ulcerations after being treated for one month with cimetidine. In contrast, Kennedy et al. [16] and Wastell [17] could not document a significant effect of cimetidine on healing of recurrent ulcer after vagotomy and/or gastric operations (Table III). Our results and the data of other investigations [11–15] demonstrate that cimetidine is effective in healing recurring ulcers after gastric surgery.

We have shown that even jejunal ulcerations, which have in the past been considered to be an indication for surgery, can be healed by cimetidine in a percentage as high as that previously demonstrated for duodenal ulcers. The percentage of ulcers healed on an intensive antacid regimen (33%) is lower than that reported in hospitalized patients and in outpatients with duodenal ulcer (52–100%) [7, 8, 18]. This decrease in efficacy of antacids can only be explained by rapid gastric emptying, as it occurs otherwise only in fasting ulcer patients [19]. The results of maintenance treatment in the present study are promising, although the numbers of patients were small. Cimetidine prevented relapse in all patients during a one-year trial, whereas 2 patients relapsed while taking antacids only. There was no asymptomatic recurrence in the patients enrolled in the trial, as documented by repeated endoscopic examinations. Our long-term results are in good agreement with recently published data by Festen et al. [12], who found an incidence of relapse of 15% during maintenance treatment. Still, the question remains as to whether recurrent ulcer means inappropriate surgery and that patients would be best reoperated (i.e., completion of vagotomy, re-resection) or be on long-term cimetidine therapy.

Now that the efficacy of cimetidine has been proven in patients with jejunal ulcers following B II gastrectomy, prospective studies comparing cimetidine treatment with surgery should answer this question.

Summary

In order to assess the efficacy of cimetidine or an antacid in patients with endoscopically proven jejunal ulcers after Billroth II gastrectomy, 18 such patients entered a randomized clinical trial. After 4 weeks of treatment within the hospital, 8 of 9 patients treated with 1 g of cimetidine per day had healed ulcers, compared to 3 of 9 patients receiving antacids, the difference being statistically significant (p < 0.05). There was no significant difference between the 2 groups with regard to pain relief. During a 1-year maintenance trial in 11 patients using cimetidine in a dose of 800 mg/day or an antacid, none of the patients taking cimetidine relapsed. In contrast, 2 of 5 patients receiving antacids developed recurrent ulcers and symptoms after 3 and 5 months, respectively. The results of the present study demonstrate a beneficial effect of

Table III: Results of cimetidine therapy in patients with recurrent ulcers following gastric surgery.

Study	Type of gastric surgery*		Number of patients	Duration of therapy (weeks)	Healing of ulcers	
					Cimetidine	Control
Delle Fave et al.	B II gastrectomy		10	8	9/10	–
Festen et al.	B I / B II gastrectomy	(4/17)	21	4	8/12	1/9
Gugler et al.	B I / B II gastrectomy	(8/ 7)	15	8	7/7	1/8
Hoare et al.	PGV Vagotomy + pyloroplasty B II gastrectomy	(1) (14) (5)	20	6	17/20	–
Holtermüller et al.	B II gastrectomy		18	4	8/9	3/9
Kennedy et al.	PGV Vagotomy + gastrojejunostomy Vagotomy + pyloroplasty Gastrectomy	(8) (7) (6) (3)	24	6	7/12	5/12
Saunders et al.	Vagotomy + pyloroplasty Vagotomy + gastrojejunostomy B II gastrectomy	(8) (1) (4)	13	4	10/13	–
Wastell	PGV SVP PGVP	(6) (1) (1)	8	6	4/8	–

* Figures in parentheses refer to numbers of patients. PGV = proximal gastric vagotomy; PGVP = proximal gastric vagotomy and pyloroplasty; SVP = selective gastric vagotomy and pyloroplasty; B I/B II gastrectomy = Billroth I or Billroth II gastrectomy.

cimetidine on the healing of jejunal ulcers, a disease which has been considered to be an indication for surgery.

References

1. Postlethwait, R.W. (1973): Five year follow-up results of operations for duodenal ulcer. *Surg. Gynecol. Obstet. 137*, 387.
2. Wychulis, A.R., Priestley, J.T. and Foulk, W.T. (1966): A study of 360 patients with gastrojejunal ulceration. *Surg. Gynecol. Obstet. 122*, 89.
3. Stabile, B.E. and Passaro, E. (1976): Recurrent peptic ulcer. *Gastroenterology 70*, 124.
4. Multicentre trial (1979): Comparison of two doses of cimetidine and placebo in the treatment of duodenal ulcer: A multicentre trial. *Gut 20*, 68.
5. Peter, P., Kiene, K., Gonvers, J.J. et al. (1978): Cimetidin in der Behandlung des Ulcus duodeni. *Dtsch. Med. Wochenschr. 103*, 1163.
6. Binder, H.J., Cocco, A., Crossley, R.J. et al. (1978): Cimetidine in the treatment of duodenal ulcer: A multicenter double blind study. *Gastroenterology 74*, 380.
7. Peterson, W.L., Sturdevant, R.A.L., Frankl, H.D. et al. (1977): Healing of duodenal ulcer with an antacid regimen. *N. Engl. J. Med. 297*, 341.
8. Kunert, H. and Ottenjann, R. (1978): Effekt eines Mg-Al-hydroxidhaltigen Antazidums auf die Heilungsdauer von Ulcera duodeni — randomisierte Doppelblindstudie. *Z. Gastroenterol. 22*, 630.
9. Malchow, H., Sewing, K.-F., Albinus, M. et al. (1978): Cimetidin in der stationären Behandlung des peptischen Ulkus. I. Wirkung auf die Heilung des Ulcus duodeni. *Dtsch. Med. Wochenschr. 103*, 149.
10. Deering, T.B., Carlson, G.L., Malagelada, J.-R. et al. (1979): Fate of oral neutralizing antacid and its effect on postprandial secretion and emptying. *Gastroenterology 77*, 986.
11. Delle Fave, G.F., Paoluzzi, P., Bergonzi, L. et al. (1977): Cimetidine and postgastrectomy recurrent ulcer. *Rend. Gastro-enterol. 9*, 150.
12. Festen, H.P.M., Lamers, C.B.H., Driessen, W.M.M. and Van Tongeren, J.H.M. (1979): Cimetidine in anastomotic ulceration after partial gastrectomy. *Gastroenterology 76*, 83.
13. Gugler, R., Lindstaedt, H., Miederer, S. et al. (1979): Cimetidine for anastomotic ulcers after partial gastrectomy: A randomized controlled trial. *N. Engl. J. Med. 301*, 1077.
14. Hoare, A.M., Jones, E.L. and Hawkins, C.F. (1978): Cimetidine for ulcers recurring after gastric surgery. *Br. Med. J. 1.*, 1325.
15. Saunders, J.H.B., Cargill, J.M., Peden, N.R. and Wormsley, K.G. (1978): Cimetidine for ulcers recurring after surgery. *Br. Med. J. 1*, 1619.
16. Kennedy, T. and Spencer, A. (1978): Cimetidine for recurrent ulcer after vagotomy or gastrectomy: A randomised controlled trial. *Br. Med. J. 1*, 1242.
17. Wastell, C. (1978): The treatment of recurrent ulceration after vagotomy with cimetidine. In: *Cimetidine: The Westminster Hospital Symposium.* Eds: C.

Wastell and P. Lance. Churchill Livingstone, Edinburgh-London-New York.
18. Ippoliti, A.F., Surdevant, R.A.L., Isenberg, J.I. et al. (1978): Cimetidine versus intensive antacid therapy for duodenal ulcer. *Gastroenterology 74*, 393.
19. Holtermüller, K.H., Sinterhauf, K. and Büchler, R. (1975): Die Wirkung von oralem Calcium und Magnesium auf die Magensäuresekretion und Gastrinfreisetzung bei Patienten mit Ulcus duodeni. *Verh. Dtsch. Ges. Inn. Med. 81*, 1237.

Management of Zollinger-Ellison Syndrome

S. Bonfils and M. Mignon
Unité de Recherches de Gastroentérologie, INSERM, Unité 10, Paris and Chaire de Clinique des Maladies de l'Appareil Digestif, Hôpital Bichat, Paris, France

For more than 10 years, total gastrectomy has been the treatment of choice in managing patients with the Zollinger-Ellison Syndrome (ZES). This was largely because other approaches had failed to satisfactorily control the morbidity and mortality from associated gastric hypersecretion and related complications.

However, total gastrectomy, although often followed by minimum discomfort, is a drastic and purely symptomatic treatment. Furthermore, surgery is often disappointing in relation to the following: the multiplicity of pancreatic lesions makes it difficult to perform curative tumoral excision; there is a high postoperative risk in patients in a poor condition due to acute symptoms (vomiting, diarrhea, hemorrhage); and in the case of hepatic metastases, nutritional problems related to total gastrectomy have to be avoided.

The efficacy of H_2-receptor antagonists in the treatment of ZES was first supported by a series of case reports commencing in 1974 [1–3]. The replacement of metiamide with cimetidine was determined on the basis of drug toxicity and particularly agranulocytosis. Although cimetidine has few side effects, they could lead to a discontinuance of the drug and hence a need for surgery.

Studies of prolonged follow-up with cimetidine are now available [4–7], and these confirm our earlier remarks concerning 2 interesting phenomena: escape and prolonged secretory inhibition. As regards the first, the disappearance of adequate acid secretion control, despite an increasing cimetidine dosage, is another reason for considering surgery.

In general one could say that surgery is still an alternative to cimetidine treatment [6]. Since controlling acid secretion with cimetidine is, for various reasons, questionable in some patients, any attempt at a definitive or prolonged cure of ZES is justified, i.e. tumor excision should be considered in each case.

Finally, medical treatment of ZES should not be limited to the use of cimetidine. Other antisecretory drugs should be used, either in combination with cimetidine (e.g. pirenzepine) or as a full substitute (e.g. ranitidine).

Cimetidine treatment in ZES

Rationale and methods

The route of administration should be adapted to the clinical condition. Oral administration is the most common route but in acute ZES intravenous infusion is usually necessary, at least when starting treatment.

The dosage should be adapted to the rate of gastric hypersecretion: there is a dose-response correlation between cimetidine blood concentration and secretory inhibition [8]. Moreover, increasing the dosage (and hence the cimetidine blood concentration) above that necessary to obtain maximal acute secretory inhibition results in a prolongation of the drug activity [8], which could increase the therapeutic efficiency. Blood cimetidine measurement could be helpful for theoretical estimation of the dosage required by the patient.

Efficiency criteria should be correctly defined according to the initial clinical and biological status of the patient. Reliable markers, sensitive enough to allow the physician to conclude that control of the patient's hypersecretion is reached, are needed in order to feel secure in implementing long-term treatment.

According to our experience both disappearance and reappearance of diarrhea are very important criteria. Ulcer healing should be endoscopically controlled and repeatedly checked even in symptom-free patients.

Basal acid output (BAO) measurement during the second hour following cimetidine administration at the usual fractional dose (thus defining acute inhibition) only allows assessment of the pharmacological drug efficiency. However, measurement 24 hours after discontinuing the drug is more important, since it then characterizes the 'prolonged secretory inhibition' which results in optimal therapeutic activity [6, 7].

Cimetidine administration is purely treatment of the symptom 'gastric hypersecretion' and does not act on the 'tumoral gastrin' disease. Hence, it is useless to have iterative measurements of serum gastrin.

A surgery devoted to the gastrinoma itself is therefore justified and definitive or temporary cure in 10–15% of the cases has been obtained. The usefulness of cimetidine for antisecretory coverage in the postoperative period and/or in the case of tumor relapse is obvious.

Chronic ZES

Chronic ZES includes clinical pictures of long duration (many years) and usually a positive history of duodenal ulcer and diarrhea. In chronic ZES, there is no evidence of excessive virulence that could not be controlled, at least for a time, by standard medical treatment: initially these patients are often treated as ordinary ulcer patients without suspicion of ZES. However, the clinician still has time to make the correct diagnosis when suspicion arises.

Is cimetidine a valuable substitute for total gastrectomy in chronic ZES? We administered cimetidine orally in various doses, depending upon the clinical and biological information, to 10 patients. Initially, low dosages were used (0.8–1.2 g/day) and these produced occasional successes. We now suggest 1.6 g/day as a starting dose as used in 5 out of 10 of our patients.

In 2 cases cimetidine treatment was ineffective. In one patient severe diarrhea continued and in the other a gastric ulcer developed during treatment. Total gastrectomy was performed in both cases.

Prolonged inhibition, as described below, was observed in 2 cases, accompanied by stable improvement of the clinical condition. In each of these patients an isolated duodenal-wall tumor was found at laparotomy; its excision resulted in cure of the syndrome with regard to clinical symptoms and serum gastrin. In another case cimetidine was stopped after surgery – partial pancreatic tumor excision – resulting in a dramatic regression of symptoms.

In 2 other cases, who have been treated for more than 30 months, ulcer healing and disappearance of diarrhea are stable. However, BAO values remain elevated and acute secretory inhibition with 400 mg of cimetidine, orally, is only 50%. This poor correlation between clinical symptoms and endoscopy on the one hand and gastric secretion on the other, suggests that ulcer(s) could acutely relapse at any moment and possibly without any pain or other premonitory signs [6].

In 3 cases, the escape phenomenon was observed; hence, ranitidine was used instead of cimetidine. The escape phenomenon can be very generally described as a secondary therapeutic inefficacy rather than as a 'specific' resistence to cimetidine. However, we have presented elsewhere the changes observed in acid secretion inhibition that were induced by a standard dose of cimetidine (100-mg bolus) according to time (65% inhibition before treatment and 51% inhibition after 260 days' cimetidine administration) [6]. We consider symptomatic (pain, diarrhea) and/or endoscopic (ulcer) relapse as the 'escape' in patients successfully treated by a given dose of cimetidine. This results in the neccesity to increase the cimetidine dosage, which is not always successful.

The 8 cases entering the ranitidine trial were obvious 'escape from cimetidine' patients.

A prolonged inhibition of gastric secretion during continuous treatment with H_2-receptor antagonists was first observed in ZES patients after metiamide. The valid observation of this prolonged secretory inhibition needs a one-hour basal secretion study more than 12 hours after the last therapeutic dose. In a recent cooperative study, a Danish and a French group collected 23 ZES patients, all of whom had been treated daily with 1–3 g of cimetidine for periods longer than 3 months [7]. During the period under cimetidine treatment, a significant decrease in BAO was noted by comparison with the precimetidine value (62% during the 6–9 month period and 56% during the 9–12 month period). Out of 7 patients tested daily for 3 successive days after drug discontinuation (mean period of treatment: 45 weeks), 3 presented a nearly total secretory inhibition, over 60 hours. At the same time, no measurable amounts of cimetidine were found in plasma.

Although the nature of this prolonged secretory inhibition is difficult to explain at the present time, recognition of the phenomenon may be important for the proper interpretation of clinical data; its frequency is unknown and seems partly related to the duration of treatment.

Acute ZES

Acute ZES includes conditions of major emergency that could threaten the patient's life: severe metabolic disturbances, dehydration, electrolytic losses, fistula, acute ulcer complications [6].

All of these, in some way, are related to gastric hypersecretion. The virulence of the syndrome is obvious and the patient will require hospitalization with intensive medical treatment; without control of acid secretion surgical intervention will be necessary. This type of patient still remains an immediate challenge for the clinician: if the manner of presentation is primary, there is a burst of intricate problems related to diagnosis and treatment; if it appears as an evolutive aspect of chronic ZES, prior suspicion or diagnosis is helpful, but does not decrease the difficulty of treatment.

Of 6 personal cases, only one represented a secondary acute evolution in a formerly diagnosed ZES patient. In the other 5 cases, surgery for common duodenal ulcer was undertaken in 2, and was immediately followed by increased acid hypersecretion and severe complications. In the other 3 patients, jejunal perforation, iterative hemorrhages and acute dehydration due to vomiting and diarrhea were the initial symptoms.

Cimetidine infusion in the usual daily dosage of 2.4 g adjunctive to intensive medical treatment and care brought about an improvement in the patients' condition, and hence allowed time in order to obtain diagnostic certitude. But the final problem concerns the right time at which to choose total gastrectomy: in acute ZES we consider the virulence of the disease as irreversible. In our experience antisecretory drugs, even in combination (H_2-receptor antagonists + anticholinergics), are never a substitute for total gastrectomy, but are indispensable for minimizing the lethal risk of surgery [9].

Ranitidine treatment in ZES

Ranitidine is a new specific H_2-receptor antagonist without the imidazol ring of histamine and cimetidine. Comparative studies have shown that on a molar basis ranitidine is a stronger inhibitor of gastric acid secretion than cimetidine. Evaluation of the therapeutic benefit in duodenal ulcer is in progress in many countries.

Thanks to the courtesy of our colleagues*, our personal experience (3 cases) of ranitidine treatment in ZES has been broadened and we are able to present preliminary data from 8 patients, 2 females and 6 males, of whom 2 were operated upon. Of the 6 not operated all had multiple duodenal ulcers and 4 suffered from diarrhea.

These cases are fully representative of the variety of clinical and biological findings (BAO range: 21.5–77.6 mEq/hr; serum gastrin range 315–3,800 pg/ml). In the 8 cases, inclusion in the trial was decided after demonstration of an escape from cimetidine, the final and inefficacious dosage used being 2 g in 3 cases and 2.4 g or more (up to 3 g) in the others. Furthermore, 3 out of the 8 cases presented untoward effects of the drug: gynecomastia and sexual impotency [10], psychiatric disorders, and severe renal insufficiency that was considered as cimetidine-induced since it regressed after discontinuance of the drug.

The comparative effect of ranitidine and cimetidine upon 24 hours' intragastric acidity allowed us to select the dosage and regimen for ranitidine treatment [11]. This was done in 2 personal cases and in 3 others. In short, during 2 separate 24-hour periods, a combined glass electrode was introduced into the stomach to monitor continuously the pH of the gastric contents: ranitidine (150 or 200 mg) or cimetidine (600 mg) were given with the meal at 8

---

* J.P. Galmiche, F. Hagenmuller, S.J. Konturek, J.C. Rambaud, F.P. Ryan and P Zeitoun.

a.m. 1 p.m. and 8 p.m.; an additional dose of the drug was administered at 1 a.m. and results were analyzed according to Peterson et al. [12].

With a daily dosage of 400–900 mg adequate control of acid secretion was obtained, with disappearance of symptoms (ulcer and diarrhea). Over follow-up periods ranging from one to more than 6 months escape was observed in 3 patients but was easily controlled by increasing the drug dosages. Cimetidine side effects disappeared and no specific problems relating to ranitidine have been observed so far [10].

Combined antisecretory treatment

As mentioned above, there are conditions in ZES where H_2-receptor antagonists are incapable of achieving a profound and stable reduction of acid secretion, even with increasing dosages. In the case of escape as well as primary inefficacy, there is no theoretical justification to administer cimetidine, whatever the route, in a dosage above 2.4 g/day. This is documented with dose-response studies and measurements of cimetidine blood levels [8].

Longer and greater secretory inhibition has been obtained by combining anticholinergic drugs with H_2-receptor antagonists, however, the additional inhibitory effect of anticholinergics was obtained only when submaximal doses of cimetidine were used [13].

A combined treatment using pirenzepine, an antisecretory agent of the trycyclic antidepressant series, and cimetidine gave favorable results in some cases of ZES [14]. A continuous record of intragastric pH over 24-hour periods allows significant comparison between cimetidine alone and cimetidine + pirenzepine (Table). Although cimetidine alone was effective in inhibiting acid secretion, the combined treatment offered the advantage of producing achlorhydria more often and for longer periods of time: pH levels higher than 3 were found 58% of the time during combined treatment but only 7% of the time during treatment with cimetidine alone.

Encouraging clinical results were observed in acute ZES cases, i.e. cessation of diarrhea, relief of pain, ulcer healing and suppression of acid secretion. Assessment of a combination of H_2-receptor antagonists and pirenzepine in the treatment of chronic ZES is in progress.

A better understanding of the mechanism of action of pirenzepine was recently obtained. At the level of the gastric mucosa it can simply be explained by a pure antimuscarinic action [15]. Binding to muscarinic receptors showed a greater affinity for some organs (among them gastric mucosa) explaining the absence of side effects generally observed with antimuscarinic drugs [16].

Table: Continuous intragastric pH record over 2 consecutive 24-hour periods in a case of ZES.

	1–2	2–3	3–4	4–5	5–7	
Period 1 cimetidine	7	86	5	1	1	100%
Period 2 cimetidine + pirenzepine	8	34	33	17	8	100%

Period 1: cimetidine 2.4 g orally.
Period 2: cimetidine 2.4 g orally + pirenzepine 1 mg/kg orally.
Results are expressed in per cent duration for each intragastric pH range over the 24-hour period.

Conclusion

So far, cimetidine has been the most commonly used drug in ZES medical treatment. In spite of indisputable successes, it is difficult to believe that cimetidine could be a routine treatment in all gastrinomas in view of the following: the extremely high level of acid secretion observed in many cases; the unforseeable possibility of an escape, and the individual risk of side effects that may increase with the duration of treatment [4]. All these problems could occur in operated patients, whatever the surgical gesture (partial gastrectomy, truncal vagotomy, or parietal cell vagotomy).

The respective indications for surgery and cimetidine could be appreciated in view of curing the gastrinoma or suppressing acid secretion either by drug action or by total gastrectomy.

In acute ZES, we believe that antisecretory drugs are never a substitute for total gastrectomy, even if they dramatically reduce acid secretion (with subsequent diarrhea improvement and ulcer(s) healing). But these drugs do minimize the mortality risk of total gastrectomy.

In chronic ZES, the successive stages in therapeutic decision-making are: assessment of cimetidine efficacy on the basis of clinical, endoscopic and biologic criteria – in this stage, procedures for diagnosis and tumor localization are performed; if therapeutic results are satisfactory, surgery for gastrinoma is undertaken; if excision of the gastrinoma is considered complete and followed by normalization of acid secretion and serum gastrin, cimetidine is stopped and gastric secretion is repeatedly measured; if complete cure of the gastrinoma is not obtained, cimetidine is considered as a substitute for total gastrectomy as long as no clinical and/or biologic signs of escape appear; total gastrectomy is performed if the response to cimetidine is not satisfactory, if the escape phenomenon appears, or if strict medical control of the disease cannot be obtained on a long-term basis.

References

1. Bonfils, S., Mignon, M. and Accary, J.P. (1974): Inhibiteurs des récepteurs H_2 à l'histamine et syndrome de Zollinger Ellison. *Nouv. Presse Méd. 3*, 1883.
2. Bonfils, S., Mignon, M., Kloeti, G. and Jian, R. (1977): Therapeutic assessment of histamine H_2 blockers in 10 cases of Zollinger Ellison syndrome. *Gastroenterology 72*, A3, 813.
3. Bonfils, S., Bernier, J.J., Mignon, M. et al. (1977): Metiamide treatment in five patients with Zollinger Ellison syndrome. *Digestion 15*, 43.
4. McCarty, D.M. (1978): Report of the United States experience with cimetidine in Zollinger Ellison and other hypersecretory states. *Gastroenterology 74*, 453.
5. Stage, J.G., Stadil, F. and Fischerman, K. (1978): New aspects in the treatment of the Zollinger Ellison syndrome. In: *Cimetidine. Proceedings of an International Symposium on Histamine H_2-Receptor Antagonists* p. 137. Editor: W.E. Creutzfeldt. Excerpta Medica, Amsterdam-Oxford.
6. Bonfils, S., Mignon, M. and Gratton, J. (1979): Cimetidine treatment of acute and chronic Zollinger Ellison syndrome. *World J. Surg. 3*, 597.
7. Stage, J.G., Bonfils, S., Mignon, M. and Stadil, F. (1980): Prolonged secretory inhibition during cimetidine treatment in Zollinger Ellison patients. *Scand. J. Gastroenterol.* (Submitted for publication.)
8. Bonfils, S., Mignon, M., Jian, R. and Kloeti, G. (1977): Biological studies during long-term cimetidine administration. In: *Cimetidine. Proceedings of the Second International Symposium on Histamine H_2-Receptor Antagonists* p. 311. Editors: W.L. Burland and M. A. Simkins. Excerpta Medica, Amsterdam-Oxford.
9. Fox, P.S., Hoffman, J.W. and Wilson, S.D. (1974): Surgical management of the Zollinger Ellison syndrome. *Surg. Clin. North Am. 54*, 395.
10. Mignon, M., Vallot, T., Mayeur, S. and Bonfils, S. (1980): Un cas de syndrome de Zollinger Ellison traité par la ranitidine; comparaisons sécrétoires et thérapeutiques avec la cimétidine. *Gastroentérol. Clin. Biol.* (In press).
11. Mignon, M., Vallot, T., Mayeur, S. and Bonfils, S. (1980): Ranitidine and cimetidine in Zollinger Ellison syndrome. *Br. J. Clin. Pharmacol. 10*.
12. Peterson, W.L., Barnett, C., Feldman, M. and Richardson, C.T. (1979): Reduction of twenty-four-hour gastric acidity with combination drug therapy in patients with duodenal ulcer. *Gastroenterology 77*, 1015.
13. Blackwood, W.S. and Northfield, T.C. (1977): Nocturnal gastric acid secretion: effect of cimetidine and interaction with anticholinergics. In: *Cimetidine. Proceedings of the Second International Symposium on Histamine H_2-Receptor Antagonists* p. 124. Editors: W.L. Burland and M. A. Simkins. Excerpta Medica, Amsterdam-Oxford.
14. Mignon, M., Vallot, T., Galmiche, J.P. et al. (1980): Interest of a combined anti-

secretory treatment, cimetidine and pirenzepin in the management of severe forms of Zollinger Ellison syndrome. *Digestion 20*, 56.

15. Sachs, G., Kasbekar, D.K. and Berglindh, T. (1979): The mechanism of action of pirenzepin on gastric secretion. In: *Die Behandlung des Ulcus pepticum mit Pirenzepin*, p. 18. Editors: A.L. Blum and R. Hammer. Karl Demeter Verlag, Gräfelfing.

16. Hammer, R., Berrie, C.P., Birdsall, N.J.M. et al. (1980): Pirenzepine distinguishes between different subclasses of muscarinic receptors. *Nature 283*, 90.

Side effects of the histamine H$_2$-receptor antagonists and their implication for ulcer therapy

H. Goebell and J. Hotz

Medical Department, Division of Gastroenterology, University of Essen, Essen, Federal Republic of Germany

Introduction

The safety and the risks of cimetidine have been the topic of some earlier articles [1–3]. The present paper will give an overview of current knowledge concerning the unwanted effects of cimetidine outside the gastrointestinal tract, and will therefore not cover such events as ulcer perforation, hypergastrinemia, hyperplasia of G-cells, or the overlooking of a gastric carcinoma.

A number of sources contribute to our knowledge on the side effects of cimetidine. Controlled clinical trials have the great advantage of scientifically based observations and of the presence of controls, but their number is limited in relation to the estimated number of patients that have been or are being treated with cimetidine. In 1979, this estimated number was approximately 11 million for the U.S.A. and the U.K., and much higher for the whole world [4]. Very rare side effects are probably not discovered in clinical trials with a defined number of patients. They are reported in single observations, which in many cases have the disadvantage of being incomplete and incorrect. Nevertheless, these reports are necessary and form the basis for important conclusions.

Subjective symptoms

Subjective symptoms related to cimetidine treatment, such as headache, tiredness, dizziness, diarrhea, rash, muscular pain and constipation, have been reported with a frequency ranging from 1% to approximately 4% in controlled trials (Table I). However, there is no significant difference from the

Table I: Subjective symptoms (> 1% incidence) with short-term cimetidine treatment.

Symptoms	Cimetidine (%)	Placebo (%)
Headache	3.6	5.0
Tiredness	2.6	3.1
Dizziness	1.7	1.5
Diarrhea	2.0	0.8
Rash	1.9	0.8
Muscular pain	2.0	0.4
Constipation	1.1	2.7
Total numbers withdrawn from trial	9/643 (1.4%)	3/259 (1.2%)

Reproduced with permission from [1].

number of events occurring in the placebo groups. Very rarely, these symptoms have been the cause of withdrawal of cimetidine [1, 2].

Renal disorders

A slight increase in plasma creatinine can occur early during cimetidine therapy, without a concomitant rise in plasma urea and without proteinuria [2]. A steady state is reached or the phenomenon is reversible during treatment. A reduction in high dosage might be advisable. There seems to be no nephrotoxicity and no reproducible impairment of creatinine clearance. Recently, it has been demonstrated that the renal clearance of cimetidine itself is diminished with age [5], and this might be related to reduced renal function in the older patient. Five reports of interstitial nephritis have appeared, one of which is very well documented and was confirmed by rechallenge after 5 months, with the drug again leading to the same symptoms [4].

Endocrine disorders

Mild gynecomastia in men and galactorrhea in women taking cimetidine have been reported [6–8]. The total frequency was estimated by the advisory board to the Food and Drug Administration (FDA), with 2 cases occurring per million patients treated in the U.S.A. and 20 in the U.K. [4]. Generally, these patients had been taking the drug for 3 months or longer, and received higher doses of the drug, for instance in Zollinger-Ellison syndrome. It was argued that this symptom may be due to a cimetidine-induced increase in serum prolactin [7, 9], although this causal connection has not been proved. Plasma prolactin rises 15–30 minutes after intravenous injection of cimetidine (300–400 mg) [9–11] and returns to normal 75–90 minutes after injection [11]. In contrast, single oral doses do not influence serum prolactin levels [11–14]. In 7 patients with Zollinger-Ellison syndrome on long-term treatment with 1.2–2.4 g of cimetidine for more than 6 months, the plasma prolactin levels before and during treatment did not change significantly [15].

There have also been a number of reports on reproductive disorders, with impotence or libido loss [16, 17]. Van Thiel et al. [13] reported a 30% reduction in sperm count in 7 men who were taking a dose of 1.2 g for 9 weeks (with counts of 134 ± 17 million/ml before and 94 ± 13 million/ml after 9 weeks of treatment). This finding is very important. On the other hand, this study was carried out without controls, taking no account of normal fluctuations in the sperm count, and the sperm values found with cimetidine were still within the normal range [18].

Detailed endocrine studies have been prompted by recent clinical observations [13, 14]. The results are somewhat conflicting (Table II). After respectively 6 and 9 weeks of oral treatment with cimetidine, plasma testosterone levels were found to be elevated [13] or normal [14]. The luteinizing hormone (LH) response to LH-releasing hormone (LRH) was reduced [13] or normal [14]. The response of other hormones to thyrotropin-releasing hormone (TRH) was normal, as well as the basal levels of most other hormones.

Table II: Cimetidine and the endocrine system [13, 14].

Testosterone	Elevated [13], normal [14]
LH response to LRH	Reduced [13], normal [14]
Thyrotropin response to TRH Growth hormone (GH) response to TRH Thyroxine response to TRH Prolactin response to TRH	Normal [13, 14]

Basal levels of
  follicle-stimulating hormone,
  LH, GH, TSH, thyroxine
	Normal

Sperm count	Reduced 43% [13]*

* 134 ± 17 million/ml before treatment; 94 ± 13 million/ml after 9 weeks.

In summary, cimetidine seems to be a mild anti-androgenic drug [19], but without really relevant side effects during short-term treatment; the long-term effects are still open to further investigation.

One report has been published on the use of cimetidine during pregnancy [20]. A dose of 1 g/day of cimetidine produced no unwanted effects in either the mother or the fetus.

Mental disorders

Mental disorders, including confusion, psychosis, hypomania, hallucination or agitation, can occur unequivocally with cimetidine treatment. These problems have been observed mainly in patients older than 65 years of age, and in otherwise very ill patients [2, 21]. The advisory board to the FDA had, up until 1979, registered 22 cases of central/peripheral nervous system disorders per million treated patients in the U.S.A. and 88 in the U.K. [4].

Animal experiments had shown that cimetidine does not cross the blood-brain barrier, but later reports in patients with uremia and with severe liver disease have demonstrated significant concentrations in the cerebrospinal fluid [21, 22]. Blockade of H₂-receptors in the central nervous system may be the cause of the disorders.

Fever has also been reported as a side effect of cimetidine [23, 24]. In experiments with adult fowls, the microinfusion of cimetidine into the third ventricle aroused an intensive hyperthermic response [25]. Cimetidine might thus block H₂-receptors in thermoregulatory areas of the hypothalamus.

A report has been published of a 2-month old boy who received 40 mg/kg/day of cimetidine and became severely obtunded. He regained his normal mental state after withdrawal of the drug. It was concluded that the dose of 40 mg/kg/day, although the dose advised for adults, might be too high in children [26].

Blood cell disorders

Blood cell disorders, especially disorders of white blood cells, have been of great interest in observations of patients receiving cimetidine, bearing in mind the problems experienced with metiamide. These disorders have been found to be very rare with cimetidine, both with short-term and with long-term treatment (Table III). A total of 102 cases had been registered up until 1979, with only 63 displaying a temporal relationship to the drug and only 17 cases with white blood cell counts below 1,000 [4]. Bone marrow depression was found to be the cause when this was investigated [27–29]. In many cases,

Table III: White blood cell disorders with cimetidine; 102 cases reported, 63 cases with temporal relationship to the drug [4].

Incidence	Cases/million patients	
	U.S.A.	U.K.
White blood cell disorders	13	9
Red blood cell disorders	6	6
Platelet/clot disorders	4	7

Very low incidence in long-term treatment.
Seventeen cases with granylocytes $< 1,000/mm^2$ and possible relationship.

other factors which could contribute to the white cell disorder were present. Most of the observed damage to the white blood cells occurred during the first month of treatment, after which it was very rare [4]. A few cases of cimetidine-associated thrombocytopenia have also been observed [30, 31]. It seems to be the rule that blood cell alterations are fully reversible after withdrawal of the drug. In contrast to metiamide, which contains a thiourea group in its molecule, the replacement of this group by a cyanoguanidine radical in the cimetidine molecule has obviously abolished the toxicity of the drug on the blood system. Considering the fact that approximately 3 cases per million of the normal population develop agranulocytosis each year, cimetidine is shown to be a safe drug with respect to the blood system [32, 33].

Cardiovascular disorders

H_2-receptors are present in the heart and therefore it is not surprising that some cases of disturbed heart rate have been reported [34–38]. Both arrhythmias and bradycardias have been described. The overall incidence has been registered as 4–6 cases/million patients [4]. Engel et al. [39] carried out electrophysiological studies on 10 unmedicated patients before and after infusion of 300 mg of cimetidine. The drug did not affect heart rate, sinus node recovery time or sinoatrial conduction time. At present, therefore, direct evidence of a connection between cimetidine and cardiac disorders is lacking, but special care should be taken when patients are treated intravenously in intensive care situations [40].

Interaction of cimetidine with other drugs

Cimetidine interferes with the action of the anticoagulant warfarin. The prothrombin time may rise by about 20% and a reduction in the dosage of the coagulant may therefore be needed [41–43]. The kinetics of warfarin and the effects of cimetidine have been studied in detail [44]. The single-dose clearance of warfarin and of phenazone was reduced by cimetidine, presumably by interference with the microsomal drug metabolism [44].

Cimetidine also prolongs the elimination half-time of diazepam [45]. This should be taken into account when prescribing both drugs together to ulcer patients.

Elevation of transaminases and interaction with the pancreas

Transient elevation of transaminases has been observed with cimetidine, although such increases also occurred to a comparable extent in the placebo groups in controlled trials [1, 2]. The elevations seem to be dose-related, and mild centrolobular necrosis has been seen in the liver biopsy specimens of 2 patients receiving 1.6 g for 42 days [2]. The overall impression is that of a rare and mild side effect, and it is not considered to be sufficiently severe to warrant drug withdrawal.

Recently, 2 cases with drug hepatitis who showed a hypersensitivity type of reaction following 2 reexposures to the drug were published [46, 47].

A double-blind study on the use of cimetidine in the treatment of acute alcoholic pancreatitis has also recently been published [49]. Surprisingly, the amylase levels in the blood rose after the introduction of cimetidine (300 g intravenously 4 times a day), and remained higher than in the placebo group over the following 3 days. Serum creatinine was not increased in these patients, so that a diminished clearance of amylase did not seem to be the cause.

It is not clear whether cimetidine itself can damage the pancreas in any way. In rats, a high incidence of acute pancreatitis was observed (21 of 44 organs) when cimetidine was administered orally together with a gastric secretagogue (pentagastrin or carbachol), but not with the secretagogues or with cimetidine alone [49]. The history of a 78-year-old female patient with an acute pancreatitis in connection with the intake of cimetidine because of a duodenal ulcer has been published [50].

Careful observations of serum amylase levels in patients in intensive care units who receive intravenous cimetidine are needed, and should help to clarify the possible interrelationship between cimetidine and the pancreas.

Augmentation of delayed hypersensitivity

This phenomenon was observed in skin tests on 8 patients with ulcer disease who received cimetidine for 6 weeks [51]. A significant increase in both erythema and induration occurred in the treated patients, but not in 8 controls. Blockade of feedback inhibition of histamine on regulatory T-lymphocytes could be an explanation, but other explanations are possible. An increased responsiveness of lymphocytes to phytohemagglutinin has been reported [52]. The implications of these findings for patients treated with cimetidine are not known.

Improvement of acne and of psoriasis

Occasional observations have been made of a positive effect of cimetidine on psoriasis [53] and on acne [54], although others found no influence on psoriasis [55, 56]. The secretion of sebum seems to be inhibited by cimetidine [54].

Intoxication with cimetidine

One case of a 35-year-old man who took 120 tablets of cimetidine (24 g) together with forty 10-mg tablets of oxazepam has been reported [57]. The patient was unconscious, restless, and with brisk reactions to painful stimuli. Pulse rate, blood pressure and reflexes were normal. On gastric lavage 3 hours after ingestion of the tablets, only a few tablets were discovered. The patient was treated with forced diuresis and recovered after 6 hours. In another report on 4 children and 14 adults who had taken an overdose of cimetidine, it is stressed that no toxicity of the drug was observed [58]. None of the 4 children showed any symptoms. Three of the 7 adults remained completely symptom-free following 20 g of cimetidine. In most cases, a variety of other drugs had been taken together with cimetidine. The authors do not advise forced diuresis for cases of overdose with cimetidine alone.

Similar observations with a lack of severe symptoms following an overdose of the drug have also been published by others [48].

Conclusions

The following conclusions can be drawn; cimetidine is one of the best studied drugs; severe side effects are rare; in short-term treatment the benefits outweigh the risks; in long-term treatment, continued observation of side effects is needed, but here too they seem to be rare.

Summary

Following cimetidine, subjective symptoms may occur but rarely result in withdrawal of the drug. Among objective symptoms, renal disorders (increase of plasma creatinine), endocrine disorders (gynecomastia, reproductive disorders), mental disorders, depression of blood cells, cardiovascular events (arrhythmia, bradycardia), and elevation of transaminases and amylase must be considered. Cimetidine may interact with other drugs, mainly with anticoagulants; overdoses very rarely seem to give rise to serious symptoms. Severe side effects of the drug are very rare, and in short-term treatment the benefits clearly outweigh the risks. In long-term treatment continued observation of side effects is needed, but here too they seem to be rare.

References

1. Sharpe, P.C. and Hawkins, B.W. (1977): Efficacy and safety of cimetidine. Long-term treatment with cimetidine. In: *Cimetidine, Proceedings of the Second International Symposium on Histamine H₂-Receptor Antagonists*, pp. 358–366. Eds: W.L. Burland and M.A. Simkins. Excerpta Medica, Amsterdam.
2. Burland, W.L. (1978): Evidence for the safety of cimetidine in the treatment of peptic ulcer disease. In: *Cimetidine, Proceedings of an International Symposium on Histamine H₂-Receptor Antagonists*, pp. 238–255. Ed: W. Creutzfeldt. Excerpta Medica, Amsterdam.
3. Kruss, D.M. and Littman, A. (1978): Safety of cimetidine. *Gastroenterology 74*, 478–483.
4. Report to FDA (1979).
5. Gugler, R. and Somogyi, A. (1979): Reduced cimetidine clearance with age. *N. Engl. J. Med. 301*, 435.
6. Hall, W.H. (1976): Breast changes in males on cimetidine. *N. Engl. J. Med. 295*, 841.
7. Delle Fave, G.F., Tamburrano, G., De Magistris, L. et al. (1977): Gynaecomastia with cimetidine. *Lancet I*, 1319.
8. Bateson, M.C., Browning, M.C.K. and Maconnachie, A. (1977): Galactorrhoea with cimetidine. *Lancet II*, 247–248.
9. Carlson, H.E. and Ippoliti, A.F. (1977): Cimetidine, an H₂-histamine, stimulates prolactin secretion in man. *J. Clin. Endocrinol. Metab. 45*, 367–369.
10. Daubresse, J.C., Meunier, J.C. and Ligny, G. (1978): Plasma-prolactin and cimetidine. *Lancet I*, 99.
11. Rowley-Jones, D. (1978): Cimetidine and serum-prolactin. *Lancet II*, 635.
12. Valcavi, R., Bedogni, G., Dall'Asta, A. et al. (1978): Single oral dose of cimetidine and prolactin. *Lancet II*, 528.
13. Van Thiel, D.H., Gavaler, J.S., Smith, W.I. and Gwendolyn, P. (1979): Hypothalamic-pituitary-gonadal dysfunction in men using cimetidine. *N. Engl. J. Med. 300*, 1012–1015.

14. White, M.C., Gore, M. and Jewell, D.P. (1979): Endocrine function after cimetidine. *N. Engl. J. Med. 301*, 502.
15. Spiegel, A.M., Lopatin, R., Peikin, S. and McCarthy, D. (1978): Serum-prolactin in patients receiving chronic oral cimetidine. *Lancet I*, 881.
16. Peden, N.R., Cargill, J.M., Browning, M.C.K. et al. (1979): Male sexual dysfunction during treatment with cimetidine. *Br. Med. J. 1*, 659.
17. Peden, N.R., Browning, M.C.K., Cargill, J.M. et al. (1978): Reproductive abnormalities in male duodenal ulcer patients during long term treatment with cimetidine. *Acta Hepato-Gastroenterol. 25*, 501.
18. Fuentes, R.J. and Dolinsky, D. (1979): Endocrine function after cimetidine. *N. Engl. J. Med. 301*, 501.
19. Winters, S.J., Banks, J.L. and Loriaux, L. (1979): Cimetidine is an antiandrogen in rats. *Gastroenterology 76*, 504–508.
20. Zulli, P. and Di Nisio, Q. (1978): Cimetidine treatment during pregnancy. *Lancet II*, 945–946.
21. Schentag, J.J., Cerra, F.B., Calleri, G. et al. (1979): Pharmacokinetic and clinical studies in patients with cimetidine-associated mental confusion. *Lancet I*, 177–181.
22. Edmonds, M.E., Ashford, R.F.U., Brenner, M.K. and Saunders, A. (1979): Cimetidine: does neurotoxicity occur? Report of three cases. *J.R. Soc. Med. 72*, 172.
23. Ramboer, C. (1978): Drug fever with cimetidine. *Lancet I*, 330–331.
24. Corbett, C.L. and Holdsworth, S.D. (1978): Fever, abdominal pain, and leucopenia during treatment with cimetidine. *Br. Med. J. 1*, 753–754.
25. Nistico, G., Rotiroti, D., De Sarro, A. and Naccari, F. (1978): Mechanism of cimetidine-induced fever. *Lancet II*, 265–266.
26. Thompson, J. and Lilly, J. (1979): Cimetidine-induced cerebral toxicity in children. *Lancet I*, 725.
27. Druart, F., Frocrain, C., Metois, P. et al. (1979): Association of cimetidine and bone-marrow suppression in man. *Dig. Dis. Sci. 24*, 730–731.
28. Lopez-Luque, A., Rodriguez-Cuartero, A., Perez-Galvez, N. et al. (1978): Cimetidine and bone-marrow toxicity. *Lancet I*, 444.
29. Gouffier, E., Schnurmann, D., Durepaire, H. and Vernant, J.B. (1978): Aplasie médullaire transitoire au cours d'un traitement par la cimetidine. *Nouv. Presse Méd. 7*, 2660.
30. McDaniel, J.L. and Stein, J.J. (1979): Thrombocytopenia with cimetidine therapy. *N. Engl. J. Med. 300*, 864.
31. Idvall, J. (1979): Cimetidine-associated thrombocytopenia. *Lancet II*, 159.
32. Langman, M.J.S. (1978): Cimetidine for gastric and duodenal ulcer? *Am. J. Med. 65*, 885–887.
33. Finkelstein, W. and Isselbacher, K.J. (1978): Cimetidine. *N. Engl. J. Med. 299*, 992–996.
34. Jeffreys, D.B. and Vale, J.A. (1978): Cimetidine and bradycardia. *Lancet I*, 828.
35. Bournerias, F., Ganeval, D. and Danan, G. (1978): Trouble du rythme cardiaque mortel au cours d'un traitement par la cimetidine. *Nouv. Presse Méd. 7*, 2069.
36. Ligumsky, M., Shochina, M. and Rachnilewitz, D. (1978): Cimetidine and arrhythmia suppression. *Ann. Intern. Med. 89*, 1008–1009.
37. Reding, P., Devroede, C. and Barbier, P. (1977): Bradycardia after cimetidine. *Lancet II*, 1227.

38. Cohen, J., Weetman, A.P., Dargie, H.J. and Krikler, D.M. (1979): Life-threatening arrhythmias and intravenous cimetidine. *Br. Med. J. 2*, 768.

39. Engel, T.R. and Luck, J.C. (1979): Histamine H_2-receptor antagonism by cimetidine and sinus-node function. *N. Engl. J. Med. 301*, 591–592.

40. Levi, R. and Trzeciakowski, J.P. (1980): Cimetidine and sinus node function. *N. Engl. J. Med. 302*, 235.

41. Flind, A.C. (1978): Cimetidine and oral anticoagulants. *Br. Med. J. 2*, 1367.

42. Silver, B.A. and Bell, W.R. (1979): Cimetidine potentiation of the hypoprothrombinemic effect of warfarin. *Ann. Intern. Med. 90*, 348.

43. Hetzel, D., Birkett, D. and Miners, J. (1979): Cimetidine interaction with warfarin. *Lancet II*, 639.

44. Serlin, M.J., Sibeon, R.G., Mossman, S. et al. (1979): Cimetidine: interaction with oral anticoagulants in man. *Lancet II*, 317–319.

45. Klotz, U., Anttila, V.J. and Reimann, I. (1979): Cimetidine/Diazepam interaction. *Lancet II*, 699.

46. Züchner, H. (1977): Cholestatische Hepatose unter Cimetidin. *Dtsch. Med. Wochenschr. 102*, 1788.

47. Villeneuve, J.P. and Warner, H.A. (1979): Cimetidine hepatitis. *Gastroenterology 77*, 143–144.

48. Illingworth, R.N. and Jarvie, D.R. (1979): Absence of toxicity in cimetidine overdosage. *Br. Med. J. 1*, 453–454.

49. Meshkinpour, H., Molineri, M.D., Gardner, L. et al. (1979): Cimetidine in the treatment of acute alcoholic pancreatitis. A randomized, double blind study. *Gastroenterology 77*, 687–690.

50. Arnold, F., Doyle, P.J. and Bell, G. (1978): Acute pancreatitis in a patient treated with cimetidine. *Lancet I*, 382–383.

51. Avella, J., Madsen, J.E., Binder, H.J. and Askenase, P.W. (1978): Effect of histamine H_2-receptor antagonists on delayed hypersensitivity. *Lancet I*, 624–626.

52. Robertson, A.J., Peden, N.R., Saunders, J.H.B. et al. (1979): Cimetidine and the immune response. *Lancet II*, 420–421.

53. Giacosa, A., Farris, A. and Cheli, R. (1978): Cimetidine and psoriasis. *Lancet II*, 1211–1212.

54. Lyons, F., Cook, J. and Shuster, S. (1979): Inhibition of sebum excretion by an H_2 blocker. *Lancet I*, 1376.

55. Raffle, E.J. (1978): Cimetidine and psoriasis. *Lancet II*, 1314.

56. Rai, G.S. and Webster, S.G.P. (1979): Cimetidine and psoriasis. *Lancet I*, 50.

57. Van Rijthoven, A.W.A.M. (1979): Cimetidine intoxication. *Lancet II*, 370.

58. Meredith, T.J. and Volans, G.N. (1979): Management of cimetidine overdose. *Lancet II*, 1367.

Pharmacological basis and clinical use of antacids*

J.-R. Malagelada and G.L. Carlson**
Gastroenterology Unit, Mayo Clinic and Mayo Foundation, Rochester, Minnesota, U.S.A.

Introduction

Despite major advances in antiulcer pharmacology led by the development of potent gastric antisecretory agents, antacids, the older and more traditional form of therapy for ulcer disease remains a viable approach. Antacids have also evolved over the years, thanks to improvements in their physicochemistry and formulation. The basis of antacid action, however, remains unchanged. Antacids aim at reducing the acidity of gastric contents and the load of acid into the duodenum and, secondarily, they diminish peptic activity by increasing the luminal pH above that optimal for proteolysis. We will discuss here the physicochemical and pharmacological basis of antacid therapy, its effect on gastric function, and its efficiency in achieving the above goals. We will also refer to other properties of common antacids, which may be of clinical value in special circumstances: bile acid binding and effects on pancreatic, gallbladder, and intestinal function.

Common commercially available antacids consist of sodium bicarbonate, calcium carbonate, magnesium hydroxide, or aluminium hydroxide, either alone or in combination. Because there are significant chemical and physical differences between these compounds and the products of their reaction with hydrochloric acid, the chemistry and pharmacology of each will be reviewed. Many of these concepts also apply to a variety of other compounds incorporated into some commercial antacid preparations, but due to space limitations these cannot be discussed individually.

* This work was supported in part by Research Grant AM 6908 from the National Institutes of Health, Bethesda, Maryland.
** Dr. Malagelada is the recipient of Research Career Development Award AM 00330 from the National Institutes of Health.

Pharmacology of typical antacids

Sodium bicarbonate

Sodium bicarbonate is the salt of a weak acid (carbonic acid) and a strong base (sodium hydroxide). The compound is soluble in water (6.9 g/dl at 0°C) and reacts with HCl to form NaCl, H_2O, and CO_2. Loss of CO_2 makes this reaction irreversible under physiologic conditions. The reaction product, NaCl, is very water-soluble (35.7 g/dl, 0°C), and no hydrolysis to NaOH is observed.

Sodium bicarbonate or baking soda is one of the oldest known and utilized antacids. It reacts almost instantaneously with acid. Simmons et al. have recently shown that bicarbonate administered postprandially in conventional doses raises the intragastric pH to 7 to 8, explaining the immediate symptomatic benefit experienced by many patients [1]. However, as expected, the effects are of short duration because the antacid is rapidly consumed and new acid is secreted rapidly, lowering intragastric pH. Further, bicarbonate produces CO_2 which increases gaseous feeling and has a high sodium content, which may be contraindicated in some patients. Ingestion of sodium bicarbonate produces a base excess equivalent to the amount ingested because of the failure of NaCl to react with carbonate, phosphate, or hydroxide ions later in the gastrointestinal tract. Thus there is a risk of significant alkalosis from its frequent and prolonged use. Sodium bicarbonate is not an optimal antacid form chronic use.

Calcium carbonate

Calcium carbonate is analogous to sodium bicarbonate, but is much less soluble (0.0015 g/dl). Reaction with HCl yields CO_2, H_2O, and $CaCl_2$, again a highly water-soluble salt. Unlike sodium, however, the divalent Ca ion will reform (and precipitate) calcium carbonate in the presence of aqueous carbonate or bicarbonate (from which carbonate can be formed by reaction with hydroxide ion). Calcium phosphate may also be precipitated if phosphate ion is present; in both cases, the reaction is driven to the right by the low solubility product of the calcium carbonate or phosphate. Thus the essential difference between sodium and calcium carbonate is that the reaction of $CaCO_3$ with HCl is effectively reversible under physiologic conditions; it must be emphasized, however, that the forward and reverse reactions occur at different times, in anatomically-distinct organs, and in different chemical milieus. To the extent that calcium is reconverted to the carbonate or phosphate in the gut, an equal amount of acid and base will have been used. Alkalosis will therefore be of lesser magnitude than with sodium bicarbonate. However, since some calcium will be absorbed by the proximal small bowel, the reverse reaction cannot be equal to the neutralization and, furthermore, hypercalcemia may become a problem in chronic users [2, 3].

Calcium carbonate is a potent antacid with a rapid onset of action and a relatively prolonged effect. The main disadvantage of calcium carbonate is that it causes acid rebound [4, 5]. This is due to the effect of calcium ion which has the capacity of stimulating the parietal cells directly [6] through gastrin release [7] and indirectly by causing hypercalcemia [8]. The magnitude of the acid rebound is not great and its effects might theoretically be counteracted by frequent administration of the antacid. However, there still would be concern about the effects of prolonged stimulation of parietal cells.

Magnesium hydroxide

Magnesium hydroxide is another antacid derived from a group-II metal. Like calcium carbonate, $Mg(OH)_2$ is poorly soluble (0.0009 g/dl, 18°C); the chloride produced is quite soluble (54.25 g/dl, 20°C) and both the carbonate and the phosphate are insoluble. Because the reaction to form $MgCl_2$ produces only water, the reaction is theoretically reversible; in practice, the hydrolysis of Mg^{2+} requires a pH above 8 [9] and so may be ignored in the bowel. Presumably magnesium behaves like calcium in the bowel and reacts with phosphate or bicarbonate to produce the insoluble magnesium salts which are excreted. However, about one-third to one-fourth of the total amount of magnesium ingested is absorbed. In patients with renal failure (thus with limited ability to excrete magnesium), this poses a significant risk.

Aluminium hydroxide

Aluminium hydroxide is the only antacid derived from a group-III element, and therefore differs from all the others. $Al(OH)_3$ is amphoteric and relatively insoluble in water. Although $AlCl_3$ is water soluble, the hydrated trivalent cation is quite acidic and hydrolysis becomes significant in the physiologic pH range, leading to the formation of various intermediate chlorohydroxides. The situation is further complicated by the slow approach to equilibrium and because the cation may form complex hydrated ions such as $[Al_2 (OH)_2]^{4+}$ and $[Al_{13} (OH)_{32}]^{7+}$, both of which are known to exist in basic crystalline salts [10]. This pH-dependent formation of intermediate chlorohydroxides thus lowers the effective acid-neutralizing capacity of $Al(OH)_3$ gels (to about 80%

of the theoretical value) in a complex, pH-sensitive fashion [11]. The situation is further complicated by the probable formation of the insoluble phosphate in the gut. Aluminium ion is poorly absorbed by the small bowel but detectable plasma aluminium concentrations after aluminium-containing antacids have been reported [12]. Circulating aluminium is cleared by the normal kidney; increased deposition in tissues has been observed in chronic renal failure [13].

Current formulations

Aluminium and magnesium hydroxides constitute the basis of most commercial antacids currently available. There is no evidence that these subtances cause significant acid rebound. The relative proportion of magnesium and aluminium are adjusted by different pharmaceutical manufacturers to lean either toward causing looser stools or constipation. The characteristics of gel on which aluminium and magnesium hydroxides are incorporated also vary depending on the manufacturer and this may perhaps influence its capacity to mix with gastric contents and react with acid. Older preparations of magnesium and aluminium hydroxides tended to contain large quantities of sodium. This posed the risk of causing sodium overload in susceptible patients. Many modern commercial preparations are low in sodium and can be used more broadly. Calcium carbonate remains a popular ingredient of self-prescribed antacid tablets in the United States. Magnesium trisilicate is another common ingredient of commercial antacid mixtures, but it adds little neutralizing power.

Other ingredients are sometimes found in commercial antacid mixtures. Alginic acid is claimed to produce a foam which floats on top of gastric contents and carries the antacid to the esophagus during reflux, sticking to the mucosal surface. It is unclear, however, whether it adds any advantage to antacids alone. Bismuth salts are also present in some proprietary mixtures. Whereas they have no significant acid-neutralizing activity, they are claimed to coat and help protect the ulcer from injurious acid-peptic action. This is unsubstantiated. However, there is some evidence that bismuth salts may enhance cytoprotective activity by the gastric mucosa, although more work is needed in this area. Dimeticone, an antifoaming silicone derivative which reduces surface tension, is also present in some antacid mixtures. It is claimed to have an antiflatulence effect. At least one clinical trial supports its effectiveness in relieving dyspeptic symptoms [14], but more data is clearly needed to substantiate this effect. Another common ingredient of commercial antacids is peppermint oil, which is a strong antispasmodic and reduces lower esophageal sphincter pressure [15].

Liquid antacids are more effective than tablets in lowering gastric acidity. In part this is due to the relatively large quantities of active ingredient which can be ingested as liquid in usual doses, i.e., 1 oz or more, but also to the greater dispersion and reactivity achieved by liquid preparations in the stomach. Tablets are usually preferred by patients because of convenience.

Principles of clinical utilization

Antacids for clinical use should be employed, taking into account their chemical composition, as outlined earlier, time of administration, and dose.

It has long been recognized that antacids ingested on an empty stomach are quickly evacuated and only partially utilized. Thus their acid-neutralizing effects are brief [16]. In contrast, administration of antacid after a meal leads to better utilization of the antacid and a more prolonged action [17]. For this reason, antacids are clinically prescribed according to schedules linking their administration to the time of ingestion of a meal.

The dose of antacid to be administered has been a subject of controversy. Obviously the more antacid and the higher its neutralizing power the better, but limitations exist on the amount that patients accept as convenient or even bearable. For most commercial preparations of aluminium and magnesium hydroxides, 1 oz, 1 and 3 hours after meals and on retiring is about as much as most patients will tolerate. Higher or more frequent doses risk poor compliance, a common problem with antacid therapy [18], and increase the risk of unpleasant side effects. Fordtran et al. have proposed tailoring the dosage of antacid to acid secretory capacity [19]. This, however, is not practical since patients with duodenal ulcer are not invariably subjected to gastric secretory tests. Furthermore, as we expressed earlier, the efficacy of the neutralizing process depends on gastric emptying of the antacid as well as on gastric acid secretion, and measuring the former is not feasible in routine clinical practice.

Evaluation of antacids

'In-vitro' evaluation

Several years ago Fordtran and coworkers popularized a standardized procedure for testing antacids 'in vitro'. This test was based on the capacity of an antacid solution to neutralize acid added to it at a constant rate, so that the pH of the solution would be maintained constant at 3.0. At this pH, 99% of a 100 mM solution of HCl would have been neutralized. The conditions for the test were chosen arbitrarily but they were felt to reflect 'in vivo' measurements more closely than would a simple determination of the total neutralizing capacity by end-point titration. This may be due to the fact that it evaluates the speed with which the antacid combines with acid, as well as the total neutralizing capacity (to pH 3.0 as end point). As we will discuss later, an antacid which reacts too rapidly with acid will have an intense but also transient neutralizing effect in contrast to the sustained effect of a slower one. However, it is important to recognize that no form of 'in-vitro' testing can actually approximate the real behavior of antacids in the stomach, which depends as much on gastric emptying as it does on neutralizing kinetics.

'In-vivo' evaluation

The development of new methodology has allowed us to evaluate the 'in-vivo' effects of antacids beyond simple determinations of gastric pH and titratable acidity. It is now possible to quantify the action of antacids on postprandial gastric secretion and emptying and to closely monitor the neutralizing reaction in the stomach. Measuring the effect of antacids on duodenal acid load is particularly important since reduction of duodenal acid load is the major aim of antacid therapy in duodenal ulcer. Further, duodenal acid load depends not only on the efficiency of neutralization but also on gastric secretion and emptying. Thus, it is possible to measure the fraction of ingested antacid consumed by neutralization with gastric acid and the fraction emptied from the stomach before it has had a chance to react with acid. This is a quantitative assessment of the utilization of antacid. Such measurements are only available to date for a combination of aluminium and magnesium hydroxides studied in our laboratory [9, 20]. Indirect data are also available for other antacids [19].

When an antacid mixture of aluminium and magnesium hydroxides is given to patients after a meal, it produces a rather sustained, though somewhat fluctuating, increase of intragastric pH (Fig. 1; [20]). The time of administration should be carefully chosen, for it is necessary to take advantage of the elevation of intragastric pH produced by the diluting and buffering action of the meal itself. By the end of the first postprandial hour, the intragastric pH is rapidly declining and at that time ingestion of a dose of antacid will be utilized most efficiently to reduce gastric acidity. Because of the slower neutralization process, the gastric pH, in contrast to what is observed with sodium bicarbonate, does not get up to 7 or 8 but, on the other hand, the effect is more prolonged. By the end of the third postprandial hour the pH is declining again since the first dose of antacid has already been partially consumed or

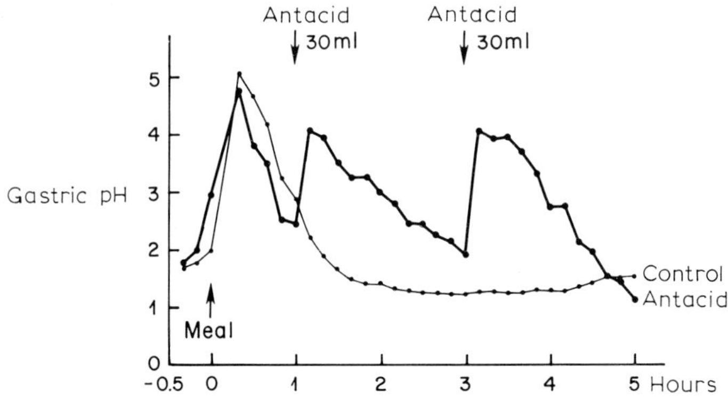

Fig. 1: Effect of liquid aluminium and magnesium hydroxides (antacid) on post-prandial gastric pH in patients with duodenal ulcer. Modified from [20].

emptied. At this time, a second dose of the antacid raises the pH again for at least another hour — a total of 4 hours after the meal. During daytime, it would be expected that another meal and another cycle of antacid administration would follow at regular intervals, thus keeping the intragastric pH almost continuously elevated.

Simultaneous measurements of duodenal acid load (Fig. 2) show that for about one hour after ingestion of a meal, negligible amounts of H^+ ion enter

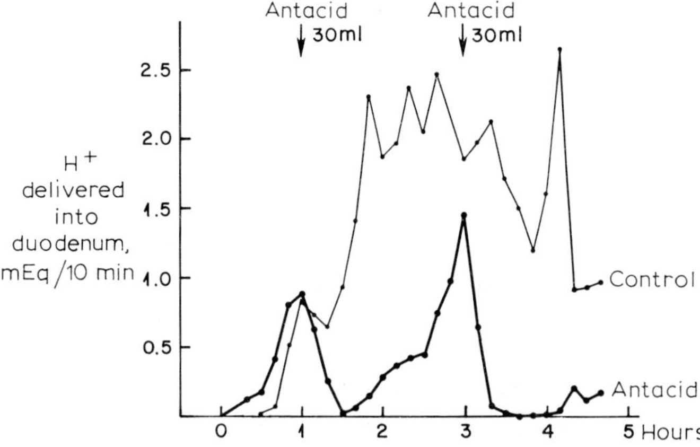

Fig. 2: Effect of liquid aluminium and magnesium hydroxides (antacid) on post-prandial delivery of H ion into the duodenum in patients with duodenal ulcer. Modified from [20].

the duodenum. Although this would, of course, depend a great deal on the type of meal and patient studied, it probably applies to some extent to most common therapeutic situations. The low duodenal H^+ ion load is due to buffering and dilution of acid by meal protein. In other words, acid which leaves the stomach during the early postprandial period does so combined with food. Buffered H^+ probably has little injurious effect on the duodenal mucosa. After the first hour the effect of the meal is rapidly diminishing and if no therapy is given, duodenal acid load sharply rises and will remain high for the next several hours. However, the 2 doses of aluminium and magnesium hydroxides spaced one and 3 hours after the meal produce a marked reduction in H^+ duodenal load. As observed with the intragastric pH, there is some fluctuation with the least effect being observed during the second half of the third hour, and the maximum effect immediately after administering each dose.

The efficiency of antacid therapy, as measured concomitantly in these studies, is remarkable. A mean 127 mEq of antacid was consumed in the stomach (range 93–138 mEq) out of a possible total 162 mEq given (60 ml of liquid antacid). This represents a mean utilization of about 80%. The first dose of antacid, given one hour after the meal, was utilized more efficiently and emptied more slowly than the second dose given 3 hours after the meal. These results suggest that a further 20% of total antacid capacity could be utilized if antacid could be prevented from leaving the stomach before it has completely reacted with acid. Others have suggested that simultaneous administration of anticholinergic agents, which delay gastric emptying as well as decreasing gastric secretion, would potentiate the action of antacids and increase their utilization. Some experimental support for this concept exists, but further evidence would be needed before it could be recommended for routine clinical practice.

Effect of therapy on gastric function

The effects of antacids on gastric function are an important aspect of antacid pharmacology. Since intragastric and intraduodenal pH play a key role in regulating gastric secretion and emptying, it is not unexpected that changes in gastric and duodenal acidity induced by antacid therapy would affect gastric secretion and emptying as well as gastrin release [21]. Additional effects might be due to certain constituents of the antacids, such as calcium, magnesium, or aluminium ions.

In our laboratory, we have recently measured the effects of aluminium and magnesium hydroxides on postprandial gastric secretion and emptying [9].

We found that administration of 1 oz of liquid aluminium and magnesium hydroxides one and 3 hours after a meal significantly increased gastric acid output, by 16% on average (Fig. 3). This means that the quantity of acid available for neutralization after the antacid was greater than if no antacid had been given, further evidence that the actual conditions on which antacids act cannot easily be predicted 'in vitro' or by measurements of gastric acidity. In the case of aluminium and magnesium hydroxides this increase in gastric secretion is mostly due to abolition of pH-dependent feedback inhibition of gastric secretion stimulated by the meal. The same would apply to sodium bicarbonate [21]. There is no evidence that the aluminium ion has any direct stimulatory effect on gastric secretion. In contrast, intraluminal calcium is a well-known stimulus to gastric secretion and it is known to cause acid rebound. Although not yet quantified, it seems likely that postprandial gastric secretion after calcium carbonate increases relatively more than with aluminium and magnesium hydroxides since one should add the direct stimulatory effects of the calcium ion to the decrease in acid feedback inhibition. Intragastric magnesium might have some weak stimulatory effect [22, 23], although intravenous magnesium appears to inhibit calcium-induced gastric secretion. Nevertheless, the addition of magnesium to a calcium solution does not modify the stimulatory effect of calcium alone on gastric secretion [24].

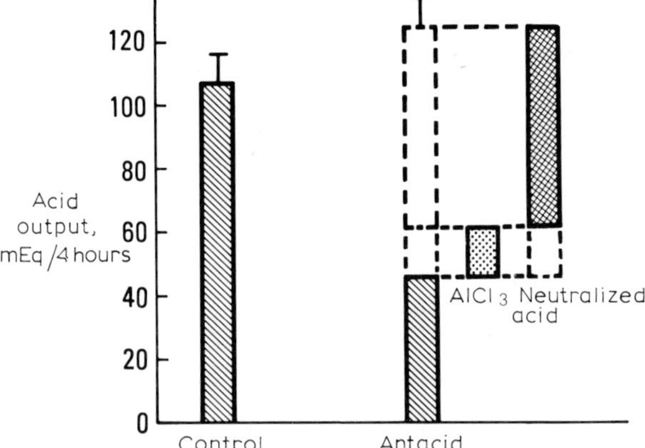

Fig. 3:   Postprandial gastric acid output after meal (control) and meal plus an antacid suspension. The dashed bar above the antacid label indicates the total acid secreted by the stomach in 4 hours, which was significantly higher than control (p < 0.05). The hatched bar on the extreme right plus the dashed appendix at its lower end indicates the total amount of secreted gastric acid which was neutralized by the antacid. The dashed bar labeled $AlCl_3$ in the middle indicates the titratable acid derived from hydrolysis of aluminium chloride. Reproduced with permission from [62].

The increase in gastric secretion produced by antacids means not only an increase in the amount of acid available for neutralization but also a parallel increase in the volume of gastric juice. Theoretically, the stomach confronted by an increased load of acid would have at least 2 ways to dispose of it. One way would be to increase the absolute rate of delivery of gastric contents into the duodenum so that the total volume of gastric contents remains constant. Another way would be to maintain constant the absolute rate of emptying but expand intragastric volume to accommodate temporarily the increased volume load [25]. Our studies on postprandial gastric function after administration of aluminium and magnesium hydroxides suggest that the latter hypothesis is true: intragastric volume increases whereas duodenal volume load remains constant. Hurwitz et al., employing an external gamma camera to monitor the fractional gastric emptying of a radioactive marker, found delayed evacuation after aluminium hydroxide but not after nonaluminium-containing antacids of similar or greater neutralizing power [26]. This suggests that aluminium-containing antacids have an inhibitory effect on motility besides their effect on gastric secretion. These observations are relevant to antacid pharmacology in relation to other substances administered concomitantly with antacids. One would expect that these substances would be diluted in the stomach and their emptying retarded by the effects of antacids on gastric function. Obviously, delayed emptying would influence absorption and times of peak serum levels as well as the level itself.

Just the opposite situation is observed with cimetidine administration which reduces gastric secretion with a contraction in gastric volume while maintaining a normal fractional gastric emptying [27]. This may explain why, in patients with pancreatic insufficiency, cimetidine administered together with pancreatic enzyme supplements causes much greater concentration of exogenous enzymes in the duodenum than when antacids are used as adjuvan therapy [28].

Clinical effectiveness

The effectiveness of antacid therapy in duodenal or gastric ulcer has been debated for years. Until not long ago, the tide of opinion seemed to be leaning towards skepticism about the efficacy of these agents, supported by the negative results of several studies [29–31]. Yet, more recently, data strongly supporting the effectiveness of antacids in duodenal ulcer disease have been acquired.

Peterson et al. reported the results of a double-blind controlled trial employing an intensive antacid regimen (1 oz of an aluminium and magnesium hydroxides preparation taken one and 3 hours after each meal and at bedtime) versus a placebo [32]. These investigators found that antacid therapy significantly accelerated the healing of duodenal ulcer. After 4 weeks of therapy, 78% of patients had endoscopically proven healing versus 45% for placebo, a statistically significant difference. From a prophylactic standpoint, Hastings et al. found that neutralization (pH > 3.5) of gastric contents by oral administration of relatively large quantities of antacids prevented the development of stress ulcer in critically ill patients [33]. A subsequent study from the same group was purported to show that antacid therapy was superior to intravenous cimetidine in prophylaxis of stress ulceration in seriously ill patients but, in fact, the differences between the 2 therapies appear to be small, if any [34]. One further study from another group suggested that the combination of cimetidine and antacids was more effective in this setting than antacids alone [35]. There have been, to our knowledge, no recent studies reevaluating the use of antacids in healing of gastric ulcer.

Several reasons may explain the apparent discrepancies between the results of these recent studies which tend to support the efficacy of antacid therapy and the older studies which did not. First, many of the early studies utilized doses of antacid which were smaller than that needed to obtain the degree of reduction in acidity apparently required for a full therapeutic effect. Secondly, they might have employed preparations like calcium carbonate which, despite an excellent neutralizing capacity, cause acid rebound. Thirdly, proper dosage schedule is critically needed to coordinate antacid administration with meals and taking optimal advantage from them. Fourthly, techniques for designing and carrying out therapeutic controlled trials have improved with time; most particularly, the use of fiberoptic endoscopy allows an accurate verification of ulcer healing.

Remarkably, whereas most modern studies with antacids support their efficacy in healing duodenal ulcer, no convincing evidence that they relieve ulcer pain has been brought forward. Sturdevant et al. failed to show any significant difference between a liquid antacid and placebo in the relief of duodenal ulcer pain [36]. However, it has been pointed out that such a difference might have existed but could have been obscured by the presence of peppermint oil (see page 379) in both antacid and placebo mixtures [37]. Even in the study of Peterson et al., where antacids proved more efficacious than placebo in healing duodenal ulcer, it could not be proven that they were better than placebo in relieving symptoms [32]. Earlier studies by Littman et al. showed equivocal results [38]. Some tests showed an advantage of antacid (aluminium hydroxide gel) over placebo for relief of ulcer pain and other tests did not. In gastric ulcer, Butler and Gersh could not show an advantage of antacid over placebo for pain relief [30].

The failure of most controlled studies to demonstrate the efficacy of antacid for relief of ulcer pain appears to contradict individual testimony of individual patients and their physicians in a clinical practice setting. The truth may lie somewhere in between, for one of the interpretations of the results of the controlled trials could be that the 'placebo effect' in ulcer pain is so strong that an advantage of the antacid could not be statistically shown. Further, as pointed out earlier, some placebos employed in control trials contain ingredients that may have effects on gastrointestinal motility and other functions perhaps involved in the production of pain. At this time the question of antacid effects on ulcer pain remains open and only further studies may provide an answer.

Antacids versus other therapeutic agents in duodenal ulcer

Antacids, of course, neutralize acid which has already been secreted, as opposed to other agents, such as cimetidine or anticholinergics, which inhibit acid secretion. Despite different mechanisms, as far as duodenal ulcer is concerned, all these different therapies have a common goal, namely, to reduce duodenal acid load. Comparisons between them may be referred to this parameter as a normalizing index.

We have examined the effect of accepted therapeutic doses of cimetidine and an antacid on postprandial acid delivery into the duodenum in patients with duodenal ulcer. We found that either 400 mg of cimetidine administered with a meal or an ounce of aluminium and magnesium hydroxides, given one and 3 hours after the meal, would produce a similar reduction in duodenal acid load during the first 4 postprandial hours. The results of this study should, of course, be taken only as a guideline since the results are highly dependent on the dosage employed for either agent. However, it provides a reference to help interpreting the results of clinical trials.

The study of Peterson et al. showed that duodenal ulcer in patients on intensive antacid therapy healed at the same rate as observed in patients treated with cimetidine alone [32]. In a subsequent controlled trial, Ippoliti et al. compared the effect of intensive antacid therapy and cimetidine, finding a similar healing rate of duodenal ulcer for both treatment modalities [39]. However, follow-up studies of patients after the trial had terminated suggest that antacids may be less effective than cimetidine in patients with severe, long-standing duodenal ulcer.

Other considerations besides healing rates are important when deciding whether to use antacids or cimetidine for the treatment of duodenal ulcer. Intensive antacid therapy, employing even, well-balanced aluminium and magnesium hydroxides combinations, has a high incidence of unpleasant side effects, mostly diarrhea. Cimetidine, in contrast, is better tolerated by the majority of patients but, being a systemic drug and relatively new, has potentially unrecognized side effects, which might become apparent as experience with this drug increases. Patient acceptance and compliance are probably greater for cimetidine than for antacids, which require cumbersome liquid administration and a rather rigid schedule. Also, nocturnal acidity is reduced more conveniently by cimetidine than by antacids which would require frequent administration during the night. Because of these advantages and disadvantages for each therapy, choosing one or the other must remain, for the present time, an individualized decision for the physician and his patient.

Similar comparative data do not exist for anticholinergics versus antacids. Anticholinergics are less potent inhibitors of acid secretion than cimetidine [40]. Further, the evidence that anticholinergics alone enhance the healing of peptic ulcer is equivocal, even when the drugs are given in a maximally tolerated dose which causes bothersome side effects [41]. However, Feldman et al. have shown that the acid inhibitory actions of cimetidine and anticholinergics are additive, even when the latter are given at well-tolerated, submaximal doses [42]. The slowing in gastric emptying produced by anticholinergics could potentially improve the efficiency of antacids administered simultaneously.

Despite these encouraging hints, the therapeutic opportunities offered by combinations of available agents are yet to be fully explored. The concept is sound because these drugs have different mechanisms of action and thus their effects may be additive or even synergistic. Thus greater efficacy might be achieved with lower doses and a lesser risk of side effects than if each drug were used independently. Clinical trials should now be designed to test the validity of these assumptions.

Adsorbent properties

Antacids, apart from their neutralizing properties, are known to possess adsorbant properties for endogenous secretions such as bile acids or pepsin, certain drugs [43–45], or bacteria. Bile acid binding by antacids initially reported by Wenger and Heymsfield [46] has been recently characterized 'in vitro' in our laboratory [47]. We tested the binding properties of various commercial antacids for the bile acids present in human gallbladder bile obtained at surgery. Aluminium hydroxide was a potent binding agent similar in affinity and capacity to colestyramine. With aluminium hydroxide, dihydroxy bile acid conjugates were bound more strongly than trihydroxy bile acid conjugates; pH had no effect per se on binding. Magnesium hydroxide and magnesium trisilicate bound bile acids much more weakly. It was also found that aluminium phosphate had a poor bile-acid binding capacity. Since ingested aluminium hydroxide is eventually precipitated, at least in part, as aluminium phosphate in the intestine, aluminium hydroxide ingestion may not influence the concentration of bile acids in solution in the small intestinal lumen.

Bile acids produce both functional and structural damage to the gastric mucosa. Reflux of bile into the stomach has been shown to be increased in patients with gastric ulcers, esophagitis, or gastritis, and it is considered to be important in the pathogenesis of these conditions. The finding that aluminium hydroxide is an effective binder of antacids is of potential therapeutic value. Further, bile acids have been shown to be most damaging to the gastric mucosa in the nonionized state (e.g., at pH < 3) [48]. Use of aluminium hydroxide alone or in combination with colestyramine would have the additional advantage of raising intragastric pH which would enhance ionization and, in turn, increase binding. The value of antacids as bile acid binding deserves further investigation 'in vivo'.

Binding of pepsin by antacids, on the other hand, is of unclear significance since the amounts bound are small relative to the quantities of the enzyme secreted. Binding of drugs is relevant in that bioavailability of medications given concomitantly with antacids may be diminished.

Pancreatic, biliary, and intestinal effects

Calcium and magnesium ions, present in many antacids, have intestinal effects. Calcium is a powerful stimulant of pancreatic enzyme secretion and gallbladder contraction [49]. These effects may be due to cholecystokinin release but no direct proof for this exists as yet. Magnesium shares some of the stimulatory properties of calcium but it is less potent [50]. On the other hand, magnesium, a poorly absorbed ion, inhibits water and electrolyte secretion from the intestine and at higher concentration induces water secretion. Thus, diarrhea frequently develops after the ingestion of magnesium salts. The mechanism responsible for the intestinal effects of magnesium is poorly characterized. It appears to be, in some aspects, dissociated from the effects on pancreas and gallbladder, because $MgSO_4$ causes much greater net luminal accumulation of fluid than $MgCl_2$ (as opposed to similar stimulatory potency of both magnesium salts on the pancreas and gallbladder when infused in equimolar amounts). Thus, the intestinal secretory effect appears to be at least in part 'osmotic' and based on sodium diffusion gradients: poorly absorbable ions (Mg^{2+}, SO_4^{2-}) replacing intraluminal sodium and causing net water transport into the lumen [51, 52]. However, it is also possible that magnesium directly stimulates secretion and motility of the gut [53]. In contrast, trivalent aluminium inhibits gastrointestinal motility [54] and aluminium-containing antacids have a delaying effect on bowel transit. The pathogenesis of the effects of these compounds on the gut is poorly understood and clearly deserves further investigation.

Side effects and complications of therapy

The most frequent side effects of modern antacids, particularly when ingested in large doses, are alterations in bowel movement pattern. We have already alluded to the laxative action of magnesium-containing antacids and to the constipating effect of those incorporating aluminium. Combinations of magnesium and aluminium hydroxides are employed in many commercial preparations to offset the opposite effects of each of these compounds on bowel habit.

Chronic ingestion of sodium bicarbonate or other well-absorbed alkalis may cause metabolic alkalosis, and hypokalemia. The milk alkali syndrome (hypercalcemia, alkalosis and elevated serum creatinine) may develop in patients ingesting large quantities of calcium carbonate, sodium bicarbonate, milk, or combinations of all of these [55, 56]. However, the syndrome has become distinctly less frequent since magnesium and aluminium hydroxide gels are increasingly prescribed for long-term therapy, and milk is less enthusiastically recommended as a panacea to ulcer patients. The possibility of sodium overload from some antacid preparations rich in sodium has already been alluded to earlier.

Phosphorus depletion due to binding by aluminium salts is uncommon because most diets are rich enough in phosphorus to make it unlikely [57]. However, it can develop with chronic ingestion of strong phosphorus-binding antacids [58]. Supplemental phosphate should probably be administered concomitantly to such patients. Absorption of small quantities of magnesium, and to a lesser extent aluminium, is known to occur but may become clinically significant only in patients with advanced renal insufficiency in whom it has been implicated without strong proof in the syndrome of 'dialysis dementia' [59, 60]. The binding properties of aluminium hydroxide may interfere with the absorption of tetracycline, warfarin, digoxins, quinidine, and other drugs, reducing their bioavailability [43–45]. The slight elevation in blood and urinary pH resulting from chronic use of many antacids may increase blood levels of quinidine and acetylsalicylic acid by decreasing their renal excretion [61]. Intestinal obstruction from impacted antacid has been reported [52].

Conclusion

What is the role of antacids in modern therapy of ulcer disease? The practical usefulness of intensive antacid therapy to treat symptomatic ulcer relapses is, in our opinion, limited, in spite of the traditional enthusiasm on this side of the Atlantic for massive antacid medication. As alternative safe therapies are developed and gradually become available for prescription, the appeal of antacid therapy with its inconveniences and troublesome bowel disturbance becomes less attractive. Perhaps newer preparations at reduced doses will prove effective. However, antacids are over-the-counter drugs which can and will continue to be used rather freely by patients. The probability that this self-medication with modern antacid preparations causes harmful effects is quite small. From the point of view of availability and symptomatic benefit, antacids remain useful drugs.

References

1. Simmons, T.C., Hogan, D.L., Isenberg, J.I. and Grossman, M.I. (1978): Sodium bicarbonate versus aluminum-magnesium antacid on postprandial gastric acidity. *Gastroenterology 74*, 1095.
2. Ivanovich, P., Fellows, H. and Rich, C. (1967): The absorption of calcium carbonate. *Ann. Intern. Med. 66*, 917.
3. Morrissey, J.F. and Barreras, R.F. (1974): Drug therapy. Antacid therapy. *N. Engl. J. Med. 290*, 550.
4. Barreras, R.F. (1970): Acid secretion after calcium carbonate in patients with duodenal ulcer. *N. Engl. J. Med. 282*, 1402.
5. Fordtran, J.S. (1968): Acid rebound. *N. Engl. J. Med. 279*, 900.
6. Holtermüller, K.H., Goldsmith, R.S., Sizemore, G.W. and Go, V.L.W. (1974): Dissociation of gastric acid and serum gastrin responses to intraluminal calcium in man: influence of calcitonin and parathyroid hormone. *Gastroenterology 67*, 1101.
7. Levant, J.A., Walsh, J.H. and Isenberg, J.I. (1973): Stimulation of gastric secretion and gastrin release by single oral doses of calcium carbonate in man. *N. Engl. J. Med. 289*, 555.
8. Malagelada, J.-R., Holtermüller, K.H., Sizemore, G.W. and Go, V.L.W. (1976): The influence of hypercalcemia on basal and cholecystokinin-stimulated pancreatic, gallbladder, and gastric functions in man. *Gastroenterology 71*, 405.
9. Derek, L. (1963): Studies on the hydrolysis of metal ions. The hydrolysis of magnesium in chloride self-medium. *Acta Chem. Scand. 17*, 1891.

10. Aveston, J. (1965): Hydrolysis of the aluminium ion: ultracentrifugation and acidity measurements. *J. Chem. Soc. part III*, 4438.

11. Deering, T.B., McCall, J.T., Carlson, G.L. and Malagelada, J.-R. (1977): Acid reduction by H_2-receptor antagonist vs neutralizing antacid in duodenal ulcer (Abstract). *Gastroenterology 72*, 1046.

12. Kaehny, W.D., Hegg, A.P. and Alfrey, A.C. (1977): Gastrointestinal absorption of aluminum from aluminum-containing antacids. *N. Engl. J. Med. 296*, 1389.

13. Recker, R.R., Blotcky, A.J., Leffler, J.A. and Rack, E.P. (1977): Evidence for aluminum absorption from the gastrointestinal tract and bone deposition by aluminum carbonate ingestion with normal renal function. *J. Lab. Clin. Med. 90*, 810.

14. Bernstein, J.E. and Karich, A.M. (1974): A double-blind trial of simethicone in functional disease of the upper gastrointestinal tract. *J. Clin. Pharmacol. 14*, 617.

15. Sigmund, C.J. and McNally, E.F. (1969): The action of a carminative on the lower esophageal sphincter. *Gastroenterology 56*, 13.

16. Grossman, M.I. (1956): Duration of action of antacids. *Am. J. Dig. Dis. 1*, 453.

17. Fordtran, J.S. and Collyns, J.A. (1966): Antacid pharmacology in duodenal ulcer. Effect of antacids on postcibal gastric acidity and peptic activity. *N. Engl. J. Med. 274*, 921.

18. Roth, H.P. and Berger, D.G. (1960): Studies on patient cooperation in ulcer treatment. I. Observation of actual as compared to prescribed antacid intake on a hospital ward. *Gastroenterology 38*, 630.

19. Fordtran, J.S., Morawski, S.G. and Richardson, C.T. (1973): In vivo and in vitro evaluation of liquid antacids. *N. Engl. J. Med. 288*, 923.

20. Deering, T.B. and Malagelada, J.-R. (1977): Comparison of an H_2-receptor antagonist and a neutralizing antacid on postprandial acid delivery into the duodenum in patients with duodenal ulcer. *Gastroenterology 73*, 11.

21. Walsh, J.H., Richardson, C.T. and Fordtran, J.S. (1975): pH dependence of acid secretion and gastrin release in normal and ulcer subjects. *J. Clin. Invest. 55*, 462.

22. Brodie, M.J., Ganguli, P.C., Fine, A. and Thomson, T.J. (1977): Effects of oral calcium gluconate on gastric acid secretion and serum gastrin concentration in man. *Gut 18*, 111.

23. Christiansen, J., Rehfeld, J.F. and Stadil, F. (1975): Interaction of calcium and magnesium on gastric acid secretion and serum gastrin concentration in man. *Gastroenterology 68*, 1140.

24. Holtermüller, K.H. (1977): Does oral magnesium hydroxide prevent the calcium carbonate induced acid rebound in patients with duodenal ulcer? (Abstract). *Gastroenterology 72*, 1071.

25. Malagelada, J.-R., Longstreth, G.F., Summerskill, W.H.J. and Go, V.L.W. (1976): Measurement of gastric functions during digestion of ordinary solid meals in man. *Gastroenterology 70*, 203.

26. Hurwitz, A., Robinson, R.G., Vats, T.S. et al. (1976): Effects of antacids on gastric emptying. *Gastroenterology 71*, 268.

27. Longstreth, G.F., Go, V.L.W. and Malagelada, J.-R. (1977): Postprandial gastric, pancreatic, and biliary response to histamine H_2-receptor antagonists in active duodenal ulcer. *Gastroenterology 72*, 9.

28. Regan, P.T., Malagelada, J.-R., DiMagno, E.P. et al. (1977): Comparative effects of antacids, cimetidine and enteric coating on the therapeutic response to

oral enzymes in severe pancreatic insufficiency. *N. Engl. J. Med. 297*, 854.

29. Hollander, D. and Harlan, J. (1973): Antacids vs placebos in peptic ulcer therapy. *J. Am. Med. Assoc. 226*, 1181.

30. Butler, M.L. and Gersh, H. (1975): Antacid vs placebo in hospitalized gastric ulcer patients: a controlled therapeutic study. *Am. J. Dig. Dis. 20*, 803.

31. Baume, P.E. and Hunt, J.H. (1969): Failure of potent antacid therapy to hasten healing in chronic gastric ulcers. *Australas. Ann. Med. 18*, 113.

32. Peterson, W.L., Sturdevant, R.A.L., Frankl, H.D. et al. (1977): Healing of duodenal ulcer with an antacid regimen. *N. Engl. J. Med. 297*, 341.

33. Hastings, P.R., Skillman, J.J., Bushnell, L.S. and Silen, W. (1978): Antacid titration in the prevention of acute gastrointestinal bleeding: a controlled, randomized trial in 100 critically ill patients. *N. Engl. J. Med. 298*, 1041.

34. Priebe, H.J., Skillman, J.J., Bushnell, L.S. et al. (1980): Antacid versus cimetidine in preventing acute gastrointestinal bleeding. *N. Engl. J. Med. 30*, 425.

35. Terés, J., Bordas, J.M., Rimola, A. et al. (1980): Cimetidine in acute gastric mucosal bleeding: results of a double-blind randomized trial. *Dig. Dis. Sci. 25*, 92.

36. Sturdevant, R.A.L., Isenberg, J.I., Secrist, D. and Ansfield, J. (1977): Antacid and placebo produced similar pain relief in duodenal ulcer patients. *Gastroenterology 72*, 1.

37. Morris, T. and Rhodes, J. (1979): Antacids and peptic ulcer – a reappraisal. *Gut 20*, 538.

38. Littman, A., Welch, R., Fruin, R.C. and Aronson, A.R. (1977): Controlled trial of aluminum hydroxide gels for peptic ulcer. *Gastroenterology 73*, 6.

39. Ippoliti, A., Elashoff, J., Cooney, C. et al. (1978): Duodenal ulcer (DU) relapse after cimetidine withdrawal (Abstract). *Gastroenterology 74*, 1047.

40. Richardson, C.T., Bailey, B.A., Walsh, J.H. and Fordtran, J.S. (1975): The effect of an H_2-receptor antagonist on food-stimulated acid secretion, serum gastrin, and gastric emptying in patients with duodenal ulcer. *J. Clin. Invest. 55*, 536.

41. Ivey, K.J. (1975): Anticholinergics: do they work in peptic ulcer? *Gastroenterology 68*, 154

42. Feldman, M., Richardson, C.T., Peterson, W.L. et al. (1977): Effect of low-dose propantheline on food-stimulated gastric acid secretion. *N. Engl. J. Med. 297*, 1427.

43. Chulski, T. and Forist, A.A. (1958): The effects of some solid buffering agents in aqueous suspension on prednisolone. *J. Am. Pharmaceut. Assoc. (Scientific Edition) 47*, 553.

44. Paul, H.E. and Harrington, C.M. (1952): Absorption characteristics of aureomycin and terramycin on aluminum hydroxide gel and on bismuth subsalicylate preparation. *J. Am. Pharmaceut. Assoc. (Scientific Edition) 41*, 50.

45. Grote, I.W. and Woods, M. (1953): Studies on antacids; absorption effects of various aluminum antacids upon simultaneously administered anticholinergetic drugs. *J. Am. Pharmaceut. Assoc. (Scientific Edition) 42*, 319.

46. Wenger, J. and Heymsfield, S. (1974): Adsorption of bile by aluminum hydroxide. *J. Clin. Pharmacol. 14*, 163.

47. Clain, J.E., Malagelada, J.-R., Chadwick, V.S. and Hofmann, A.F. (1977): Binding properties in vitro of antacids for conjugated bile acids. *Gastroenterology 73*, 556.

48. Eastwood, G.L. (1975): Failure of cholestyramine to prevent bile salt injury to mouse gastric mucosa. *Gastroenterology 68*, 1466.

49. Holtermüller, K.H., Malagelada, J.-R., McCall, J.T. and Go, V.L.W. (1976): Pancreatic, gallbladder, and gastric responses to intraduodenal calcium perfusion in man. *Gastroenterology 70*, 693.

50. Malagelada, J.-R., Holtermüller, K.H., McCall, J.T. and Go, V.L.W. (1978): Pancreatic, gallbladder, and intestinal responses to intraluminal magnesium salts in man. *Am. J. Dig. Dis. 23*, 481.

51. Fordtran, J.S., Rector, F.C. Jr. and Carter, N.W. (1968): The mechanisms of sodium absorption in the human small intestine. *J. Clin. Invest. 47*, 884.

52. Potyk, D. (1970): Brief recordings: intestinal obstruction from impacted antacid tablets. *N. Engl. J. Med. 283*, 134.

53. Wanitschke, R. and Ammon, H.V. (1976): Effects of magnesium sulfate on transit time and water transport in the human jejunum (Abstract). *Gastroenterology 70*, 949.

54. Hava, M. and Hurwitz, A. (1973): The relaxing effect of aluminum and lanthanum on rat and human gastric smooth muscle in vitro. *Eur. J. Pharmacol. 22*, 156.

55. McMillan, D.E. and Freeman, R.B. (1965): The milk-alkali syndrome: a study of the acute disorder with comments on the development of the chronic condition. *Medicine 44*, 485.

56. Kyle, L.H., Canary, J.J., Mintz, D.H. and Deleon, A. (1962): Inhibitor effects of induced hypercalcemia on secretion of parathyroid hormone. *J. Clin. Endocrinol. Metab. 22*, 52.

57. Robitscher, T. (1968): Antacids and phosphorus absorption. *N. Engl. J. Med. 279*, 328.

58. Dent, C.E. and Winter, C.S. (1974): Osteomalacia due to phosphate depletion from excessive aluminium hydroxide ingestion. *Br. Med. J. 1*, 551.

59. Kaehny, W.D., Hegg, A.P. and Alfrey, A.C. (1977): Gastrointestinal absorption of aluminum from aluminum-containing antacids. *N. Engl. J. Med. 296*, 1389.

60. Alfrey, A.C., LeGendre, G.R. and Kaehny, W.D. (1976): The dialysis encephalopathy syndrome: possible aluminum intoxication. *N. Engl. J. Med. 294*, 184.

61. Levy, G., Lampman, T., Kamath, B.L. and Garrettson, L.K. (1975): Decreased serum salicylate concentrations in children with rheumatic fever treated with antacid. *N. Engl. J. Med. 293*, 1975.

62. Deering, T.B., Carlson, G.L., Malagelada, J.-R. et al. (1979): Fate of oral neutralizing antacid and its effect on postprandial gastric secretion and emptying. *Gastroenterology 77*, 986.

Anticholinergics in the treatment of ulcer disease

M. Ström, R. Gotthard, G. Bodemar and A. Walan
*Department of Internal Medicine, Linköping University Medical School,
Linköping, Sweden*

Introduction

Anticholinergic and antimuscarinic agents are drugs that inhibit the action of
acetylcholine on the autonomic effectors innervated by postganglionic
cholinergic nerves and on the smooth muscles that lack cholinergic
innervation. They have very little effect on the action of acetylcholine at
nicotinic receptor sites.

Anticholinergic agents are of 2 types. The first group is comprised of the
tertiary ammonium compounds, the predominant activity being antimuscarinic. Atropine, the prototype of this group, which also includes
belladonna and the synthetic compound oxyphencyclimine, is the racemic
form of D, L-hyoscyamine. The antimuscarinic activity is almost wholly due to
the naturally-occurring L-form.

The second group comprises the quaternary ammonium compounds which
make up the majority of the synthetic compounds. The main activity of the
quaternary ammonium compounds is also antimuscarinic but they also exhibit
varying degrees of ganglionic blocking activity.

Absorption

The tertiary ammonium agents are well and rapidly absorbed. Beermann et al.
found atropine to be absorbed almost 100% after oral administration whereas
they found a much lower degree of absorption (15–25%) for the quaternary
ammonium drugs studied, such as ammonium-methyl-atropine, propantheline and methylscopolamine [1, 2]. The absorption of butylscopolamine
was less than 5%.

After oral administration of the quaternary compounds absorption was not
only less but also more variable. These compounds are not only less well

absorbed but they also penetrate some organs more slowly, where they exhibit their effect, e.g., in the eye. In ordinary therapeutic doses, they have no central effects as they do not readily cross the blood-brain barrier.

In most experimental situations in which the effects of anticholinergics are studied, for example when studying the effect on gastric secretion, the drugs are given on an empty stomach. To see whether concomitant administration of food would affect absorption we have investigated the effect of the tertiary ammonium compound hyoscyamine (in ordinary tablet form, and as a sustained-release tablet) and of the quaternary compound propantheline, on salivation, when the tablets were given on an empty stomach and together with a small meal [3].

All 3 preparations had a pronounced effect on salivation when taken during fasting. With both hyoscyamine tablet forms the inhibitory effect on salivation was unchanged when the tablets were taken with food, whereas no effect on salivation could be observed after administration of propantheline when this drug was given with food. Later we performed a similar study with another quaternary drug, benzilonium bromide [4]. The results in this study were similar to those in the previous study, with no effect on salivation after benzilonium bromide when the drug was taken with food, in contrast to the inhibitory effect on salivation when the drug was taken while fasting.

Selectivity

In the clinical use of anticholinergic drugs only one effect is generally desired and in the treatment of peptic ulcer what is required is an inhibitory effect on gastric secretion. Much effort has been devoted towards developing antimuscarinic agents with a selective effect on gastric secretion. Recently some evidence has been published that demonstrates the presence of receptor subtypes which show different affinity for different antimuscarinic drugs [5]. In this study by Hammer et al. pirenzipine exhibited a greater heterogeneity of binding sites to muscarinic receptors than did N-methylscopolamine. The binding properties of pirenzepine to the muscarinic receptors in the parietal cells of the gastric mucosa were, however, not investigated. Thus it remains to be investigated whether this drug inhibits gastric secretion at doses which do not inhibit salivation. This has not yet been clearly established.

The detection of subclasses of muscarinic receptors is, however, exciting and we look forward to the development of drugs with a selective effect on various organs and especially the parietal cell.

The rationale for the use of anticholinergic drugs in the treatment of peptic ulcer disease is based upon the known vagal control of acid secretion. The main aim of therapy is thus to reduce acid secretion; another aim is to decrease the rate of gastric emptying and thus prolong the effect of drugs acting locally in the stomach, e.g., antacids.

Effect on acid secretion

When studying the effects of anticholinergic drugs on acid secretion in experimental conditions it is essential that they are administered in the same way and in the same doses as are recommended in the ordinary clinical situation. This is true for most drugs but especially true for the anticholinergic agents as there is a great variation in the degree of absorption.

Despite the great number of anticholinergic drugs on the market, only a few have conclusively been shown to reduce acid secretion after oral administration in ordinary doses.

In these studies basal acid output (BAO) has been reduced by about 40–50%. Maximal acid output (MAO), as measured with the ordinary pentagastrin test or the augmented histamine test, can be reduced by 30–40% 2–4 hours after oral administration. Controlled studies on stimulated acid output several hours after intake of the drug have not been performed despite the presence of several so-called long-acting drugs on the market. Food-stimulated gastric secretion can also be reduced by about 30%, although in some studies no effect at all has been seen. As an example it can be mentioned that, although the mean inhibition of the 3-hour food-stimulated secretion by poldine was 32% in the study by Bieberdorf et al., the individual responses of the 5 subjects studied varied widely, from 0–60% inhibition [6]. There is great individual variation in sensitivity to anticholinergic drugs, which does not necessarily depend on the degree of absorption. This was the basis for the suggestion, by Sun and Shay in 1956, to administer anticholinergic drugs in an 'optimal effective dose' which has since been widely accepted [7]. Normally the dose given is one increment below that which can cause intolerable side effects.

The importance of using an optimal effective dose has not been adequately tested. In a recent study by Feldman et al. no difference was found in the decrease in food-stimulated acid secretion measured by the Fordtran technique after a 15-mg dose of propantheline compared to that after the optimal effective dose, which varied between 15 and 90 mg [8]. As we know that propantheline is absorbed in varying degrees, it might well be that the special experimental conditions with intragastric titration of food-stimulated secretion affected the absorption in another way than when the tablets were given for titration of the dose. The mean decrease in food-stimulated acid secretion was 29% with both the optimal effective dose and with the 15-mg dose. This is probably the mean maximal decrease of intragastrically-titrated food-stimulated acid secretion that can be achieved. In the long-term study with hyoscyamine by Walan there was wide individual variation in the optimal effective dose [9]. The mean decrease in both BAO and MAO was, however, equal in patients with high and low optimal effective doses. The possible advantage of an optimal effective dose over smaller doses needs to be investigated further, with regard to effect on acid secretion and on peptic ulcer disease. There is also some evidence that anticholinergic agents as well as prostaglandins and cimetidine can have an ulcer-preventive effect that is brought about by another mechanism than by a decrease in acid output [10].

Anticholinergic drugs can also decrease the rate of gastric emptying, which could give a prolongation of the effect of antacids. There are only a few experimental studies in which the influence of a combination of antacid and anticholinergic therapy has been studied. In one early study, Lennard-Jones found the acidity in the stomach during the day to be halved by poldine administered in optimal effective doses whereas no prolongation of the effect of the sucked antacid tablets was observed [11]. Fordtran and Collyns who studied the effect of calcium carbonate given one hour after a steak meal found no significant influence on acidity of optimal effective doses of glycopyrronium given half an hour before the meal, although the mean values for acidity at all observations were lower when glycopyrronium was given [12]. However, in a study with a rather small antacid dose we found a statistically significant prolongation of the time (from 29 to 71 minutes) during which the pH was above 3 when the patients were given an optimal effective dose of hyoscyamine [13]. Similar results have been published by Keyriläinen and Uusitalo [14].

Effect on ulcer healing

Despite the fact that we have had anticholinergics for several decades we know much less about their effect on healing than we know of cimetidine's. The main reason for this is that at the time when anticholinergics were introduced healing could only be measured radiologically, which definitely is not suitable for assessment of duodenal ulcer healing, although it may be used for assessing gastric ulcer.

A well-known study on gastric ulcer was performed by Doll who, using a rather large dose of belladonna given 3 times a day, found no significant advantage over the control group [15]. A preparation with a very short duration of action was, however, used. In another double-blind study on gastric ulcer Baume et al. investigated the effect of glycopyrronium given in optimal effective doses for 3 weeks [16]. After a period of bed rest during which time the patients also avoided salicylates and smoking, significantly more patients on glycopyrronium compared to the placebo group had healed their ulcers completely and the mean decrease in ulcer area had also diminished more in patients taking glycopyrronium. The recent interest in pirenzepine has resulted in endoscopically controlled studies on gastric ulcer, in which significant benefit over placebo has sometimes been seen [17]. Very few studies have been published where the effect of anticholinergic drugs on healing of duodenal ulcer has been endoscopically assessed.

Cheli and coworkers compared a fixed dose of phentonium with cimetidine and placebo [18]. Phentonium produced no significant effect on healing whereas cimetidine was significantly better than placebo. Recent interest in pirenzepine has resulted in several studies, mainly from Italy [19, 21], in which significant differences were found compared to placebo, however, others have not found any significant differences although most of these studies have been in favor of the anticholinergic drug. A high placebo healing rate was, as usual, found in Switzerland although there was no significant difference between the groups treated with pirenzepine, cimetidine or placebo [22].

Combinations with other drugs

A combination of an antacid and an anticholinergic will give low acid concentrations for a longer period than with an antacid alone and may be of value in the treatment of duodenal ulcer [23]. We have compared cimetidine and placebo against such a combination − a rather low (70 ml) daily volume of antacid together with a daily dose of 1.2 mg of hyoscyamine in sustained release tablets − in patients with duodenal ulcer [38]. After 6 weeks' treatment, 33% in the placebo group had healed compared to 83% in the cimetidine group and 100% in the antacid-anticholinergic group. Nocturnal pain decreased at an earlier point with cimetidine.

In the first studies on the effect of a combination of an anticholinergic drug and a histamine H_2-receptor antagonist, Tjodleifsson and Wormsley found that atropine augmented and prolonged the effect of metiamide [24]. Pounder, however, did not find any greater inhibition with a combination of cimetidine and atropine than with cimetidine alone [25]. Blackwood and Northfield found only a small additional effect of combination of poldine and cimetidine compared with cimetidine alone [26]. More pronounced and long-lasting inhibition of such a combination was, however, found by Feldman et al. using propantheline [8], and by Scholten et al. [27] and Londong et al.

[28], both groups using pirenzepine together with cimetidine. We also have found a greater inhibition with a combination of cimetidine and hyoscyamine than with either drug alone. In a preliminary study, Venables et al. found a combination of cimetidine and poldine to be more effective than cimetidine alone in patients whose ulcers had not healed after 4 weeks' cimetidine therapy [29]. However, more and longer-term studies into various combinations of anticholinergics and cimetidine in duodenal and gastric ulcer arc needed.

Long-term clinical trials with anticholinergics

Gastric ulcer

A long-term study was performed by Baume et al., who investigated the effect of optimal effective doses of glycopyrronium in 40 patients with gastric ulcer [16]. After 6 months, recurrences had occurred in 2 out of 18 patients in the glycopyrronium group compared to 10 recurrences among the 22 patients in the placebo group. After one year, recurrences had occurred in 5 out of 17 patients given glycopyrronium compared to 15 recurrences in the 21 patients in the placebo group; this is a significant difference.

Duodenal ulcer

There are several controlled studies into the long-term effect of anticholinergic drugs in duodenal ulcer disease. The studies, which have lasted for one year or more, and shorter studies which have been much quoted in the literature are summarized in the Table. A cross-over study by Lennard-Jones showed no beneficial effect of poldine, but the study covered a very short time period and a small number of patients [11]. In the study by Trevino et al., no significant difference between the groups was found but the overall trend was towards 'improvement', suggesting that the total therapy was of benefit to the patients [34]. The study by Kaye et al. showed no significant effect of anticholinergic therapy on pain, vomiting, antacid consumption or the patients' own assessment of their well-being [35]. Only one hemorrhage occurred in the whole group of 92 patients. At the end of the trial 80% felt that they had improved, suggesting that the total therapy excluding the anticholinergic drugs had been of benefit or that the good result obtained was a reflection of the natural course of the disease in these patients.

In several other studies, however, clear differences have been observed, for example, in the very large study by Ruffin and Cayer comprising 1,034

Table: Influence of long-term anticholinergic treatment on peptic ulcer disease. Summary of different studies.

Study	Number of patients	Treatment	Duration	Results				Significance
Lennard-Jones 1961 [11]	11 11	Poldine OED Placebo	3 months					NS
Melrose and Pinkerton 1961 [30]	31 27	Poldine OED Placebo	9 months					NS
Ruffin and Cayer 1962 [31]	705 226 103	Anticholinergics Atropine Placebo	—	good	74% 53% 48%	bleeding	3% 2% 10%	Significant Significant Significant
Sun 1962 [32]	25 20	Tricyclamol OED Placebo	2 years	recurrences	2 9	complications	2 6	Significant
Sun 1964 [33]	20 17	Glycopyrronium OED Placebo	18 months	recurrences	3 12	complications	1 10	Significant
Trevino et al. 1967 [34]	26 27	Glycopyrronium OED Placebo	18–27 months					NS
Kaye et al. 1970 [35]	28 31 32	Glycopyrronium OED Hyoscyamine OED Placebo	1 year					NS
Sun and Ryan 1970 [36]	18 16	Propantheline 15 mg x 4 Placebo	1 year	recurrences	7 12			$0.05 < p < 0.1$
Walan 1970 [9]	29 29	Hyoscyamine OED Placebo	2 years	complications recurrences sick-listing sick-listing/year pain	0 5 4 12 3 12 0.8 9.4 15 14			$p < 0.02$ $p < 0.02$ $p < 0.01$ $p < 0.01$ NS
Cocking 1972 [37]	31 30	Propantheline 75 mg/day	48 weeks					NS

OED = optimal effective dose.
NS = not significant.

patients, which reported a much higher incidence of hemorrhage in the placebo group than in the anticholinergic group [31]. A lower incidence of recurrences was seen in patients treated with tricyclamol or glycopyrronium in the first studies by Sun [32, 33]. Anticholinergic-treated patients also had fewer complications, 8% and 5%, respectively, compared to the placebo groups, in which complications were seen in 45% and 50% respectively.

In the study by Walan with hyoscyamine in sustained-release tablets and placebo, patients on hyoscyamine had fewer recurrences, fewer complications and fewer days lost from work, however there was no difference between groups as regards the occurrence of pain [9]. In the few patients with recurrence during long-term treatment with hyoscyamine this drug had less effect on both basal and stimulated secretion and these patients also had higher initial secretory values. An interesting observation was that low optimal effective doses of hyoscyamine were as effective as high optimal effective doses in inhibiting basal and stimulated acid output.

During the last decade we have seen new drugs with quite different modes of action introduced in the treatment of peptic ulcer disease. During the years to come we will see still more such drugs, perhaps anticholinergic drugs with selectivity for the parietal cell. It will then be the duty of gastroenterologists to perform clinical studies comparing the new and old drugs alone and in combination, to find the best combination, with minimal side effects, tailored to the individual patient.

Summary

Anticholinergic agents consist of tertiary and quaternary ammonium compounds. Tertiary ammonium agents are fully and rapidly absorbed. Quaternary ammonium agents are slowly and incompletely absorbed but do not pass the blood-brain barrier. There may be subclasses of cholinergic receptors and anticholinergic agents with different affinity for these. Anticholinergics can reduce BAO by about 40–50%, pentagastrin-stimulated secretion by about 30–40% and food-stimulated secretion by about 30%. The importance of using an optimal effective dose has not been adequately tested. Combined therapy with antacids and anticholinergics will give a more long lasting decrease in acidity than with either drug alone. Anticholinergics can hasten healing of duodenal and gastric ulcer. Combined therapy with antacids and anticholinergics will give equally good results as with cimetidine alone. Cimetidine and anticholinergics will give a more long lasting and pronounced inhibition of acid secretion than will either drug alone. Long-term treatment with anticholinergics can decrease recurrences and complications of peptic ulcer disease.

References

1. Beermann, B., Hellström, K. and Rosen, A. (1971): The gastrointestinal absorption of atropine in man. *Clin. Sci. 40*, 95.
2. Beermann, B., Hellström, K. and Rosén, A. (1973): The effect of long-term administration on the absorption of methylscopolamine in man. *Acta Med. Scand. 193*, 35.
3. Ekenved, G., Magnusson, A., Bodemar, G. and Walan, A. (1977): Influence of food on the effect of propantheline and l-hyoscyamine on salivation. *Scand. J. Gastroenterol. 12*, 963.
4. Post, C. and Walan, A. (1977): Influence of food on the effect of l-hyoscyamine and benzilonium-bromide. *Scand. J. Gastroenterol. 12, Suppl. 45*, 72.
5. Hammer, R., Berrie, C.P., Birdsall, N.J.M. et al. (1980): Pirenzepine distinguishes between different subclasses of muscarinic receptors. *Nature 283*, 90.
6. Bieberdorf, F.A., Walsh, J.H. and Fordtran, J.S. (1975): Effect of optimum therapeutic dose of poldine on acid secretion, gastric acidity, gastric emptying and serum gastrin concentration after a protein meal. *Gastroenterology 68*, 50.
7. Sun, D.C.H. and Shay, H. (1956): Optimal effective dose of anticholinergic drug in peptic ulcer therapy. *Arch. Intern. Med. 97*, 442.
8. Feldman, M., Richardson, C.T., Peterson, W.L. et al. (1977): Effect of low-dose propantheline on food-stimulated gastric acid secretion. Comparison with an 'Optimal Effective Dose' and interaction with cimetidine. *N. Engl. J. Med. 297*, 1472.
9. Walan, A. (1970): Studies on peptic ulcer disease with special reference to the effect of l-hyoscyamine. *Acta Med. Scand. (Suppl.)*, 516.
10. Guth, P.H., Aures, D. and Paulsen, G. (1979): Topical aspirin plus HCl gastric lesions in the rat. *Gastroenterology 76*, 88.
11. Lennard-Jones, J.E. (1961): Experimental and clinical observations of poldine in treatment of duodenal ulcer. *Br. Med. J. 1*, 1071.
12. Fordtran, J.S. and Collyns, J.A. (1966): Antacid pharmacology in duodenal ulcer. Effect of antacids on postcibal gastric acidity and peptic activity. *N. Engl. J. Med. 274*, 921.
13. Dotevall, G. and Walan, A. (1967): Antacids in the treatment of peptic ulcer. *Acta Med. Scand. 182*, 529.
14. Keyriläinen, O. and Uusitalo, A. (1978): The influence of an anticholinergic agent on the duration of the effect of antacids. In: *Abstracts of Papers from the XIIth Scandinavian Conference on Gastroenterology, 24–26 August, 1978*, p. 59. Editor: I. Ihse.
15. Doll, R. (1964): Medical treatment of gastric ulcer. *Scott. Med. J. 9*, 183.
16. Baume, P.E., Hunt, J.H. and Piper, D.W. (1972): Glycopyrronium bromide in the treatment of chronic gastric ulcer. *Gastroenterology 63*, 399.
17. Schmid, E. (1978): Randomisierte Doppelblindstudie mit Pirenzepin beim Ulcus ventriculi. In: *Die Behandlung des Ulcus Pepticum mit Pirenzipin*, p. 231. Editors: A.L. Blum and R. Hammer. Karl Demeter Verlag, Gräfelfing.
18. Cheli, R., Ciancamerla, G., Giacosa, A. et al. (1978): Short-term cimetidine treatment of duodenal ulcer. Comparison with placebo and an anticholinergic drug. *Ital. J. Gastroenterol 10*, 18.

19. Chierichetti, S.M. and Giorgiconciato, M. (1978): Die Behandlung des Ulcus duodeni und -ventriculi mit Pirenzepin: Eine multizentrische Doppelblindstudie. In: *Die Behandlung des Ulcus pepticum mit Pirenzepin*, p. 178. Editors: A.L. Blum and R. Hammer. Karl Demeter Verlag, Gräfelfing.

20. Morelli, A. (1978): Treatment of gastric and duodenal ulcer with Pirenzepine. In: *Die Behandlung des Ulcus pepticum mit Pirenzepin,* p. 196. Editors: A.L. Blum and R. Hammer. Karl Demeter Verlag, Gräfelfing.

21. Bianchi Porro, G., Petrillo, M., Benassai, D. et al. (1978): Preliminary communication. Pirenzepinc vs cimetidine and placebo in the treatment of duodenal ulcer. In: *Die Behandlung des Ulcus pepticum mit Pirenzepin*, p. 194. Editors: A.L. Blum and R. Hammer. Karl Demeter Verlag, Gräfelfing.

22. Giger, M., Convers, J.-J., Weber, K.B. et al. (1978): Pirenzepin-Behandlung des Ulcus duodeni. Vergleich mit Cimetidin und Placebo. In: *Die Behandlung des Ulcus pepticum mit Pirenzepin*, p. 216. Editors: A.L. Blum and R. Hammer. Karl Demeter Verlag, Gräfelfing.

23. Bowers, J., Forbes, J. and Freston, J. (1977): Effect of night-time anisotropine methyl bromide (AMB) on duodenal ulcer (DU) healing: a controlled trial. *Gastroenterology 72*, 1032.

24. Tjodleifsson, B. and Wormsley, K.G. (1975): Aspects of the effect of metiamide on pentagastrin stimulated and basal gastric secretion of acid and pepsin in man. *Gut 16,* 501.

25. Pounder, R.E., Williams, J.G., Hunt, R.H. et al. (1977): The effect of oral cimetidine on food-stimulated gastric acid secretion on 24-hour intragastric acidity. In: *Cimetidine. Proceedings of the Second International Symposium on Histamine H_2-Receptor Antagonists*, pp. 189–204. Editors: W.L. Burland and M. A. Simkins. Excerpta Medica, Amsterdam-Oxford.

26. Blackwood, W.S. and Northfield, T.C. (1977): Nocturnal gastric acid secretion: Effect of cimetidine and interaction with anticholinergics. In: *Cimetidine. Proceedings of the Second International Symposium on Histamine H_2-Receptor Antagonists*, pp. 124–130. Editors: W.L. Burland and M. A. Simkins. Excerpta Medica, Amsterdam-Oxford.

27. Scholten, T., Hengels, K.J., Fritsch, W.P. and Hausamen, T.U. (1978): Langzeitsuppression der H^+-Sekretion durch Kombination von Cimetidine mit Methanthelinbromid und Pirenzepin-Dihydro-Chlorid. In: *Ergebnisse der Gastroenterologie 1977*, Abstract 60. Editors: W. Creutzfeldt and M. Klassen. Karl Demeter Verlag, Gräfelfing.

28. Londong, W., Londong, V., Prechtl, R. and Eversmann, T. (1978): Vergleichende Untersuchung der Pirenzepin- und Cimetidinwirkung auf Pepton-stimulierte Säuresekretion und Serumgastrin des Menschen. In: *Die Behandlung des Ulcus pepticum mit Pirenzepin*, p. 75. Editors: A.L. Blum and R. Hammer. Karl Demeter Verlag, Gräfelfing.

29. Venables, C.W., Stephen, J.G., Blair, E.L. et al. (1978): Cimetidine in the treatment of duodenal ulceration and the relationship of this therapy to surgical management. In: *Cimetidine. The Westminster Hospital Symposium*. Editors: C. Wastell and P. Lance. Churchill Livingstone, Edinburgh.

30. Melrose, A.G. and Pinkerton, I.W. (1961): Clinical evaluation of poldine methosulphate. *Br. Med. J. I,* 1076.

31. Ruffin, J.M. and Cayer, D. (1962): The role of anticholinergic drugs in treatment of peptic ulcer disease. *Ann. N.Y. Acad. Sci. 99,* 179.

32. Sun, D.C.H. (1962): The medical management of duodenal ulcer and long-term study with drug therapy in the prevention of recurrences. *Ann. N.Y. Acad. Sci.* *99*, 104.

33. Sun, D.C.H. (1964): Long-term anticholinergic therapy for recurrences in duodenal ulcer. *Am. J. Dig. Dis. 9*, 706.

34. Trevino, H., Anderson, J., Davey, P.G. and Henley, K.S. (1967): The effect of glycopyrrolate on the course of symptomatic duodenal ulcer. *Am. J. Dig. Dis. 12*, 983.

35. Kaye, M.D., Rhodes, J., Beck, P. et al. (1970): A controlled trial of glycopyrronium and l-hyoscyamine in the long-term treatment of duodenal ulcer. *Gut 11*, 559.

36. Sun, D.C.H. and Ryan, M.L. (1970): A controlled study on the use of propantheline and amylopectin sulpfate (SN-263) for recurrences in duodenal ulcer. *Gastroenterology 58*, 756.

37. Cocking, J.B. (1972): A trial of amylopectin sulphate (SN-263) and propantheline bromide in the long-term treatment of chronic duodenal ulcer. *Gastroenterology 62*, 6.

37. Ström, M., Gotthard, R., Bodemar, G. and Walan, A. (1980): Treatment of peptic ulcer disease. A comparative study between cimetidine and combined anticholinergic and antacid therapy. *Scand. J. Gastroenterol.* (In press).

Carbenoxolone in the treatment of ulcer disease

M.J.S. Langman
Department of Therapeutics, City Hospital, Nottingham, England

The value of any drug is judged by the balance between its safety and efficacy. An appraisal of carbenoxolone therefore needs a dispassionate assessment of both.

Carbenoxolone in the promotion of peptic ulcer healing

Gastric ulcer

There is ample evidence that carbenoxolone is superior to placebo treatment (except, as with other drugs, in the United States of America). A convenient method of assessment is to calculate the ratio between the proportions of ulcers healed during active drug and placebo treatment. If this is done for carbenoxolone then nearly twice as many ulcers can be expected to heal overall, as during treatment with placebo (Table I). If these findings are

Table I: Results of outpatient treatment trials with gastric ulcer.

Study	Percentage of patients with complete healing	
	Carbenoxolone	Placebo
Doll et al. [1]	37	5
Doll et al. [2]	42	27
Cocking and MacCaig [3]	47	12
Gilbert [4]	67	44
Lorber [5]	36	33
Stadelmann et al. [6]	45	33
Overall	46	26

Overall ratio 1.8:1.

compared with those obtained with other drugs then variable results are obtained. Some, such as gefarnate and deglycyrrhizinized liquorice, show a lesser degree of healing when calculated overall, but roughly equivalent findings are obtained with 2 other drugs, chelated bismuth and cimetidine (Table II).

The significance of this finding is uncertain, but it suggests that the maximum healing rate achievable is a doubling of the proportions of ulcers that will heal during a short fixed term compared with expectation. Even this conclusion may be invalid in certain geographical areas, notably the United States, where ulcer healing rates during placebo treatment may be considerably higher than rates in European communities.

Table II: Overall results of some outpatient treatment trials of gastric ulcer with carbenoxolone, chelated bismuth and cimetidine.

Drug	Percentage of patients with complete healing		Ratio
	Drug	Placebo	
Carbenoxolone [1–6]	46	26	1.8:1
Chelated bismuth [7–9]	85	32	2.6:1
Cimetidine [10–16]	68	41	1.7:1

Duodenal ulcer

Ample evidence exists to show that carbenoxolone treatment promotes duodenal ulcer healing and that the proportions of ulcers healed, as with gastric ulcer, are about twice those expected during placebo treatment. An equivalent rate of healing is achieved with cimetidine, again with the exception of the United States, and again it would seem that a doubling of the healing rate is the maximum achievable in areas where spontaneous healing rates are relatively low (Table III).

Mechanism of healing

The healing mechanism is obscure. Carbenoxolone is weakly antipeptic but is not an antisecretory drug. Following treatment there is an increase in the rate of production of mucosubstances, suggesting that these are locally protective,

Table III: Results of treatment for duodenal ulcer with carbenoxolone and cime-tidine.

Study	Percentage of patients with complete healing		Ratio
	Test	Control	
Cimetidine			
Bank et al. [17] (South Africa)	86	42	2.0:1
Blackwood et al. [18] (U.K.)	82	25	3.3:1
Bodemar and Walan [19] (Scandinavia)	93	36	2.6:1
Gray et al. [20] (U.K.)	85	25	3.4:1
Hetzel et al. [21] (Australia)	82	39	2.1:1
Bardhan et al. [22] (U.K.)	63	28	2.3:1
Malchow et al. [23] (Germany)	49	21	2.3:1
Binder et al. [24] (U.S.A.)	57	48	1.2:1
Semb et al. [25] (Scandinavia)	85	60	1.4:1
Overall	76	36	2.1:1
Carbenoxolone			
Archambault [26] (Canada)	76	55	1.4:1
Nagy [29] (Australia)	67	30	2.2:1
Davies and Reed [27] (U.K.)	81	39	2.1:1
Sahel et al. [28] (France)	65	20	3.3:1
Young et al. [30] (Australia)	60	25	2.4:1
Overall	70	34	2.3:1

though we have no direct evidence to support such activity beyond an increase in mucus output and in epithelial cell life during treatment.

Prevention of relapse

Ulcer recurrence occurs early and often in patients with duodenal ulcer, and probably in those with gastric ulcer when antisecretory treatment with cimetidine ceases, so that there is about a 75% chance of recurrence within 6 months of stopping treatment. For this reason cimetidine treatment may be continued and there is ample evidence that during 6–12 months' maintenance treatment the chances of relapse are substantially reduced. The aldosterone-like adverse effects of carbenoxolone make maintenance treatment impractical, but since the drug is not an antisecretory agent there seems at least a possibility that ulcers might be less liable to break down once treatment stops than is the case when antisecretory drug treatment is stopped. Evidence is fragmentary, but the rate of breakdown of gastric ulcers seems to be no greater on stopping treatment than might be expected after spontaneous healing (Table IV).

Since about twice as many ulcers would be expected to have healed during initial treatment with carbenoxolone than with placebo, the figures suggest

Table IV: Gastric ulcer recurrence rates after carbenoxolone and placebo treatment.

Study	Initial treatment			
	Carbenoxolone		Placebo	
	(%)	(No.)	(%)	(No.)
Horwich and Galloway [31]	44	8/18	17	1/6
Bank et al. [32]	40	–	40	–
Langman [33]	36	8/22	43	3/7
Geismar et al. [34]	38	–	38	–

(All relapse rates after 12 months except Geismar et al. after 24 months).

that if relapse rates are identical then, in patients given carbenoxolone, about twice as many ulcers remain healed after 1–2 years as might have been expected.

Adverse effects

Successful treatments are those for which the advantages outweigh the drawbacks. The major adverse effects of drugs are those which are occasional, but idiosyncratic and severe, while those which are predictable and reversible present lesser hazards. Carbenoxolone is well known to have aldosterone-like adverse effects. These occur with increasing frequency with age, with associated cardiorespiratory disease and with increasing carbenoxolone dose. Pharmacokinetic analyses show some of the reasons why this should be.

Age effects

Carbenoxolone is bound to serum albumin and elderly people tend to have

Table V: Carbenoxolone pharmacokinetics.

	Age	
	Less than 40 years	65 years or more
Average available protein binding sites	798	640*
Plasma half time in hours after a single 300 mg dose	13.3	22.9*
Percentage displacement of aldosterone from protein binding sites	2.5	3.2^{+}

Data from [35]

* Differences significant, $p < 0.02$

$^{+}$ Differences insignificant, $p < 0.1$

low serum albumin levels, thus they tend to have more available in the free active form. More important perhaps is that carbenoxolone is especially slowly metabolized in the liver of elderly people (Table V).

Aldosterone-like action

Carbenoxolone does not seem to displace important amounts of aldosterone from plasma protein binding sites, but it may well interact with intracellular binding sites in the kidney and elsewhere.

Several approaches have been made to try and mitigate these effects, and they include the following.

Thiazide diuretic treatment   Such agents will reverse the fluid retention, but have the disadvantage that they tend to accentuate any tendency to hypokalemia.

Aldosterone antagonists   Spironolactone will prevent the adverse effects of carbenoxolone, but it also inhibits ulcer healing. This finding, which was unexpected, suggests that the integrity of the gastric mucosa depends in some way upon influences which include electrolyte homeostasis. This hypothesis is testable. Spironolactone acts intracellularly, whereas amiloride, another potassium-conserving agent, acts at the cell membrane. It would therefore be of considerable interest to know whether amiloride treatment ameliorates carbenoxolone side effects but allows ulcer healing to continue. If ulcer healing under the influence of carbenoxolone depends upon changes in potassium flux it might also be that healing would occur more quickly and

Table VI: Healing of gastric ulcers during carbenoxolone treatment.

	Healing	
	Complete or at least 66% healed during 4 weeks' treatment	Less than 66% reduction in ulcer size
*Change in serum potassium levels in relation to healing**		
Serum potassium fall of 1 mmol/l or more	10	13
Serum potassium fall of less than 1 mmol/l	8	11
*Prescription of thiazide diuretics and ulcer healing**		
Thiazide diuretics prescribed	10	13
Thiazide diuretics not prescribed	20	18

* Combined data of [36 and 37].

completely in patients who tend to suffer from salt and water retention or hypokalemia.

Reanalysis of earlier data obtained about gastric ulcer healing shows in fact that those developing fluid retention or hypokalemia in our studies did not have a greater tendency for their ulcers to heal (Table VI).

Prescription of carbenoxolone analogues Carbenoxolone is the succinate ester of glycyrrhetic acid, the moiety of liquorice which also causes fluid retention. Alternative treatments which have been tried include the lauryl ester; an open chain farnesene derivative geranylfarnesyl acetate (gefarnate), and deglycyrrhizinized liquorice [38–41]. These have generally proved

Table VII: Comparative effects of succinyl and lauryl salts of glycyrrhetic acid in gastric ulcer.*

	Healing	
	Complete or at least 66% healed during 4 weeks' treatment	Less than 66% reduction in ulcer size
Succinate (carbenoxolone)	16	8
Lauryl salt	9	15

*Data from [38].

disappointing, absence of adverse effects being matched by no, or indifferent, evidence of healing properties (Table VII illustrates these for the lauryl salt). We therefore still do not know for certain if the healing and fluid retaining properties of carbenoxolone can be separated.

Use of carbenoxolone in clinical practice

Whether carbenoxolone is used depends upon an individual's appraisal of the balance between benefits and risks compared with other drugs. The importance to be attached to specific features depends upon factors which are, in great part, imponderable. Three agents, carbenoxolone sodium, chelated bismuth and cimetidine, promote ulcer healing to much the same degree but patterns of adverse effects vary greatly. Carbenoxolone is safe in short-term use provided patients are observed carefully and are watched for evidence of salt and water retention, hypokalemia and raised blood pressure. Chelated bismuth produces no adverse effects and does not seem to cause encephalopathy like other bismuth salts, however, its ammoniacal odor is unpleasant and could inhibit patient compliance. Cimetidine is substantially safe in short-term use, however, it inhibits drug metabolism [42] and so may interfere with the use of other agents; it is also antiandrogenic [43] and (usually in large doses) can cause mental confusion in the elderly [44]. Carbenoxolone cannot be used long-term because of its adverse effects, chelated bismuth has not been tested, and cimetidine clearly prevents ulcer breakdown while it is in use. However, we do not know if long-term treatment is safe. The relative achlorhydria induced by cimetidine could predispose to gastric cancer, but there is no firm evidence to support this hypothesis. There is evidence that cimetidine alters myocardial activity but there is no general evidence yet that patients taking the drug and who have frail cardiovascular systems are unduly likely to develop arrhythmias or other problems, though there is at least one suggestive report [45].

Summary

Carbenoxolone, like cimetidine and chelated bismuth, will promote the healing of gastric and duodenal ulcers. Its known and predictable adverse effects prevent its use in maintenance treatment. Its place relative to chelated bismuth and cimetidine depends upon assessment of the importance of aldosterone-like adverse effects with carbenoxolone, of patient compliance with chelated bismuth, and of the possible long-term adverse effects of cimetidine which need clearer definition.

References

1. Doll, R., Hill, I.D., Hutton, C.F. and Underwood, D.J. (1962): Clinical trial of triterpenoid liquorice compound in gastric and duodenal ulcer. *Lancet II*, 793.
2. Doll, R., Hill, I.D. and Hutton, C.F. (1965): Treatment of gastric ulcer with carbenoxolone sodium and oestrogens. *Gut 6*, 19.
3. Cocking, J.B. and MacCaig, J.N. (1969): Effect of low dosage of carbenoxolone sodium on gastric ulcer healing and acid secretion. *Gut 10*, 219.
4. Gilbert, J.A.L. (1976): Multi-centre Canadian double-blind study of carbenoxolone (Biogastrone®) in the treatment of gastric ulcer. In: *North American Symposium on Carbenoxolone,* pp. 85–92. Ed: I.T. Beck. Excerpta Medica, Amsterdam.
5. Lorber, S.H. (1976): U.S. trial of carbenoxolone (Biogastrone®) in gastric ulcer. In: *North American Symposium on Carbenoxolone*, pp. 93–97. Ed: I.T. Beck. Excerpta Medica, Amsterdam.
6. Stadelmann, O., Miederer, S.E., Werner, C. et al. (1972): Aktuelle Probleme des Magen-Duodenalulkus. *Fortschr. Med. 90*, 123.
7. Moshal, M.G. (1974): A double-blind gastroscopic study of a bismuth-peptide complex in gastric ulceration. *S. Afr. Med. J. 48*, 1610.
8. Lee, S.P. and Nicholson, G.I. (1977): Increased healing of gastric and duodenal ulcers in a controlled trial using tripotassium dicitratobismuthate. *Med. J. Austr. 1*, 808.
9. Boyes, B.E., Woolf, I.L., Wilson, R.Y. et al. (1975): Treatment of gastric ulceration with a bismuth preparation. *Postgrad. Med. J. 51 (Sup. 5)*, 29.
10. Bader, J.P., Morin, T., Bernier, J.J. et al. (1977): Treatment of gastric ulcer by cimetidine. In: *Cimetidine, Proceedings of the Second International Symposium on Histamine H_2-Receptor Antagonists*, pp. 287–292. Eds: W.L. Burland and M.A. Simkins. Excerpta Medica, Amsterdam.
11. Ciclitira, P.J., Machell, R.J. et al. (1977): Experience with cimetidine in the treatment of gastric ulceration. *Gut 18*, A419.

12. Frost, F., Rahbek, I., Rune, S.J. et al. (1977): Cimetidine in patients with gastric ulcer: a multicentre controlled trial. *Br. Med. J. 2*, 795.

13. Dyck, W.P., Belsito, A., Fleshler, B. et al. (1978): Cimetidine and placebo in the treatment of benign gastric ulcer. A multicenter double-blind study. *Gastroenterology 74*, 410.

14. Englert, E., Freston, J.W., Graham, D.Y. et al. (1978): Cimetidine, antacid and hospitalisation in the treatment of benign gastric ulcer. A multicenter double-blind study. *Gastroenterology 74*, 416.

15. Sewing, K.F., Malchow, H., Albinus, M. et al. (1978): Cimetidin in der stationären Behandlung des peptischen Ulkus. II. Doppelblindstudie bei Ulcus ventriculi. *Dtsch. Med. Wochenschr. 103*, 152.

16. Smith, P.M., Edwards, J.L. and Aubrey, D.A. (1978): Gastric secretory studies and cimetidine treatment in gastric ulcers. In: *Cimetidine: The Westminster Hospital Symposium*, pp. 258–272. Eds: C. Wastell and P. Lance. Churchill Livingstone, Edinburgh.

17. Bank, S., Barbezat, G.O., Novis, B.H. et al. (1976): Histamine H_2 receptor antagonists in the treatment of duodenal ulcers. *South Afr. Med. J. 50*, 1781.

18. Blackwood, W.S., Maudgal, D.P., Pickard, R.G. et al. (1976): Cimetidine in duodenal ulcer. *Lancet II*, 161.

19. Bodemar, G. and Walan, A. (1976): Cimetidine in the treatment of active duodenal and pre-pyloric ulcers. *Lancet II*, 161.

20. Gray, G.R., MacKenzie, I., Smith, I.S. et al. (1977): Oral cimetidine in severe duodenal ulceration. *Lancet I*, 4.

21. Hetzel, D.J., Hansky, J., Shearman, D.J.C. et al. (1978): Cimetidine treatment of duodenal ulceration. Short-term clinical trial and maintenance study. *Gastroenterology 74*, 389.

22. Bardhan, K.D., Saul, D.M., Edwards, J.L. et al. (1979): Comparison of two doses of cimetidine and placebo in the treatment of duodenal ulcer: a multicentre trial. *Gut 20*, 68.

23. Malchow, H., Sewing, K.F., Albinus, M. et al. (1978): Cimetidin in der stationären Behandlung des peptischen Ulkus. *Dtsch. Med. Wochenschr. 103*, 149.

24. Binder, H.J., Cocco, A., Crossley, R.J. et al. (1978): Cimetidine in the treatment of duodenal ulcer. A multicenter double-blind study. *Gastroenterology 74*, 380.

25. Semb, L.S., Berstad, A., Myren, J. et al. (1977): A double blind multicentre comparative study of cimetidine and placebo in short term treatment of active duodenal ulceration. In: *Cimetidine, Proceedings of the Second International Symposium on Histamine H_2-Receptor Antagonists*, pp. 248–253. Eds: W.L. Burland and M.A. Simkins. Excerpta Medica, Amsterdam.

26. Archambault, A. (1976): The Canadian study of carbenoxolone (Duogastrone) in the treatment of duodenal ulcers. In: *North American Symposium on Carbenoxolone*, pp. 150–157. Ed: I.T. Beck. Excerpta Medica, Amsterdam.

27. Davies, W.A. and Reed, P.I. (1977): Controlled trial of Duogastrone in duodenal ulcer. *Gut 18*, 78.

28. Sahel, J., Sarles, H., Baisson, J. et al. (1977): Carbenoxolone sodium capsules in the treatment of duodenal ulcer. *Gut 18*, 717.

29. Nagy, G.S. (1978): Evaluation of carbenoxolone sodium in the treatment of duodenal ulcer. *Gastroenterology 74*, 7.

30. Young, G.P., St. John, D.J.B. and Coventry, D.A. (1978): A double-masked endoscopic evaluation of carbenoxolone in duodenal ulcer: further evidence for a beneficial effect. In: *Peptic Ulcer Healing – Recent Studies on Carbenoxolone*, pp. 117–125. Eds: F. Avery Jones, M.J.S. Langman and R.D. Mann. MTP Press, Lancaster.

31. Horwich, L. and Galloway, R. (1965): Treatment of gastric ulcer with carbenoxolone sodium. Clinical and radiological evaluation. *Br. Med. J. 2*, 1272.

32. Bank, S., Marks, I.N., Palmer, P.E.S. et al. (1967): A trial of carbenoxolone sodium in the treatment of gastric ulceration. *South Afr. Med. J. 41*, 297.

33. Langman, M.J.S. (1968): The medical treatment of gastric and duodenal ulcer. *Postgrad. Med. J. 44*, 603.

34. Geismar, P., Mosbech, J. and Myren, J. (1973): A double-blind study of the effect of carbenoxolone sodium in the treatment of gastric ulcer. *Scand. J. Gastroenterol. 8*, 251.

35. Hayes, M.J., Spackling, M.E. and Langman, M.J.S. (1977): Changes in the plasma clearance and protein binding of carbenoxolone with age, and their possible relationship to adverse drug effects. *Gut 18*, 1054.

36. Doll, R., Langman, M.J.S. and Shawdon, H.H. (1968): Treatment of gastric ulcer with carbenoxolone: antagonistic effect of spironolactone. *Gut 9*, 42.

37. Langman, M.J.S., Knapp, D.R. and Wakley, E.J. (1973): Treatment of chronic gastric ulcer with carbenoxolone and gefarnate: a comparative trial. *Br. Med. J. 3*, 84.

38. Fraser, P.M., Doll, R., Langman, M.J.S. et al. (1972): Clinical trial of a new carbenoxolone analogue BX-24, zinc sulphate and vitamin A in the treatment of gastric ulcer. *Gut 13*, 459.

39. Smith, P.M., Sladen, G.E., Beck, E.R. et al. (1975): A double-blind trial of carbenoxolone and geranyl farnesyl acetate in gastric ulcer. *Scand. J. Gastroenterol. 10*, 753.

40. Montgomery, R.D. and Cookson, J.B. (1972): Comparative trial of carbenoxolone and a deglycyrrhizinated liquorice preparation (Caved-S). *Clin. Trials J. 9*, 33.

41. Wilson, J.A.C. (1972): A comparison of carbenoxolone sodium and deglycyrrhizinated liquorice in the treatment of gastric ulcer in the ambulant patient. *Br. J. Clin. Prac. 26*, 563.

42. Serlin, M.J., Sibeon, R.G., Mossman, A.S. et al. (1979): Cimetidine: interaction with oral anticoagulants in man. *Lancet II*, 317.

43. Van Thiel, D.H., Govaler, J.S., Smith, W.I. and Paul, G. (1979): Hypothalamic-pituitary-gonadal dysfunction in men using cimetidine. *N. Engl. J. Med. 300*, 1012.

44. Schentag, J.J., Cerra, F.B., Calleri, G. et al. (1979): Pharmacokinetic and clinical studies in patients with cimetidine-associated mental confusion. *Lancet I*, 177.

45. Cohen, J., Weetman, A.P., Dargie, H.J. and Krikler, D.M. (1979): Life-threatening arrhythmias and intravenous cimetidine. *Br. Med. J. II*, 768.

Prostaglandins: pharmacologic principles

J. I. Isenberg
*Department of Medicine, University of California at San Diego, San Diego,
California, U.S.A.*

The prostaglandins are a group of long chain, oxygenated fatty acids
discovered in seminal fluid by von Euler in Sweden in 1933 and by Goldblatt
in England [1]. These 20 carbonated oxygenated fatty acids are present in
almost all organs, and probably formed in every mammalian cell [2]. The
prostaglandins are synthesized from essential fatty acid, the main precursor
being arachidonic acid. Arachidonic acid is first transformed by cyclo-
oxygenase into endoperoxides. The endoperoxides are rapidly converted by
prostaglandin synthetases into specific prostaglandins (such as prostaglandin
E_2 (PGE_2), PGD_2, $PGF_{2\alpha}$, PGI_2, and thromboxane) [3].

In animals and man, intravenous infusions of either natural PGE_1 or
natural PGA_1 significantly inhibit resting and stimulated gastric acid secretion
[4, 5]. The degree of inhibition is dose-related. However, the natural
prostaglandins are not orally effective. This is probably due to 15-hydroxy-
prostaglandin dehydrogenase present in gastric juice, which rapidly
inactivates the natural prostaglandins. Therefore, to prevent oral inactivation
of the prostaglandins a number of analogues have been synthesized. The
principal modifications were the addition of one or more methyl groups at
either the carbon-15 or carbon-16. These modifications prevent rapid
intragastric inactivation by dehydrogenation at carbon-15.

In man, oral 16,16-dimethyl PGE_2, 15(S)-15-methyl PGE_2, and 15(R)-15-
methyl PGE_2 markedly inhibit basal and all forms of stimulated gastric acid
secretion [6]. At doses which are free of significant untoward side effects,
basal and stimulated gastric acid secretions are inhibited by approximately
80–90%, which is similar to the inhibitory effect of a 300-mg dose of cimetidine [7].

Of potential clinical importance is the fact that the 15(R)-15-methyl PGE_2 is
not active when administered intravenously or intrajejunally, but is active
when given orally [8]. However, the 15(S)-15-methyl PGE_2 is active both

intravenously and orally. At an acid pH, the 15(R)-form epimerizes to the active 15(S)-form. At pH 1, approximately 50% is in the S-form and 50% in the R-form. In theory, this conversion to and from an active inhibitor of acid secretion in the presence of gastric acid could effectively modulate gastric acid secretion; i.e. it is activated in the presence of acid and inactivated in the absence of acid.

The mechanism(s) of action of the prostaglandins on gastric acid secretion is not fully understood. They clearly have a direct inhibitory effect on the gastric mucosa of animals and man, and recent evidence indicates that many forms (e.g. 16,16-dimethyl PGE_2) are also effective intravenously [9]. Of interest is that oral 16,16-dimethyl PGE_2, 15(S)-15-methyl PGE_2 methyl ester, and 15(R)-15-methyl PGE_2 methyl ester are potent inhibitors of meal-stimulated gastrin release [10, 11]. The 15(R)-15-methyl PGE_2 administered orally, however, failed to inhibit meal-stimulated gastrin release [12]. Therefore, it appears that the slight modification of the prostaglandin molecule can alter its effect on inhibiting gastrin release. Ippoliti and associates observed that equivalent doses of intravenous and oral 16,16-dimethyl PGE_2 produce comparable inhibition of both gastric acid secretion and gastrin release in response to a meal (unpublished data). Recently, Konturek reported that the addition of an anticholinergic plus 15(R)-15-methyl PGE_2 prostaglandin abolished the inhibitory effect of that prostaglandin on meal-stimulated gastrin release [12]. The explanation for this observation is unclear, but suggests that cholinergic innervation may be involved in the effect of PGE_2 on gastrin release.

The prostaglandins do not have any apparent anticholinergic effect. Measurements of gastric mucosal blood flow indicate that the ratio of blood flow to secretory flow does not fall, and may increase (as occurs, for instance, with infusion of PGI_2) during prostaglandin-induced inhibition of gastric acid secretion [13]. This indicates that their inhibitory effect on gastric acid secretion is not secondary to their effect on gastric mucosal blood flow. Whether or not the prostaglandins inhibit gastric acid secretion via the adenylate cyclase systems is not known and requires further study on isolated parietal cells.

Clinical and experimental trials with prostaglandins

PGI, PGE_2 and $PGF_{2\beta}$ have been thoroughly studied by Robert and others in the inhibition of a multitude of forms of experimentally induced ulcer, even at doses which do not inhibit gastric acid secretion. It has been postulated that this effect is due to an inherent 'cytoprotective' effect of prostaglandins [14].

The ancient Chinese are said to have used seminal fluid to treat patients with peptic ulcer. Unfortunately, only a few studies have examined the effect of prostaglandins in patients with acid peptic diseases. 15(R)-15-methyl PGE_2 was more effective than placebo in expediting gastric ulcer healing, as measured endoscopically under double-blind conditions [14]. Gastric mucus production was reported to be greater in the prostaglandin-treated group, according to endoscopic observations. PGE_2 plus antacid was also reported to be more effective than antacid alone in relieving gastric and duodenal ulcer pain [15, 16]. Recent studies in Europe have examined the effect of 15(R)-15-methyl PGE_2 in duodenal ulcer. The gastroenterologic community is anxiously awaiting the results of this important study.

16,16-dimethyl PGE_2 has also been shown to be a potent inhibitor of gastric acid secretion in patients with Zollinger-Ellison syndrome, comparable in effect to cimetidine (Ippoliti et al., unpublished data). No long-term therapeutic studies with prostaglandin have so far been conducted in Zollinger-Ellison patients.

Untoward effects

One of the major limiting factors in the use of prostaglandins is their inherent toxicity at high doses. Many of the prostaglandins produce diarrhea, which is of a secretory type [17]. This is due mainly to profuse secretion of fluid by the small intestine, probably secondary to stimulation of intestinal mucosal adenosine $3',5'$-phosphate. In addition, some of the prostaglandins (such as $PGF_{2\alpha}$, PGE_1 and thromboxane) have inherent effects on gastrointestinal smooth muscle. The prostaglandins also have a multitude of other effects, including inhibition of platelet aggregation, uterine contraction, alteration of pulse and blood pressure, and bronchial contraction [2]. Large-scale clinical studies are needed to determine whether long-term prostaglandin therapy has any significant untoward effects in man.

The future

Acetylsalicylic acid and indometacin, and other nonsteroidal anti-inflammatory agents inhibit prostaglandin synthetase and are associated with erosions and ulcers of the stomach and duodenum [18, 19]. Studies should be conducted to determine whether prostaglandin treatment prevents gastric lesions in patients who require chronic acetylsalicylic acid and indometacin treatment. Studies are also needed to carefully evaluate the effect of prostaglandins on the healing of gastric and duodenal ulcers under double-blind conditions.

The formulation of a stable prostaglandin tablet has been a problem. Gelatin capsules have been used, but these are impractical. The development of an effective, stable tablet form of prostaglandin is much needed. Finally, the role of prostaglandins in other 'acid peptic' diseases such as gastroenterologic reflux and gastrointestinal bleeding should be examined and the long-term toxicity of chronic prostaglandin therapy needs to be explored.

References

1. Wilson, D. (Ed) (1974): Symposium on prostaglandins. *Arch. Intern. Med. 133*, 29.
2. Robert, A. (1979): Prostaglandins: Their effect on the digestive system. *Viewpoints Dig. Dis. 2*.
3. Samuelson, B. and Paoletti, R. (Eds) (1976): *Advances in Prostaglandin and Thromboxane Research*, Vol. 2. Raven Press, New York.
4. Horton, E.W., Main, I.H.M., Thompson, C.F. et al. (1968): Effect of orally administered prostaglandin E_1 on gastric secretion and gastrointestinal motility in man. *Gut 9*, 655.
5. Karim, S.S.M., Carter, D.C., Bhana, D. et al. (1973): Effect of orally administered prostaglandin E_2 and its 15-methyl analogues on gastric secretion. *Br. Med. J. 1*, 143.
6. Nylander, B. and Anderson, S. (1974): Gastric secretory inhibition induced by three methyl analogs of prostaglandin E_2 administered intragastrically to man. *Scand. J. Gastroenterol. 9*, 751.
7. Konturek, T., Radecki, T., Demitrescu, N. et al. (1974): Effect of synthetic 15-methyl analog of prostaglandin E_2 on gastric secretion and peptic ulcer formation. *J. Lab. Clin. Med. 84*, 716.
8. Robert, A. (1977): Prostaglandins and the digestive system. *The Prostaglandins*, Vol. 3. Ed: P.B. Ramwell. Plenum Publishing Company, New York.
9. Konturek, S.J., Oleksy, J., Biernat, J. et al. (1976): Effect of 15-methyl analog of PGE_2 on gastric acid and serum gastrin response to peptone meal, pentagastrin, and histamine in duodenal ulcer patients. *Am. J. Dig. Dis. 21*, 291.
10. Ippoliti, A.F., Isenberg, J.I., Maxwell, V. et al. (1976): The effect of 16,16-dimethyl prostaglandin E_2 on meal-stimulated gastric acid secretion and serum gastrin in duodenal ulcer patients. *Gastroenterology 70*, 488.
11. Konturek, S.J., Swiecen, N., Swierczek, J.S. et al. (1976): Comparison of methylated prostaglandin E_2 analogues given orally in the inhibition of gastric responses to pentagastrin and peptone meal in man. *Gastroenterology 70*, 683.
12. Konturek, S.J., Swierczek, J.S., Kwiecien, W. et al. (1979): Effect of orally administered 15(R)-15 methyl prostaglandin E_2 and/or an anticholinergic drug on meal-induced gastric acid secretion and serum gastrin level in patients with duodenal ulcers. *Scand. J. Gastroenterol. 14*, 813.
13. Way, L. and Durbin, R.P. (1969): Inhibition of gastric acid secretion in vitro by prostaglandin E_1. *Nature (London) 221*, 874.
14. Robert, A. (1980): Prostaglandins as cytoprotective factors. (This publication, pp. 72–77).

15. Fung, W.P. and Karim, S.M.M. (1976): Effect of 15(R)-methyl prostaglandin E_2 on healing of gastric ulcers: A double blind endoscopic study. *Med. J. Aust. 2*, 127.
16. Fung, W.P., Lee, S.K. and Karim, S.M.M. (1974): Effect of prostaglandin 15(R) methyl-E_2-methyl ester on the gastric mucosa in patients with peptic ulceration – an endoscopic and histological study. *Prostaglandins 14*, 465.
17. Rybicka, J. and Gibinski, K. (1978): Methyl-prostaglandin E_2 analogues for healing of gastroduodenal ulcers. *Scand. J. Gastroenterol. 13*, 155.
18. Robert, A., Nezamis, J.E., Lancaster, C. et al. (1976): Enteropooling assay. A test for diarrhea produced by prostaglandins. *Prostaglandins 11*, 809.
19. Sivosos, G.R., Ivey, K.J., Butt, J.H. et al. (1979): Incidence of gastric lesions in patients with rheumatic disease on chronic aspirin therapy. *Ann. Intern. Med. 91*, 517.
20. Kauffman, G.L. and Grossman, M.I. (1978): Prostaglandins and cimetidine inhibit the formation of ulcers produced by parenteral salicylates. *Gastroenterology 75*, 1099.

E$_2$ prostaglandins – potential agents in peptic ulcer treatment

C. Johansson and B. Kollberg
Gastroenterology Unit, Department of Medicine, Karolinska Hospital, Stockholm, Sweden

The development of E$_2$ prostaglandins (PG) in the treatment of peptic ulcer was initiated by the demonstration by Robert that i.v. PGE$_2$ suppressed gastric acid secretion in the dog [1]. When given orally to dog and man natural PGE$_2$ was ineffective [2, 3], as opposed to its methyl analogues. Oral methyl PGE$_2$ inhibit, dose-dependently, the basal acid secretion and the acid and pepsin response to various stimuli, including food, in healthy subjects and in patients with duodenal ulcer [4–6]. Studies in dogs with gastric pouches suggest that methyl PGE$_2$ have local effects on the gastric mucosa (Figs 1 and 2) [2, 7]. Thus, systemic absorption should not be required for effective acid inhibition. This may be important in regard to the uterotonic actions of PGE$_2$ and should be further explored together with studies of their metabolism and pharmacokinetics in man.

Of the different methyl PGE$_2$, 15(R)-15-methyl PGE$_2$ is clinically the most promising due to its wider dose interval (Fig. 3) and lower frequency of side-effects. This analogue is presently used in clinical trials [8].

To make use of the acid antisecretory action of the PG in peptic ulcer treatment is in line with the traditional concept of anti-ulcer agents as substances which reduce the 'aggressive attack' on the gastric mucosa. PG also have properties which may be described in terms of mobilization of the gastric mucosal 'defense force'. PG protect the mucosa against induced damage in experimental animals as originally shown by Robert [9]. The PG protection is not secondary to gastric acid inhibition, since doses below the acid anti-secretory threshold are effective, as are PG devoid of inhibitory actions on gastric acid secretion [9].

The protective ability has also been demonstrated in man [10–12]. We found that the indometacin-induced gastrointestinal bleeding in patients with rheumatic diseases was reduced to normal by concomitant oral supplementation with a methyl PGE$_2$-analogue or PGE$_2$, which later should not affect gastric acid secretion (Fig. 4). Even at the low dose of 0.33 mg 3 times a day PGE$_2$ was effective [11].

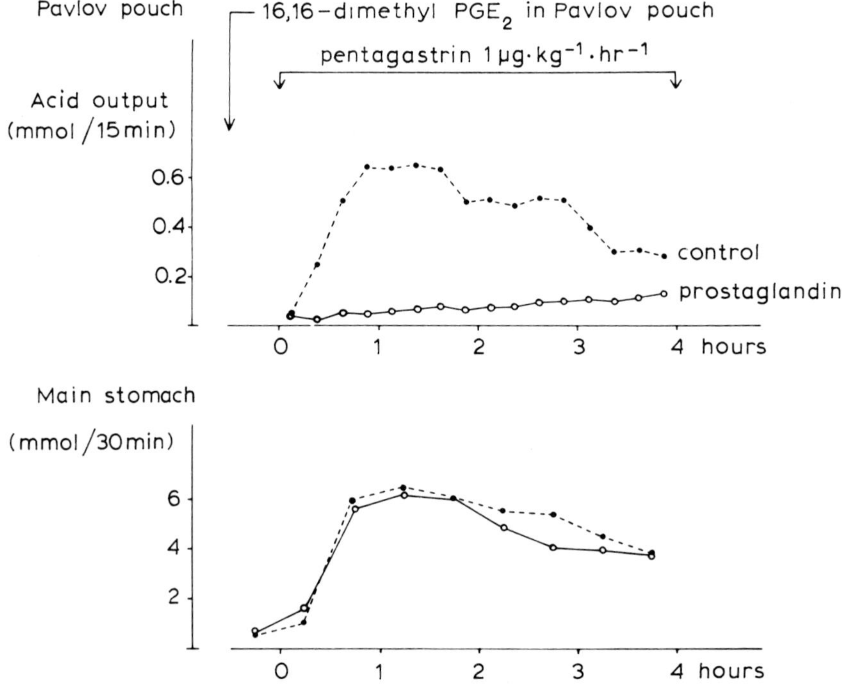

Fig. 1:   Topical administration of 40µg of 16,16-dimethyl PGE₂ into a Pavlov pouch of a dog inhibits the gastric acid secretory response to pentagastrin in the pouch but not in the main stomach. (Reproduced with permission from Dr. B. Nylander, Stockholm).

The mechanisms by which PG protect the gastric mucosa are unknown, although a connection has been made to their stimulatory effect on gastric alkaline and mucus secretions [13–15].

The concept of gastric nonparietal secretions serving as a protective barrier against the gastric luminal contents is not new [16], but is again attracting interest due to the increased understanding of the structure and properties of gastric mucus [17] and the recent observation that bicarbonate secretion from the gastric mucosa is an active process [18].

The gastric surface epithelial cells secrete bicarbonate, which is separated from the intraluminal acid by a layer of mucus, which limits the diffusion rate of pepsin and hydrogen ions from the lumen [19] and, assumedly, of bicarbonate form the epithelial surface. A pH-gradient exists across the mucus layer, along which slowly diffused acid is neutralized by bicarbonate [17], the viscosity of mucus being maximal at the point of the highest water concentration

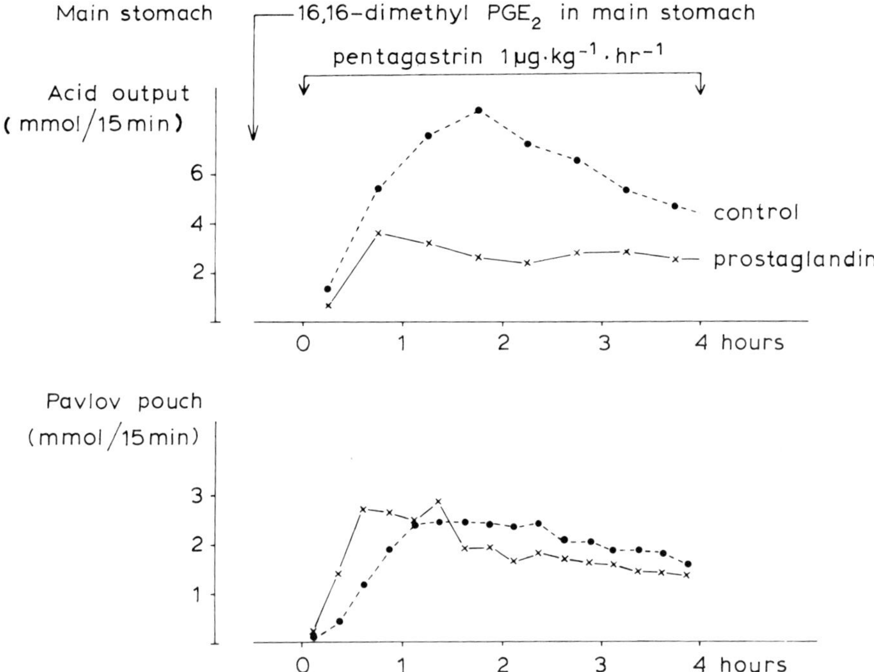

Fig. 2:   Topical 16,16-dimethyl PGE₂ in the main stomach of a dog inhibits the gastric acid secretory response in the main stomach but not in the Pavlov pouch. (Reproduced with permission from Dr. B. Nylander, Stockholm).

[20]. This should of course be regarded as a simplified model.

Exogenous PG stimulates the secretion of bicarbonate from the gastric mucosa in vitro [21] and in vivo [22], and increases the gastric mucus output in the dog [13] and in man (Fig. 5) [14]. The association of these stimulatory properties of PG with their protective effect is still speculative. Compatible with this hypothesis is a recent finding that inhibition of the alkaline secretion by small doses of acetazolamid eliminates the protective effect of PGE₂ on the gastric mucosa in the rat [23]. Further there is the observation that compounds, which suppress the biosynthesis of PG, inhibit gastric alkaline and mucus secretions [21, 22] and have ulcerogenic actions.

Clinical trials are now being carried out to examine the effects of PG on both peptic ulcer healing and prevention using methyl PGE₂, which combines acid inhibitory and protective properties. The natural PG are also being tried [23] and such studies will provide information on the usefulness of protection alone as a therapeutic principle.

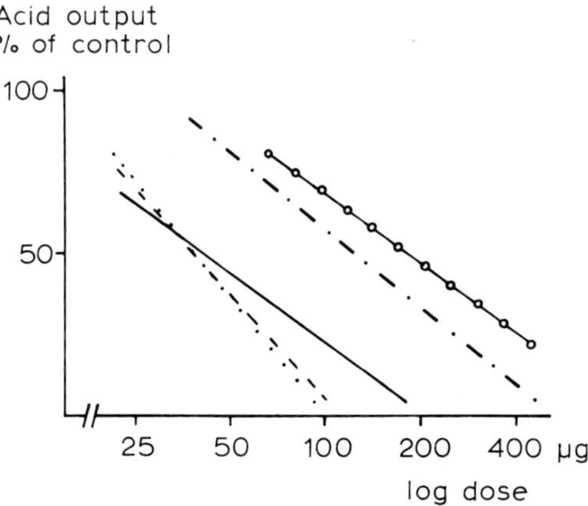

Fig. 3:   Dose response relationships for inhibitory effects of different methyl PGE_2 on the gastric acid response to pentagastrin in healthy subjects. Methyl PGE_2 given orally 45 minutes prior to pentagastrin infusion for 2 hours (0.6 $\mu g \cdot kg^{-1} \cdot min^{-1}$). Three to four dose levels of each analogue tested in 4–6 subjects. ——— = 16,16-dimethyl PGE_2; ———— = 16,16-dimethyl PGE_2Me; ...... = 15(S)-15-methyl PGE_2Me; —·— = 15(R)-15-methyl PGE_2Me; o—o—o = 15(R)-15-methyl PGE_2.

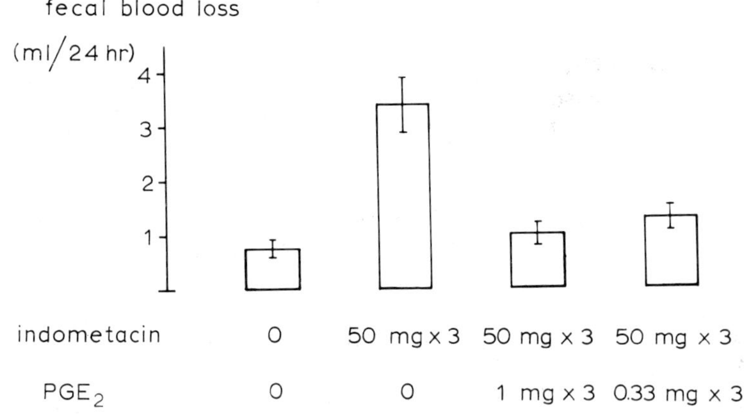

Fig. 4:   Gastrointestinal bleeding induced by indometacin in patients with rheumatic diseases was prevented by concomitant oral supplementation with PGE_2 1 mg 3 times a day (n = 10, p < 0.01) or PGE_2 0.33 mg 3 times a day (n = 6, p < 0.05).

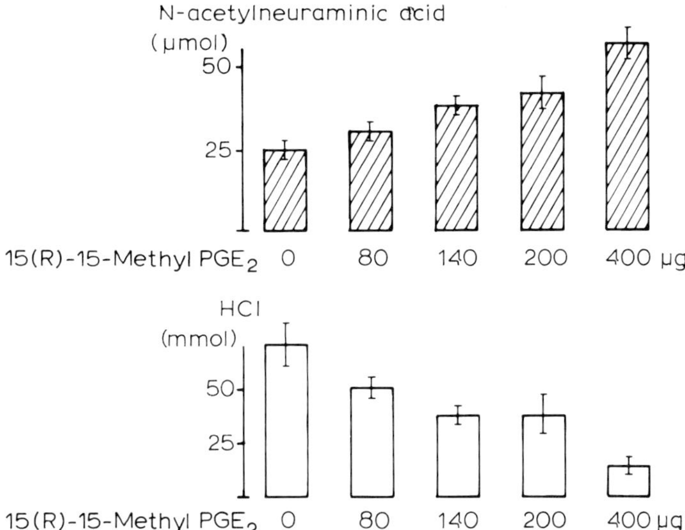

Fig. 5:   Oral methyl PGE₂ increased dose-dependently the gastric output of N-acetyl-neuraminic acid (index of gastric mucus) and inhibited the gastric acid secretion during a 2.5 hours' infusion of pentagastrin. Mean ± SEM from 5 experiments in each of 5 healthy subjects.

References

1. Robert, A., Nezamis, J.E. and Phillips, J.P. (1968): Effect of prostaglandin E, on gastric secretion and ulcer formation in the rat. *Gastroenterology* **55**, 481.

2. Robert, A., Schultz, J.R., Nezamis, J.E. and Lancaster, C. (1976): Gastric antisecretory and antiulcer properties of PGE₂, 15-methyl PGE₂ and 16,16-dimethyl PGE₂. *Gastroenterology* **70**, 359.

3. Karim, S.M.M., Carter, D.C., Bhana, D. and Ganesan, P.A. (1973): Effect of orally administered prostaglandin E₂ and its 15-methyl analogues on gastric secretion. *Br. Med. J. I*, 143.

4. Nylander, B. and Andersson, S. (1974): Gastric secretory inhibition induced by three methyl analogues of prostaglandin E₂ administered intragastrically to man. *Scand. J. Gastroenterol.* **9**, 751.

5. Konturek, S.J., Kwiecien, N., Swierczek, J. et al. (1976): Comparison of methylated prostaglandin E₂ analogues given orally on the inhibition of gastric responses to pentagastrin and peptone meal in man. *Gastroenterology* **70**, 683.

6. Ippoliti, A.E., Isenberg, J.I., Maxwell, V. and Walsh, J.H. (1976): The effect of 16,16 dimethyl prostaglandin E₂ on mealstimulated gastric acid secretion and serum gastrin in duodenal ulcer patients. *Gastroenterology* **70**, 488.

7. Nylander, B. (1975): *Effects of some methyl analogues of prostaglandin E₂ on*

    gastric secretion and gastrointestinal motility in man and dog. Thesis, Karolinska Institutet.

8. Gibinski, K., Rybicka, J., Mikos, E. and Nowak, A. (1977): Double-blind clinical trial of gastroduodenal ulcer healing with prostaglandin E_2 analogues. *Gut 18*, 636.

9. Robert, A. (1975): Antisecretory, antiulcer, cytoprotective and diarrheogenic properties of prostaglandins. In: *Advances in Prostaglandin and Thromboxane Research.* pp. 507–520. Eds: B. Samuelsson and R. Paoletti. Raven Press, New York.

10. Cohen, M.M. (1978): Mucosal cytoprotection by prostaglandin E_2. *Lancet II*, 1253.

11. Johansson, C., Kollberg, B. and Bergström, S. (1979): Protection of gastrointestinal mucosa by E_2 prostaglandins. *Lancet I*, 317.

12. Johansson, C., Kollberg, B., Nordemar, R. et al. (1980): Protective effect of prostaglandin E_2 in the gastrointestinal tract during indometacin treatment of rheumatic diseases. *Gastroenterology 78*, 479.

13. Bolton, J.P. and Cohen, M.M. (1978): Stimulation of non-parietal cell secretion in canine Heidenhain pouches by 16,16-dimethyl prostaglandin E_2. *Digestion 17*, 291.

14. Johansson, C. and Kollberg, B. (1979): Stimulation by intragastrically administered E_2 prostaglandins of human gastric mucus output. *Eur. J. Clin. Invest. 9*, 229.

15. Garner, A. and Heylings, J.R. (1979): Stimulation of alkaline secretion in amphibian-isolated gastric mucosa by 16,16-dimethyl PGE_2 and PGF_2'. *Gastroenterology 76*, 497;

16. Heatley, N.G. (1959): Mucosubstance as a barrier to diffusion. *Gastroenterology 37*, 313.

17. Allen, A. and Garner, A. (1980): Mucus and bicarbonate secretion in the stomach and their possible role in mucosal protection. *Gut 21*, 249.

18. Flemström, G. (1977): Active alkalinization by amphibian gastric fundic mucosa in vitro. *Am. J. Physiol. 233*, E1–E12.

19. Williams, S.E. and Turnberg, L.A. (1979): Studies of the 'protective' properties of gastric mucus. *Gut 20*, A922.

20. Clamp, J.R., Allen, A. Gibbons, R. and Roberts, G.P. (1978): Chemical aspects of mucus. *Br. Med. Bull. 34*, 29.

21. Garner, A., Flemström, G. and Heylings, J.R. (1979): Effects of anti-inflammatory agents and prostaglandins on acid and bicarbonate secretions in the amphibian-isolated gastric mucosa. *Gastroenterology 77*, 451.

22. Kauffman, G.L. and Grossman, M.I. (1979): Gastric alkaline secretion: Effect of topical and intravenous 16,16-dimethyl prostaglandin E_2. *Gastroenterology 76*, 1165.

23. Kollberg, B., Aly, A., Rubio, C. and Johansson, C. (1980): Acetazolamid interferes with protective effect of prostaglandin E_2 in the rat gastric mucosa. *Scand. J. Gastroenterol.* (Accepted for publication).

Newly developed drugs: modes of action and clinical experience

W.-P. Fritsch, T. Scholten, J. Müller and K.-J. Hengels
Medizinische Klinik und Poliklinik, Klinik D, Universität Düsseldorf, Düsseldorf, Federal Republic of Germany

Although peptic ulcer disease exhibits a high rate of spontaneous healing, more and more new drugs said to be effective in treating peptic ulcerations have been introduced by the pharmaceutical industry. New drugs are developed in spite of the availability of effective therapeutic means for treating acute peptic ulcers, and in spite of a declining incidence of peptic ulcer disease, at least in central Europe.

Colloidal bismuth (tripotassium dicitrate bismuthate, TDB)

TDB is a stable colloidal bismuth salt complex. Colloidal bismuth acts on proteins in an acid medium to form a bismuth-proteinate coagulum at the site

Table I: Effect of colloidal bismuth in the healing rate of peptic ulcers: results of controlled double-blind studies after 4–6 weeks.

	TDB		Placebo	
	Healed (n)	Not healed (n)	Healed (n)	Not healed (n)
Duodenal ulcer				
Salmon et al. [4]	7	1	1	7
Shreeve [5]	14	5	4	15
Moshal [3]	27	3	4	16
Total	48 (84%)	9	9 (19%)	38
Gastric ulcer				
Boyes et al. [2]	9	1	3	10

of the ulcer crater, and this is said to protect the ulcer from further acid and pepsin digestion [1]. All bismuth salts have a marked ability to fix chloride ions in the gastric juice, with formation of insoluble bismuth chloride. Thus, the diffusion of the bismuth ion into the circulation and subsequent toxic effects are prevented. Nevertheless, it is not recommended in severe renal disease. Colloidal bismuth has also been shown to have pepsin-binding properties.

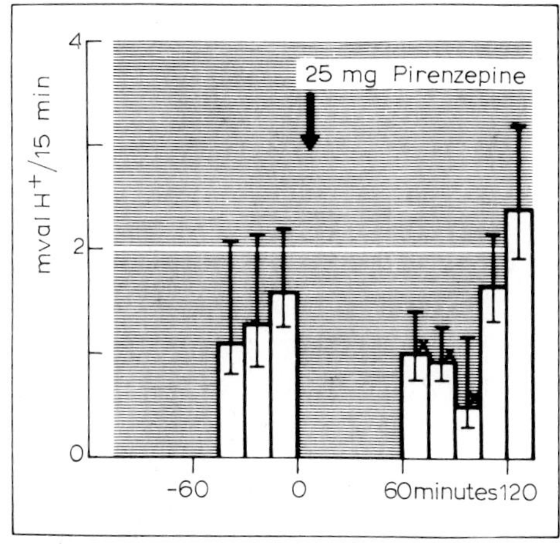

Fig. 1:   Inhibition of basal acid secretion after an oral dose of 25 mg pirenzepine (duodenal ulcer patients, n = 5). X: p< 0.05.

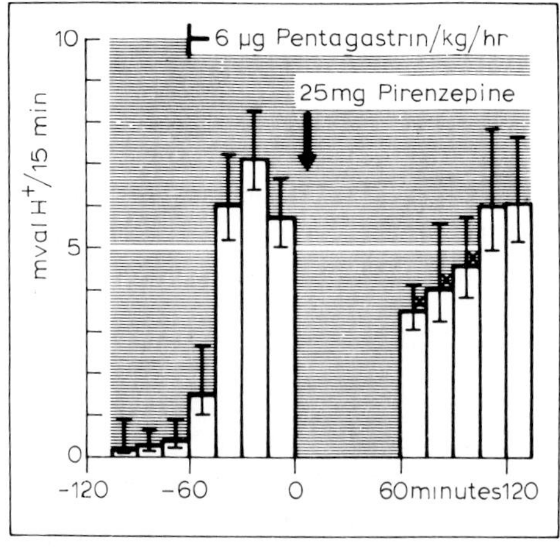

Fig. 2:   Inhibition of pentagastrin-stimulated acid secretion after an oral dose of 25 mg pirenzepine (duodenal ulcer patients, n = 5). X: p< 0.05.

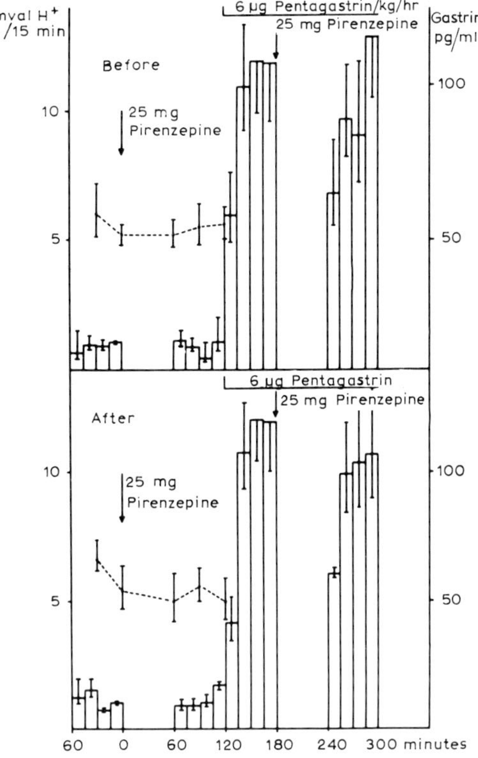

Fig. 3:   Effect of an oral dose of 25 mg of pirenzepine on basal serum gastrin, and on basal and pentagastrin-stimulated acid secretion before and after one week of treatment with 2 × 25 mg pirenzepine per day (duodenal ulcer patients, n = 4).

The effectiveness of colloidal bismuth compounds in the treatment of gastric and duodenal ulceration in double-blind, endoscopically monitored trials of 4–6 weeks' duration has been confirmed (Table I) [2–5]. The colloidal bismuth compounds have the disadvantage, however, of causing black stools and, in some patients, a black tongue.

Pirenzepine

An oral dose of 25 mg of pirenzepine will inhibit basal acid secretion by 50% (Fig. 1) and pentagastrin-stimulated acid secretion by 30–40% (Fig. 2). After doubling the dose, there is an additional inhibition of 10% [6]. Pirenzepine does not influence the basal serum gastrin level (Fig. 3). There is no difference in pentagastrin- or peptone-stimulated acid secretion before and after one

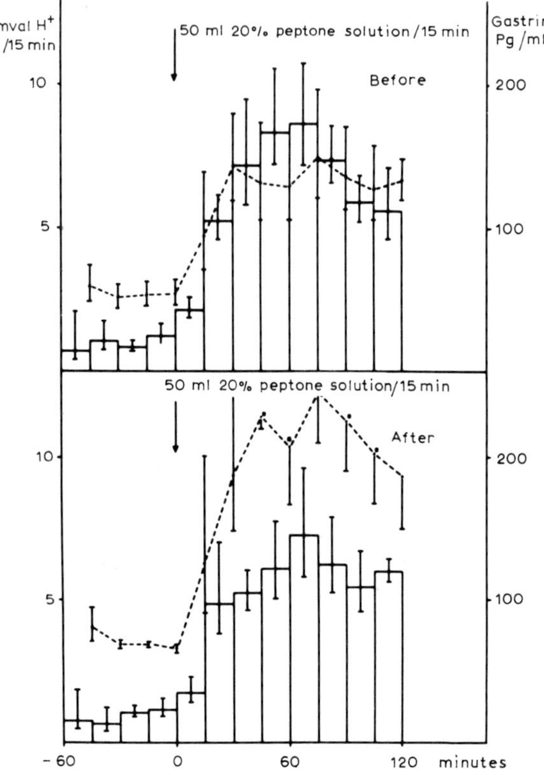

Fig. 4: Peptone (10%)-stimulation of acid secretion and gastrin before and after one week of treatment with 2 × 25 mg pirenzepine per day (duodenal ulcer patients, n = 4).

week of treatment with pirenzepine, 25 mg 2 times a day (Figs. 3 and 4). After pretreatment with pirenzepine, peptone causes a further significant elevation of serum gastrin levels.

After an intravenous injection of pirenzepine there is a dose-response relationship for basal acid secretion as well as for pentagastrin-stimulated acid secretion (Fig. 5). Basal secretion is inhibited by more than 90%, and stimulated secretion by about 50% when 0.32 mg/kg body weight is given. There is also a dose-response relationship for the inhibition time (Fig. 6). The duration of inhibition seems to be longer during peptone stimulation (Fig. 7) [7].

Atropine and pirenzepine will inhibit pentagastrin-stimulated secretion to an equal extent when 10 times as much pirenzepine as atropine is used (Fig. 8). Neither drug markedly influences acid concentration. The inhibition is caused

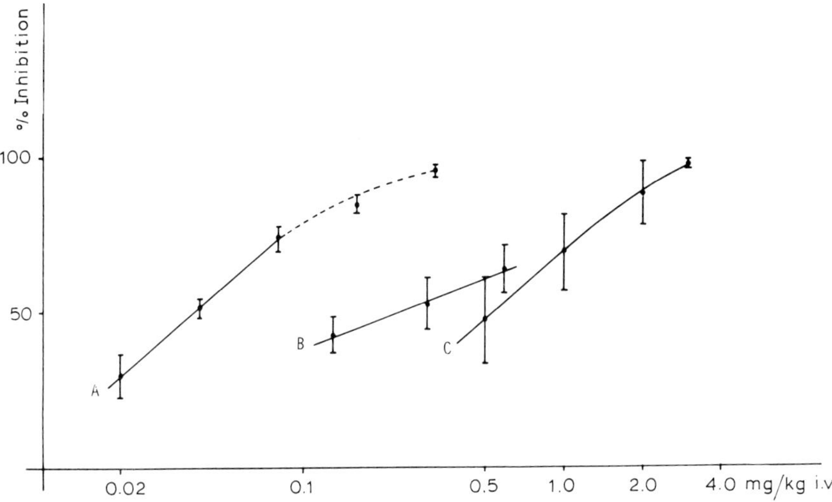

Fig. 5: Inhibition of basal (A) and pentagastrin (0.15 µg/kg/hr)-stimulated (B + C) acid secretion by various doses of intravenous pirenzepine (A + B) and cimetidine (C) (duodenal ulcer patients, n = 4).

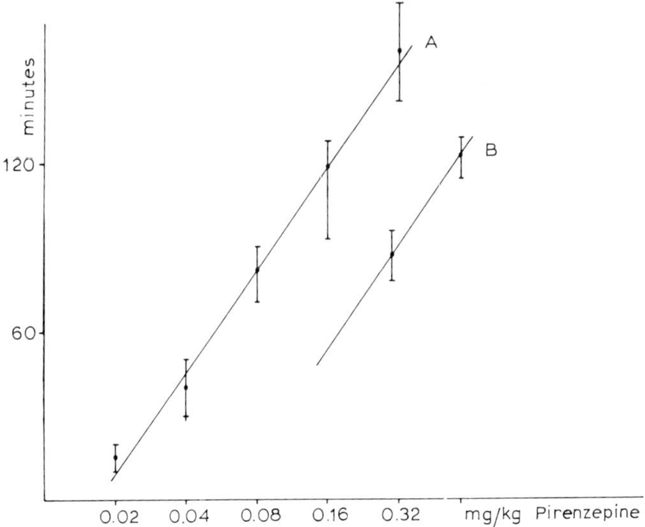

Fig. 6: Time-period for inhibition in relation to various doses of intravenous pirenzepine: basal (A) and pentagastrin (0.15 µg/kg/hr)-stimulated (B) acid secretion (duodenal ulcer patients, n = 4).

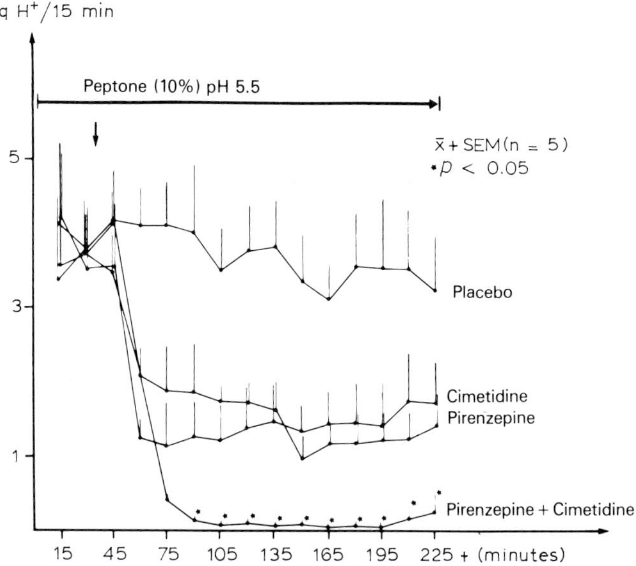

Fig. 7:   *Peptone-stimulated acid secretion in normal subjects (n = 5) after intravenous placebo, cimetidine (3.0 mg/kg), pirenzepine (0.3 mg/kg) and pirenzepine + cimetidine [7].*

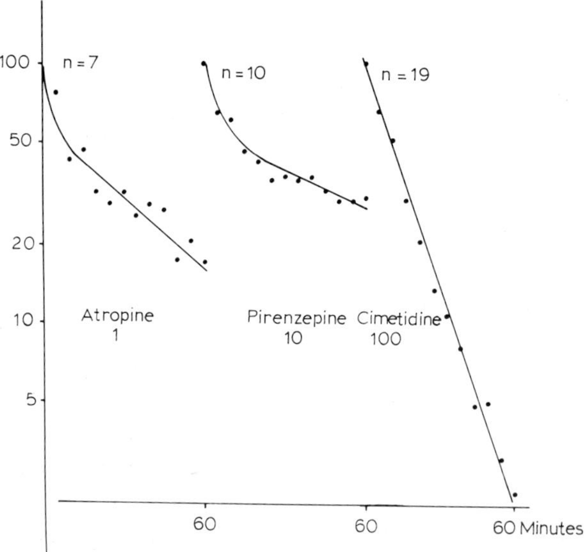

Fig. 8:   *Inhibition of pentagastrin (0.15 µg/kg/hr)-stimulated acid secretion after atropine (1 mg, 30 µg/kg/hr), pirenzepine (5 mg, 0.24 mg/kg/hr) and cimetidine (50 mg, 2.4 mg/kg/hr) in duodenal ulcer patients.*

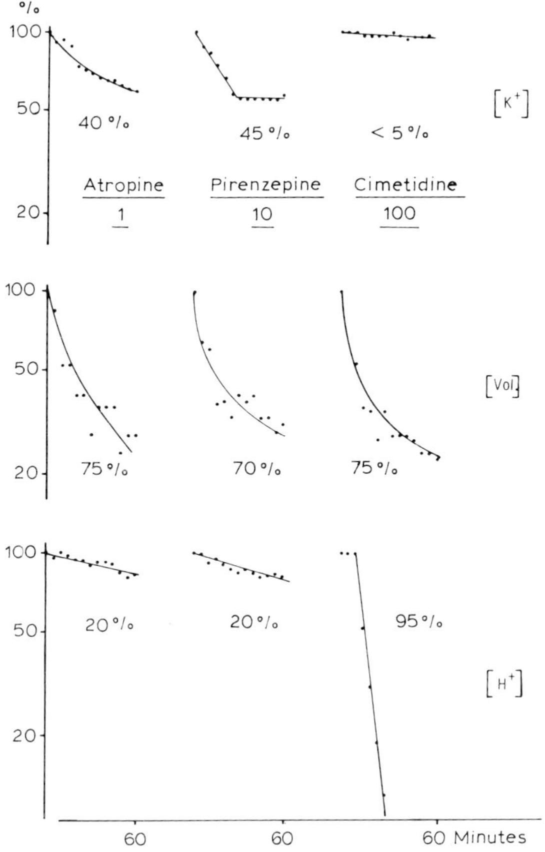

Fig. 9: *Potassium, volume and acid concentration after atropine, pirenzepine and cimetidine.*

mainly by volume reduction. Atropine and pirenzepine decrease the potassium concentration of gastric juice, in contrast to cimetidine (Fig. 9).

Pirenzepine, as well as classical anticholinergic drugs, will increase the duration and extent of acid inhibition when given in combination with H_2-receptor antagonists (Fig. 10). The more gastric acid secretion is sensitive to electrical vagal stimulation the less is the effect of H_2-receptor antagonists; inhibition tends to approach zero when the extent of vagal stimulation is equal to the pentagastrin-stimulated secretion. In contrast, inhibition of vagus-stimulated secretion by pirenzepine as well as by atropine averages 45%, independently of the extent of stimulation (Fig. 11).

In-vitro studies on isolated gastric mucosa showed a pure anticholinergic

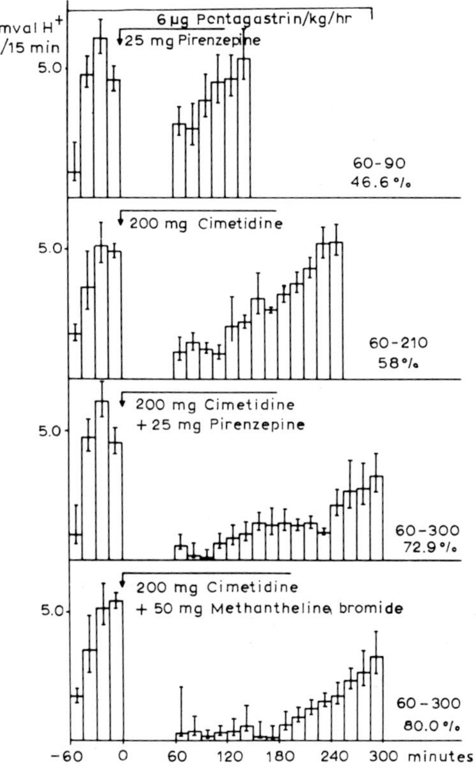

Fig. 10: Inhibition of pentagastrin (6 µg/kg/hr)-stimulated acid secretion after an oral dose of 25 mg pirenzepine, 200 mg cimetidine, 200 mg cimetidine + 25 mg pirenzepine and 200 mg cimetidine + 50 mg methantheline bromide (duodenal ulcer patients, n = 3).

effect of pirenzepine [8]. Pirenzepine has also been shown to act as an anticholinergic drug on human gastric mucosa [9–12].

Hammer et al. [13] showed that pirenzepine, in contrast to other anticholinergic drugs, has varying affinity constants for different subclasses of muscarinic receptors. The affinity profile of pirenzepine is characterized by a low affinity to smooth muscle as well as to heart muscle, and by a considerably higher affinity to exocrine glands. High doses of pirenzepine will inhibit salivary secretion (Strub, personal communication), motility of the lower esophageal sphincter (Wienbeck, personal communication) and motility of the colon [14]. Interestingly, heart rate tends to decrease, in contrast to the effect of other anticholinergics.

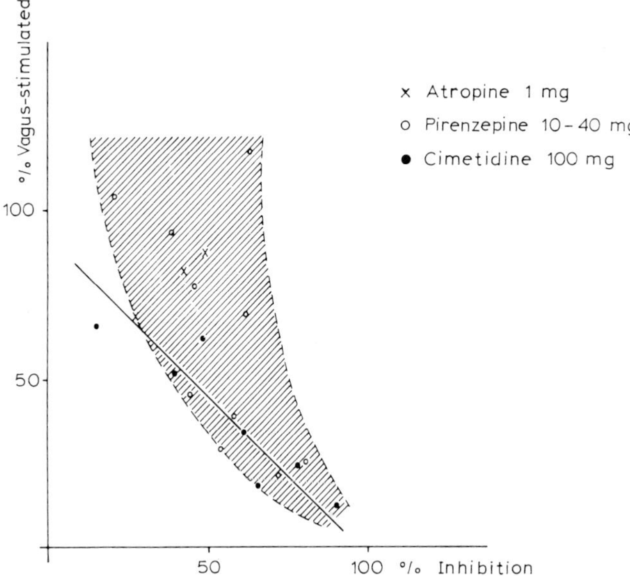

Fig. 11: Inhibition of vagus-stimulated (300 mA, 30"/min) acid secretion after atropine, pirenzepine and cimetidine in relation to the extent of secretion as percentage of the pentagastrin-stimulated acid output.

After oral administration, about 20–30% of pirenzepine is absorbed under basal conditions. Maximal plasma serum levels are measured 3 hours later. After an initial dose of 50 mg followed by 50 mg every 12 hours, plasma levels of between 30 and 45 ng/ml are measured for several days.

Pirenzepine is eliminated in equal amounts by the kidney and the liver. Elimination is completed 4 days after a single dose [15]. Less than 10% is excreted as a metabolite.

The chemical structure of pirenzepine dihydrochloride is very similar to that of tricyclic psychotropic compounds and serotonin antagonists (Fig. 12). In contrast to the tricyclic antidepressives, however, only a very small amount of pirenzepine passes the blood-brain barrier, because of its marked hydrophilic property. Stacher et al. [16] demonstrated marked central effects of an anticholinergic reaction type after injection of 0.3 mg/kg body weight of pirenzepine.

According to published studies, pirenzepine probably fails to exhibit an effect on healing rates of duodenal ulcers using 50–75 mg/day [17–21]. Using 100–150 mg/day, however, the drug seems to be effective (Table II) [19, 21–24]. This should be confirmed in other countries.

Table II: Treatment of duodenal ulcer with pirenzepine: results of controlled double-blind studies (healing after 4 weeks).

	Pirenzepine (50–75 mg/day)			Placebo		
	Healed (n)	Not healed (n)	Healed (%)	Healed (n)	Not healed (n)	Healed (%)
Chierichetti et al. [18]	23	21	52	12	23	34
Oselladore et al. [21]	9	6	60	6	9	40
Bourry [17]	10	11	48	8	16	33
Gassmann et al. [19]	15	15	50	10	18	35
Giger et al. [20]	11	5	69	11	7	61
Total	68	58	(54)	47	73	(39)

	Pirenzepine (100–150 mg/day)			Placebo		
	Healed (n)	Not healed (n)	Healed (%)	Healed (n)	Not healed (n)	Healed (%)
Chierichetti et al. [18]	32	14	70	15	31	32
Oselladore et al. [21]	12	2	87	6	9	40
Bianchi Porro et al. [22]	19	6	76	10	13	44
Morelli [24]	11	3	79	2	13	13
Dal Monte [23]	9	1	90	5	5	50
Total	83	26	(76)	38	71	(35)

The treatment of gastric ulcer with pirenzepine cannot be analyzed because of a lack of sufficient data (Table III) [18, 19, 21, 24–26].

The study by Matthes et al. [27] using a prospective controlled design but with a small number of cases showed a protective effect for stress-induced

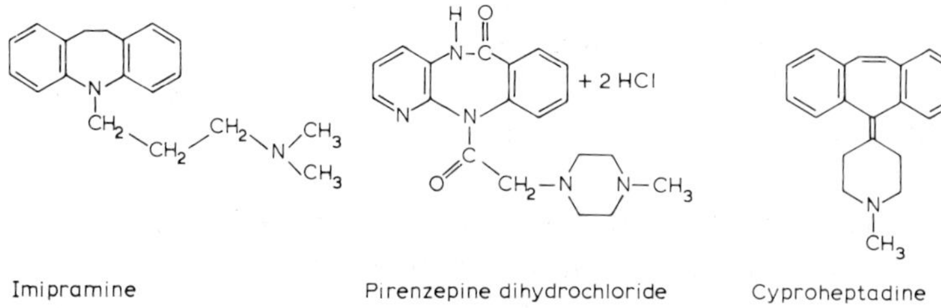

Fig. 12: Structures of imipramine, pirenzepine and cyproheptadine.

Table III: Treatment of gastric ulcer with pirenzepine: results of controlled double-blind studies (healing after 4 weeks).

	Pirenzepine (50–75 mg/day)		Placebo	
	Healed (n)	Not healed (n)	Healed (n)	Not healed (n)
Chierichetti et al. [18]	2	9	–	–
Oselladore et al. [21]	6	4	–	–
Gassman et al. [19]	5	5	2	5
Kunert [26]	11	9	9	7
Total	24 (47%)	27	11 (33%)	12

	Pirenzepine (100–150 mg/day)		Placebo	
	Healed (n)	Not healed (n)	Healed (n)	Not healed (n)
Chierichetti et al. [18]	5	0	–	–
Morelli [24]	9	1	5	5
Huchzermeyer [25]	8	4	4	6
Total	22 (81%)	5	9 (45%)	11

bleeding, as well as for the number and degree of stress lesions. Further studies are under way.

H_2-receptor antagonists and pirenzepine have been successfully combined in clinical practice for the treatment of Zollinger-Ellison syndrome. Mignon et al. [28] reported successful treatment of gastric, duodenal and jejunal ulcers in 3 of 4 patients with Zollinger-Ellison syndrome.

Dryness of the mouth is the most commonly reported side effect. Such possible side effects as pruritus, diarrhea, obstipation, difficulty with accommodation, impairment of erection and increased appetite have been observed, but need further evaluation.

Tritiozine

Tritiozine was introduced into clinical practice in 1977 in Italy, Spain and Portugal. Chemically, tritiozine has the structure of thiobenzoyl oxazin (Fig. 13). The drug is metabolized rapidly by oxidation and hydrolysis; the metabolite trioxazine is pharmacologically active and acts as a tranquilizer.

Table IV: Tritiozine in the treatment of duodenal ulcer: results of controlled double-blind studies (healing after 4 weeks).

	Tritiozin		Placebo	
	Healed (n)	Not healed (n)	Healed	Not healed (n)
Bereti [30]	3	17	0	20
Alberdi Frias et al. [43]	9	7	3	14
Catalano et al. [45]	12	5	3	18
Belsasso et al. [44]	6	3	2	9
Herrerias Gutierrez et al. [36]	8	7	5	12
Ponti et al. [46]	38 (50%)	39	13 (15%)	73

An oral dose of 1200 mg will decrease basal acid secretion by 44% [29–38], histamine-stimulated secretion (25 μg/kg histamine intramuscularly) by 10% [33, 34], pentagastrin-stimulated secretion (6 μg/kg intramuscularly) by 20% [31, 39], and insulin-stimulated acid output by 20% [34, 39]. The mechanism of action is not clear. Tritiozine does not influence pepsin secretion [38]. Acid secretion is not increased after the cessation of medication [40]. Serum gastrin levels are unchanged during therapy [41].

There is neither an effect on motility of the stomach nor on pancreatic secretion [32, 42].

Most of the controlled clinical trials have been carried out with small numbers of patients [30, 36, 43–45]. Ponti et al. [46] showed healing of duodenal ulcers in 50% of patients treated for 4 weeks, compared to 15% in the placebo group (Table IV). No effect has so far been demonstrated in patients with gastric ulcer. However, the number of patients in the reported studies is very small [36, 43, 45]. Further studies will be necessary to demonstrate the effectiveness of this new drug, especially on account of the high spontaneous healing rate observed in some other countries.

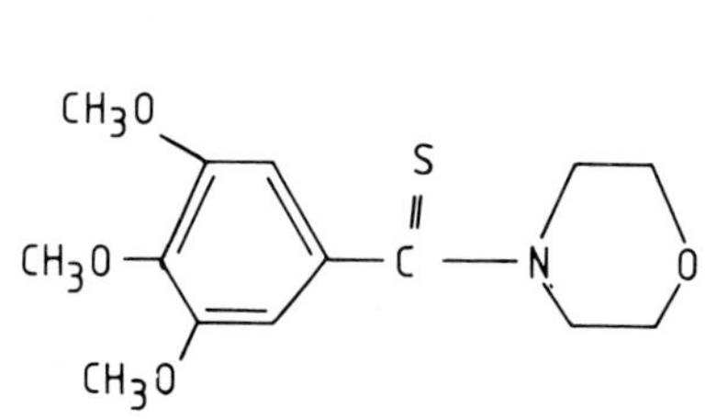

Fig. 13:   Structure of tritiozine.

No important side effect, apart from a discrete transient increase of serum glutamic oxaloacetic transaminase and serum glutamic pyruvic transaminase and tiredness, was observed.

Trimipramine

Trimipramine – a combination of imipramine, a tricyclic antidepressant, and levomepromazine – inhibits basal and stimulated acid and pepsin secretion only slightly, similar to the anticholinergics [47, 48]. After a meal or insulin-induced hypoglycemia, the increased gastrin levels are further augmented by trimipramine treatment [26].

Although based on small numbers of treated subjects, results of controlled studies have shown trimipramine to be more effective in healing peptic ulcers than placebos [49, 50].

The effectiveness of this drug has, however, yet to be confirmec.. Because of its well-known central depressant effect, treatment of nondepressive ulcer patients with trimipramine seems to be questionable. Side effects noted have been drowsiness and dryness of the mouth.

Sucralfate

Sucralfate, a sulphated disaccharide (Fig. 14), is a new antipepsin allegedly without adverse effects on the blood-clotting mechanism. An ingested sucralfate tablet disintegrates in the stomach and forms a suspension in the gastric juice. Most of the sucralfate binds to the wall of the gastrointestinal tract, and a small quantity dissolves. The soluble portion is believed to contribute minimally to the ulcer-healing properties of the compound.

Sucralfate may promote healing of peptic ulcers by forming a chemical complex that binds to the ulcer site to establish a protective barrier, directly

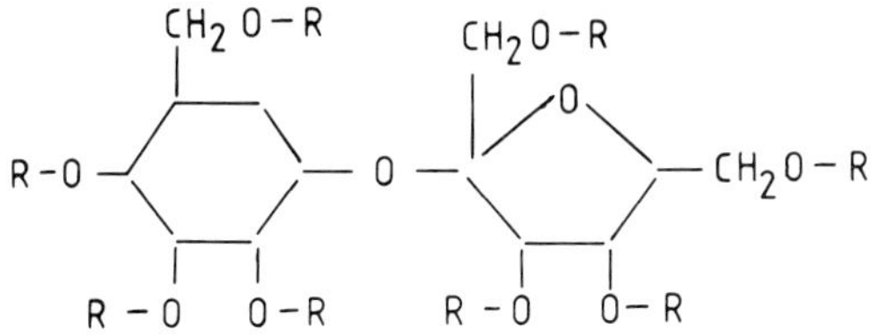

$$R = -SO_3[Al_2(OH)\cdot(H_2O)y]$$

Fig. 14: Structure of sucralfate.

inhibiting the action of pepsin and bile, and blocking the diffusion of gastric acid across the barrier. Since sucralfate is insoluble in aqueous solutions, it is minimally absorbed and has no systemic effects [51].

The first controlled double-blind studies demonstrated a more rapid healing of duodenal ulcers with sucralfate than with placebo (Table V) [52–54]. Comparative studies with sucralfate and cimetidine showed nearly similar results with both substances in the healing of gastric as well as of duodenal ulcers. The effectiveness cannot yet be fully accepted, however.

Secretin

Secretin would be expected to be a therapeutic agent for the treatment of duodenal ulcers because of its known, experimentally well-documented effects on the human gastrointestinal tract. Among these are alkalinization of the duodenal bulb, inhibition of acid secretion, inhibition of gastric emptying, and decrease of basal and stimulated serum gastrin concentrations.

On the other hand, however, there are no experimental data demonstrating a lack of secretin in patients with ulcer disease. Using a synthetic depot secretin, a long-lasting action of secretin following a single injection can be shown.

After subcutaneous injection of 10 clinical units of depot secretin per kilogram body weight, a stimulation of bicarbonate output and inhibition of acid secretion lasting 9–10 hours was demonstrated in men. Serum gastrin was decreased for 6–8 hours.

The results of a multicenter, controlled, double-blind study [55] showed healing of the duodenal ulcer in 68% of patients after 3 weeks of treatment, as compared to 64% for patients treated with placebo. Because the drug had to be injected twice a day, the study was carried out on inpatients. This may be the reason for the very high healing rate in the placebo group after 3 weeks.

Proglumide

Proglumide, chemically a derivative of isoglutamic acid (Fig. 15), is said to be a gastrin receptor antagonist, because of its gastrin-like molecular structure and because of the dose-dependent inhibition of pentagastrin-stimulated acid secretion after 15 days of treatment. Histamine-stimulated acid secretion is inhibited by an average of 50%. There is no dose-dependency [56]. The cellular metabolism of gastric mucosa appears from experimental data to be influenced favorably [57]. The mode of action of this compound is unclear.

Clinical data from various small studies in Japan and Germany, observing

Table V: *Sucralfate treatment in peptic ulcer disease: results of controlled double-blind studies after 4–6 weeks.*

Duodenal ulcer	Weeks	Sucralfate			Cimetidine			Placebo		
		Healed (n)	Not healed (n)	Healed (%)	Healed (n)	Not healed (n)	Healed (%)	Healed (n)	Not healed (n)	Healed (%)
Marks [53]	6	21	3	88	18	6	75	–	–	–
McHardy and Fisher [52]	4	82	26	76	–	–	–	69	107	69
Moshal et al. [54]	6	18	12	60	–	–	–	7	22	24

Gastric ulcer	Weeks	Sucralfate (n = 24)		Cimetidine (n = 24)	
		Healed (n)	Not healed (n)	Healed (n)	Not healed (n)
Marks [53]	6	16	8	18	6

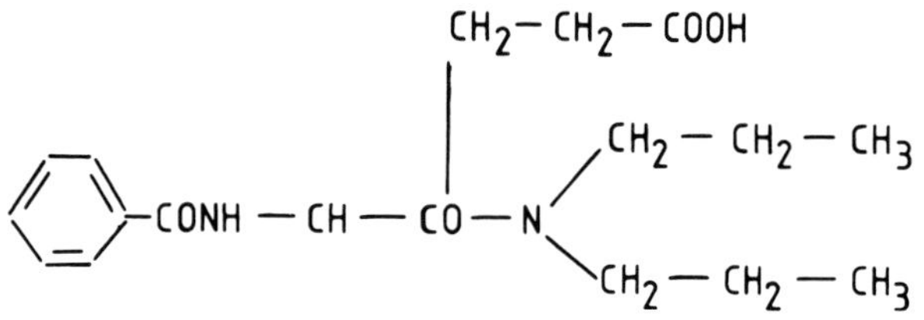

$$CH_2-CH_2-COOH$$

Proglumide: N-benzoyl-N, N-di-n-prophyl-DL-isoglutamatic acid

Fig. 15:   Structure of proglumide.

the rate of peptic ulcer healing, differ so much that the efficiency of this drug cannot be assessed [58–66].

Metoclopramide

Metoclopramide stimulates gastric emptying. Duodenogastric reflux is considered to be an important factor in the etiology of gastric ulcers, and metoclopramide would thus seem to be a possible therapeutic agent for the treatment of gastric ulcers. A controlled study by Hoskins [67] compared the effect of metoclopramide with that of carbenoxolone sodium on the healing of gastric ulcers. Among 15 patients with gastric ulcers treated with 30 mg of metoclopramide per day for 5 weeks, 10 recovered, compared with 7 of 13 treated with carbenoxolone sodium. Because of the small number of patients studied, there was no statistical difference between the 2 groups.

Metoclopramide has a theoretically unfavorable effect in the treatment of duodenal ulcer disease, and its effectiveness has not been demonstrated in any peptic disease.

Sulpiride

Sulpiride stimulates gastric emptying only moderately. In man, sulpiride is less effective than an equal dose of metoclopramide. Sulpiride exhibits no influence on basal or on histamine-, insulin- or pentagastrin-stimulated acid secretion in patients with or without duodenal ulcer [68, 69].

By injecting 2.0–2.5 mg/kg body weight, blood circulation of the stomach and duodenum is increased in the mucosa as well as in the muscularis layer of the intestinal wall. Two controlled double-blind studies by Molle [70] and Lam et al. [71] did not demonstrate any effect on the healing of duodenal ulcer. To date there are no convincing data to support the treatment of peptic ulcers with sulpiride.

Salmefamol

In dogs salmefamol, a new adrenergic β_2 agonist, inhibits maximal acid output stimulated by pentagastrin (0.8 μg/kg/min). The mean inhibition for the maximal dose is 89%. The pulse rate is increased. Practolol prevents tachycardia, but does not affect the inhibitory effect on gastric acid output.

Kinetic studies indicate that the inhibition follows a noncompetitive mechanism [72]. The use of this drug in the treatment of bronchial asthma has shown a smaller effect on pulse rate in man. Therefore its clinical use is feasible. Clinical use of this drug in duodenal ulcer patients is presently being assessed.

Conclusions

With pirenzepine, an effective anticholinergic agent, therapy is possible without severe side effects. Sucralfate effectively supports the protective components of the gastric mucosa. Thus, an alternative principle of therapy to acid inhibition might prove useful in the future. Some of these newer compounds may therefore become important in combined therapy with conventional drugs. Nevertheless, none of the available data indicate that any of the newer drugs are superior to common therapeutic regimens.

Summary

Pirenzepine has been shown to act as an anticholinergic drug on human gastric mucosa. In contrast to the case with other anticholinergics, side effects are rare. Pirenzepine distinguishes between the different subclasses of muscarinic receptors. The drug will probably fail to exhibit an effect on the healing rates of duodenal ulcers with doses lower than 100 mg/day. Using higher doses, however, pirenzepine seems to be effective.

Tritiozine moderately inhibits acid secretion. The mechanism of action is not clear. In a clinical trial in which sufficiently high numbers of patients were studied, healing rates for treated duodenal ulcers were significantly higher than those in the placebo group. The healing rate in patients receiving placebo was only 15%. With the exception of a discrete transient increase of serum glutamic oxaloacetic transaminase and serum glutamic pyruvic transaminase, there were no important side effects.

The effectiveness of colloidal bismuth compounds in the treatment of gastric and duodenal ulceration has been confirmed in some double-blind studies. This compound has the disadvantage of causing black stools and a black tongue.

Sucralfate may promote healing of peptic ulcers by forming a chemical complex that binds to the ulcer site to establish a protective barrier. Comparative studies with sucralfate and cimetidine showed nearly similar results for the healing of gastric ulcers as well as for duodenal ulcers.

On the basis of a few clinical trials it would appear that secretin, metoclopramide and sulpiride are not effective in the treatment of peptic ulcer disease. The efficiency of proglumide cannot be assessed because of the varying data from various small clinical studies.

Of the newer compounds, some will probably achieve importance in combined therapy with conventional drugs.

Acknowledgment

We gratefully acknowledge the skillful technical assistance of Mrs. Gerda Berti.

References

1. Bank, S. and Marks, I.N. (1973): Evaluation of new drugs for peptic ulcer. *Clin. Gastroenterol. 2*, 379.
2. Boyes, B.E., Woolf, I.L., Wilson, R.Y. et al. (1975): Treatment of gastric ulceration with a bismuth preparation. *Postgrad. Med. J. 51, Sup. 5*, 29.
3. Moshal, M.G. (1975): The treatment of duodenal ulcers with TDB: a duodenoscopic double-blind cross-over investigation. *Postgrad. Med. J. 51*, Sup. 5, 36.
4. Salmon, P.R., Brown, P., Williams, R. and Read, A.E. (1974): Evaluation of colloidal bismuth (De-Nol) in the treatment of duodenal ulcer employing endoscopic selection and follow up. *Gut 15*, 189.
5. Shreeve, D.R. (1975): A double-blind study of tri-potassium di-citrato bismuthate in duodenal ulcer. *Postgrad. Med. J. 51, Sup. 5*, 33.
6. Stockbrügger, R., Jaup, B., Dotevall, D. and Bozler, G. (1979): Inhibition of gastric acid secretion by pirenzepine in man. In: *Die Behandlung des Ulcus pepticum mit Pirenzepin*, pp. 66–72. Eds: A.L. Blum and R. Hammer. Karl Demeter Verlag, Gräfelfing.
7. Londong, W., Londong, V., Prechtl, R. and Eversmann, T. (1979): Vergleichende Untersuchungen der Pirenzepin- und Cimetidinwirkung auf Pepton-stimulierte Säuresekretion und Serumgastrin des Menschen. In: *Die Behandlung*

des Ulcus pepticum mit Pirenzepin, pp. 239–241. Eds: A.L. Blum and R. Hammer. Karl Demeter Verlag, Gräfelfing.

8. Sachs, G., Kasbekar, D.K. and Berglindh, T. (1979): The mechanism of action of pirenzepine on gastric secretion. In: *Die Behandlung des Ulcus pepticum mit Pirenzepin*, pp. 18–23. Eds: A.L. Blum and R. Hammer. Karl Demeter Verlag, Gräfelfing.

9. Fritsch, W.-P. (1978): Andere Sekretionshemmer und Medikamente zur Förderung des Schleimhautresistenz. In: *Ulcus-Therapie*, pp. 137–154. Eds: A.L. Blum and J.R. Siewert. Springer, Berlin-Heidelberg-New York.

10. Fritsch, W.-P. (1979): Anticholinerge Sekretionshemmung mit Atropin, Methantelinbromid und Pirenzepin. In: *Die Behandlung des Ulcus pepticum mit Pirenzepin*, pp. 110–115. Eds: A.L. Blum and R. Hammer. Karl Demeter Verlag, Gräfelfing.

11. Fritsch, W.-P., Schacht, U., Scholten, Th. et al. (1979): Hemmung der Vagus-und Pentagastrin-stimulierten Säuresekretion durch Cimetidin, Atropin und Pirenzepin-Dihydrochlorid. *Verh. Dtsch. Ges. Inn. Med. 85*, 1267.

12. Fritsch, W.-P., Schacht, U., Scholten, Th. et al. (1979): Hinweise für einen cholinergen Rezeptor an der Belegzelle. *Gastroenterologie 17*, 624.

13. Hammer, R., Berrie, C.P., Birdsall, N.J.M. et al. (1980): Pirenzepine distinguishes between different subclasses of muscarinic receptors. *Nature (London) 283*, 90.

14. Stacher, G., Steinringer, H., Bauer, P. et al. (1979): Die Wirkung von intramuskulärem Pirenzepin, Atropin und Placebo auf die mahlzeitstimulierte Motilität des Kolons. Eine Doppelblindstudie. In: *Die Behandlung des Ulcus pepticum mit Pirenzepin*, pp. 139–144. Eds: A.L. Blum and R. Hammer. Karl Demeter Verlag, Gräfelfing.

15. Hammer, R. and Koss, R.W. (1979): Pharmakokinetik an Tier und Mensch nach oraler und parenteraler Gabe von Pirenzepin. In: *Die Behandlung des Ulcus pepticum mit Pirenzepin*, pp. 53–60. Eds: A.L. Blum and R. Hammer. Karl Demeter Verlag, Gräfelfing.

16. Stacher, G., Steinringer, H., Bauer, P. et al. (1979): Zentralnervöse Wirkungen von intramuskulär verabreichtem Pirenzepin. Eine Doppelblindstudie. In: *Die Behandlung des Ulcus pepticum mit Pirenzepin*, pp. 145–150. Eds: A.L. Blum and R. Hammer. Karl Demeter Verlag, Gräfelfing.

17. Bourry, J. (1979): Treatment of duodenal ulcer with pirenzepine: A double-blind controlled clinical trial. In: *Die Behandlung des Ulcus pepticum mit Pirenzepin*, pp. 192–193. Eds: A.L. Blum and R. Hammer. Karl Demeter Verlag, Gräfelfing.

18. Chierichetti, S.M. and Giorgi Conciato, M. (1979): Die Behandlung des Ulcus duodeni und -ventriculi mit Pirenzepin: eine multizentrische Doppelblindstudie. In: *Die Behandlung des Ulcus pepticum mit Pirenzepin*, pp. 178–184. Eds: A.L. Blum and R. Hammer. Karl Demeter Verlag, Gräfelfing.

19. Gassmann, R., Baumgartner, R., Leuthold, E. et al. (1979): Behandlung des Ulcus duodeni und des Ulcus ventriculi mit Pirenzepin: Erfahrungen im Doppelblindversuch in der ambulanten Fachpraxis. Vorläufige Ergebnisse. In: *Die Behandlung des Ulcus pepticum mit Pirenzepin*, pp. 203–206. Eds: A.L. Blum and R. Hammer. Karl Demeter Verlag, Gräfelfing.

20. Giger, M., Gonvers, J.-J., Weber, K.B. et al. (1979): Pirenzepin-Behandlung des Ulcus duodeni: Vergleich mit Cimetidin und Placebo. In: *Die Behandlung des*

Ulcus pepticum mit Pirenzepin, pp. 216–220. Eds: A.L. Blum and R. Hammer. Karl Demeter Verlag, Gräfelfing.

21. Oselladore, D. (1979): Doppelblindstudie mit Pirenzepin beim Ulcus duodeni und Ulcus ventriculi. In: *Die Behandlung des Ulcus pepticum mit Pirenzepin*, pp. 185–190. Eds: A.L. Blum and R. Hammer. Karl Demeter Verlag, Gräfelfing.

22. Bianchi Porro, G., Petrillo, M., Benassai, D. et al. (1979): Preliminary communication: Pirenzepine vs. cimetidine and placebo in the treatment of duodenal ulcer. In: *Die Behandlung des Ulcus pepticum mit Pirenzepin*, p. 194. Eds: A.L. Blum and R. Hammer. Karl Demeter Verlag, Gräfelring.

23. Dal Monte, P.R., D'Imperio, N., Giuliani Piccari, G. et al. (1979): Double blind study in the treatment of duodenal ulcer: Pirenzepine against placebo. In: *Die Behandlung des Ulcus pepticum mit Pirenzepin*, pp. 208–214. Eds: A.L. Blum and R. Hammer. Karl Demeter Verlag, Gräfelfing.

24. Morelli, A. (1979): Treatment of gastric and duodenal ulcer with pirenzepin. In: *Die Behandlung des Ulcus pepticum mit Pirenzepin*, pp. 196–202. Eds: A.L. Blum and R. Hammer. Karl Demeter Verlag, Gräfelfing.

25. Huchzermeyer, H. (1979): Pirenzepin-Placebo-Doppelblindstudie beim Ulcus ventriculi. In: *Die Behandlung des Ulcus pepticum mit Pirenzepin*, pp. 226–227. Eds: A.L. Blum and R. Hammer. Karl Demeter Verlag, Gräfelfing.

26. Kunert, H. (1979): Kontrollierte klinische Studie über Pirenzepin-Therapie beim Ulcus ventriculi. In: *Die Behandlung des Ulcus pepticum mit Pirenzepin*, pp. 228–230. Eds: A.L. Blum and R. Hammer. Karl Demeter Verlag, Gräfelfing.

27. Mattes, P., Belohlavek, D., Peros, G. et al. (1969): Kontrollierte prospektive Studie über die Wirkung von Pirenzepin beim Streß-Ulkus. In: *Die Behandlung des Ulcus pepticum mit Pirenzepin*, pp. 239–242. Eds: A.L. Blum and R. Hammer. Karl Demeter Verlag, Gräfelfing.

28. Mignon, M., Vallot, T., Galmiche, J.P. et al. (1980): Interest of a combined antisecretory treatment, cimetidine and pirenzepin, in the management of severe forms of Zollinger-Ellison syndrome. *Digestion 20*, 56.

29. Barbara, L., Corinaldesi, R., Miglioli, M. et al. (1975): Efficacia terapeutica della tritiozina (ISF 2001) nelle affezioni gastroduodenali. *Minerva Gastroenterol. 21*, 169.

30. Bereti, I. (1976): Effects of trithiozine (ISF 2001) on duodenal ulcer: a controlled double blind trial. *Farmaco Ed. Prat. 31*, 495.

31. Bereti, I. (1977): Comparison between the activities of trithiozine (ISF 2001) and atropine on human gastric secretion. *Riv. Farmacol. Ter. 8*, 139.

32. Corinaldesi, R., Luchetta, L., Ricci, P. et al. (1977): Valutazione dell tollerabilità, a lungo termine, della tritiozina (ISF 2001). *Farmaco Ed. Prat. 32*, 25.

33. Corinaldesi, R., Luchetta, L., Ricci, P. et al. (1977): Cross-over clinical comparison between antisecretory activity of propantheline bromide and trithiozine (ISF 2001). *Panminerva Med. 19*, 339.

34. Corinaldesi, R., Miglioli, M., Cornelli, U. et al. (1977): Effect of trithiozine on 24-hour gastric acidity in duodenal ulcer patients. *Rend. Gastro-enterol. 9*, 20.

35. Fichera, G., Calliera, M., Maroni, G.C. and Mirelli, E. (1976): La tritiozina (ISF 2001) nell duodenopatie. Studio clinico, endoscopico e funzionale. *Arch. Ital. Mal. Appar. Dig. 37*, 201.

36. Herrerias Gutierrez, J.M. and Carrido Peralta, M. (1979): La tritiozina nell'ulcera peptica: studio clinico controllato. *Clin. Ter. 88*, 363.

37. Knego, Z. (1976): Vagotomia superselettiva e trattamento con ISF 2001 (tritiozina) confronto degli effetti sulla secrezione gastrica. *Arch. Ital. Mal. Appar. Dig. 37*, 213.

38. Van Trappen, G. and Peeters, T. (1978): Gastric antisecretory effect of tritiozine in normal volunteers. *Riv. Gastroenterol. 30*, 21.

39. Corinaldesi, R., Luchetta, L., Ricci, P. et al. (1977): Effects of trithiozine (ISF 2001) on gastric secretion in man. *Riv. Farmacol. Ter. 8*, 113.

40. Bertaccini, G. (1978): Effects of thritiozine on histamine H_2-receptors. *Ber.J.S.F.*

41. Cheli, R., Giacosa, A. and Perasso, A. (1979): Tritiozine and gastrinemia. *Clin.Ther. 2*, 106.

42. Dobrilla, G., Filippini, M., Valentini, M. et al. (1977): Effect of a new gastric antisecretory compound, trithiozine, on pancreatic secretion in control subjects and patients affected by duodenal ulcer. *Acta Ther. 3*, 247.

43. Alberdi Frias, J., Guemes Diaz, F. and Perez Mota, A. (1978): A double blind study of trithiozine in peptic ulcer. *Clinical Therapeutics 1*, 251.

44. Belsasso, E., Caenazzo, E. and Visintini, E. (1978): Efficacia terapeutica della tritiozina nell'ulcera duodenale. Ricera controllata in doppio cieco. *Clin. Europea 17*, 3.

45. Catalano, F., Brogna, A. and Blasi, A. (1977): Tritiozina e ulcera peptica: ricerca clinica in doppio cieco. *Minerva Dietol. Gastroenterol 23*, 1.

46. Ponti, V., Pera, A. and Verme, C. (1979): Ricerca clinica comparativa sulla tritiozina e la cimetidina nell'ulcera duodenale. *Clin. Ter. 89*, 299.

47. Bohmann, T., Schrumpf, E. and Myren, J. (1977): The effect of trimipramine (Surmontil) on gastric secretion and the serum gastrin release in healthy young students. *Scand. J. Gastroenterol. 10, Sup. 43*, 7.

48. Roland, M., Berstad, A., Myren, J. and Liavag, I. (1977): The effect of trimipramine (Surmontil) on gastric secretion of acid and pepsin in man. *Scand. J. Gastroenterol. 10, Sup. 43*, 19.

49. Nitter, L., Haraldsson, A., Holek, P. et al. (1977): The effect of trimipramine on the healing of peptic ulcer. A double-blind study. Multicentre investigation - G.P. *Scand. J. Gastroenterol. 12, Sup. 43*, 39.

50. Wetterhus, S., Aubert, E., Berg, C.E. et al. (1977): The effect of trimipramine on the healing of peptic ulcer. A double-blind study. *Scand. J. Gastroenterol., 10, Sup. 43*, 33.

51. Bighley, L.D. and Giesing, D. (1979): Sucralfate: A new concept in ulcer therapy. In: *Peptic Ulcer Disease: An Update*, pp. 307–319. *3rd International Symposium on Gastroenterology*. BMI Publications, Kansas City.

52. McHardy, G. and Fisher, R.S. (1980): Sucralfate in duodenal ulcer disease: Account of a double blind, randomised, multicenter endoscopically controlled evaluation of ulcer response. (In press).

53. Marks, I.N. (1980): Kontrollierte klinische Prüfung von Sucralfate im Vergleich zu Cimetidin. *S. Afr. Med. J. 57*, 567.

54. Moshal, M.G., Spitaels, J.M. and Khan, F. (1980): A double-blind endoscopically-controlled trial of Ulsanic (sucralfate) in the treatment of duodenal ulcers. *S. Afr. Med. J. 57*, 742.

55. Scholten, Th., Fritsch, W.-P., Classen, M. et al. (1980): Die Behandlung des Ulcus duodeni mit Depot-Sekretin: eine multizentrische Doppelblindstudie. (In press).

56. Weiss, J. (1972): Double-blind clinical evaluation of the antihypersecretive activity of proglumide in gastric secretion induced by pentagastrin and other stimulants (Abstract). In: *9th International Congress of Gastroenterology*, Paris.
57. Rovati, A.L. (1976): Inhibition of gastric secretion by anti-gastrinic and H_2-blocking agents. *Scand. J. Gastroenterol. 11, Sup. 42,* 113.
58. Asano, T. (1969): Study of gastric blood flow. In: *VI. Congress Ther. Res. New Drugs, Osaka*, Rep. Vol., p. 108.
59. Bergemann, W., Consentius, K., Braun, H.E. et al. (1978): Multizentrische Doppelblindstudie bei Patienten mit Ulcera duodeni (Abstract). In: *6. Weltkongress für Gastroenterologie, Madrid.*
60. Enoch, W. (1980): Die Wirkung von Proglumid (Milid) auf Magen- und Zwölffingerdarmgeschwüre. Vergleich mit einer kombinierten Antazida-Anticholinergika-Behandlung. *Inform. Arzt. 8,* 64.
61. Hogita, K., Okundo, T., Igiri, Y. and Tosa, M. (1970): Erfahrungen mit Proglumid bei Magenerkrankungen, Nachweis der Wirkung auf Magenulcera mittels der Doppelblindmethode. *Shinyaku to Rinsho 19,* 1185.
62. Miederer, S.E., Lindstaedt, H., Kutz, K. and Wuttke, H. (1979): Wirksame ambulante Therapie des Ulcus ventriculi mit Proglumid. *Dtsch. Med. Wochenschr. 104,* 313.
63. Shinagawa, F., Fujita, R. and Hasegawa, Y. (1972): Klinische Erfahrungen mit Proglumid (Milid) bei der Behandlung von peptischen Ulzera (Abstract). In: *9. Internationaler Kongress für Gastroenterologie, Paris.*
64. Suga, S., Shimochi, H., Koide, K. et al. (1970): Therapeutische Wirkung von Proglumid bei gastroduodenalen Ulzera. *Clinical Report 4,* 2703.
65. Takeo, W., Katsuni, S. and Satoru, O. (1970): Medizinische Behandlung des Magenulcus. Doppelblindstudie über die klinische Anwendung von Proglumid. *Nihon Rinsho 28,* 2498.
66. Tete, R. (1975): Stellung von Proglumid bei der Behandlung pathologischer Zustände im Magen und Duodenum. *Actual. Therap. 51,* 1227.
67. Hoskins, E.O.L. (1973): Metoclopramide in benign gastric ulceration. *Postgrad. Med. J. 49, Sup. 4,* 95.
68. Cornet, A. and Grivaux, M. (1968): Recherches physiopathologiques sur le sulpiride en gastroenterologie. *Bull. Mem. Soc. Med. Hôp. 119,* 753.
69. Masuda, M. (1969): Results of a national scale statistical study of a double blind study. *VI. Congress Ther. Res. New Drugs, Osaka*, pp. 1–8.
70. Molle, M. (1975): Sulpirid bei der Behandlung von Gastroduodenalgeschwüren. *Fortschr. Med. 93,* 1077.
71. Lam, S.K., Lam, K.C., Lai, C.L. et al. (1979): Treatment of duodenal ulcer with antacid and Sulpiride. A double-blind controlled study. *Gastroenterology 76,* 315.
72. Gottrup, F. and Ornsholt, J. (1979): Effects of a β_2-sympathomimetic on histamine-stimulated gastric acid secretion in dogs. *Scand J. Gastroenterol. 14,* 321.

The impact of medical therapy on the natural history of ulcer disease*

J. Hansky
*Monash University Department of Medicine and Gastroenterology Unit,
Prince Henry's Hospital, Melbourne, Australia*

Review of the impact of medical therapy on the natural history of ulcer
disease demands as a prerequisite, knowledge of the natural history of
untreated ulcer disease. Unfortunately such knowledge is scarce but there is
some data available. Duodenal and gastric ulcers have somewhat different
rates of spontaneous exacerbation and remission and will be considered
separately.

The natural history of duodenal ulcer

The clinical spectrum of duodenal ulcer disease is variable. Some patients
have frequent exacerbations, few remissions and proceed to intractable
disease. In others, there is the advent of complications superimposed on a
history of chronic disease; complications such as scarring leading to outlet
obstruction, hemorrhage, penetration and perforation. These complications
often lead to surgery. Some patients present initially with hemorrhage or
perforation, may then remain symptom free or have further recurrent
hemorrhage or perforation. There is a small group who have an acute
exacerbation, and healing is followed by a prolonged remission. In 1964 Fry
attempted to determine the natural history of ulcer disease [1]. He found in
general practice in South England that duodenal ulcer patients peaked
symptomatically at about 8 years after diagnosis but that symptoms, and
possibly the ulcer, tended to disappear after a mean of 10 years. He stated that
the tendency toward spontaneous remission was not influenced by medical
treatment as then available. In another study consisting of hospital patients,

* These studies were aided by grants from Smith Kline & French (Australia) and Parke,
Davis Australia.

Greibe et al. reviewed 227 patients with duodenal ulcer [2]. Of these 22% had died during the 13-year follow-up period, not more than expected from the general population. Fifteen per cent had undergone surgery in the period, 37% had no symptoms, 29% had mild symptoms, 12% had severe symptoms and over half the patients had few symptoms at the end of 13 years. The highest mortality rate appears to be within the first 2 years after diagnosis but the most important aspect of the study was that diagnosis made in hospital, as opposed to general practice, led to a more serious prognosis. Complications are the major causes of mortality and although precise estimates of complication rates are difficult to obtain, the rate is about one per cent per annum after diagnosis.

The natural history of gastric ulcer

Gastric ulcer is a recurrent disease and it is estimated that about 50% recur within 2 years of the initial diagnosis. However, it differs from duodenal ulcer in that frequent recurrences over a prolonged period are uncommon. The reasons for this are that patients with 2 or more recurrences are often treated surgically or there may be a spontaneous cure. Fenger et al. studied 701 patients and found a 40% mortality rate with 7% dying in the first admission and 21% in the first 5 years [3]. Of the survivors, 50% had surgery. In the United States Veterans Administration study, Hanscom and Buchman followed 565 patients after healing or surgery and of the 377 healed medically, 42% had one or more recurrences in 2 years [4]. They also noted that slow initial healers had a high recurrence rate.

The mortality and morbidity of gastric ulcer is higher than for duodenal ulcer. Although the complications of hemorrhage, perforation and obstruction occur as in duodenal ulcer, patients are older and in addition there is the question of malignant change supervening on a previously benign chronic gastric ulcer.

Factors which influence natural history

As little is known about the factors which influence the natural history as of the natural history itself. Some of the factors which influence the natural history of ulcer disease are shown in Table I. Acid secretory rates may influence healing and the higher the acid secretory rate, the greater the chances of exacerbation, the most extreme example of this being the

Table I: Factors which may influence the natural history of ulcers.

Inherent:	Acid secretory rates
	Serum pepsinogens
	Mucosal defence
	Genetic − family history
Exogenous:	Salicylates in gastric ulcer
	Cigarette smoking
	Occupational
	Geographic
	Personality traits
	Dietary factors

Zollinger-Ellison syndrome. Some families with ulcer disease have high serum pepsinogen which may lead to continued disease. In others there is a strong family history of ulcer which may also be a factor. Salicylates have certainly been implicated in gastric ulcer and continued ingestion leads to continued disease. Stressful occupations are associated with development of ulcers and there are certainly geographic areas where ulcers are prevalent, e.g., Scotland and Southern India. Personality traits such as anxiety may make exacerbation more common. In terms of dietary factors, ingestion of coffee or carbonated beverages may be factors in continued ulcer disease but alcohol has not been implicated. One of the most powerful factors in both the development of ulcer and lack of healing is heavy cigarette smoking. Data is accumulating that smokers have more ulcers and continued smoking may lead to less healing and more frequent relapses. Removal of all of these factors may alter the natural history and response to medical therapy.

Can natural history be altered by medical therapy?

Until the mid 1970's, the answer to this question was no. This was due to the fact that medical therapy, apart from removal of exogenous factors and bed rest, did not lead to ulcer healing. With the advent of more powerful modes of therapy, such as H_2-receptor antagonists, prostaglandins, powerful antacids, carbenoxolone sodium and bismuth, healing of ulcers can now occur. However, the key question is whether healing of the ulcer alters the natural history of the disease. In short, the answer in 1980 again remains no. The remainder of this paper will examine the evidence for this statement and attempt to extrapolate for the future.

Effect of short-term cimetidine on the natural history of duodenal ulcer

Since the advent of histamine H_2-receptor antagonists in the treatment of duodenal ulcer, numerous controlled studies have shown that there is no doubt that they produce healing rates of between 65–85% compared to the placebo rate of 30–50% [5–9]. Cessation of therapy following healing of an ulcer and suppression of symptoms is associated with a relapse rate of around 75% within 6 months, the majority within 3 months [10–12]. Thus we can conclude that a short healing course of cimetidine in duodenal ulcer does not influence the natural history of ulcer recurrence in the majority of patients so treated.

Effect of long-term (maintenance) cimetidine on the natural history of duodenal ulcer

In an attempt to influence the relapse rate of duodenal ulcer, long-term maintenance therapy has been evaluated after an initial course of treatment designed to heal the ulcer. Doses of cimetidine employed have been 400 mg twice daily or 400–800 mg as a single bedtime dose. In one study, 800 mg of cimetidine given at bedtime was associated with an endoscopically-proven relapse rate of 24% at the completion of 6 months [13]. At the end of this period patients who remained healed were randomly allocated to either placebo or 400 mg of cimetidine at night [14]. On either regime, a further 66% had relapsed at the end of 6 weeks. In our studies with maintenance cimetidine, 40 patients with duodenal ulcer who had healed on a 6-week course of 1 g of cimetidine daily were randomly allocated to placebo or 400 mg of cimetidine twice daily and were followed for 12 months when they were endoscoped at relapse or at 12 months. The results are shown in Table II. Ninety-five per cent of patients on active treatment remained symptomatically and endoscopically healed at 12 months while 90% of the placebo-treated group had relapsed [12]. In another study, forty-one patients who had remained healed (endoscopically) after 12 months of maintenance cimetidine therapy, 400 mg twice daily, were then allocated to either placebo or continu-

Table II: Symptomatic and endoscopic relapse after 12 months of cimetidine or placebo.

	Relapse	No relapse
Cimetidine (400 mg twice daily)	1	19
Placebo	18	2

ation of the cimetidine dose and endoscoped on relapse or at 6 months [15]. Twenty-six patients received placebo and 15 patients active cimetidine. One of the 15 patients on active cimetidine had relapsed at 6 months while 20 of the 26 patients allocated to placebo had relapsed by 6 months. The cumulative relapse rates at 1, 2, 3 and 6 months are shown in Table III.

Comparison of cumulative relapse rates at 6 months after 6 weeks' and 12 months' cimetidine therapy is shown in the Figure. The relapse rates are similar, suggesting that 12 months' continuous cimetidine does not alter the natural history of duodenal ulcer disease.

The following conclusions can be drawn from these and other studies:
— Cimetidine heals duodenal ulcers.
— Long-term maintenance therapy keeps about 75–80% of patients symptom free when employed for at least 12 months at a dose of 800 mg daily.
— There is a high relapse rate after cessation of either short- or long-term therapy which approaches 90% within 12 months of cessation.
— Up to 15% of patients who remain symptom free may have ulcers demonstrated at endoscopy. This is seen more often in patients on no treatment than in patients having active treatment.

Does cimetidine therapy make the ulcer more prone to recurrence: that is, does it adversely affect the natural history?

To answer this question, one needs information about the natural relapse rate of duodenal ulcer and this is not known. Certainly, early relapse does occur following cessation of cimetidine and some studies have also reported perforation of the ulcer [16–19]. Bardhan has summarized the situation very precisely [20]. The majority of patients treated with cimetidine have such a sense of well being that even the slightest recurrence of symptoms leads them to seek further attention and endoscopy invariably finds an ulcer. It is not known how many such episodes occurred prior to the introduction of cimetidine and perhaps these patients merely treated themselves with antacids, bed rest etc.

Table III: Cumulative numbers of patients who have relapsed up to 6 months after one year of maintenance cimetidine therapy.

Treatment	Number entered	Total number relapsed at (months)			
		1	2	3	6
Cimetidine	15	1	1	1	1
Placebo	26	7	12	14	20

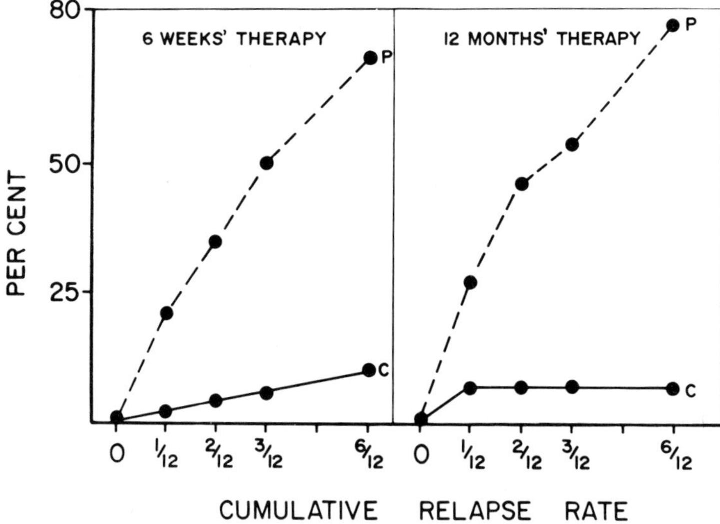

Figure: Cumulative relapse rates in duodenal ulcer treated with cimetidine (C) or placebo (P) for 6 weeks and 12 months.

and did not seek medical advice. Two theoretical considerations could account for early relapse – hypergastrinemia consequent upon protracted hypochlorhydria and acid rebound. We and others have shown an increase in the integrated gastrin response to food during cimetidine therapy [21, 22]. The increase tends to remain static between 6 and 12 months' cimetidine [23] and on cessation the gastrin response may remain abnormal for a few weeks [24]. In terms of acid rebound, numerous studies indicate no increase in acid secretion above pretreatment values. Thus it is unlikely that early relapse is due to rebound acid hypersecretion but return of acid secretion to pretreatment levels may be sufficient to account for relapse.

In summary, the relapse time after cessation of cimetidine is often early but no inferences can be drawn because of lack of data pre-cimetidine. The possibility remains that cimetidine given in short courses may adversely affect the natural history.

Effect of high-dose antacid therapy on the natural history of duodenal ulcer

High-dose antacid therapy has been shown to heal duodenal ulcers at the same rate as cimetidine [25]. In a recently completed double-blind 6-week trial, we have shown that high-dose dimeticone does not heal as many patients as cimetidine although the differences were not statistically significant. The results are shown in Table IV and it was noted that cigarette smoking adversely affected healing rates with both modes of therapy. At the completion of the study, all patients who had healed were followed, at monthly intervals, and endoscoped at clinical relapse or at 6 months. The relapse rates are shown in Table V and there were no differences between cimetidine and dimeticone, although the time to relapse was earlier after cessation of cimetidine than after cessation of dimeticone. There were no differences in relapse rates between smokers and nonsmokers but the numbers were very small.

To my knowledge, maintenance therapy with high-dose dimeticone (or other antacids) has not been reported. The high incidence of diarrhea (70% in the above study) would probably preclude patient compliance with this regime.

Effect of carbenoxolone, bismuth and prostaglandins on the natural history of duodenal ulcer

Controlled trials of carbenoxolone and bismuth have indicated a high healing rate with short treatment courses of these agents. There are no reports of maintenance studies and at least for carbenoxolone, relapse rates are similar after cessation of therapy to those obtained with H_2-receptor antagonists [26].

Table IV: Double-blind trial of dimeticone and cimetidine on healing of duodenal ulcer: influence of smoking.

Drug	Number treated	Number healed/Total (%)		
		Smokers	Nonsmokers	Total
Cimetidine	25	5/10 (50)	15/15 (100)	20/25 (80)
Dimeticone	25	5/13 (39)	8/12 (67)	13/25 (52)

Table V: Relapse rate of duodenal ulcer after healing with cimetidine or dimeticone at 6 months.

Drug	Total entered	Relapsed	Still healed	Mean time to relapse (months)
Cimetidine	18	17	1	2.8
Dimeticone	13	9	4	3.9

Thus these agents do not appear to influence the natural history of duodenal ulcer disease.

Effect of medical therapy on the natural history of gastric ulcer

Before the advent of histamine H_2-receptor antagonists, the only factors shown to heal gastric ulcer were bed rest, cessation of smoking and carbenoxolone sodium [27]. Certainly carbenoxolone sodium healed gastric ulcers in patients treated on an outpatient basis but it is doubtful whether such treatment influenced the natural history of the ulcer to recur. Long-term maintenance therapy with carbenoxolone has not been acceptable because of the increased incidence of side effects seen with the drug.

Cimetidine has been used in the treatment of gastric ulcer but the efficacy compared with placebo or intensive antacid therapy has been quite variable. What is clear from various studies is that the healing rate of 60–75% within 6 weeks is less than that achieved for duodenal ulcer disease.

Freston has reviewed the role of cimetidine in gastric ulcer based on 6 reported studies [28]. Although cimetidine was shown to be effective in the healing of gastric ulcer, there were marked differences in the United States and European trials; the latter showing a much greater effect while the former showed little difference between antacid- and cimetidine-treated groups. This difference was ascribed to a higher antacid consumption in the United States trials.

Information about relapse rates following cessation of therapy is scarce in gastric ulcer. Wulff and Rune have reported a maintenance trial of cimetidine and placebo in 23 patients healed with cimetidine [29]. Four patients withdrew, 10 patients treated for 12 months with 400 mg of cimetidine twice daily remained healed, and 5 of 9 patients on placebo relapsed from 7 to 18 weeks after initial healing. In another study, Machel studied 31 patients healed with cimetidine and followed for 11 months [30]. Five patients defaulted, one died of a cerebrovascular accident and of the remaining 25, 14 had placebo and 11 cimetidine. Two of the 11 cimetidine-treated patients relapsed while 12 of the 14 placebo-treated patients relapsed.

Thus the relapse rates of gastric ulcer are similar to those of duodenal ulcer treated with cimetidine, and maintenance therapy keeps the majority of gastric ulcers healed. We can conclude that one course of cimetidine (and presumably antacids and carbenoxolone sodium) does not positively influence the natural history of gastric ulcer to recur. Whether treatment adversely affects the natural history is problematical because the true healing and relapse rate of untreated ulcers is not known.

Does the initial healing rate influence the subsequent relapse rate?

The ease of healing a duodenal ulcer does not appear to influence its subsequent relapse rate but a recent study by Scobie suggests that it may influence the relapse of gastric ulcers [31]. He concluded that in a study based on 80 healed chronic gastric ulcers, those taking longer than 8 weeks to heal with medical therapy relapse earlier and more frequently than those more readily healed. This suggests that certain ulcer patients have different natural histories to others and thus the ease of healing may influence future management.

Does cessation of smoking lead to a lower relapse rate?

As shown in our studies on the effect of smoking on healing of ulcers, cigarette smoking adversely affects healing rate. However, there were no differences in relapse rates between smokers and nonsmokers. This does not answer the question of whether cessation of smoking decreases the natural relapse rate but it may be worthwhile stopping patients smoking to try and answer this question. It seems that some patients who stop smoking once the ulcer is healed appear to have more prolonged remissions.

Summary

Review of the available literature and our own experience indicate that medical therapy consisting of one healing course of the currently available agents does not favorably alter the natural history of ulcer disease. Because the precise natural history is not known, it is uncertain whether healing of the ulcer with one course of cimetidine or antacids leads to earlier and more frequent recurrence and thus an adverse effect on the natural history.

In duodenal ulcer and probably in gastric ulcer, maintenance therapy with cimetidine keeps a majority of the ulcers healed and the patients symptom-free. By continued therapy, the natural history can be positively influenced but this has to be tempered by factors such as patient compliance and the unknown side effects of long-term acid suppression or effects of the drugs themselves. Whether intermittent long-term therapy can achieve a low relapse rate remains to be proven but there are some patients in whom only one to 2 courses of treatment yearly are all that is required. Perhaps frequent relapsers, in whom the disease is obviously severe, can be culled from the general ulcer population and treated either surgically or with long-term therapy depending on age, concurrent diseases and compliance. The advent of powerful ulcer-healing agents has created as many problems as benefits and we are left with the fact that 'these agents heal the ulcer but do not cure the disease'.

References

1. Fry, J. (1964): Peptic ulcer: A profile. *Br. Med. J. 2*, 809.
2. Greibe, J., Bugge, P., Gjorup, T. et al. (1977): Long term prognosis of duodenal ulcer: follow up study and survey of doctor's estimates. *Br. Med. J. 2*, 1572.
3. Fenger, C., Amdrup, E., Christiansen, P. et al. (1973): Gastric ulcer. I. Analysis of 701 patients. *Acta Chir. Scand. 139*, 455.
4. Hanscom, D.H. and Buchman, E. (1971): The follow up period. *Gastroenterology 61*, 585.
5. Bodemar, G. and Walan, A. (1976): Cimetidine in the treatment of active duodenal and prepyloric ulcers. *Lancet II*, 161.
6. Blackwood, W.S., Maudgal, D.P., Pickard, R.D. et al. (1976): Cimetidine in duodenal ulcer. *Lancet II*, 176.
7. Hetzel, D.J., Taggart, G.J., Hansky, J. et al. (1977): Cimetidine in the treatment of duodenal ulcer. *Med. J. Aust. 1*, 317.
8. Bardhan, K.D., Saul, D.M. and Balmforth, G.V. (1977): The effect of cimetidine on duodenal ulceration. In: *Cimetidine: Proceedings of the Second International Symposium on Histamine H_2-Receptor Antagonists*, pp. 260–271. Eds: W.L. Burland and M.A. Simkins. Excerpta Medica, Amsterdam.
9. Gray, G.R., McKenzie, I., Smith, I.S. et al. (1977): Oral cimetidine in severe duodenal ulceration. *Lancet I*, 4.
10. Bardhan, K.D., Blum, A., Gillespie, G. et al. (1977): Long term treatment with cimetidine in duodenal ulceration. *Lancet I*, 900.
11. Hetzel, D.J., Shearman, D.J.C., Hecker, R. and Sheers, R. (1979): Prevention of duodenal ulcer relapse by cimetidine: a one year double blind trial. *Med. J. Aust. 1*, 529.
12. Hansky, J. and Korman, M.G. (1979): Long term cimetidine in duodenal ulcer disease. *Dig. Dis. Scis. 24*, 465.
13. Blackwood, W.S., Maudgal, D.P. and Northfield, T.C. (1978): Prevention of bedtime cimetidine by duodenal ulcer relapse. *Lancet I*, 626.
14. Fitzpatrick, W.J.F., Blackwood, W.S. and Northfield, T.C. (1979): Does cimetidine alter subsequent natural history of duodenal ulcer? *Gut 20*, A905.
15. Korman, M.G., Hetzel, D.J., Hansky, J. et al. (1980): The relapse rate of duodenal ulcer after cessation of long term cimetidine: A double blind controlled study. *Dig. Dis. Scis.* (In press).
16. Gill, M.J. and Saunders, J.B. (1977): Perforation of chronic peptic ulcers after cimetidine. *Br. Med. J. 2*, 1149.
17. Keighley, B.D. (1977): Perforation of peptic ulcer after withdrawal of cimetidine. *Br. Med. J. 2*, 1022.
18. Saunders, J.H.B. and Wormsley, K.G. (1977): Long term effects and after effects of treatment of duodenal ulcer with metiamide. *Lancet I*, 765.
19. Wallace, W.A., Orr, C.M.E. and Bearn, A.R. (1977): Perforation of chronic

peptic ulcer after cimetidine. *Br. Med. J. 2*, 865.

20. Bardhan, K.D. (1978): Cimetidine in duodenal ulceration. In: *Cimetidine. The Westminster Hospital Symposium,* p. 31. Eds: C. Wastell and P. Lance. Churchill Livingstone, Edinburgh-London-New York.

21. Hansky, J., Stern, A.I. and Korman, M.G. (1979): Effects of long term cimetidine on serum gastrin in duodenal ulcer. *Dig. Dis. Scis. 24*, 468.

22. Spence, R.W., Celestin, L.R., McCormick, D.A. et al. (1977): Effects of one year's treatment with cimetidine on fasting and oxo stimulated serum gastrin in duodenal ulcer patients. *Gut 18*, A949.

23. Hansky, J., Stern, A.I., Korman, M.G. and Waugh, J. (1979): Serum gastrin after 12 months continuous cimetidine therapy for duodenal ulcer. *Aust. N.Z. J. Med. 9*, 637.

24. Bank, S., Barbezat, G.O., Vinik, A.I. et al. (1977): Cimetidine and serum gastrin levels in man. In: *Cimetidine: Proceedings of the Second International Symposium on Histamine H_2-Receptor Antagonists,* pp. 155–162. Eds: W.L. Burland and M.A. Simkins. Excerpta Medica, Amsterdam.

25. Ippoliti, A.F., Sturdevant, R.A.L., Isenberg, J.I. et al. (1978): Cimetidine versus intensive antacid therapy for duodenal ulcer. A multicenter trial. *Gastroenterology 74*, 393.

26. Brown, P., Salmon, P.R., Neumann, C.S. et al. (1979): Comparison of carbenoxolone sodium and cimetidine in duodenal ulceration. *Gut 20*, A904.

27. Sircus, W. (1972): Progress report: carbenoxolone sodium. *Gut 13*, 816.

28. Freston, J.W. (1978): Cimetidine in the treatment of gastric ulcer. Review and commentary. *Gastroenterology 74*, 426.

29. Wulff, H.R. and Rune, S.J. (1978): A comparison of studies in the treatment of gastric ulceration with cimetidine. In: *Cimetidine. The Westminster Hospital Symposium,* pp. 281–288. Eds: C. Wastell and P. Lance. Churchill Livingstone, Edinburgh-London-New York.

30. Machel, R.J. (1979): The prevention of gastric ulcer relapse with cimetidine. *Gastroenterology 76*, 1191.

31. Scobie, B.A. (1979): Prognosis of completely healed gastric ulcer. *N.Z. Med. J. 89*, 344.

Discussion

The discussion centered around the aim of medical therapy and the means to increase the therapeutic efficacy of drug treatment. The goal of medical therapy should be to control ulcer disease characterized by a 10- to 15-year course of recurrences. This type of ulcer disease which represents an appreciable fraction of the disease entity should be considered on the basis of the length and the severity of the disease for long-term treatment. Future studies comparing the efficacy of medical and surgical therapy in reducing the recurrence rate, the incidence of complications, the death rate, the days off work, etc. will be necessary to allow us a judgment about the effect of treatment with H_2-blockers on the long-term outcome of ulcer disease. The therapeutic efficacy of medical treatment should be increased by enhancing the time period during which the concentration of the drug in the blood is optimal for achieving the desired effects. This enhancement of the therapeutic window might help to decrease the impact of compliance on the therapeutic results.

Pharmacokinetic studies have shown that cimetidine disposition is an age-dependent process (Figure). Total plasma clearance was 659–797 ml/min in patients aged 28–45 years but was only 259–441 ml/min in patients 53–64 years of age. When comparing nonresponders to cimetidine therapy with responders no significant differences were found (Table) [1].

H_2-receptor antagonists

The following part of the discussion dealt with the role of H_2-receptor antagonists in ulcer disease as well as with the side effects of these drugs. To evaluate new drugs it will be very important to compare the relative potency of cimetidine with other H_2-receptor antagonists. The relative potency of cimetidine and ranitidine calculated on the molar basis seems to depend on the model being used. Using the human model one way to compare the drugs would be to calculate the IC_{50}* for each drug in the same subject, then use these subjects as comparisons. Using intragastric titration there is a ratio of 1:10, ranitidine to cimetidine. There is no indication at the moment that

* IC_{50} is the dose necessary to achieve 50% inhibition of acid secretion.

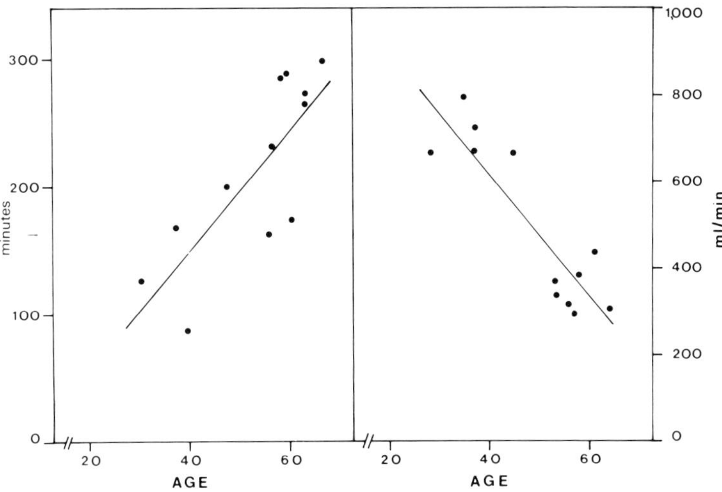

Figure: Age dependency of cimetidine plasma clearance (right) and time period of effective (above 0.5 µg/ml) plasma concentration (left).

ranitidine has a different length of action compared with cimetidine. The affinity of the receptors for ranitidine versus cimetidine was 1:5 (Lewin). Analyzing the effect of both compounds on 24-hour gastric acidity there was a difference in hydrogen ion activity between 8 a.m. and 12 p.m. The explanation might be that there was more ranitidine still circulating after the nocturnal dose. Furthermore, there seems to be an escape in terms of intragastric

Table: Pharmacokinetic data of cimetidine and gastric acid secretion values after 6 weeks' treatment with cimetidine 1 g daily. Tests were performed during cimetidine treatment in 6 patients with healed ulcers and in 6 patients with unhealed ulcers.

	Responders	Non-responders
Lowest level before morning dose (µg/ml)	0.24 ± 0.14	0.23 ± 0.26
Area under plasma level curve (morning dose)	179 ± 72	208 ± 76
Plasma levels above 0.5 µg/ml (min)	156 ± 105	157 ± 131
Cimetidine excretion (mg)	68 ± 25	80 ± 12
Basal acid output* (mEq/hr)	1.6 ± 2.1	0.6 ± 1.0
Peak acid output° (mEq/hr)	22.7 ± 16.1	23.3 ± 21.9

* 2 hours after morning dose.

° 3 hours after morning dose.

hydrogen ion activity at any rate from both drugs, ranitidine and cimetidine, in the afternoon, despite adequate blood levels (Misiewicz and Bonfils).

Long-term treatment with cimetidine in patients with duodenal ulcer reduces significantly the recurrence rate and was shown to decrease the incidence of complications and the need for elective surgery in a small number of patients. Confirmation of these results in a larger population and longer observation periods will be necessary to evaluate the efficacy of maintenance therapy on the natural course of the disease. The recently proposed intermittent therapy with cimetidine in patients with duodenal ulcer might be of benefit for patients with sporadically occurring ulcers ('ulcer episodes') [2]. Patients with repeated attacks of recurring ulcers ('ulcer disease') might be selected for cimetidine maintenance therapy or surgery. Again these therapeutic implications derived from the results of previously published studies must be put to the test.

In the studies available on gastric ulcer rarely a differentiation between the different types of gastric ulcer has been made. Only Frost et al. [3] analyzed the response to cimetidine in patients with prepyloric ulcers and corpus ulcers. Prepyloric ulcers seemed to be less responsive in regard to ulcer healing and symptomatic relief than ulcers located in the body of the stomach, but there were too few patients to provide conclusive results [3]. In a prospective double-blind study including 84 patients with severe hemorrhage from gastric or duodenal ulcers, cimetidine did not reduce the severity of bleeding nor the incidence of emergency surgery. Furthermore, treatment did not improve the mortality rate [4]. Based on these results one may conclude that patients with severe bleeding – needing immediate blood transfusion at admission – will not benefit from immediate treatment with intravenous cimetidine (1,200 mg/24 hour).

Zollinger-Ellison syndrome

In patients with Zollinger-Ellison syndrome, once cimetidine efficacy has been documented and metastases have been excluded, tumor resection might be considered. Transhepatic catheterizations with gastrin determinations in the venous outflow have been proposed to localize gastrinomas [5]. In the majority of patients curative surgery will not be feasible and these patients should be treated with cimetidine alone or in combination with other antisecretory drugs and chemotherapy when indicated. The combination of pirenzepine (72 mg/day intramuscularly) with cimetidine may be useful in controlling hypersecretion in patients with acute Zollinger-Ellison syndrome based on preliminary observations [6]. In long-term treatment this combination has no advantage over cimetidine alone due to the side effects (dryness of the mouth, blurring of the vision) of high dosages of pirenzepine. The appropriate surgical treatment should be total gastrectomy when cimetidine treatment fails. The recently published suggestion based on observations in 3 patients of combining vagotomy with cimetidine therapy [7] to control the Zollinger-Ellison syndrome will need confirmation in a larger group of patients.

Side effects

The discussion centered around the immunological effects and their possible implications. A subpopulation of T lymphocytes is known to have H_2-receptors and therefore concern has arisen about enhancement of delayed hypersensitivity by cimetidine. In dogs, cimetidine increased rejection of renal allografts. The onset of rejection occurred earlier with higher doses of cimetidine (300 mg twice daily) than with lower doses (150 mg twice daily) [8]. In a well-defined transplantation model of inbred mice there was no influence of cimetidine on the rejection of skin grafts, even if histo-incompatibility was weak [9]. Although there may be a certain immunological effect of cimetidine, its clinical relevance is not yet established and deserves further investigation.

In regard to drug interaction it should be noted that the imidazole ring is a general interferer with drug metabolism. Cimetidine interferes with hydroxylation and with methylation. In the United Kingdom, Professor Langman together with other centers is following 10,000 patients who have taken cimetidine and 10,000 controls in a long-term study to assess mortality and morbidity experience. Data will be produced for one, 2 and in due course possibly 3 or 4 years and results will be available from this ongoing study in the future.

Antacids

Should the choice of antacids in ulcer treatment take into consideration the possibility of an acid rebound when the buffering activity disappears? Comparing calcium carbonate and magnesium salts, rebound is greater for the first one [10] but there is no clinical evidence that decreased therapeutic activity results.

Concerning consequences of mixing antacids with food, theoretical considerations were presented suggesting a balance between advantages and disadvantages: food prolongs the intragastric presence of the drug by slowing gastric emptying and adds its own buffering capacity; contrariwise, intragastric food can modify the solubility of antacids and thus decrease their efficacy.

In stress ulcer prevention, the use of antacid appeared controversial, in spite of successful results reported by various groups. Criticisms were related to: difficulties in performing endoscopy repeatedly; disturbance in systemic acid/bases balance when administering large amounts of alkalins; and diarrhea and renal loss of calcium with magnesium salts. The optimal intragastric pH for stress ulcer prevention remains undefined. Empirically, several groups use titration to pH 3.5 as the lowest with therapeutic value.

In the treatment of chronic peptic ulcer, one could consider that antacids are able to cure ulcer attacks; but simplification of drug regimen, better compliance, greater efficacy favor the use of H_2-antagonists. Antacids could be combined with cimetidine in long-term treatment for covering diurnal acid secretion. Recent results suggesting that low dose antacid regimens are effective in the treatment of duodenal ulcer are of interest [11, 12]. Even with lower dose regimens, marked side effects such as diarrhea and significant changes in serum electrolyte levels and urinary electrolyte excretions will occur during a 4-week treatment period when compared to placebo [13].

Anticholinergics

Although new and more efficacious anticholinergic drugs are available for ulcer treatment, the use of anticholinergics remains controversial. Side effects are not minor and poor absorbability may limit their effectiveness.

One possible indication could be the combination of low doses of anticholinergics with low doses of cimetidine, administered either simultaneously at bedtime or, alternatively, over 24 hours. Theoretically anticholinergics could be useful in the prevention or treatment of stress ulcer. This is currently being investigated by clinical trials but data are not yet available.

Carbenoxolone

The mechanism of action of carbenoxolone was discussed. Carbenoxolone may inhibit prostaglandin-degrading enzymes in the gastric mucosa, as shown in vitro by Peskar et al. [14]. No in vivo data are available. Reduced degradation of prostaglandins may increase symptoms of glycosaminoglycans and glycoproteins, enhancing cytoprotection (see Chapter II, Dousa, pages 128–136).

Side effects of carbenoxolone therapy remain a concern. The possibility of combining carbenoxolone with a potassium-sparing diuretic, like triamterene, is a possibility but no controlled clinical data on its value are available.

Prostaglandins

Prostaglandins have been demonstrated potent inhibitors of gastric acid secretion. Are they of therapeutic value? Among the numerous natural and synthetic prostaglandins, which of them deserves a clinical trial? Do they have untoward effects in man?

Professor Konturek presented impressive results in man with different methyl analogues administered orally, either in alcohol solution or in capsules (16,16-dimethyl PGE_2, 15(S)-15-methyl PGE_2, 15(R)-15-methyl PGE_2). After a single oral dose of 1 μg/kg body weight inhibition of meal-induced gastric secretion can last for 5 or 6 hours. Professor Konturek confirmed Professor Isenberg's observation of suppression of postprandial gastrin release after oral prostaglandins. This important observation should be modulated by the results observed in dog using natural or methylated prostaglandins. In these studies it was observed that PGE_2 had no effect on gastrin release and PGI_2 even increased the gastrin response.

In man, prostaglandins seem to be unable to suppress the increase in post-prandial gastrin release induced by the anticholinergic scopolamine methyl bromide; this suggests inefficacy of prostaglandins towards the removal of the vagal inhibitory effect of vagal release. Practically, this has to be taken into consideration in case of combined administration of prostaglandins and anticholinergics.

Untoward effects concern mainly diarrhea. The difference between the dosage inhibiting gastric secretion and that inducing diarrhea as a side effect is small. Furthermore, methyl analogues of prostaglandins given in multiple daily doses result in a marked accumulation frequently causing diarrhea. On the other hand, if changes in stimulated pancreatic secretion are insignificant, duodenogastric reflux is often observed and could introduce a bias in the assessment of prostaglandin antisecretory activity, particularly when using intragastric titration.

A recent European multicenter trial assessed the effect of 15(R)-15-methyl PGE_2 (100 μg 4 times a day) and placebo on ulcer healing in 105 patients with duodenal ulcer. Complete ulcer healing occurred within 28 days in 62.8% of treated patients compared to 38.9% in the placebo group. Gastrointestinal side effects, usually diarrhea, were reported by 9 patients in the treated group [15].

Concerning prostaglandin-ulcer relationships various suggestions were discussed: assessment of prostaglandin level in the duodenal bulb in normals and in ulcer patients hypothesizing that duodenal ulcer could be related to local prostaglandin defect, use of very low doses of prostaglandins for distinguishing cytoprotection from secretion inhibition (needing very much higher dose) in the therapeutic efficacy, and use of prostaglandins to prevent ulcer relapses.

Professor Johansson presented evidence that when patients are treated with oral doses of an antisecretory prostaglandin derivative 15(R)-15-methyl PGE_2, which suppresses gastric secretion, fecal blood loss induced by simultaneous indometacin administration is reduced to control levels [16]. N-acetylneuraminic acid production (an index of mucus production) was increased at the same time that acid output declined. However, fecal blood loss is also reduced to control levels by low doses of PGE_2 which has no effect on gastric acid secretion.

In a study performed at the Karolinska Institute, and reported by Professor Johansson, prostaglandins were applied locally to the main stomach of dogs provided with gastric Pavlov pouches. It was then observed that gastric acid output was reduced in the main stomach whereas secretion in the Pavlov pouch was unaffected. When the reverse experiment was carried out, prostaglandins applied to the Pavlov pouch decreased acid secretion in the pouch but not in the main stomach. These results suggest that absorption of locally applied prostaglandins into the systemic circulation is not a prerequisite to their inhibitory effect upon gastric secretion. This would imply that prostaglandins applied locally can penetrate the mucosa to an extent that enables them to exert their effects. At higher doses, however, local prostaglandins may be absorbed locally and produce systemic effects. For instance, Professor A. Robert reported on some experiments in which 16,16-dimethyl PGE_2 was administered to a Heidenhain pouch in a dog which had 2 Heidenhain pouches. There was stimulation by histamine intravenously, so both pouches were secreting. When the 16,16-dimethyl PGE_2 was put into one of the 2 pouches at a particular dose, only that pouch was inhibited. When the dose was increased, however, both pouches were inhibited.

Newly developed drugs

Several points of interest were discussed. Side effects due to prolonged pancreatic response to secretin have not been observed. Sucralfate binds bile acids in vitro but is only one-fourth as potent as colestyramine on a molar basis. Colloidal bismuth was discussed without mentioning possible severe neurologic toxicity occasionally observed with other bismuth salts (myoclonic encephalopathy). Clearly any form of bismuth therapy needs to be carefully controlled for possible bismuth absorption and toxicity.

Other drugs currently under evaluation or development need to be considered.

Nolinium bromide is a newly synthetized compound that exhibits strong smooth muscle spasmolytic effects but appears to be deprived of systemic anticholinergic effects. Animal and human studies indicate that this substance inhibits gastric acid secretion stimulated by exogenous secretagogues [17]. However, recent studies in patients with duodenal ulcer (unpublished observations) failed to demonstrate any significant reduction in meal-stimulated gastric acid secretion although gastric emptying was markedly delayed. At this point it is uncertain whether this drug will play any significant role in future therapy of patients with ulcer disease.

Substituted benzimidazoles have shown strong inhibitory effects upon gastric acid secretion both in vitro and in vivo [18, 19]. In dogs provided with gastric fistula these compounds have been shown to block gastric acid responses to pentagastrin, histamine, vagal activation and meal. Compared with classic H_2-receptor antagonists they exhibited a remarkably long duration of inhibitory action. These compounds are devoid of any anticholinergic or H_2-blocking effects and appear to block selectively K^+-dependent ATPase in the parietal cell, an enzyme critical to H^+ transport into the canaliculi (see Chapter III, Sachs et al., pages 139–146). Studies are in progress to determine whether these interesting compounds can be applied to human therapy of ulcer disease.

Natural history

There is a lack of comparative data among countries or continents. Geographic factors involve a large variety of parameters: nature and condition of social assistance to the patient; amount of health expenses, medical habits, and particularly for deciding endoscopy; political or social conditions in the country resulting possibly in mental or physical stress; sampling of patients as representative (or not representative) of identical conditions of employment and richness among the countries; acceptance or reluctance of smoking in the patients' environment; psychic influence of negative prescriptions such as prohibition of cigarettes, salicylates, etc.

Individual factors are also very important. For each patient there is a particular rhythm for relapses: seasonal, annual or sometimes related to occasional environment. The key problem indeed is to determine to what extent is the natural history of peptic ulcer disease effectively altered by prolonged administration of drugs.

References

1. Somogyi, A., Rohner, H.G. and Gugler, R. (1980): Pharmacokinetics and bioavailability of cimetidine in gastric and duodenal ulcer patients. *Clin. Pharmacokin. 5*, 84.
2. Bardhan, K.D. (1980): Intermittent treatment of duodenal ulcer with cimetidine. *Br. Med. J. 2*, 20.
3. Frost, F., Rahbek, I., Rune, S.J. et al. (1977): Cimetidine in patients with gastric ulcer: a multicentre controlled trial. *Br. Med. J. II*, 795.
4. Carstens, H.E., Bulow, S., Hart-Hansen, O. et al. (1980): Cimetidine for severe gastroduodenal hemorrhage: a randomized controlled trial. *Scand. J. Gastroenterol. 15*, 103.
5. Burcharth, F., Stage, G., Stadil, F. et al. (1979): Localization of gastrinomas by transhepatic portal catheterization and gastrin assay. *Gastroenterology 77*, 444.
6. Mignon, M., Vallot, T., Galmiche, J.P. et al. (1980): Interest of a combined antisecretory treatment, cimetidine and pirenzepin, in the management of severe forms of Zollinger-Ellison syndrome. *Digestion 20*, 56.
7. Richardson, C.T., Feldmann, M., McClelland, R.N. et al. (1979): Effect of vagotomy in Zollinger-Ellison syndrome. *Gastroenterology 77*, 682.
8. Zammit, M. and Toledo-Pereyra, L.H. (1979): Increased rejection after cimetidine treatment in kidney transplants. *Transplantation 27*, 358.
9. Festen, H.P.M., Berden, J.H.M. and Koene, R.A.P. (1980): Cimetidine does not accelerate skin graft rejection in mice. *Clin. Exp. Immunol. 40*, 193.
10. Holtermüller, K.H. (1977): Does oral magnesium hydroxide prevent the calcium carbonate induced acid rebound in patients with duodenal ulcer? (Abstract.) *Gastroenterology 77*, 1071.
11. Kunert, H. and Ottenjann, R. (1979): Effekt eines Magnesium-Aluminium hydroxidhaltigen Antazidums auf die Heilungsdauer von Ulcera duodeni — randomisierte Doppelblindstudie. *Z. Gastroenterol. 27*, 630.
12. Lam, S.K., Lam, K.C., Lai, C.L. et al. (1979): Treatment of duodenal ulcer with antacid and sulpiride. *Gastroenterology 76*, 315.
13. Herzog, P., Grendahl, T., Linden, J. et al. (1980): Veränderungen der Serum- und Urinelektrolyte unter langfristiger Einnahme von Antacida. In: *Abstracts of the XI International Congress of Gastroenterology*, Hamburg, June 8–13, 1980; p. 208, Georg Thieme Verlag, Stuttgart-New York.
14. Peskar, B.M., Holland, A. and Peskar, B.A. (1976): Effect of carbenoxolone on prostaglandin synthesis and degradation. *J. Pharm. Pharmacol. 28*, 146.
15. Vantrappen, G., Popiela, T., Tytgat, D.N.J. et al. (1980): A multicenter trial of 15(R)-15-methylprostaglandin E_2 in duodenal ulcer. (Abstract.) *Gastroenterology 78*, 1283.
16. Johansson, C., Kollberg, B., Nordemar, R. et al. (1980): Protective effect of prostaglandin E_2 in the gastrointestinal tract during indomethacin treatment of rheumatic diseases. *Gastroenterology 78*, 479.
17. Larach, J.R., Dozois, R.R. and Malagelada, J.-R. (1980): Nolinium bromide: a new antisecretory agent in duodenal ulcer. (Abstract.) *Gastroenterology 78*, 1204.
18. Sundell, G., Sjostrand, S.E. and Olbe, L. (1977): Gastric antisecretory effects of

H 83/69, a benzimidozolyl-pyridyl methyl-sulphoxide. *Acta Pharmacol. Toxicol. 41, Suppl. 4*, 77.
19. Olbe, L., Berglindh, T., Elander, B. et al. (1979): Properties of a new class of gastric acid inhibitors. *Scand. J. Gastroenterol. 14, Suppl. 55*, 131.

Chapter VI: Surgery for ulcer disease

Rationale of surgical therapy in ulcer disease

E.H. Farthmann
Chirurgische Universitätsklinik, Freiburg im Breisgau, Federal Republic of Germany

Introduction

By definition, according to the Oxford dictionary [1], a rationale for surgical therapy in ulcer disease is a reasoned exposition, a statement of reasons, the fundamental reasons, or the logical basis for such therapy. In reality, however, the history of ulcer surgery has been dominated as much by rationality as by empiricism. This dualism extends to the present day.

A discussion of 'surgical therapy' requires a review of a wide spectrum of procedures for use in ulcer disease. They range from diverting procedures, such as gastroenterostomy, to ablative procedures such as gastrectomy and functional operations such as vagotomy. For the purpose of this review of the whys and wherefores of surgery in ulcer disease, a simplified approach seems justified.

The title of this paper also refers to surgery in 'ulcer disease', and not in one of the many other facets of peptic lesions. Again, the review should be wide enough to include acute gastric mucosal lesions of the stressed individual as well as the fibrotic ulcer near the cardia of the elderly.

Obviously it is as yet impossible to give a rational reason for every kind of operation in every type of ulcer disease, since despite all that has been discovered concerning the etiology and pathogenesis of ulcer, it is still a disease of unknown cause. And, as Sir Heneage Ogilvie has stated in this context, there is no rational treatment of a disease without knowledge of its cause [2].

Nevertheless, patients cannot be denied treatment only because the cause of their disease is still unknown. The therapist cannot be blamed for this lack of knowledge. He must do his best, and in doing so he must keep a record of what he is doing, since he may in this way contribute to the elucidation of pathogenic principles. It is for this reason that a review is again being made of the history of the development of surgical procedures for ulcer disease, which is in part a story of trial and error.

Development of surgical therapy

Gastric surgery on a scientific level began with the treatment of gastric cancer. Anton Wölffler developed gastroenterostomy and Theodor Bilroth gastrectomy for this disease [3]. It was left to Ludwig Rydygier to perform these procedures for the first time for benign obstructing ulcer—gastrectomy on November 11, 1881 and gastroenterostomy on March 3, 1884. The report of the first successful partial gastrectomy for ulcer prompted the reviewer to add the terse, if somewhat unprophetic footnote, 'Hoffentlich auch die letzte' (hopefully, also the last) [4]. This incident is cited not for anecdotal reasons, but to warn against the making of premature definitive judgments. New developments in this field must be evaluated with caution.

The proliferation of new procedures continued, and not a few of the variations of gastroenterostomy were invented for purely technical reasons, especially to overcome the problem of the vicious circle. Some did, however, have a rational background, if one is willing to consider it rational to base one's thinking on the knowledge available at the time.

It was generally believed that in order to neutralize the destructive influence of gastric juice, as much alkaline duodenal content as possible should be delivered into the stomach. Schmilinsky, in 1918, perfected this theory by what he termed 'Innere Apotheke' − internal pharmacy [5]. He transected both the pylorus and the first jejunal loop, whose limbs were separately anastomosed to the stomach (Fig. 1). There was virtually nothing the alkaline contents could do but bathe the antral mucosa. Viewed ex post facto, jejunal ulcers resulting from permanent antral stimulation had to be the rule, and they served to elucidate this mechanism.

In 1895, von Eiselsberg developed the antral exclusion operation (Fig. 2) to exclude stenosing nonresectable cancers from the food passage [6]. The operation was adopted for low-lying ulcers in the hope that they would heal when excluded from the acid stream. An epidemic of stomal ulcers followed, and the stage was set to clarify the role of the excluded antrum as a source of continuous humoral stimulation of acid secretion. The operation was abandoned and Edkins published his paper on the chemical mechanism of gastric secretion in 1905 [7].

Obviously, the development of surgical procedures and the increase in understanding of ulcer disease were by no means synchronous. Surgeons were

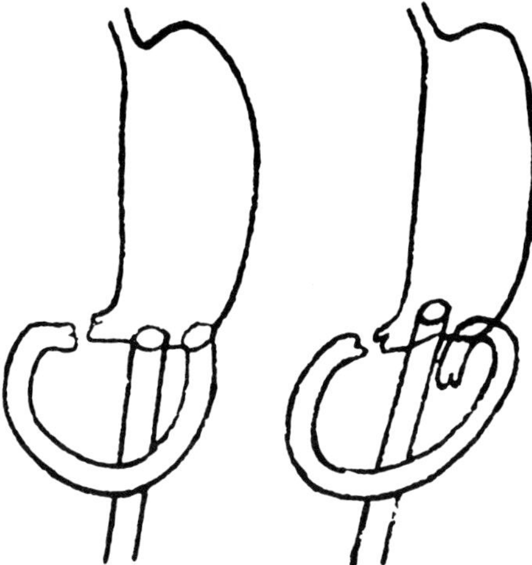

Fig. 1: Original drawing of Schmilinsky's operation to direct the duodenal contents through the stomach. Reproduced with permission from [3].

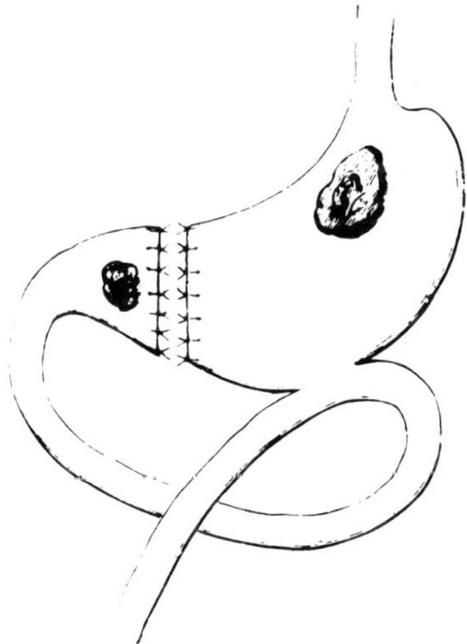

Fig. 2: Original drawing of von Eiselberg's antral exclusion operation for unresectable pyloric stenosis. Reproduced with permission from [3].

forced to treat patients, mainly for so-called absolute indications, and they did their best, but this was not necessarily what turned out to be the best. One should, however, refrain from criticism. If empiricism was further advanced than rational knowledge, it had to be transformed into therapeutic action as soon as it became available.

It was apparent to Charles Mayo that the means of helping the patient medically or surgically had far outstripped the knowledge of the cause of disease [8]. This dualism of empiricism and rationality extends to the present day, since patients require treatment, whether one can completely rationalize the approach used or not.

Present situation

To summarize the aims of ulcer surgery one has to distinguish acute from chronic ulcer disease, since each requires a different strategy.

Surgical strategy

In acute ulcer disease, it is essential that the intervention be well-timed. A short period of intensive preoperative preparation is as mandatory as the avoidance of undue delay.

Since it is the ulcer itself that makes an emergency procedure necessary, the primary goal of the operation is to attack the morphological lesion, be it by excision, closure, underrunning or another such procedure. Usually, this is the first step of the operation. But in the long run the procedure should eliminate the ulcer diathesis and prevent recurrences. There are a few exceptions to this rule, one being simple closure of a perforation in a patient with no previous ulcer history.

In chronic ulcer disease, the order of priorities is different. An elective procedure requires careful preparation of the patient and the exclusion of contraindications, assuming that the indication to operate has been thoroughly evaluated and validated.

The primary strategic goal of an elective operation is to cure ulcer disease. This does not necessarily imply dealing with the ulcer itself, since this is merely the morphological substrate of disturbed function. Instead, the operation is primarily directed against structures that control function. The aim is to install a new balance that leaves the patient ulcer-free.

This goal should be attained with the least possible interference with unrelated functions, in other words with minimal side effects. This is obviously true for all kinds of therapy, but is especially true in surgery, since side effects may assume the magnitude of diseases in their own right.

The risk of mortality following surgery is difficult to evaluate, but some points seem clear: there is no operation which carries no risk of patient death; everything possible must be done to minimize this risk, including implementation of lesser procedures; the risk for the individual patient is not calculable, since operations are performed on individual patients and not on randomized groups; and one should not strive for the unattainable, that is for zero mortality, since this would mean abstaining from operating altogether, and thus denying the patient the possible benefit of surgery.

Indications for surgery

Indications for surgery have commonly been subdivided into absolute and relative indications. These terms are now obsolete, since there is virtually no manifestation of ulcer disease that cannot be handled in some cases by nonsurgical means. It is only in large groups of patients that the risk-benefit ratio is in favor of the one or the other modality. Perforation can be treated in the elderly, debilitated patient conservatively, and the same holds true for most complications formerly regarded as absolute. But it can be difficult in the individual situation to transpose data gained from prospective or retrospective studies to a given patient.

Surgical procedures

Schwarz was indisputably right when he wrote in 1910: 'Ohne sauren Magensaft kein peptisches Geschwür', which, translated epigrammatically, means 'No acid, no ulcer' [9].

It seems only rational, therefore, that acid be reduced by decreasing the number of parietal cells, by eliminating humoral stimulation from the antrum and/or by sectioning the vagal nerves. The only question that remains is how this should be done, in what combination, and how much of it is necessary to start off with.

Motility is the other side of the coin. Acid-pepsin secretion has received much, maybe too much, attention in the past. However, 'the rate at which the corrosive juice is delivered to susceptible tissues is also a key factor in the development of ulceration' [10]. It seems essential to find again a synthesis between purely secretory and motility aspects of ulcerogenesis and to regard the ulcer as the net result of disturbed coordination between secretion and motility. If both delayed and accelerated emptying can lead to the formation of ulcers, both abnormalities should be amenable to surgery when looking for the rational basis of an operation.

It is generally agreed that gastric stasis should be corrected if present and responsible for ulcer formation. This can be done by either bypassing the gastric outlet, enlarging it by a plastic procedure, or by removing it. This, however, incurs the risk of duodenogastric reflux, with all its undesirable sequelae. A preventive procedure must therefore be performed at the same time; a discussion of the technicalities will not be given here.

A gastric denervating procedure that spares the antrum will have quite different effects. Highly selective vagotomy should be regarded as antral-saving vagotomy where gastric motility is concerned.

It is surprising to realize for how long the pylorus has been regarded as being merely a ring-like structure at the end of the stomach. Many surgical strategies were based on this concept, such as the procedure of cutting it lengthwise and suturing it transversely, which is called pyloroplasty. Actually, the pylorus proper is only part of a rather complex structure comprising the whole of the antrum and closely connected to its neighboring structures.

When looking at the gastric musculature in a cleared specimen, it is quite obvious that the pyloric ring is situated obliquely and forms only the end of a segment starting at the angular incisure where the nerves of Latarjet intersect (Fig. 3). The peculiar structure of this segment becomes even more obvious when the essential features are abstracted in a diagram (Fig. 4). The whole of the antrum is a structural and functional entity, with its own nerve supply. It is encircled by spiraling muscle fibers that always contract together [11].

Comparative anatomy also shows that the antrum with the pylorus is a

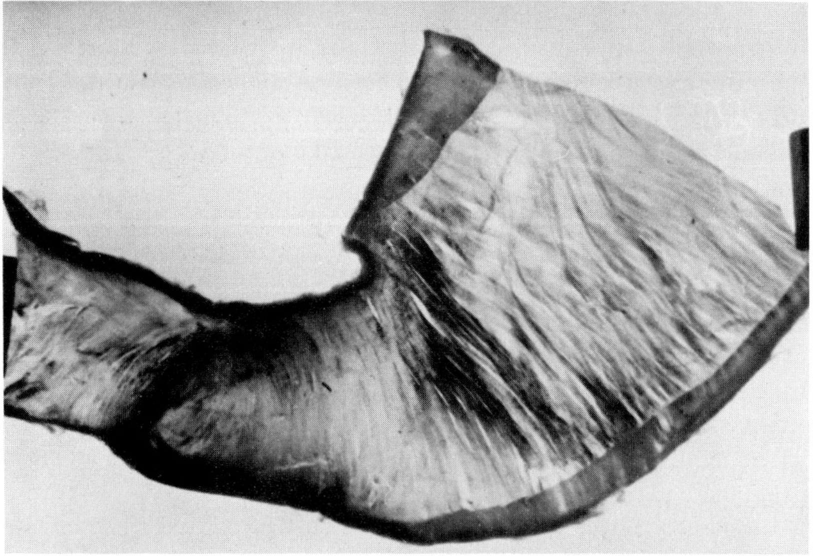

Fig. 3: Polarized view of gastric musculature in a cleared specimen, showing boundaries and structure of muscular antrum.

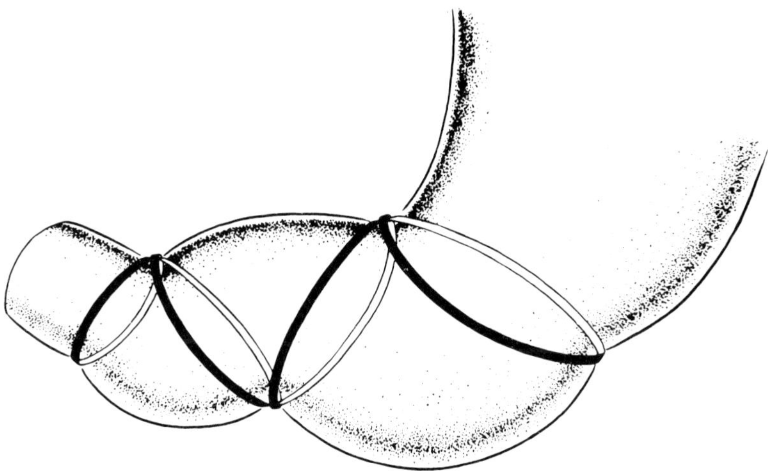

Fig. 4:   Diagram of functional muscular structure of human antrum.

segment in its own right. The simple-appearing human stomach contains all the elements of the rather complex stomach of ruminants (Fig. 5).

Where a rationale for ulcer surgery is concerned, the antrum and the pylorus should be respected for their importance in gastric motility. Obviously, this is the case when highly selective vagotomy is performed. The distal stomach plus the duodenum down to the papilla should be regarded as a functional entity. There is direct and circumstantial evidence of this, including the classification of gastric ulcers.

Conclusion

In conclusion it can be said that ulcer surgery, although having an empirical background, has now attained a high degree of rationality. Current procedures are based on a sound knowledge of their mode of action. Although designed for a disease of unknown cause, they selectively eliminate pathogenic principles responsible for the development of ulcers. There are surgical options for all types of ulcer manifestations.

The dualism of empiricism versus rationality will exist as long as the cause of a disease remains unknown. It can, however, be resolved by substituting wisdom for rationality which, according to William Mayo, can be gained by translating knowledge into proper action [12].

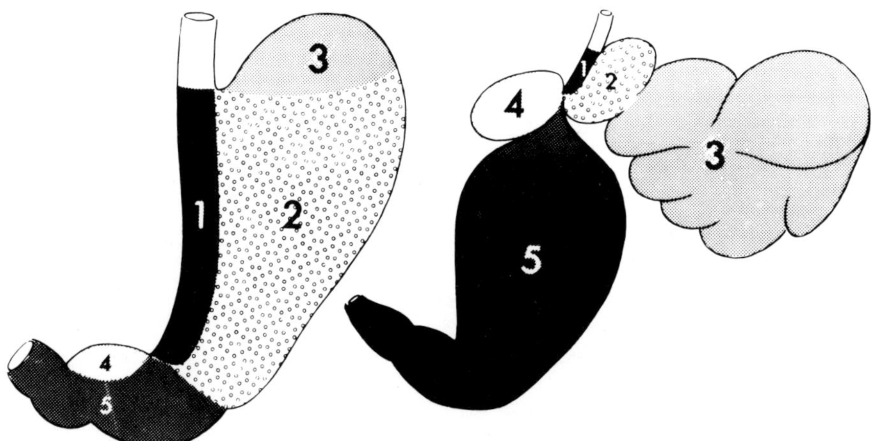

Fig. 5:   Homology of human and ruminant stomach: 1. ventricular groove — magenstrasse; 2. corpus — reticulum; 3. fundus — rumen; 4, 5. antrum — omasum/abomasum.

Summary

To define a rationale for surgical therapy in ulcer disease requires abstraction of the varied scale of ulcer operations as well as of the broad spectrum of ulcer manifestations. It must be kept in mind that the cause of ulcer disease is still unknown. This fact gives ulcer surgery an empirical background from which the various procedures have arisen, sometimes through trial and error. Some operations, although rightly claiming a rational basis at their time of origin since they were based on the then available knowledge, served to further elucidate the pathogenesis of ulcers due to their untoward effects. At present, surgical strategies can be formulated for various acute or chronic manifestations of ulcer disease. The tactical means available have a rational approach in that they reduce acid secretion and/or correct motility disturbances.

Acknowledgments

Figures 3, 4 and 5 are reproduced with permission from Farthmann, E.H. (1973): Die Faserstruktur des Muscularis propria des menschlichen Magens. In: *Gastorenterologie und Stoffwechsel*, Vol. 3, pp. 1–36. Thieme, Stuttgart.

References

1. J.B. Sykes (Ed.) (1976): *The Concise Oxford Dictionary of Current English*, 6th edition. Clarendon Press, Oxford.
2. Ogilvie, H. (1952): The surgery of peptic ulceration. *Br. Med. J. 2*, 299.
3. Schumpelick, V., Farthmann, E.H. and Schreiber, H.W. (1976): Chirurgie des Magens. *Med. Welt 27*, 2349 and 2440.
4. Rydygier, L. (1881): Die erste Magenresektion beim Magengeschwür. *Zentralbl. Chir. 9*, 190.
5. Schmilinsky, H. (1918): Die Einleitung der gesamten Duodenalsäfte in den Magen (innere Apotheke). *Zentralbl. Chir. 25*, 416.
6. Eiselsberg, A. von (1895): Über Ausschaltung inoperabler Pylorusstrikturen nebst Bemerkungen über die Jejunostomie. *Langenbecks Arch. Klin. Chir. 50*, 919.
7. Edkins, J.S. (1905): On the chemical mechanism of gastric secretion. *Proc. R. Soc. (London) Ser. B. Biol. Sci. 76*, 376.
8. Mayo, C.H. (1920): Surgery in the kidney. *Ann. Surg. 7*, 123.
9. Schwarz, K. (1910): Ueber penetrierende Magen- und Jejunalgeschwüre. *Brun's Beitr. Klin. Chir. 67*, 96.
10. Kelly, K.H. (1971): Gastric motility and ulcer surgery. *Surg. Clin. North Am. 51*, 927.
11. Farthmann, E.H. (1973): Die Faserstruktur des Muscularis propria des menschlichen Magens. In: *Gastroenterologie und Stoffwechsel*, Vol. 3, pp. 1–36. Eds: H. Bartelheimer, H.A. Kühn, V. Becker and F. Stelzner. Thieme, Stuttgart.
12. Mayo, W. (1920): American College of Surgeons, Annual Meeting October 20–24, 1919, Presidential Address. *Surg. Gynecol. Obstet. 30*, 98.

Effect of surgical procedures on gastric secretory and motor function*

K.A. Kelly

Section of Gastroenterologic and General Surgery, Mayo Clinic, Rochester, Minnesota, U.S.A.

Two general types of operations are being employed currently in the surgical treatment of gastroduodenal peptic ulcer; viz., vagotomy and gastric resection. Each type has specific effects on gastric secretion and motility.

Vagotomy

Three varieties of vagotomy are in use today: proximal gastric vagotomy, total gastric vagotomy, and truncal vagotomy. In proximal gastric vagotomy the vagal branches to the gastric fundus and corpus are divided, while those to the antrum and pylorus (the nerves of Latarjet) and to the remaining abdominal viscera are left intact. Total gastric vagotomy consists of division of all the vagal nerves to the stomach, but not those to the other abdominal viscera. In truncal vagotomy not only the vagal nerves to the stomach are divided, but those to all other abdominal viscera are severed as well. The latter 2 vagotomies are usually combined with a so-called 'drainage' operation, such as pyloroplasty or gastroenterostomy. In contrast, proximal gastric vagotomy does not require any additional operative procedure.

Proximal gastric vagotomy

Gastric secretion – HCl Proximal gastric vagotomy interrupts the extrinsic vagal drive to the oxyntic cells and so decreases gastric output of HCl. Vagal nerve impulses originating in the central nervous system as a result of the anticipation, sight, smell, and taste of food ordinarily bring about stimulation

* Supported in part by USPHS NIH Grant AM18278. K.A. Kelly is the Roberts Professor of Surgery, Mayo Medical School, Rochester, Minnesota, U.S.A.

of gastric secretion, the so-called cephalic phase of gastric secretion [1]. These neural impulses never reach the oxyntic cells after proximal gastric vagotomy. Proximal gastric vagotomy also interrupts reflexes originating in the proximal stomach (oxynto-oxyntic reflexes) or distal stomach (pyloro-oxyntic reflexes) that augment gastric secretion [2, 3]. Moreover, the vagotomy results in a decreased responsiveness of the oxyntic cells to other stimuli such as histamine and gastrin. Acetylcholine potentiates the response of the oxyntic cells to histamine and gastrin. Division of the vagal nerves impairs the release of acetylcholine from postganglionic neurons, and so decreases the response to the other first messengers.

The net result of proximal gastric vagotomy on HCl secretion is a decrease in basal acid output of about 90% and a decrease in betazole or pentagastrin-stimulated output of about 50% (Fig. 1). These effects appear immediately after the operation, and persist for years, although there is some slight recovery over time [4, 5].

Gastric secretion – pepsinogen Proximal gastric vagotomy decreases the amount of pepsinogen secreted. In one study, pepsinogen secretion decreased greater than 2-fold in response to pentagastrin stimulation [6], while in another study the secretion in response to insulin-induced hypoglycemia decreased 9-fold [7]. The decreased secretion of pepsinogen, combined with

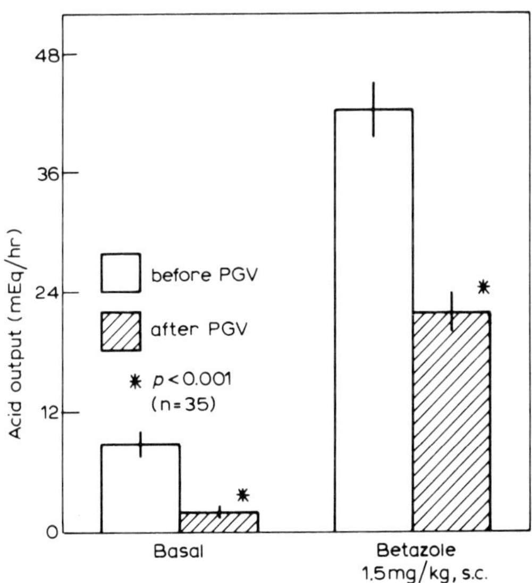

Fig. 1:   Effect of proximal gastric vagotomy (PGV) on basal and betazole-stimulated gastric secretion of HCl. Reproduced with permission from [4].

the lessened output of acid, reduces markedly the corrosive properties of gastric juice.

Gastric secretion – gastrin   The 'G' cell population in the antrum increases after proximal gastric vagotomy. Not only are greater numbers of 'G' cells found, but the mean tissue concentration of gastrin within the antrum, as determined by radioimmunoassay, is greater than in control stomachs [8]. The concentration of gastrin in the serum during fasting and after eating is also greater after proximal gastric vagotomy (Table) [9]. The mechanism for the increased basal and postprandial serum gastrin is not known, but may be related to a lack of suppression of antral release of gastrin by acid. Acid bathing the antrum ordinarily blocks the release of gastrin by the 'G' cells. After proximal gastric vagotomy, less acid is secreted, and so acid inhibition of antral release of gastrin may not occur. Other explanations for the increased serum gastrin after proximal gastric vagotomy might be impaired secretion of a hormonal inhibitor of gastrin release or the disruption of vagal inhibition of gastrin release.

Gastric motility – proximal stomach   Proximal gastric vagotomy abolishes gastric receptive relaxation and impairs accommodation and storage in the proximal stomach. The proximal stomach of healthy subjects relaxes with the onset of swallowing and prior to the entrance of the bolus of food from the esophagus into the stomach. This receptive relaxation is mediated via the vagal nerves [10], and is abolished by proximal gastric vagotomy.

Accommodation to distention is also impaired by proximal gastric vagotomy. Accommodation is that property of the proximal stomach that

Table: Effect of vagotomy on serum gastrin.

Vagotomy	Serum gastrin (pg/ml)	
	Basal	45-min post protein meal
Before	10	90
After		
Proximal gastric	46	170
Total gastric + pyloroplasty	50	120
Total abdominal + pyloroplasty	84	230

Reproduced with permission from [9].

allows it to adapt to distention without greatly increasing intragastric pressure. Accommodation is, in part, vagally mediated [11, 12]. After proximal gastric vagotomy, intragastric pressure increases to larger values with gastric distention compared to before vagotomy (Fig. 2). As a consequence, the ability of the stomach to store chyme is diminished.

The loss of receptive relaxation and the impaired ability to accommodate and store food after proximal gastric vagotomy result in a feeling of easy fullness and gastric distention during eating among patients who have had the operation. These complaints improve with time, but persist to some extent indefinitely.

The larger increases in intragastric pressure that occur with gastric filling lead to more rapid gastric emptying of liquids in the period immediately after their ingestion. The rate of emptying of liquids is ordinarily carefully controlled to facilitate digestion and absorption in the small intestine. The rate (dv/dt) depends on the gradient between the pressure in the stomach (P_S) and that in the duodenum (P_D), and varies with the resistance to flow across the pylorus (R_P):

$$dv/dt = \frac{P_S - P_D}{R_P}.$$

With larger increases in intragastric pressure during gastric filling after vagotomy, the gradient is larger and the rate of emptying faster [11, 13].

The more rapid emptying of liquids after proximal gastric vagotomy is not

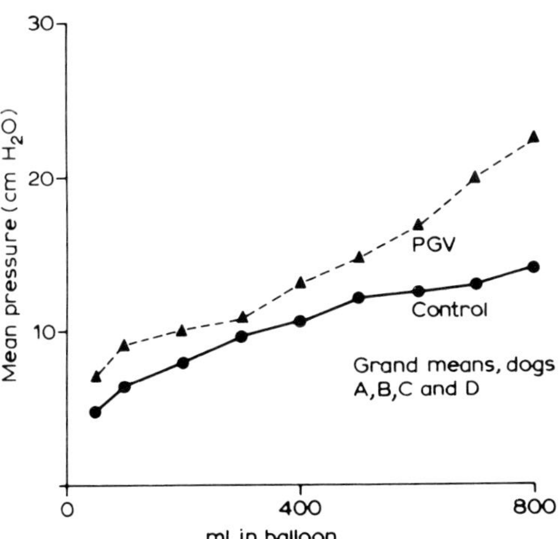

Fig. 2:   Effect of proximal gastric vagotomy on the canine gastric pressure-volume response. Reproduced with permission from [12].

only due to disturbed receptive relaxation and accommodation. The ability of gastrin and probably other hormones to relax the proximal stomach and so decrease intragastric pressure and the rate of gastric emptying is also impaired after proximal gastric vagotomy [14]. Moreover, the negative feedback from small intestinal receptors to the stomach that slows gastric emptying via neural pathways is also disturbed. The stomach empties more rapidly in the upright position after vagotomy than in the supine position, probably because the neural inhibition of the gravitationally-induced rapid gastric emptying in the upright position is not as effective postvagotomy [15]. Fortunately, the rate of gastric emptying after proximal gastric vagotomy is seldom great enough to result in dumping and/or diarrhea in patients undergoing the operation.

Gastric motility – distal stomach   Proximal gastric vagotomy does not greatly disturb the oral corporeal gastric pacemaker or the distal propagation of the cyclic changes in potential generated by the pacemaker. The cyclic changes in potential still appear at a frequency of about 3 cycles/minute, and the cycles are still propagated in a distal direction [16]. Moreover, the strength of antral peristaltic contractions is likely not greatly altered. Gastric trituration and emptying of digestible solids and gastric emptying of indigestible solids are normal [11, 13]. Also, duodenal-gastric reflux, and, hence, nausea, bilious vomiting, and alkaline gastritis, are rarely found after proximal gastric vagotomy. The distal gastric and pyloric mechanisms that maintain gastric continence for solids and prevent duodenal-gastric reflex are not impaired by the operation.

Total gastric vagotomy and truncal vagotomy

Gastric secretion – HCl and pepsinogen   Total gastric vagotomy and truncal vagotomy have effects on gastric secretion of HCl and pepsinogen which are similar to those found after proximal gastric vagotomy. Basal and post-stimulation secretion of HCl are decreased to a similar extent by these operations and proximal gastric vagotomy [17].

Gastric secretion – gastrin   The 'G' cell population is also increased by dividing the vagal innervation to the entire stomach, just as after division of the vagal nerves to the proximal stomach [18, 19]. There are more 'G' cells identified in the antral mucosa by immunofluorescent staining techniques after truncal vagotomy compared to before the vagotomy. Moreover, the amount of immunoreactive gastrin in the antral mucosa is increased after truncal vagotomy, although the density index of the G-cell granules in the 'G' cells is decreased. Increases in both basal and postprandial concentrations of gastrin in the serum are also found after the more extensive vagotomies, just as after proximal gastric vagotomy (Table). The cephalic phase of gastrin secretion, which is disputed after total gastric vagotomy, is apparently not required for basal or postprandial gastrin secretion.

Gastric motility – proximal stomach   Total gastric and truncal vagotomy have effects on proximal gastric motility similar to those found after proximal gastric vagotomy. Receptive relaxation, accommodation, and storage is impaired, increases in intragastric pressure with distention are greater, and gastric emptying of liquids more rapid [11].

Gastric motility – distal stomach   In contrast to proximal gastric vagotomy, total gastric and truncal vagotomy weaken the strength of distal gastric peristalsis, impair trituration, and markedly slow gastric emptying of solid food. In fact, gastric emptying of solid food is so slow after total gastric and truncal vagotomy, that symptoms of bloating, nausea, vomiting, and a feeling of gastric fullness often appear.

Indigestible solids are also emptied poorly after the total gastric vagotomies. Materials left over after meals, such as indigestible fiber, are ordinarily emptied by cyclically recurring bursts of indigestive contractions that appear in the stomach at about 2-hour intervals during fasting [20]. The vagal nerves have a role in regulating these cycles. After truncal vagotomy, the cycles are more irregular in rhythm, the periods are shorter, and the bursts of contractions briefer or even absent [21, 22]. As a consequence, gastric emptying of debris left over after a meal is slowed or abolished. Patients may note that indigestible portions of foods can be regurgitated from the stomach days after their ingestion.

The gastric stasis for digestible and indigestible solids after total gastric or truncal vagotomy requires an additional operative maneuver designed to speed gastric emptying. Pyloroplasty and gastroenterostomy have been the 2 procedures usually employed in this situation. They decrease resistance to outflow from the stomach and so usually speed gastric emptying of solids [23]. Unfortunately, the uncontrolled speeding in gastric emptying they produce can lead to dumping and diarrhea. Moreover, the bypass or destruction of the pylorus they entail sometimes results in small intestinal-gastric reflux with its attendant nausea, belching, bilious vomiting, and alkaline gastritis [24].

Gastric resection

Two types of gastric resection are being employed as surgical therapies for gastroduodenal peptic ulcer. The first type consists of resection of the distal stomach and pylorus with either gastroduodenal or gastrojejunal reconstruction. The resection includes the pylorus, all of the antrum and a variable portion of the gastric corpus, depending on the intent of the resection. The second type of resection preserves the pylorus and the distal 1.5 cm of antrum, while excising the remaining antrum and a portion of the gastric corpus. Reconstruction is by an end-to-end gastrogastrostomy. This procedure has been called the 'pylorus-preserving' gastrectomy [25].

Subtotal distal gastrectomy

Gastric secretion – HCl   Gastric secretion of HCl is decreased after subtotal distal gastric resection by 2 main mechanisms. The resection of the antrum removes a major source of gastrin and so reduces the gastrin drive of the oxyntic cells. Gastrin not only stimulates the oxyntic cells to produce acid, but it also exerts a trophic effect on the gastric mucosa that enhances the ability of the cells to produce the acid [26]. In addition, the withdrawal of gastrin, like the withdrawal of acetylcholine after vagotomy, decreases the sensitivity of the cells to the other first messengers of gastric secretion. Distal gastric resection also removes oxyntic cells, the quantity removed depending on the proximal extent of the resection. The more proximal the resection, the more acid-secreting cells are removed, and the greater is the resulting postoperative decrease in acid secretion.

The overall net effect of distal gastric resection is to reduce gastric secretion of HCl by about 75% in the resting stomach and about 50% in the stimulated stomach, effects similar to those after the vagotomies.

Gastric secretion – pepsinogen   Subtotal distal gastric resection decreases the output of pepsinogen by the stomach. Pepsinogens are produced both in the antrum and the corpus, so that removal of the antrum and a portion of the corpus lessen the capacity of the stomach to secrete pepsinogens.

Gastric secretion – gastrin   Distal subtotal gastrectomy excises a major source of gastrin production. The concentration of gastrin in the serum is lower after the operation, providing the reconstruction of gastrointestinal continuity after the gastrectomy is via gastrojejunostomy [17]. However, basal and postprandial serum gastrins are changed little after subtotal distal gastric resection when reconstruction is via gastroduodenostomy and truncal vagotomy is also done [17]. Apparently, enough gastrin is released from duodenal 'G' cells in the basal and postprandial period with the gastroduodenal reconstruction to compensate for the loss of antral gastrin production and release. The duodenal source is bypassed with gastrojejunostomy.

Gastric motility – proximal stomach   Proximal gastric motility is changed little after small distal gastric resections. Receptive relaxation, accommodation, and storage are not much impaired, and intragastric pressure is still satisfactorily regulated. The rate of gastric emptying of liquids is not greatly altered [27]. The slight speeding that does occur may be related to some decrease in gastric resistance to outflow after the distal gastric resection. With larger resections of the distal stomach, however, accommodation and storage are impaired, and liquids are emptied rapidly [28, 29]. The loss of inhibition of proximal gastric contractions brought about by gastrin in those patients with resection of the entire antrum and gastrojejunostomy likely contributes to the more rapid gastric emptying.

Gastric motility – distal stomach   Antral trituration of solids is abolished after both small and more extensive distal subtotal gastrectomies, and solids empty prematurely and rapidly from the stomach (Fig. 3) [23, 27, 28]. Such rapid emptying sometimes results in dumping and diarrhea. The loss of the gastroduodenal junction also destroys the distal gastric mechanism preventing

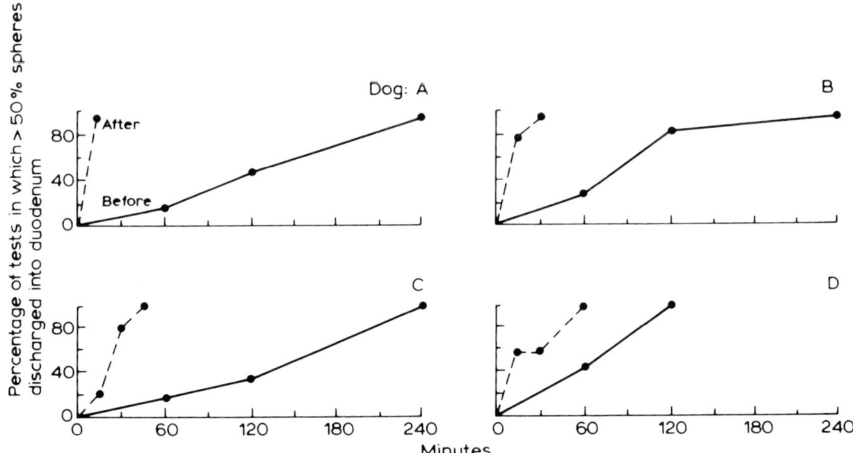

Fig. 3:   Effect of distal antrectomy on canine gastric emptying of 15 solid spheres 1 cm in diameter inserted at time 0. Reproduced with permission from [27].

duodenal-gastric reflux. Small intestinal content readily enters the stomach after the operation and can sometimes produce belching, nausea, vomiting and alkaline gastritis.

Pylorus-preserving gastrectomy

Gastric secretion   Pylorus-preserving gastrectomy has an effect on gastric secretion of HCl similar to that of subtotal distal gastrectomy [30]. The influence of the operation on the secretion of pepsinogen and gastrin has as yet not been reported.

Gastric motility   Pylorus-preserving gastrectomy has motor advantages over distal gastric resection, in that gastric continence for solids is maintained by preserving the gastroduodenal junction. Moreover, duodenal-gastric reflux is uncommon after the operation, again because the pylorus is preserved. However, gastric trituration of solids is impaired by the resection of the antral grinding mechanism. As a consequence, gastric emptying of solids is slow. Some have reported no evidence of clinical gastric stasis after the operation [25], but others have raised this concern [31].

Combined vagotomy and resection

Combining vagotomy and distal gastric resection produces alterations in gastric secretion and motility that are a net result of the 2 procedures. Gastric secretion of HCl and pepsinogen are decreased to levels even greater than those found with either procedure alone [17]. The net effect on serum gastrin is midway between the increase caused by the vagotomy and the decrease resulting from the resection. Both proximal gastric and distal gastric motor functions are impaired [31]. Patients may have easy filling, bloating, and rapid emptying of liquids from proximal gastric motor alterations, as well as rapid emptying of solids and small intestinal-gastric reflux from distal gastric motor alterations. Symptoms suggestive of gastric motor disturbances occur in about 25% of patients [24].

Summary

Both vagotomy and gastric resection decrease the secretion of acid and pepsinogen by the stomach. Vagotomy also increases the serum gastrin, but gastric resection does not. Both vagotomy and resection speed gastric emptying of liquids, but only proximal gastric vagotomy preserves gastric emptying of solids and the barricade to duodenal-gastric reflux.

References

1. Pavlov, I.P. (1902): *Work of the Digestive Glands*. Translated by W.H. Thompson. Charles Griffin, London.
2. Grossman, M.I. (1962): Secretion of acid and pepsin in response to distention of vagally innervated fundic gland area in dogs. *Gastroenterology 42*, 718.
3. Debas, H.T., Konturek, S.J., Walsh, J.H. and Grossman, M.I. (1974): Proof of a pyloro-oxyntic reflex for stimulation of acid secretion. *Gastroenterology 66*, 526.
4. van Heerden, J.A., Kelly, K.A., Dozois, R.R. et al. (1980): Proximal gastric vagotomy. Initial experience. *Mayo Clin. Proc. 55*, 10.
5. Johnston, D., Wilkinson, A.R., Humphrey, C.S. et al. (1973): Serial studies of gastric secretion in patients after highly selective (parietal cell) vagotomy without a drainage procedure for duodenal ulcer. I. Effect of highly selective vagotomy on basal and Pentagastrin-stimulated maximal acid output. *Gastroenterology 64*, 1.
6. Roland, M., Berstad, A. and Liavag, I. (1974): Acid and pepsin secretion in duodenal ulcer patients in response to graded doses of pentagastrin or pentagastrin and carbacholine before and after proximal gastric vagotomy. *Scand. J. Gastroenterol. 9*, 511.
7. Hallenbeck, G.A. and Gleysteen, J. (1974): Proximal gastric vagotomy without 'drainage': an experimental study. *Ann. Surg. 179*, 608.
8. Dunn, D.H., Decanini, C., Bonsack, M.E. et al. (1979): Gastrin cell populations after highly selective vagotomy in the dog. *Am. J. Surg. 137*, 111.
9. Hansky, J. and Korman, M. (1973): Immunoassay studies in peptic ulcer. *Clin. Gastroenterol. 2*, 275.
10. Cannon, W.B. and Lieb, C.M. (1911): The receptive relaxation of the stomach. *Am. J. Physiol. 29*, 270.
11. Wilbur, B.G. and Kelly, K.A. (1973): Effect of proximal gastric, complete gastric, and truncal vagotomy on canine gastric electric activity, motility and emptying. *Ann. Surg. 178*, 295.
12. Kelly, K.A. (1974): Gastric motility after gastric operations. *Surg. Annu. 6*, 103.
13. Lavigne, M.E., Wiley, Z.D., Martin, P., Vay, L.W., Meyer, J.H., Sleisenger, M.H. and MacGregor, I.L. (1979): Gastric, pancreatic and biliary secretion and the rate of gastric emptying after parietal cell vagotomy. *Am. J. Surg. 138*, 644.
14. Okike, N. and Kelly, K.A. (1977): Vagotomy impairs pentagastrin-induced relaxation of the canine gastric fundus. *Am. J. Physiol. 1*, E504.
15. McKelvey, S.T.D. (1970): Gastric incontinence and postvagotomy diarrhea. *Br. J. Surg. 57*, 741.
16. Hinder, R.A. and Kelly, K.A. (1977): Human gastric pacesetter potential. Site of origin, spread and response to gastric transection and proximal gastric vagotomy. *Am. J. Surg. 133*, 29.
17. Thompson, J.C., Fender, H.R., Villar, H.V. and Watson, L.C. (1977): The effects of gastrin and gastric secretion of five current operations for duodenal ulcer. *Gastroentrology 72*, 825.
18. Becker, H.D., Arnold, R., Boerger, H.W. et al. (1977): Influence of truncal vagotomy on serum and antral gastrin and G-cells. *Gastroenterology 72*, 811.
19. Dunn, D.H., Decanini, C.O., Eisenberg, M.M. et al. (1979): Mechanism for gastrin cell hyperplasia after truncal vagotomy. *Surg. Forum 30*, 376.

20. Mroz, C.T. and Kelly, K.A. (1977): The role of the extrinsic antral nerves in the regulation of gastric emptying. *Surg. Gynecol. Obstet. 145*, 369.
21. Marik, F. and Code, C.F. (1975): Control of the interdigestive myoelectric activity in dogs by the vagus nerves and pentagastrin. *Gastroenterology 69*, 387.
22. Diamant, N.E., Mui, H., El-Sharkawy, T.Y. and Hall, K. (1979): The vagus controls the lower esophageal sphincter and gastric components of the migrating motor complex in the dog. *Gastroenterology 76*, 1122.
23. MacGregor, I.L., Martin, P. and Meyer, J.H. (1977): Gastric emptying of solid food in normal man and after subtotal gastrectomy and truncal vagotomy with pyloroplasty. *Gastroenterology 72*, 206.
24. Goligher, J.C., Pulvertaft, C.N., DeDombal, F.T. et al. (1968): Five- to eight-year results of Leeds/York controlled trial of elective surgery for duodenal ulcer. *Br. Med. J. 2*, 781.
25. Maki, T., Shiratori, T., Hatafuku, T. and Sugawara, K. (1967): Pylorus-preserving gastrectomy as an improved operation for gastric ulcer. *Surgery 61*, 838.
26. Johnson, L.R. (1977): New aspects of the trophic action of gastrointestinal hormones. *Gastroenterology 72*, 788.
27. Dozois, R.R., Kelly, K.A. and Code, C.F. (1971): Effect of distal antrectomy on gastric emptying of liquids and solids. *Gastroenterology 61*, 675.
28. Heading, R.C., Tothill, P., McLaughlin, G.P. and Shearman, D.J.C. (1976): Gastric emptying rate measurement in man. A double isotopic scanning technique for simultaneous study of liquid and solid components of a meal. *Gastroenterology 71*, 45.
29. MacGregor, I., Parent, J. and Meyer, J.H. (1977): Gastric emptying of liquid meals and pancreatic and biliary secretion after subtotal gastrectomy or truncal vagotomy and pyloroplasty in man. *Gastroenterology 72*, 195.
30. Hennessy, T.P.J., Weir, D.G. and D'Auria, D. (1972): Pylorus-preserving gastrectomy in the treatment of duodenal ulcer. *Br. J. Surg. 59*, 27.
31. Isono, K. and Kelly, K.A. (1979): Proximal gastric vagotomy and suprapyloric antrectomy: experimental evaluation in the dog. *Arch. Surg. 114*, 623.

Surgical options for the treatment of duodenal ulcer disease

D. Johnston
University Department of Surgery, The General Infirmary, Leeds, England

I do not intend to discuss the indications for surgical treatment, except to say that these remain the failure of medical treatment or the occurrence of severe complications such as hemorrhage, perforation or pyloric stenosis.

The 3 traditional, or 'standard' options for the treatment of duodenal ulcer were a two-thirds Polya (type) partial gastrectomy (PG), truncal vagotomy (TV) combined with either antrectomy or hemigastrectomy (TV + A) and finally TV and pyloroplasty or gastroenterostomy (TV + P; TV + GJ). Each of these 3 modalities of treatment has its fervent advocates. Since each has been in use for at least 20 years we have available many excellent clinical assessments of their value. Of particular importance are the prospective randomized controlled trials, such as those organized by Goligher et al. in Leeds and York [1–3], by Jordan and Condon [4] and the Veterans Administration (VA) study reported by Postlethwait [5] (See Tables I and II). The results of these controlled trials have shown that TV with a drainage (D) procedure does not yield better clinical results in the long term than the results obtained after PG or TV + A. In fact, in both the Leeds-York trial and the VA study, gastric resection, with or without TV, emerged as slightly, though

Table I: Results of Leeds-York trials. Visick gradings 5–8 years after operation for duodenal ulcer.

Visick grade	TV + GJ (% of 119)	TV + A (% of 116)	Polya 2/3 (% of 107)	TV + P (% of 164)
1. Perfect	44 ⎫ 70	50 ⎫ 78	49 ⎫ 77	45 ⎫ 68
2. Very good	26 ⎭	28 ⎭	28 ⎭	23 ⎭
3. Fair	19	14	17	18
4. Poor	11	8	6	14

Table II: Veterans   Administration   Study.   Five-year   results   of   operations   for duodenal ulcer.

	TV + P/GJ	TV + A	PG
Number of patients	337	674	346
Operative mortality (%)	0.6	0.8	1.8
Recurrent ulceration (%)	7	2	5
Overall results good-excellent (%)	84	90	90

Recurrence: TV + P, 10%; TV + GJ, 6%; TV + BI, 4% and RV + BII, 1%.

not significantly, superior to TV + D after 5–10 years of follow-up. For example, after both TV + GJ and TV + P in Leeds, only about 70% of patients were judged to have achieved good or excellent clinical results after 5–8 years' follow-up, whereas, after PG or TV + A approximately 80% of patients had achieved good or excellent results (Visick grades I and II). Similarly in the VA study, about 90% of patients had good or excellent results after resection with or without TV compared with about 84% after TV + D. I would like to make it perfectly clear that I do not deduce from these results that PG is a better operation to offer a patient with a duodenal ulcer than TV + D, for 2 reasons. The first is that the operative mortality of gastric resection averages between 1 and 2% whereas the operative mortality of TV + D is about 0.7%. In other words the operative risk of TV + D is half that of PG. The other reason is that even these excellent prospective trials have their weaknesses and one is that they do not go on for long enough to tell us in detail about the long-term nutritional disadvantages of PG, which are almost certainly greater than those of TV + D.

Furthermore, there is good evidence that in the very long term, PG predisposes to the development of gastric carcinoma, whereas there is no convincing evidence as yet that there is any increased risk of gastric carcinoma after TV + D. For these reasons, I think that the merits of PG are approximately the same as those of TV + D and I would find it difficult to say which was the better option for a patient with a duodenal ulcer. As will be seen, however, I think that both these procedures are now outmoded, excessively radical and should not be used in the elective surgical treatment of patients with duodenal ulcer.

Selective vagotomy

In selective vagotomy (SV) the hepatic and celiac vagal fibers are carefully preserved but the stomach itself is completely deprived of its vagal innervation from cardia to pylorus. This means that the nerves of Latarjet to the antral region are cut so that the 'antral mill' is deprived of its motor nerve supply, loses its propulsive power and gastric stasis ensues unless P or GJ is added. A number of surgeons, notably Burge, Kirk, Kennedy and Alexander-Williams have experimented with the use of SV without D, but although some patients did well, an unacceptably high proportion developed gastric retention and sometimes gastric ulceration followed. Thus SV must always be complemented by D of some sort.

The claims made for SV by its proponents, such as Burge in Britain and Griffith in the United States, were that by its greater precision it led to a more complete gastric vagotomy and hence to a lower incidence of recurrent ulceration than was found after TV + D, that it decreased the incidence of postvagotomy diarrhea and finally that it was likely to yield better overall clinical results than the standard operative procedures. These claims have been subjected to careful scientific scrutiny by means of controlled trials [6, 7], and the following conclusions have been reached.

Firstly, there is absolutely no doubt that the use of SV rather than TV significantly diminishes the incidence of postvagotomy diarrhea. After TV + D, the incidence is about 20% and after SV + D it is about 10%. Diarrhea of such severity as to be a social or occupational disadvantage occurs in 2–4% of patients after TV + D and in only about 1–2% of patients after SV + D. The claim that SV leads to a more complete vagotomy of the stomach is not convincingly supported by the evidence [8]. Admittedly, expert surgeons performing SV can achieve very low incidences of incomplete vagotomy and in consequence the incidences of recurrent ulceration in their series are low. On the other hand, we found in Leeds and Sheffield that the incidence of incomplete vagotomy after SV was as high as after TV and that after both types of vagotomy, there was a much stronger correlation with the individual surgeon performing the vagotomy than with the particular type of vagotomy that had been used [8]. This is also true for highly SV (HSV). In short, it is the surgeon doing the vagotomy rather than the type of vagotomy which determines the completeness of the vagal denervation.

As for the overall clinical results of SV + D, they have not been shown to be convincingly better than those of TV + D. The long-term incidence of recurrent ulceration is about the same and the only real improvement is in the incidence of diarrhea. Indeed in some series the incidence of dumping is higher after SV + D than after TV + D.

The need for change

It will be seen therefore that neither TV + D nor SV + D yields clinical results after 5–10 years that are significantly better than those of PG. These were puzzling and surprising findings, which led one to speculate about the reasons for the comparatively disappointing results of vagotomy, which at the time of its reintroduction by Dragstedt and Owens had seemed such an attractive and physiological procedure. The obvious defect of both TV + D and SV + D was that they both destroyed or bypassed the pylorus, or more accurately the antropyloroduodenal segment, which controls gastric emptying and prevents regurgitation of duodenal content into the stomach. The main function of the stomach after all is to act as the hopper and the mill of the alimentary tract, and by denervating the antral mill and destroying the distal antrum and pylorus, vagotomy with P severely impaired the milling and grinding activities of the antral mill and led to poorly regulated gastric emptying. In particular, the stomach was rendered incontinent of liquids, as McKelvey first demonstrated [9].

It seemed therefore that if the results of gastric surgery for peptic ulcer were to be improved, it would be necessary to preserve the pylorus, and for this to be done it would also be necessary to preserve the motor nerve supply to several centimeters of prepyloric stomach. This led to a reconsideration by us in Leeds [10], and by Amdrup and Jensen in Copenhagen [11], of the earlier work in dogs by Griffith and Harkins in Seattle whereby a partial gastric vagotomy was performed in which the parietal cell mass was denervated but the antrum was left vagally innervated and the pylorus was kept intact [12]. By the late 1960's it seemed ethical to try the crucial test of preserving the vagal innervation of the gastric antrum in man, because the evidence that the antrum had to be vagally denervated was based on experiments performed in another species, the dog, and moreover not in dogs with the antrum in situ, in continuity with the acid stream from the body and fundus of the stomach, but in dogs in which the antrum was separated from the inhibitory action of endogenous HCl by some form of mucosal septum.

I would now like to compare and contrast the physiological effects of TV and HSV in man, give an account of our 11-year experience with HSV for duodenal ulcer at the Leeds General Infirmary and describe the results of some controlled trials in which unbiased comparison of this procedure has been made with the more traditional procedures.

Physiological comparison of HSV without a drainage procedure and TV + P or TV + GJ

Serum gastrin

At the physiological level, the crucial question was whether gastrin release from the innervated undrained antrum would be significantly greater than from the vagally denervated and 'drained' antrum. Before the advent of radioimmunoassay of gastrin, it had been assumed that vagal release of gastrin was important in man and that one of the major therapeutic benefits of TV or SV was to abolish such vagal release of gastrin. Now that we can measure gastrin levels, however, we find that all types of vagotomy lead to a significant increase in serum gastrin levels and that both fasting and food-stimulated gastrin levels are just as high or higher after TV as after HSV [13]. There is increasing evidence, too, that under certain circumstances the vagus may exert an inhibitory influence on gastrin release in man, while in dogs increasing degrees of vagotomy starting with HSV and going on through SV to TV lead to stepwise increases in acid output from Heidenhain pouches and increases in serum gastrin levels (Figs. 1 and 2; [14]).

It was always illogical to cut the hepatic and celiac vagal fibers when attempting to cure a duodenal ulcer. In 1980 it seems fair to conclude that it is also illogical to cut the vagal nerve supply to the antrum of the stomach. It is on that statement that the whole of gastric surgery for peptic ulcer depends, because if it is true, there is no need to destroy or bypass the pylorus, and if that is so, the traditional side effects of gastric surgery, dumping, diarrhea and bilious vomiting, can be almost abolished.

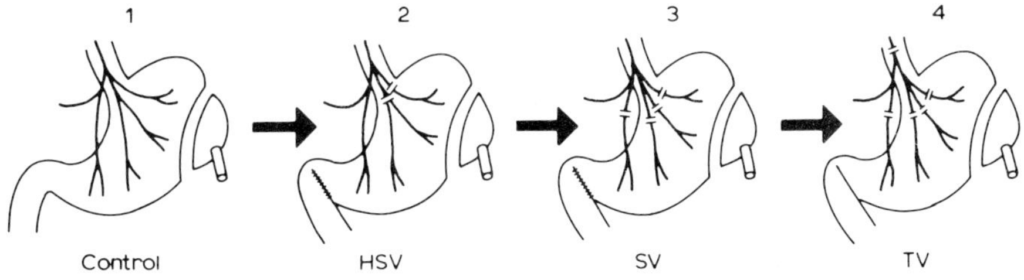

Fig. 1: Experimental preparation in dogs subjected to increasing degrees of vagotomy. The Finney P prevented gastric stasis. Reproduced with permission from [14].

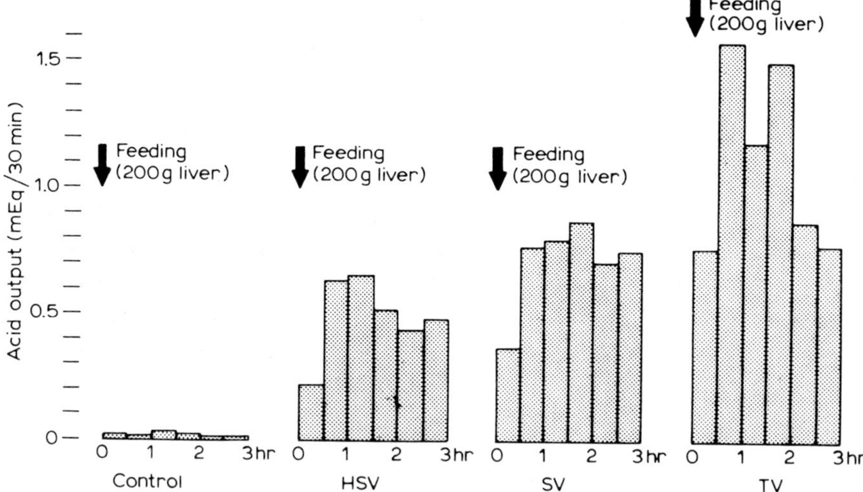

Fig. 2: Stepwise increases in Heidenhain pouch acid output as increasing numbers of vagal fibers are cut. Since antral stasis was avoided by the use of a P, the results provide evidence for vagal inhibition of gastric secretion.

Gastric secretion [15, 16]

Basal acid output (BAO) is reduced by about 80%, 5 years after HSV. This reduction in BAO is at least as great as that produced by TV or SV + D.

HSV reduces maximal acid output (MAO) by about 50% in the long term. This is approximately the same reduction as is achieved by SV + D and slightly less than the 55–60% long-term reduction after TV + D.

Insulin response [16]

Before vagotomy, peak acid response to insulin (PAO^I) minus BAO is about 30 mmol/hour in duodenal ulcer patients. One week after either HSV or TV + D, PAO^I is nil. At least, it is nil if the vagotomy has been expertly performed, but in practice the surgeon's performance is less than ideal, with the result that between 5 and 50% of patients have a Hollander-positive response to insulin one week after vagotomy. This has an important bearing on their subsequent clinical progress, because if the acid response is a large one, the chances that the patient will develop a recurrent ulcer are much higher than if there is no response at all. It is difficult to give exact figures but if there is absolutely no response to insulin one week after either type of vagotomy, the incidence of recurrent ulceration in the long term is about

2–3%, whereas if there is a large secretory response (PAO^I greater than 5 mmol/hour) the incidence of recurrence after both HSV and TV + D is between 10 and 30%. Intermediate degrees of incomplete vagotomy will lead to intermediate incidences of recurrent ulceration. Thus it is simplistic in the extreme to talk of a Hollander insulin test as 'positive' or 'negative'. As Grossman has said, it is about as useful as expressing the blood glucose as positive or negative. The key question is, how great is the response? Hence the importance of the surgeon's role in achieving a complete vagotomy of the parietal cell mass cannot be overemphasized. In this regard, it may well be that HSV is a less forgiving operative procedure than TV, because if the parietal cell mass retains some vagal innervation and the antrum also remains innervated, the patient may be at particularly high risk of developing a recurrent ulcer. Nonetheless, as will be seen, the long term incidences of recurrence after HSV and after TV + D are similar.

If the insulin test is repeated more than one year after HSV or TV + D, the incidence of positive responses is much greater than one week after operation. Between 40 and 80% of patients are then Hollander-positive but in most of them the actual amount of acid secreted is quite small, averaging about 4 mmol/hour after HSV and about 2 mmol/hour after TV + D. These low levels should be compared with the 30 mmol/hour secreted before operation. The likeliest cause of these small positive responses in the long term after vagotomy is vagal nerve regeneration, but if that is the case it would appear that only a small proportion of the parietal cell mass becomes reinnervated.

Gastric emptying

Stasis HSV does not produce gastric stasis. If patients with clinical evidence of pyloric stenosis are excluded, fewer than one per cent of patients who undergo HSV require re-operation for the relief of gastric stasis. In addition, symptoms suggestive of gastric retention, such as vomiting, are less common after HSV than after TV + D. Finally, numerous studies of gastric emptying both of liquids and of solids have failed to reveal any significant stasis after HSV without a drainage procedure in man. In fact, gastric emptying of liquids is significantly accelerated after HSV (because of the raised intragastric pressure after all types of vagotomy) (Fig. 3; [17]) and the rapid entry of liquid gastric contents into the small intestine may on occasion elicit mild early dumping. However, gastric emptying of liquids is not as fast after HSV as after TV + D (Fig. 4). Gastric emptying of solids is within normal limits after HSV whereas after TV + D it is very variable, being normal in some patients, excessively slow in some and unduly rapid in others (Fig. 5). The results of the

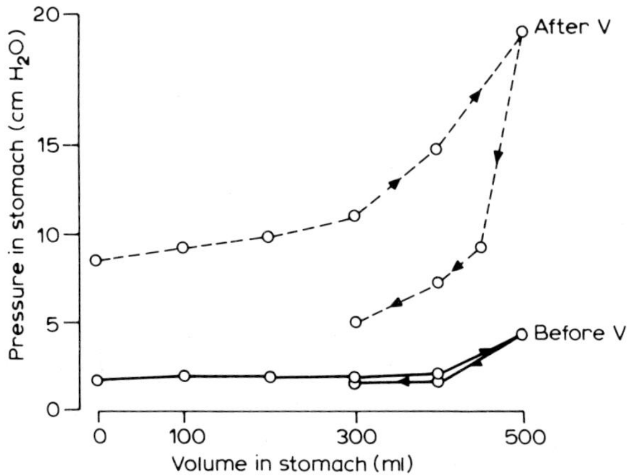

Fig. 3:   After V, the stomach's ability to accommodate increasing volumes of food with little increase in intragastric pressure is impaired. As a result, gastric emptying of liquids is accelerated. Reproduced with permission from [17].

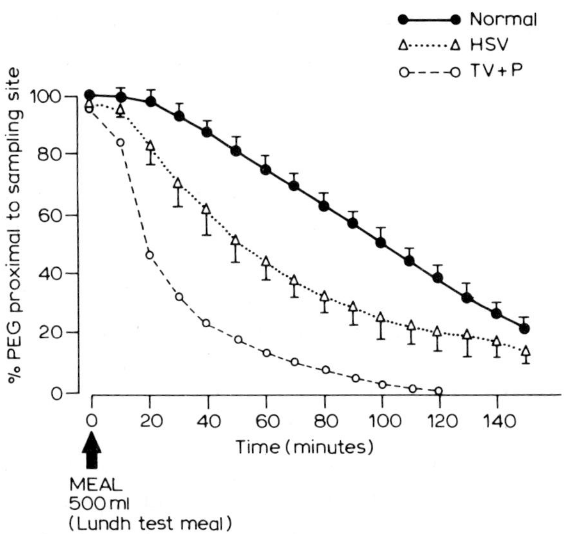

Fig. 4:   This shows the accelerated gastric emptying of a Lundh test meal after HSV and TV + P. Emptying is faster after TV + P than after HSV. Data from [19, 20]. The test meal was labeled with polyethylene glycol (PEG), recovery of which from the small intestine was measured.

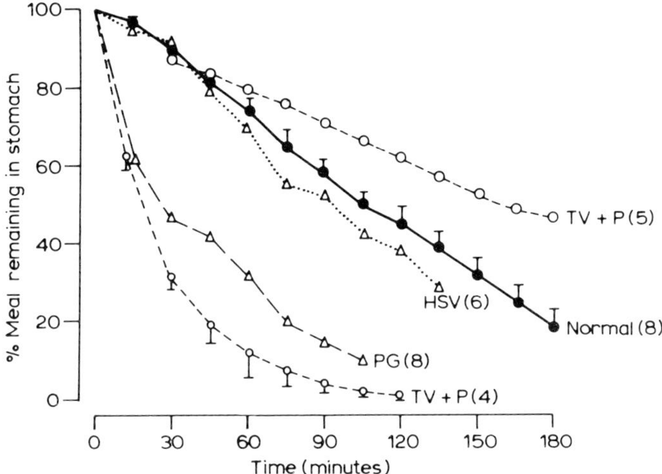

Fig. 5: Gastric emptying of a solid meal is normal after HSV, abnormally rapid after PG, and also rapid in some patients after TV + P. Data from [20].

clinical and laboratory studies can be summarized by saying that gastric emptying is under much better control after HSV than after TV + D and that, on the other hand, HSV is not followed by gastric retention.

Biliary tract

The resting gallbladder has been shown to be significantly dilated after TV + D whereas after HSV it is not dilated. Gallbladder contraction after a meal is unimpaired after both types of vagotomy [18].

Recent work by MacGregor [19] and Lavigne [20] has shown that bile salt concentrations in the upper small intestine are significantly diminished after TV + D but are within normal limits after HSV. There is some evidence from work in dogs that bile flow diminishes and bile becomes more lithogenic in composition after TV.

The effect of vagotomy on the formation of gallstones has been disputed, but evidence is steadily accumulating that TV in man predisposes to gallstone formation. For example, Csendes et al. found a 40% incidence of gallstones 3–5 years after hiatal hernia repair in which the hepatic branches of the anterior vagal trunk were severed [21]. In contrast, the incidence of gallstones was only about 7% in patients with hiatus hernia who were treated medically for the same period of time. Again, Sapala et al. found that the incidence of gallstones after PG for duodenal ulcer was 6%, whereas after PG combined with TV for duodenal ulcer the incidence of gallstones was 21% [22].

In conclusion, there is now a great deal of evidence that TV produces serious impairment of biliary tract function in man. There is no evidence that HSV does so and there is no reason to believe that it will do so.

Pancreas

It used to be believed that TV had no significant effect on pancreatic function in man but there is now convincing evidence that this procedure impairs the output of pancreatic enzymes after a meal in man. The output is diminished by about 50%, but the precipitate gastric emptying in the first hour after the meal further dilutes the enzyme concentration in the upper small intestine to levels that are only 25–30% of normal [19]. In contrast, after HSV enzyme output is within normal limits and enzyme concentrations in the upper small intestine after a meal are also normal (Fig. 6; [19, 20]).

Fecal fat excretion [23]

TV + D leads to a significant increase in fecal fat output in man and about 40% of patients develop steatorrhea. After HSV, fecal fat output is unchanged.

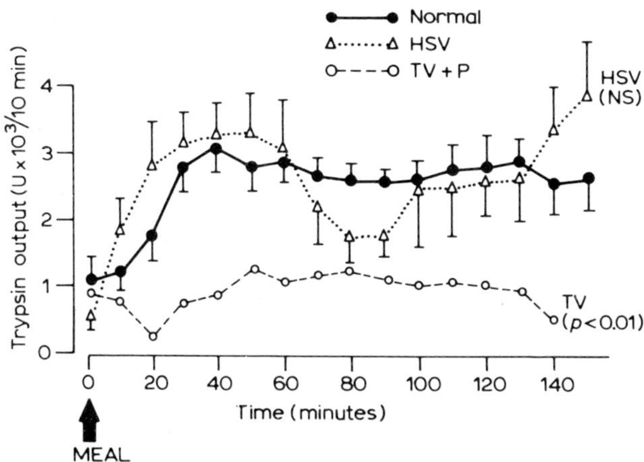

Fig. 6: TV impairs pancreatic enzyme output in response to a meal in man, whereas HSV does not. Adapted from [19, 20].

Summary of effects of HSV and TV + D on the intestinal tract

The results of the numerous tests of alimentary function after the different types of vagotomy can be summarized as follows. Each branch of the vagus nerves has a function and division of that branch impairs that function. The only type of vagal section that has been shown to be of therapeutic value is section of the vagal fibers to the parietal cell mass. Division of the vagal nerve supply to the gastric musculature, to the biliary tract, pancreas and small intestine impairs function and so has a deleterious effect in man. Hence, from the physiological point of view at least, vagotomy should be as specific and selective as possible.

Clinical results of HSV without a drainage procedure for duodenal ulcer in Leeds

HSV has now been used in the elective surgical treatment of duodenal ulcer at Leeds General Infirmary for 11 years and 3 months. The principal indication for surgical treatment was intractability or failure of medical treatment, but many of the 510 patients had previously perforated or bled. About 85 of the first 100 patients treated were operated on personally by the author but thereafter HSV became the standard method of treatment for duodenal ulcer in the University Department of Surgery and so the 11-year experience reflects the results of 3 consultant surgeons and 5 lecturers of senior registrar status. About 15% of the operations were performed by registrars under supervision.

Patients were followed up at yearly intervals at a special Gastric Follow-up Clinic where they were interviewed by a panel of 2 or 3 doctors who were not permitted to know which type of operation had been performed until they had written down the answers to a predetermined set of questions and made their collective verdict about the overall result of the operation. This clinic was attended not only by patients after HSV but by many hundreds of patients who had undergone gastric resection, TV, SV etc. for duodenal ulcer, gastric resection or vagotomy for gastric ulcer, simple closure of perforated duodenal ulcer and gastric resection for carcinoma. There was usually one physician or radiologist in the panel and so although the surgeons also took part in the assessment the results obtained are felt to be reasonably free from bias.

Operative mortality

There was one operative death (0.2%).

Morbidity

No case of lesser curve necrosis has been encountered. In general the post-operative course of these patients has been remarkably smooth and it is our routine policy to nurse them from the time of operation without either a nasogastric tube or an intravenous drip. This allows the patient to be much more mobile and to clear his chest more easily.

Side effects

One hundred patients treated by the author have now been followed up for 6–10 years and the incidence of side effects in the long term is shown in Table III. It will be seen that the incidences of diarrhea, early dumping and bilious vomiting are very low and it should be added that the severity of these side effects in the few patients affected was not great. For comparison, the incidence of diarrhea after TV + D after a comparable length of follow-up was 24%, 4% being very severe. There were no severe cases of diarrhea after HSV. After TV + P the incidence of early dumping at 5–10 years was 12% and after TV + GJ, 18%. The incidence of bilious vomiting 5–10 years after TV + P, was 10% and after TV + GJ, 15%. These large differences between HSV and TV + D cannot be claimed to be statistically significant because patients were not allotted in a random manner to one or other procedure. However, it seems very likely that they are indeed both significant and clinically very important. They are certainly borne out by the results of subsequent prospective controlled trials (vide infra).

Thus, our carefully studied but uncontrolled series has provided strong evidence that the use of HSV greatly reduces the incidence of diarrhea, early

Table III: Incidence of side effects (in per cent) more than 5 years after HSV or TV in Leeds.*

Symptom	HSV (n = 100)	TV + D (n = 280)
Diarrhea	4	24
Severe diarrhea	0	4
Dumping	2	15
Bilious vomiting	1	12
Heartburn	17	17
Early satiety	34	38

* A comparison not based on a prospective randomized trial.

dumping and bilious vomiting and does not increase the incidence of any other side effect. Vomiting and flatulence which might be suggestive of gastric retention are no more common after HSV than after TV + D. Only 2 patients out of 500 have so far required re-operation for the relief of gastric stasis.

Recurrent ulceration

By recurrence we mean symptomatic recurrence diagnosed by endoscopy or at re-operation. We do not routinely endoscope asymptomatic patients. Hence, the true incidence of recurrent ulceration is probably a little higher than that quoted, but such an objection applies equally to the incidences quoted for TV + D and other operative procedures.

Thirty patients have developed recurrent ulceration in the 11 years' follow-up. Of 225 patients who have been followed for 5–11 years, 18 have developed recurrent ulceration (8%). Six have undergone PG with good results and without operative mortality. Twelve are currently in good health, mostly on cimetidine therapy, but some on no therapy whatsoever.

Recurrence was 3 times as likely to occur if the early postoperative insulin test was Hollander-positive than if it was negative. No statistically-significant correlation was found between recurrent ulceration and pre-operative acid response to pentagastrin.

Importance of the individual surgeon

One of the most striking findings when reviewing the long term results of HSV within one surgical unit has been the correlation between the individual surgeon operating and the clinical outcome. For example, within this one unit, as in the world literature, the incidence of recurrent ulceration has varied from 2–20% depending on the surgeon who performed the operation. One surgeon had a series of 250 HSV procedures for duodenal ulcer with a recurrence rate of only 2%.

Prospective controlled trials of HSV versus other surgical procedures

HSV versus vagotomy with a drainage procedure

Several such trials have been carried out and the results of 3 of them are shown in Tables IV and V [24–26]. In Kennedy's trial side effects such as dumping and bilious vomiting were significantly less and weight gain was greater after HSV [24]. The overall clinical results were significantly better

Table IV: Results of prospective trials of SV and HSV at 1–4 years.

	Kennedy et al. [24] Belfast, 1975		Kronborg and Madsen [25] Copenhagen, 1975	
	SV + GJ	HSV	SV + P	HSV
Number of patients	50	50	50	50
Operative mortality	0	0	0	0
Positive insulin tests				
at 1 week* (%)	4	4	60	58[≠]
Recurrent ulceration (%)	2	2	8	22
Dumping[+] (%)	37	8	30	6
Diarrhea (%)	12	4	20	6
Bilious vomiting (%)	14	2	14	4
Weight gain (kg)	0.3	4.2	–	–
Clinical grading at				
1–4 years				
1. Perfect (%)	33 ⎫	60 ⎫	40 ⎫	68 ⎫
2. Good (%)	43 ⎬ 76	36 ⎬ 96	28 ⎬ 68	10 ⎬ 78
3. Fair (%)	18	2	24	2
4. Poor (%)	6	2	8	20

*   Results judged by Hollander's criteria.

[+] Dumping, diarrhea and bilious vomiting were each significantly commoner after SV + D than after HSV.

[≠] Note the much higher incidence of Hollander-positive insulin tests in the Copenhagen trial, which was associated with a 22% incidence of recurrent ulceration after HSV. All the poor results after HSV in Copenhagen were attributable to recurrence.

after HSV than after vagotomy with a drainage procedure. Similar results were found in a trial in Denmark by Kronborg and Madsen of HSV versus SV + P [25]. A remarkable feature of the latter trial was that the incidence of recurrent ulceration in the HSV group was 22% (a fact which may not have been unconnected with the incidence (58%) of positive Hollander tests in the early postoperative period), and yet in spite of this more patients achieved excellent or very good clinical results after HSV than after SV + P.

In nearly all the trials which have been carried out, there has been agreement that the side effects of operation are significantly reduced when HSV is used. Table VI summarizes the data on dumping from the Århus County Vagotomy Trial in which it can be seen that the incidence of dumping was only 4% after parietal cell vagotomy (PCV) compared with more than 20%

Table V: Indidence of side effects (per cent) in a prospective trial of HSV and TV + P.*

Symptom	HSV (n = 56)	TV + P (n = 55)	Significance
Early dumping	2	17	$p < 0.01$
Late dumping	4	17	$p < 0.05$
Flatulence	20	42	$p < 0.01$
Bile vomiting	4	18	$p < 0.02$
Postprandial distension	21	44	$p < 0.02$
Diarrhea	7	13	NS
Nausea	13	24	NS
Heartburn	16	18	NS
Dysphagia	5	5	NS
Food vomiting	7	11	NS

* From the prospective randomized trial in Sheffield by Stoddard, Vassilakis and Duthie (1978) [26]. Patients were male and were followed up for 6–66 months. NS = Not significant. The interviewer did not know which type of operation had been performed.

Table VI: Aarhus County Vagotomy Trial – incidence of dumping.

	SV + P (n = 184)		SV + A (n = 31)		PCV + P (n = 37)		PCV (n = 120)	
Dumping								
Moderate	24		41		18		4	
Severe	3.0	28%	7	48%	3	24%	0	4%*
Incapacitating	0.5		0		3		0	

* $p < 0.001$. Reproduced with permission from [27].

after the other surgical procedures [27]. In Table VII, results are shown of the trial in Nashville, Tennessee by Sawyers, Herrington and Burney in which again the incidence of dumping and diarrhea after HSV is very low compared with the incidences after SV + P and TV + A [28]. The overall clinical results after HSV were excellent, with 96% of patients recording perfect or very good results compared with 84% after SV + P and 94% after TV + A.

Table VII: Postoperative sequelae in a prospective randomized trial of HSV versus TV + A or SV + P [27].

	HSV	TV + A	HSV	SV + P
	versus		versus	
	(n = 49)	(n = 50)	(n = 37)	(n = 37)
Dumping	0	22*	3	22
Diarrhea	2	18*	0	3
Reflux gastritis	0	4	3	5
Epigastric fullness	8	0	8	8

Reproduced with permission from [28].
* Significant difference, $p < 0.05$.
Figures refer to percentages.

HSV versus TV with A

Excellent trials of these procedures have been carried out by Jordan in Houston [29] and by Dorricott et al. in England and Holland [30]. The results of both trials are fairly similar and the overall clinical results in the European trial are shown in Tables VIII and IX [31]. It can be seen that one year after operation patients were doing better after HSV than after TV + A. In both trials there were more recurrent ulcers after HSV but the re-operation rate was

Table VIII: Percentage incidence of side effects one year after operation in a prospective trial of HSV with TV + A (Billroth I)

Symptom	HSV (n = 82)	TV + A (n = 78)	Significance
Dumping	2	9	NS
Diarrhea	5	14	$p < 0.05$
Vomiting	7	19	$p < 0.05$
Epigastric fullness	10	36	$p < 0.0005$
Heartburn	10	23	$p < 0.05$
Abdominal pain	11	12	NS
Dysphagia	0	4	NS

Reproduced with permission from [30].
The interviewer did not know which type of operation had been performed.

Table IX: Visick grading after one year in 160 patients.

Visick grade	HSV	TV + A	Significance
I	5 (55%) ⎫ 82%	19 (24%) ⎫ 56%	$p < 0.001$
II	22 (27%) ⎭	25 (32%) ⎭	
III	6 (7%)	19 (24%)	$p < 0.01$
IV	9 (11%)	15 (19%)	

Reproduced with permission from [31].

Table X: Incidence of recurrent ulceration in the long term after HSV.

Study	Number of patients	Length of follow-up (years)	Recurrent ulceration (%)
De Miguel (1980)	143	5–9	10
Johnston et al. (1980)	225	5–11	8
Liavåg + Roland (1979)	210	5–7	9
Kennedy et al. (1975)	50	5–8	12
Jensen + Amdrup (1978)	100	5–8	9

about the same because more patients develop gastric retention after TV + A. Side effects of operation were significantly worse after TV + A, weight loss was greater and ability to work was poorer. Hence, so far, the preliminary results of both trials suggest that HSV is the better operation for a patient with a duodenal ulcer.

HSV with and without P

Several such trials have been carried out, the aim being to answer the crucial question as to whether a drainage procedure confers any advantage on a patient who is having HSV. In one such trial carried out by Wastell and his colleagues it was found that the incidence of recurrent ulceration was higher when P was added (14% compared with 6% after HSV alone) and the overall clinical results were better after HSV alone [32]. In that and other trials it has been shown convincingly that the addition of P increases the incidence of dumping significantly without conferring any compensatory advantage. Hence it may be concluded that HSV should be performed without a drainage procedure unless the patient has clinical pyloric stenosis.

Recurrent ulceration in the long term after HSV

The incidence of recurrent ulceration ranges from 2% to more than 20%, but averages 7–10%, which is not so good as for PG or TV + A, but is similar to the incidences of recurrence after TV + D and SV + D. The results of some of the series with the longest follow-up are shown in Table X [24, 33–35, 40].

Antrectomy for hypersecretors of acid?

'Hypersecretion' may be defined arbitrarily as a PAO to pentagastrin (PAO^{Pg}) of more than 45 mmol/hour in men and more than 35 mmol/hour in women. About 30–40% of patients who come to elective operation for duodenal ulcer are hypersecretors by these criteria, and an important question is whether they should be treated, not by V alone, but by V combined with A. The evidence is conflicting. After TV + D, both Kronborg [36] and Robbs et al. [37] found a significantly higher incidence of recurrent ulcers among hypersecretors than among normal-secretors, but 3 other groups did not. After HSV in Leeds and PCV in Århus, no significant difference was found between the incidence of recurrence in hypersecretors and that in normal-secretors [38], but not all workers would agree with these findings. Once again, it all seems to depend on the individual surgeon and his ability to completely denervate the PCM. If he can do so regularly – let us say in 90% of his duodenal ulcer patients – the incidence of recurrent ulceration will be low and hypersecretors will not need A. In contrast, if the incidence of complete vagotomy is relatively high (over 20%), the incidence of recurrent ulceration will be 10% or more, and the gross hypersecretors of acid may well be at especial risk.

Summary and conclusions

The following facts have been established:
The vagally-innervated antrum does not release excessive amounts of gastrin in man.
Gastrin levels are as high, or higher after TV as after HSV.
The vagally-innervated gastric antrum is capable of emptying the stomach satisfactorily through an intact pylorus in 99% of patients with duodenal ulcer without pyloric stenosis.
Preservation of an intact pylorus, antrum and duodenum virtually eliminates dumping, diarrhea and bilious vomiting as clinical problems.
The best operative procedure for curing duodenal ulceration is TV + A

(1% recurrence). The incidence of recurrence after both TV + D and HSV averages about 10% in the long term, but can be as low as 2–4% in the hands of experts who can denervate the PCM completely in most of their patients.

In choosing the best operation for a patient with a duodenal ulcer, we must take into account not only the operative mortality and morbidity, and the expected incidences of recurrent ulceration of the various surgical options, but also the other important end-points of treatment listed in Table XI. In addition, due weight or relative importance should be assigned to each of these end-points, by means of some type of scoring system [39] or therapeutic index such as that shown in Table XII. By these means we can truly 'weigh' and evaluate the merits of the various surgical procedures.

Thus, for example, if recurrent ulceration is given an arbitrary score, or weight, of 5, I believe that an operative death should score at least 50. I would rather have 10 patients out of 100 with recurrent ulceration and no deaths after HSV, than one death in 100 and one per cent recurrence after, say, TV + A. Likewise, the gastric cripple, with severe weight loss, anemia and perhaps bone disease or tuberculosis, after gastric resection is in a much worse state than the patient who has recurrent ulceration. If recurrence scores 5 points, the gastric cripple merits 10 or even 20 points. Likewise, the patient who develops gastric carcinoma after PG or GJ merits a high score. It is

Table XI: The main factors to be considered when choosing an elective operation for duodenal ulcer.

1. Operative mortality (and postoperative morbidity)
2. Incidence of recurrent ulceration after 5–10 years
3. Side effects of operation (dumping, diarrhea etc.)
4. Long term metabolic consequences after 5–30 years
    a. loss of weight

    b. anemia $\Big\langle$ iron deficiency / megaloblastic

    c. tuberculosis

    d. bone disease $\Big\langle$ osteomalacia / osteoporosis

5. Incidence of gastric carcinoma after 15–30 years
6. Relative ease or difficulty of second, 'salvage' operation if the first operation should fail
7. Who will perform the operation?

Table XII: Evaluation of an operation for peptic ulcer: end points and their timing; the scoring system or therapeutic index [39].

End point	Definition	Timing*	Weight≠ or score
1. Operative death	The patient dies as a result of the operation	0–3 months	50
2. Recurrent ulcer	Ulcer seen endoscopically or at re-operation	5–10 years	5
3. Side effects:			
Severe	Side effects are so bad that both patient and doctor regard the operation as a failure	2–5 years	6
Moderately severe	Side effects seriously mar the outcome and cannot be avoided	2–5 years	2
Mild	Symptoms can be controlled to a large extent by care with diet or way of life	2–5 years	0.5
None	Perfect result	2–5 years	0
4. Long-term effects:			
Very severe	Carcinoma of the stomach, pulmonary tuberculosis, osteomalacia or severe osteoporosis or patient a post-gastric surgery cripple with massive weight loss, anemia and malnutrition	5–25 years	10
Moderately severe	Weight loss of > 12 kg or Hb < 10 g/100 ml (< 9 in woman), or both	5–25 years	5
Mild	Weight loss of 5–12 kg or Hb $<$ 12.5 g/100 ml (< 11.5 in woman), or both	5–25 years	< 1
None	Weight loss of < 5 kg, Hb > 12.5 g/100 ml (> 11.5 in woman)	5–25 years	0

* Time which must elapse before it is valid to state that the end point is absent.

≠ Weight of end point: this is a numerical expression of the relative importance of the end point compared to recurrent ulceration, which is arbitrarily given the number 5.

certainly inappropriate to lump these diverse causes of failure together in one apparently-homogeneous category, commonly known as Visick grade IV. Certainly many patients with recurrent ulceration after HSV respond well nowadays to medical treatment with cimetidine, and can still be regarded, over a 10-year period, as relative successes, despite the occurrence of occasional episodes of pain. The patient with severe side effects or metabolic sequelae after PG, TV + A or TV tends to have a more miserable existence and to respond less well to medical or surgical treatment.

For these reasons, it seems to me that in 1980, we have entered an era of specificity and selectivity in the medical and surgical therapy of peptic ulcer. PG and TV + A, though more effective than HSV or TV + D in curing ulcers, should seldom be used because of their relatively high operative risk, side effects and long-term metabolic sequelae. TV, though beguilingly quick and easy to perform, needlessly destroys the antral mill and the gastric reservoir, and by making a drainage procedure necessary, needlessly creates problems of dumping, diarrhea and bilious vomiting. Finally, vagal denervation of the liver and biliary system, pancreas and small bowel has now been shown to be harmful in man. Since TV has no proved advantage over HSV, apart from the speed with which it is accomplished, its use in patients with duodenal ulcer should be discontinued, until such time as prospective controlled trials show beyond doubt that it yields better results than HSV.

To conclude, I leave you with these words of Lester Dragstedt, whose creative thinking and pioneering work have exerted such a profound influence on the evolution of surgery for peptic ulcer:

> 'Death is the worst thing that can happen to a patient with a peptic ulcer. It does not seem wise to subject *all* patients to more surgery than they need in order to prevent recurrence of peptic ulcer in a *few* patients. These are still living and can be given further treatment.'

L.R. Dragstedt (1968): *Annals of Surgery 167*, 900.

References

1. Goligher, J.C., Pulvertaft, C.N., De Dombal, F.T. et al. (1968): Five- to eight-year results of Leeds/York controlled trial of elective surgery for duodenal ulcer. *Br. Med. J. 2*, 781.
2. Goligher, J.C., Pulvertaft, C.N., De Dombal, F.T. et al. (1968): Clinical comparison of vagotomy and pyloroplasty with other forms of elective surgery for duodenal ulcer. *Br. Med. J. 2*, 787.
3. Goligher, J.C., Pulvertaft, C.N., Irvin, T.T. et al. (1972): Five- to eight-year results of truncal vagotomy and pyloroplasty for duodenal ulcer. *Br. Med. J. 1*, 7.
4. Jordan, P.H. (1974): A follow-up report of a prospective evaluation of vagotomy-pyloroplasty and vagotomy-antrectomy for treatment of duodenal ulcer. *Ann. Surg. 180*, 259.
5. Postlethwait, R.W. (1973): Five year follow-up results of operations for duodenal ulcer. *Surg. Gynecol. Obstet. 137*, 387.
6. Kennedy, T. (1974): Which vagotomy? Which drainage? *Proc. R. Soc. Med. 67*, 3.

514   D. Johnston

7. Kennedy, T., Connell, A.M., Love, A.H.G. et al. (1973): Selective or truncal vagotomy? Five-year results of a double-blind, randomized, controlled trial. *Br. J. Surg. 60*, 944.
8. Johnston, D. and Goligher, J.C. (1971): The influence of the individual surgeon and of the type of vagotomy upon the insulin test after vagotomy. *Gut 12*, 963.
9. McKelvey, S.T.D. (1970): Gastric incontinence and post-vagotomy diarrhea. *Br. J. Surg. 57*, 741.
10. Johnston, D. and Wilkinson, A.R. (1970): Highly selective vagotomy without a drainage procedure in the treatment of duodenal ulcer. *Br. J. Surg. 57, 289.*
11. Amdrup, E. and Jensen, H.-E. (1970): Selective vagotomy of the parietal cell mass preserving innervation of the undrained antrum. *Gastroenterology 59*, 522.
12. Griffith, C.A. and Harkins, H.N. (1957): Partial gastric vagotomy: an experimental study. *Gastroenterology 32*, 96.
13. Hansky, J. and Korman, M.G. (1973): Immunoassay studies in peptic ulcer. In: *Clinics in Gastroenterology*, Vol. 2, p. 275. Editor: W. Sircus. Saunders, New York and London.
14. Sakakihara, Y., Kushida, T., Katto, N. and Takita, S. (1974): Effects of various types of vagotomy with and without pyloroplasty on gastric acid secretion in the dog. In: *Vagotomy, Latest Advances*, p. 99. Editors: F. Holle and S. Andersson. Springer-Verlag, Berlin, Heidelberg and New York.
15. Johnston, D., Wilkinson, A.R., Humphrey, C.S. et al. (1973): Serial studies of gastric secretion in patients after highly selective (parietal cell) vagotomy without a drainage procedure for duodenal ulcer. I. Effect of highly selective vagotomy on basal and pentagastrin-stimulated maximal acid output. *Gastroenterology 64*, 1.
16. Johnston, D., Wilkinson, A.R., Humphrey, C.S. et al. (1973): Serial studies of gastric secretion in patients after highly selective (parietal cell) vagotomy without a drainage procedure for duodenal ulcer. II. The insulin test after highly selective vagotomy. *Gastroenterology 64*, 12.
17. Stadaas, J. and Aune, S. (1970): Intragastric pressure/volume relationship before and after vagotomy. *Acta Chir. Scand. 136*, 611.
18. Parkin, G.J.S., Smith, R.B. and Johnston, D. (1973): Gall bladder volume and contractility after truncal, selective and highly selective (parietal cell) vagotomy in man. *Ann. Surg. 178*, 581.
19. MacGregor, I.L., Parent, J. and Meyer, J.H. (1977): Gastric emptying of liquid meals and pancreatic and biliary secretion after subtotal gastrectomy or truncal vagotomy and pyloroplasty in man. *Gastroenterology 72*, 195.
20. Lavigne, M.E., Wiley, Z.D., Martin, P. et al. (1979): A study of gastric, pancreatic and biliary secretion, and the rate of gastric emptying following parietal cell vagotomy. *Am. J. Surg. 138*, 644.
21. Csendes, A., Larach, J. and Godoy, M. (1978): Incidence of gall stones development after selective hepatic vagotomy. *Acta Chir. Scand. 144*, 289.
22. Sapala, M.A., Sapala, J.A., Resto Soto, A.D. and Bouwman, D.L. (1979): Cholelithiasis following subtotal gastric resection with truncal vagotomy. *Surg. Gynecol. Obstet. 148*, 36.
23. Edwards, J.P., Lyndon, P.J., Smith, R.B. and Johnston, D. (1974): Faecal fat excretion after truncal, selective and highly selective vagotomy for duodenal ulcer. *Gut 15*, 521.
24. Kennedy, T., Johnston, G.W., MacRae, K.D. and Spencer, E.F.A. (1975):

Proximal gastric vagotomy. Interim results of a randomized controlled trial. *Br. Med. J. 2*, 301.

25. Kronborg, O. and Madsen, P. (1975): A controlled randomized trial of highly selective vagotomy and pyloroplasty in the treatment of duodenal ulcer. *Gut 16*, 268.
26. Stoddard, C.J., Vassilakis, J.S. and Duthie, H.L. (1978): Highly selective vagotomy or truncal vagotomy and pyloroplasty for chronic duodenal ulceration: a randomized, prospective clinical study. *Br. J. Surg. 65*, 793.
27. Amdrup, E., Andersen, D. and Høstrup, H. (1978): The Aarhus County vagotomy trial. I. An interim report on primary results and incidence of sequelae following parietal cell vagotomy and selective gastric vagotomy in 748 patients. *World J. Surg. 2*, 85.
28. Sawyers, J.L., Herrington, J.L. and Burney, D.P. (1977): Proximal gastric vagotomy compared with vagotomy and antrectomy and selective gastric vagotomy and pyloroplasty. *Ann. Surg. 186*, 510.
29. Jordan, P.H. (1976): A prospective study of parietal cell vagotomy and selective vagotomy-antrectomy for treatment of duodenal ulcer. *Ann. Surg. 183*, 619.
30. Dorricott, N.J., McNeish, A.R., Alexander-Williams, J. et al. (1978): Prospective randomized multi-centre trial of proximal gastric vagotomy or vagotomy and antrectomy for chronic duodenal ulcer. *Gut 17*, 831.
31. Dorricott, N.J. et al. (1978): *Br. J. Surg. 65*, 152.
32. Wastell, C., Colin, J.F., Wilson, T. et al. (1977): Prospective randomized multi-centre trial of proximal gastric vagotomy or truncal vagotomy and antrectomy for chronic duodenal ulcer: interim results. *Br. Med. J. 2*, 851.
33. De Miguel, J. (1980): Late results of proximal gastric vagotomy without drainage procedure for duodenal ulcer: 5–9 year follow-up. *Br. J. Surg.* (In press).
34. Johnston, D. et al. (1980): Unpublished data.
35. Liavåg, I. and Roland, M. (1979): A seven-year follow-up of proximal gastric vagotomy. *Scand. J. Gastroenterol. 14*, 49.
36. Kronborg, O. (1974): Gastric acid secretion and risk of recurrence of duodenal ulcer within 6–8 years after truncal vagotomy and drainage. *Gut 15*, 714.
37. Robbs, J.V., Bank, S., Mark, I.N. and Louw, J.H. (1973): Selection of operation for duodenal ulcer based on acid secretory studies: a reappraisal. *Br. J. Surg. 60*, 601.
38. Anderson, D., Høstrup, H. and Amdrup, E. (1978): The Aarhus County vagotomy trial. II. An interim report on reduction in acid secretion and ulcer recurrence rate following parietal cell vagotomy and selective gastric vagotomy. *World J. Surg. 2*, 91.
39. Johnston, D. (1976): A therapeutic index (scoring system) for the evaluation of operation for peptic ulcer. *Gastroenterology 70*, 433.
40. Jensen, H.-E. and Andrup, E. (1978): Follow-up of 100 patients five to eight years after parietal cell vagotomy. *World J. Surg. 2*, 525.

Surgical options for the treatment of gastric ulcer disease

H.D. Becker and J.R. Siewert
Department of Surgery, University of Göttingen, Göttingen, Federal Republic of Germany

Peptic ulcerations localized in the stomach still represent a therapeutic problem, since recurrences or complications are a common feature of this disease. Both surgical and medical therapy have achieved major progress in recent years through the introduction of new therapeutic principles. Apart from conventional gastric resection, various types of vagotomy have become popular in the treatment of duodenal ulcer disease, but also of chronic gastric ulcerations.

Definition

According to Johnson [1], 3 types of chronic peptic ulcerations of the stomach can be differentiated (Fig. 1).

Type I is a lesion in the corpus of the stomach without abnormalities of the duodenum or pylorus; acid secretion is mostly subnormal. Type II are gastric ulcers associated with an active duodenal ulcer or with a scarred duodenum; acid secretion is normal or high. Type III is gastric ulcer situated close to or in the pylorus: there is normal or high acid secretion.

While gastric ulcer type I was believed to be an entity in itself, types II and III were attributed to chronic duodenal ulcer disease.

Indications for surgery

Whereas gastric ulcer type III has the same indications for surgery as chronic duodenal ulcers, gastric ulcer type I must be assessed separately (Fig. 2). Following complications of chronic gastric ulcerations (massive bleeding, perforation), which are rarely not an absolute indication for surgery, the most important problem in treating chronic gastric ulcerations is to exclude malignancy. It has been well documented that ulcerating small carcinomas

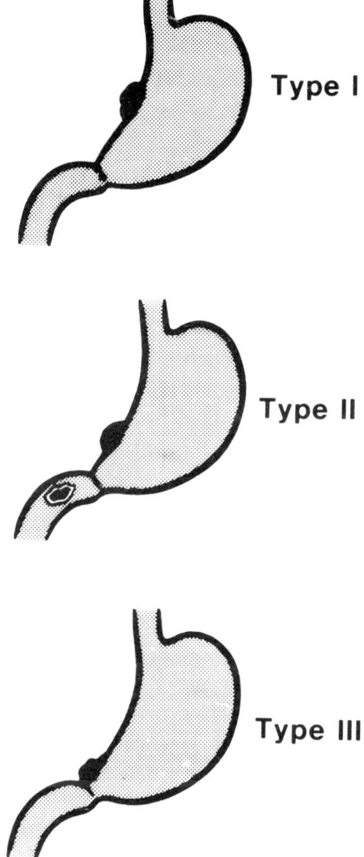

Fig. 1.   Johnson's classification of gastric ulcer.

may heal in the same way as benign ulcers [2, 3]. The tumor can be proved to be malignant only by multiple biopsies of the ulceration.

Gastric ulcer type I is characterized by a high incidence of secondary disease and a high recurrence rate [4, 5]. It may therefore be wise to perform surgical therapy in a younger patient with a progressive secondary disease (degenerative pulmonary disease, etc.), since the operative risk will later increase, and since surgery seems to be the only method proved to prevent recurrences.

Several factors claimed to affect the recurrence rate are mentioned in Figure 2, but it must be pointed out that recent data cast doubt on a number of these factors. Most of the factors listed in Figure 2 are relative indications, which have to be considered carefully [5]. No surgical treatment of gastric ulcer type I is indicated without prior medical therapy.

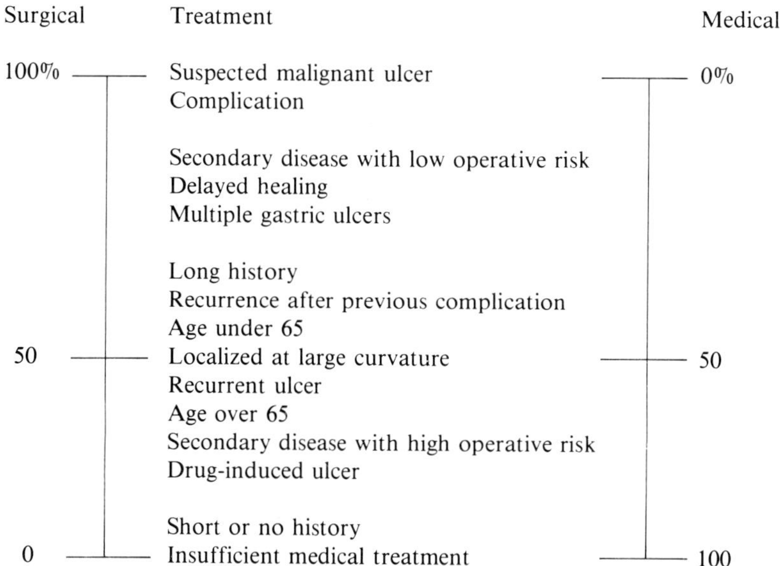

Fig. 2:   Indications for surgical or medical treatment of gastric ulcer type I.

Choice of operation

Gastric ulcer type III (Fig. 3)

Chronic prepyloric gastric ulcerations have been treated surgically following the same regimens as for chronic duodenal ulcerations (DU), since gastric acid hypersecretion is believed to be one of the major pathophysiological causes for this disease. Selective proximal vagotomy (SPV), with or without a drainage procedure, has achieved great popularity in the treatment of DU patients because of its low operative mortality, relatively few postoperative complaints and a tolerable recurrence rate.

Results on the treatment of gastric ulcer type III by SPV without drainage have been reported by Amdrup and coworkers [6]. In a prospective clinical trial (Aarhus County Vagotomy Trial), vagotomy for duodenal ulcer (DU) or prepyloric ulcer was performed in 748 patients, who were randomly allocated to selective gastric vagotomy plus drainage (SGV + D), SGV plus antrectomy (SGV + A), SPV, or SPV plus drainage (SPV + D). Calculation of the probability of ulcer recurrence suggested a 6% rate following SGV + D and an 11% rate following SPV. However, when calculations took into account the location of the primary ulcer, SPV showed a similar rate when used for

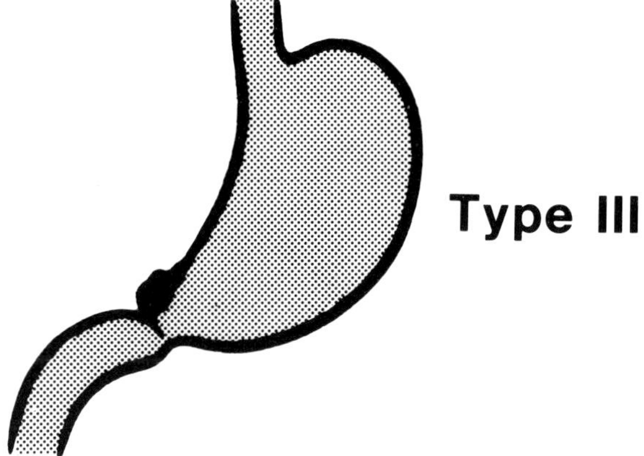

Fig. 3:   Gastric ulcer type III.

DU patients, but an incidence of 22% when used for gastric ulcer type III. The recurrence rates after SGV + D or SPV + D were lower.

Similar results were achieved in the Department of Surgery at the University of Göttingen (Table I). In a prospective study, 323 patients with chronic peptic ulcerations localized in the duodenum, pylorus, or the prepyloric antrum were treated by SPV. Preoperative examinations consisted of endoscopy, X-ray, gastric analysis (pentagastrin dose-response curve) and serum gastrin determinations. The studies were repeated postoperatively 3 months after surgery and each year up to 5 years. The follow-up period was 1.5–7 years. Forty of our 323 patients (12.3%) had a gastric ulcer type III. The recurrence rate for the whole group of patients was 6.8%, excluding the prepyloric ulcerations decreased the recurrence rate for DU patients alone to 4.9%. Patients with gastric ulcer type III developed recurrences in 20% of cases.

Table I: Results of SPV in the treatment of duodenal and prepyloric ulcer (gastric ulcer type III).

Total number of patients	323
Number of type III gastric ulcers	40 (12.3%)
Recurrences (total)	22 (6.8%)
Recurrences of duodenal ulcers	14/283 (4.9%)
Recurrences of type III gastric ulcers	8/40 (20.0%)

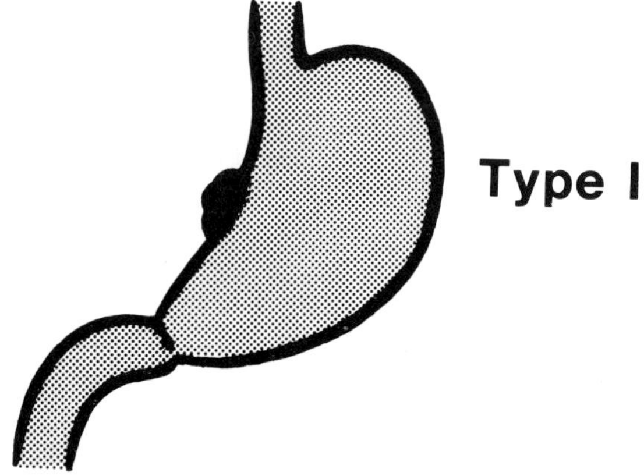

Fig. 4:   Gastric ulcer type I.

Gastric ulcer type I (Fig. 4).

Gastric resection   Gastric resection has been the standard surgical therapy for chronic gastric ulcers for many years [4, 7]. Both types of resection, Billroth I gastroduodenostomy and Billroth II gastrojejunostomy, have been widely used and give satisfactory results (Tables II, III). Postoperative mortality for both procedures is between 2 and 4%; recurrences and postgastrectomy complaints are rare in this group of patients.

The most severe postoperative sequelae of gastric resection are due to the occurrence of gastric stump cancer. After Billroth II resection for peptic ulceration, 8–13% of all patients develop a malignant tumor in the gastric remnant [16, 17] (Table IV). Analyzing the patients for their primary ulcer type indicates that patients who undergo gastric resection for gastric ulcer will develop gastric stump cancer twice as often as DU patients (Table V).

Table II: Results of Billroth I resection in uncomplicated gastric ulcer type I.

Study	Number of patients	Mortality (%)	Recurrences (%)	Postgastrectomy complaints (%)
Nielsen et al. [8]	97	6	5	4
Duthie et al.[9]	47	0	2.4	5
Mc Keown [10]	124	0.6	1.3	2.4
Salzer [11]	631	4.2	2.0	2.4
Hollender et al. [12]	228	3.0	0	8.6

Table III: Results of Billroth II resection therapy in uncomplicated gastric ulcer type I.

Study	Number of patients	Mortality (%)	Recurrences (%)	Postgastrectomy complaints (%)
Nielsen et al. [8]	158	3	5	2
Kraus et al. [13]	112	6	6	3
Welch and Burke [14]	424	4.7	1	2.4
Mc Keown [10]	80	1.2	1.3	2.4
Harvey [15]	448	2.9	1.5	1.6

Table IV: Incidence and interval before appearance of gastric stump cancer after Billroth II resection in peptic ulcer disease (Peitsch and Becker [17]).

Interval between gastric resection and death (years)	Number of patients	Number of deaths due to gastric stump cancer	Percentage deaths due to gastric cancer
5–15	96	3	3.1
16–20	76	6	7.9
21–25	52	4	7.7
26–30	50	11	22.0
31–37	28	3	10.7
Total	302	27	8.9

Table V: Incidence of gastric stump cancer with various ulcer types [17].

Ulcer type	Number of patients	Number of deaths due to gastric stump cancer	Percentage deaths due to gastric stump cancer	Median postoperative interval (years)
Gastric ulcer	91	12	13.2	19.0
Duodenal ulcer	221	15	7.1	27.4
Total	302	27	8.9	

Furthermore, it should be remembered that conservatively treated gastric ulcer patients will develop gastric cancer in up to 10% of cases during 10–15 years of follow-up.

The discussion as to which technique of gastric resection is to be preferred – Billroth I or Billroth II – has a long history. However, over the last few years there has been increasing evidence that Billroth II resection may be followed by a higher rate of gastric remnant malignancies than Billroth I. However, these preliminary data need further support.

Vagotomy (Fig. 5)   Vagotomy is a standard procedure in the surgical treatment of duodenal ulcer disease; in chronic gastric ulcer patients, however, only relatively few data are available.

As in DU patients, various types of vagotomy (truncal (TV), SGV, SPV), in each case combined with excision of the ulcer, have been used. As shown in Table VI, the number of patients treated by this procedure is still limited. However, most studies seem to indicate that the postoperative recurrence rate is clearly higher than that following gastric resection. On the other hand, postoperative mortality, which is approximately 1% following vagotomy, seems to be significantly lower.

In order to compare vagotomy and gastric resection in the surgical treatment of chronic gastric ulcer type I, several randomized prospective studies have been performed. Duthie and Kwong [7, 26] as well as Madsen et al. [27]

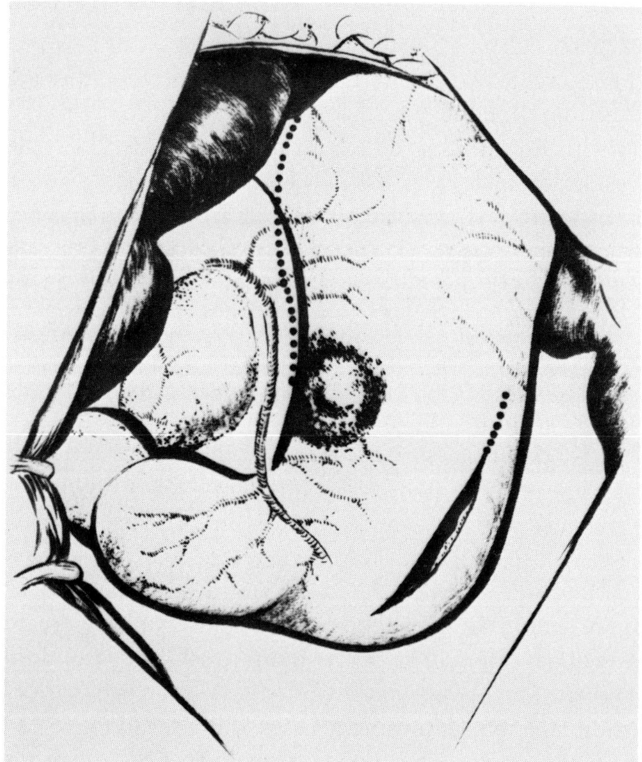

Fig. 5:   SPV in gastric ulcer type I.

Table VI: Recurrence rate following vagotomy for gastric ulcer.

Study	Type of vagotomy	Number of patients	Percentage recurrence
Kraft et al. [18]	TV	118	5
Dorton [19]	TV	30	7
Stemmer et al. [20]	TV	34	38
Sawyers et al. [21]	TV	48	15
Cade and Allan [22]	TV	90	4.5
Eastman and Gear [23]	TV	59	8
De Miguel [24]	SGV	73	18
Bauer et al. [4]	SPV + PP*	148	2.1
Duthie and Bransom [25]	SPV	26	15.0

* PP = pyloroplasty.

compared Billroth I resection with TV plus pyloroplasty. TV plus drainage was troubled by a high recurrence rate (Duthie and Kwong 14.3% [7, 26]; Madsen et al. 13% [27]). Postoperative complaints were similar following both operations, except for dumping symptoms which predominated after Billroth I resection. Randomized prospective studies comparing SPV plus ulcer excision with Billroth resection have been performed over the last few years. The results of a study performed by Duthie and Bransom [25] are summarized in Table VII. Patients seem to have a higher incidence of postoperative complaints after Billroth I resection, whereas in vagotomized patients recurrences are much more frequent. This high recurrence rate following vagotomy has been confirmed by others (Table VIII).

Another unsolved question in performing SPV in gastric ulcer patients concerns the surgical technical problems if the gastric ulcer penetrates into the liver or the lesser omentum [29]. In these cases it is sometimes impossible to perform a selective denervation of the parietal cell area without damaging the nerve of Latarjet. Another problem is the extent of vagal transection, especially if the ulceration is localized high in the lesser curvature [30]. Therefore, only in 80–90% of all gastric ulcer patients can the operation be performed.

Conclusion

Gastric ulcer disease may be a more heterogenous disease than has been suggested up to now. It is evident that in prepyloric ulcerations (gastric ulcer type III), SPV without drainage procedure is followed by a much higher

Table VII: Randomized study of surgical treatment of gastric ulcer type I (Duthie and Bransom, [25]).

	SPV + ulcer excision	Billroth I resection
No. of patients	26	30
Postoperative morbidity	8	20
Mortality	0	0
Postoperative complaints (%)		
Bile vomiting	5	19
Early dumping	5	27
Diarrhea	15	35
Recurrences (%)	15	7
Visick classification (%)		
I	61 ⎫	48 ⎫
II	17 ⎬ 78	26 ⎬ 74
III	0	15
IV	22	11

Table VIII: Recurrence rate in randomized studies on surgical treatment of gastric ulcer type I.

		Recurrence rate (%)	
Study	No. of patients	SPV + excision	Billroth I
Duthie and Bransom [25]	56	15	7
Liedberg and Oscarson [28]	36	21.1	0

recurrence rate than normal duodenal ulcer. In chronic gastric ulcer type I the surgical procedure of choice is Billroth I resection, since all types of vagotomy are troubled by a high recurrence rate.

References

1. Johnson, H.D., Love, A.H.G., Rogers, N.C. and Wyatt, A.P. (1964): Gastric ulcer, blood groups and acid secretion. *Gut 15*, 402.
2. Ottenjann, R. (1978): Notwendige Diagnostik des peptischen Ulcus. In: *Ulcus Therapie*, pp. 269–279. Eds: A.L. Blum and J.R. Siewert. Springer, Heidelberg.

3. Rösch, W. (1977): Endoskopie des Ulkus ventrikuli. In: *Ulcus ventriculi*, pp. 34–37. Eds: H.D. Becker and H.J. Peiper. Thieme, Stuttgart.

4. Bauer, H., Brückner, W., Welsch, K.H. and Holla, F. (1976): Die nicht resezierende Chirurgie des Gastro-Duodenal-Ulkus. III. Klinische Resultate. *Münch. Med. Wochenschr. 118*, 785.

5. Becker, H.D. (1977): Indikation zur Resektion in der Behandlung des Ulcus ventriculi. In: *Ulcus ventriculi*, pp. 46–53. Eds: H.D. Becker and H.J. Peiper. Thieme, Stuttgart.

6. Andersen, D., Hostrup, H. and Amdrup, E. (1978): The Aarhus County Vagotomy Trial, Part II. *World J. Surg. 2*, 91.

7. Duthie, H.L. (1977): Surgery for gastric ulcer. *World J. Surg. 1*, 29.

8. Nielsen, J., Amdrup, E., Christiansen, P. et al. (1973): Gastric ulcers surgical treatment. *Acta Chir. Scand. 139*, 460.

9. Duthie, H.L., Morre, K.T.H., Bardsley, D. and Clark, R.G. (1970): Surgical treatment of gastric ulcers. *Br. J. Surg. 57*, 784.

10. Mc Keown, K.C. (1970): A study of peptic ulcer. *Br. J. Surg. 57*, 131.

11. Salzer, G. (1967): Indikationen zur Resektion nach Billroth I und Billroth II einschließlich des hochsitzenden Ulcus. *Klin. Med. 22*, 13.

12. Hollender, L.F., Bur, F., van Peteghem, R.P. et al. (1978): Hat die Resektion nach Billroth I beim Magengeschwür an Bedeutung verloren? *Zentralbl. Chir. 103*, 329.

13. Kraus, M., Mendeloff, G. and Condon, R.E. (1976): Progonosis of gastric ulcer. *Ann. Surg. 184*, 471.

14. Welch, C.E. and Burke, J.F. (1958): An appraisal of the treatment of gastric ulcer. *Surgery 44*, 943.

15. Harvey, H.D. (1969): Twenty-five years of experience with elective gastric resection for gastric ulcer. *Surg. Gynecol. Obstet. 113*, 191.

16. Grieser, G. and Schmidt, H. (1964): Statistische Erhebung über die Häufigkeit des Carcinoms nach Magenoperation wegen eines Geschwürsleidens. *Med. Welt. 35*, 1836.

17. Peitsch, W. and Becker, H.D. (1979): Frequency and prognosis of gastric stump cancer. *Frontiers Gastrointest. Res. 5*, 170.

18. Kraft, R.O., Myers, J., Overton, S. and Fry, W.J. (1971): Vagotomy and gastric ulcer. *Am. J. Surg. 121*, 122.

19. Dorton, H.E. (1966): Vagotomy, pyloroplasty and suture for bleeding gastric ulcer. *Surg. Gynecol. Obstet. 122*, 1015.

20. Stemmer, E.A., Zahn, R.L., Hom, L. and Conolly, J.E. (1968): Vagotomy and drainage procedure for gastric ulcer. *Arch. Surg. 96*, 586.

21. Sawyers, J.L., Scott, H.W. and Graham, C. (1978): Clinical trial of vagotomy and pyloroplasty in the treatment of benign gastric ulcer. *Am. J. Surg. 121*, 119.

22. Cade, D. and Allan, D. (1979): Long term follow-up of patients with gastric ulcers treated by vagotomy, pyloroplasty and ulcerectomy. *Br. J. Surg. 66*, 46.

23. Eastman, M.C. and Gear, M.W.L. (1979): Vagotomy and pyloroplasty for gastric ulcers. *Br. J. Surg. 66*, 238.

24. De Miguel, J. (1975): Recurrence of gastric ulcer after selective vagotomy and pyloroplasty for chronic uncomplicated gastric ulcer: A 5–10 years follow-up. *Br. J. Surg. 62*, 875.

25. Duthie, H.L. and Bransom, C.J. (1979): Highly selective vagotomy with excision

of the ulcer compared with gastrectomy for gastric ulcer in a randomized trial. *Br. J. Surg. 66*, 43.

26. Duthie, H.L. and Kwong, N.K. (1973): Vagotomy or gastrectomy for gastric ulcer. *Br. Med. J. 4*, 79.

27. Madsen, P., Kronborg, O., Hart Hansen, O. and Pedersen, T. (1976): Billroth I gastric resection versus truncal vagotomy and pyloroplasty in the treatment of gastric ulcer. *Acta Chir. Scand. 142*, 151.

28. Liedberg, G. and Oscarson, J. (1979): Selective proximal vagotomy and gastric resection for gastric ulcer. In: *Selektive Proximale Vagotomie*, pp. 61–63. Eds: H. Pichlmaier and Th. Junginger. Thieme, Stuttgart.

29. Johnston, D. (1977): Rationale and results of highly selective vagotomy without a drainage procedure plus excision of the ulcer in the treatment of gastric ulcer. In: *Ulcus ventriculi*, pp. 90–100. Eds: H.D. Becker and H.J. Peiper. Thieme, Stuttgart.

30. Becker, H.D. (1978): Indikation zur chirurgischen Therapie beim unkomplizierten Ulcus ventriculi. In: *Ulcus Therapie*, pp. 298–311. Eds: A.L. Blum and J.R. Siewert. Springer, Heidelberg.

Discussion

The primary aim of elective surgery in patients with peptic ulcer is to cure the ulcer disease. The methods which will be chosen to achieve this goal are based on the pathophysiological understanding of mechanisms leading to ulcer formation and on the results of clinical trials. Following the discussion on the effect of surgical procedures on gastric secretory and motor function, the clinical relevance of the loss of receptive retardation seen after selective proximal vagotomy (SPV) was discussed. Symptoms like fullness and gastric distention seen after this operation initially in 20–30% of the patients will improve with time. Intragastric recordings repeated one year after SPV show an increase of rhythmic motility in relation to the first postoperative recording [1]. The feeling of fullness may also be related to the rapid rate of gastric emptying as part of the dumping syndrome [2].

The subsequent discussion centered around the different types of operations done nowadays in patients with duodenal ulcer disease and gastric ulcer disease. There was general agreement that the procedure of choice for uncomplicated duodenal ulcer disease should be SPV in spite of a higher recurrence rate than in SPV with antrectomy. This implies that a higher recurrence is accepted to avoid other severe sequelae of ulcer surgery such as dumping and diarrhea. This seems to be a sound approach since recurrences can be treated effectively (see Chapter V, Holtermüller et al., pages 347–356) by medical means but there is no satisfactory medical or surgical treatment for the other severe and sometimes incapacitating sequelae of ulcer surgery. The question of adequate surgical treatment for prepyloric ulcer will need to be re-examined again in view of the results of the Aarhus County vagotomy trial and those of Professor Becker (Chapter VI, pages 516–526) [3]. In regard to gastric ulcer (Johnson classification, type 1) there was no general agreement about the procedure of choice. The recent studies show that recurrence rates are higher following SPV with an excision of the ulcer than following Billroth I partial gastrectomy. Dr. Kronborg (Denmark) pointed out during the discussion that the dilemma of surgical treatment for gastric ulcer is similar to that in patients with duodenal ulcer. Recurrence rate may be kept low by doing a resection but the number of severe side effects is high. Since side effects of surgery are difficult to treat and in patients with high operative risks due to age and associated diseases it may seem reasonable, in his opinion, to consider SPV as the first surgical treatment for benign gastric ulcer. Professor Johnston (Leeds, England) supported this statement and presented as yet unpublished follow-up observations on patients with gastric ulcer being treated with SPV and excision of the ulcer. In his personal series of patients who were not part of a randomized trial the recurrence rate was 4% and the clinical response was good.

Summarizing the therapeutic reflections of many of the surgeons, SPV is the type of operation recommended in patients with duodenal ulcer disease. In regard to gastric ulcer, the issue is still open and from presently available data in controlled trials gastric resection would seem to be the more reliable procedure in regard to the postoperative ulcer recurrence rate. The frequency of gastric carcinoma following surgery for gastric and duodenal ulcer was not discussed in detail. A recently published study shows that gastrectomy or simple gastrojejunostomy for ulcer predisposed to gastric cancer. The incidence of gastric cancer was 4 times higher after surgical than after medical therapy [4].

References

1. Stadaas, J.O. (1976): Effect of vagotomy on gastric motility. *Scand. J. Gastroenterol. 2, Suppl. 42*, 85.
2. Ralphs, D.N.L., Thompson, J.P.S., Haynes, S. et al. (1978): The relationship between the rate of gastric emptying and the dumping syndrome. *Br. J. Surg. 65*, 637.
3. Andersen, D., Hostrup, H. and Amdrup, E. (1978): The Aarhus County Vagotomy Trial II. An interim report on reduction in acid secretion and ulcer recurrence rate following parietal cell vagotomy and selective gastric vagotomy. *World J. Surg. 2*, 91.
4. Papachristou, D.N., Agnanti, N. and Fortner, J.G. (1980): Gastric carcinoma after treatment of ulcer. *Am. J. Surg. 139*, 193.

Surgery for ulcer disease: comments and perspectives for the future

H.W. Schreiber and V. Schumpelick
Department of Surgery, University Clinic and Policlinic, Hamburg, Federal Republic of Germany

Ulcer surgery is the continuation of medical treatment of peptic ulcer disease by means of surgery, i.e., anatomical reconstruction or correction. The indication for surgery is strongly connected with the success of medical treatment and can therefore vary from case to case. The development of therapeutic endoscopy and the introduction of new drugs have resulted in a reduced need for emergency surgery. Elective surgery such as the heroic (for the patient *and* the surgeon) operation of the Billroth era (with its 77% mortality rate [1]) has become a procedure with a largely calculable low risk.

The rationale behind elective ulcer surgery is that it offers the possibility of reducing ulcerogenous activity. This of course assumes knowledge of the pathophysiology and pathogenesis of ulcer disease, and surgeons must therefore closely follow the results of gastric research. Surgical procedures have to mirror the present state of knowledge as well as the experience of a century of surgical treatment. Thus, ulcer surgery has to be flexible and open to changes as new procedures are proved valuable. Conservativism is as obstructive as uncritical progressiveness.

On the other hand, the results and side-effects of ulcer surgery have been very important for the understanding of gastric pathophysiology, as for example jejunal ulcer following gastroenterostomy or reflux disease of the resected stomach. Gastroenterostomy, first described by Wölffler in 1881 [2], was considered successful in the treatment of peptic ulcer disease for 4 decades, until Pribram reported on the deleterious effect of that operation on the jejunal mucosa in 1923 [3]. This marked the birth of a new gastric pathophysiology, as well as the introduction of major stomach resection as a technique in ulcer surgery [4]. From that time on, two-thirds gastric resection was the standard procedure in surgical treatment of peptic ulcer disease, but today gastric resection (at least in duodenal ulcer) seems to be heading for the same fate as gastroenterostomy met 50 years ago. Neither the mortality rate nor such side-effects as dumping, diarrhea and reflux fit the contemporary picture of an elective operation. Moreover, gastric resection potentially predisposes the patient to gastric stump carcinoma.

Farthmann pointed out in his paper (see pages 473–481) that the peptic principle is often, perhaps too often, accused in peptic ulcer disease. We totally agree with this statement. The harmful effect of acid and pepsin has been overestimated in the past, so that other valuable functions (as, for instance, that of the pylorus) were widely neglected and sacrificed by resection. Farthmann is right to stress the functional anatomy of the antrum and pyloric channel. When considering functional and morphological unity, the importance of preservation of both parts becomes evident. Therefore, any attempt to maintain pyloric function by preserving the pylorus in antrectomy will have a doubtful success. An isolated pyloric muscle, even with 1–2 cm of antrum left, cannot work as a well-coordinated gastric outlet and reflux-preventing barrier. That is the reason for the clinical discontent with the pylorus-preserving antrectomy.

However, the functional and morphological unity of antrum and pylorus emphasizes the need of sparing antral innervation in cases of vagotomy. Under this condition, i.e., preserving the intact nerve of Latarjet, a pyloroplasty is not necessary [5].

The anatomy and physiological function of the antropylorical segment needs to be studied in detail. There is a special need to understand the barrier function of the pylorus in states of health and duodenogastric disease.

Closely connected with this is the problem of duodeno-gastric reflux. How much of such reflux is physiological? Is there any circadian rhythm? Which reflux components are nocuous, and which are harmless? Is there a clearing function of the stomach? And does duodenal motility have a role in reflux? We need positive proof of acute and chronic reflux damage of the gastric mucosa without the side-effects of gastric resection or hemorrhagic shock. For clinical purposes, we need a reliable and practicable method to study pyloric function and reflux. In this way many unsolved questions regarding gastric physiology may be answered, and the state of the resected stomach may be better understood.

In a recently published study on patients with standard operations for duodenal ulcer, we investigated intragastric concentrations of bile acids and lysolecithin [6]. We demonstrated that most reflux is not only related to the width of the pyloroplasty or anastomosis, but also to the reservoir of the remaining stomach, the pH value, the acid secretion and the duodenal motility. The smallest amount of duodenal contents in the gastric cavity was found after vagotomy, even with pyloroplasty. The resected stomach showed reflux concentrations of more than 20-fold, namely in the retrocolic gastrojejunostomy (Billroth II). Even the end-to-side gastroduodenostomy (Billroth I) demonstrated bile acid and lysolecithin concentrations in the gastric juice more than 10 times those found in controls.

But what do these values mean to us? Is there any connection to destruction of gastric mucosa, to chronic atrophic gastritis or even to gastric stump carcinoma and elevated levels of duodenal contents in the stomach? Many further studies will have to be done before gastric reflux disease is fully understood. Anticipating a positive correlation between reflux and gastric mucosal damage, which seems to be very likely, it will be wise to preserve or if possible restore pyloric function. Partial gastrectomy (including pylorectomy), formerly the most frequent gastric operation, should be avoided whenever that is possible. In cases of unavoidable gastrectomy (i.e. in gastric ulcer, and especially in younger patients), a reflux-preventing procedure such as a Roux gastroenterostomy or a jejunal transposition [6] should be considered. We recently showed in an experimental and clinical study, that an interposition of 25 cm isoperistaltic jejunal segments works as well in preventing duodenogastric reflux as a Roux anastomosis [6]. This may be an effective means of reducing the side-effects of gastrectomy, at least in younger patients with long life expectancy.

After reading Kelly's excellent article (see pages 482–492), the surgeon will have to choose between injuring the proximal or the distal gastric motility by his operation. It is relatively easy to decide which damage will be more serious: either loss of receptive relaxation, accomodation and storage by denervation of the proximal stomach or distal gastric resection with dumping, diarrhea and reflux. We appreciate Kelly's exact demonstration of the side-effects of selective proximal vagotomy (SPV). Even though these consequences are relatively less serious than those accompanying gastrectomy, a better understanding of them seems desirable in the interest of more effective medical treatment. The assurances that these complaints, found after SPV in 30–40% of cases, are explainable, and, as far as we know, are without further consequences, may be comforting to the doctor's conscience, but are not particularly reassuring to the patient. The epigastric fullness following SPV can result in as much discontent as chronic ulcer disease itself. Therefore, the patient and his doctor may not trust in the success of the operation, and many control endoscopies may be done without any pathological result. From this point of view, the disturbed motility of the proximal stomach sometimes seems to be as important a handicap to vagotomy as the high recurrence rate. Low mortality and the lack of such side effects as diarrhea, dumping and reflux are convincing arguments for SPV as opposed to gastrectomy. Such arguments would be even more convincing were it not for the side effects often accompanying SPV.

Combined operation, some years ago proposed as a safe standard procedure in ulcer surgery, should be avoided. The combination of proximal and distal motility destruction and antrectomy with loss of gastrin and its trophic effect on gastric mucosa seems to be too radical a procedure in ulcer surgery, according to Kelly. The combined effect of vagotomy on gastric acid production is far more than is necessary for ulcer therapy and prevention, as too much alkalization of the stomach is not innocuous. In patients with combined gastric resection we have demonstrated that more than 90% of the gastric juices are contaminated, mostly with fecal flora. A specific role of these bacterias in stomach carcinogenesis was discussed by Deane et al. [7]. On the other hand, with increasing pH values we found a more than proportional rise in intragastric lysolecithin concentration. Above pH 6, more than 70% of the refluxed bile lecithin was hydrolized into cytotoxic lysolecithin. Therefore, hydrochloric acid in the stomach should not be totally abolished. The principle of ulcer surgery should be: as much acid depression as necessary, as much acid preservation as possible. According to present knowledge, combined operation seems to neglect this principle. Enough acid depression is attained by SPV alone or by gastric resection alone. More depression is unneccessary, and may be dangerous.

The decision between resection and SPV does not depend on secretory state, but rather on ulcer localization. Pentagastrin testing is irrelevant to the choice of surgical procedure, and it is not necessary to perform this routinely, unless it serves some specific scientific aim.

Duodenal ulceration is sufficiently managed by SPV, as Johnson has pointed out (see pages 493–517). Numerous prospective randomized trials clearly demonstrate that SPV is the best possible surgical method; its only problem is the high recurrence rate. Despite different attempts to perfect SPV, the recurrence rate remains 2–3 times that associated with gastric resection. Even with circular myotomy of the distal esophagus in addition to SPV we could not match the low recurrence rate of gastrectomy. More interesting than other short-term trials on this subject will be the late results of SPV. What about reinnervation and sprouting? What if the Hollander test becomes positive again? What about return of gastric acidity? How many late recurrences will there be? Are there any long-term side effects on the gastric mucosa? What about the rate of atrophic gastritis, carcinoma of the operated stomach, compared to the resected stomach? Is SPV only an operation with a short-term effect? On the other hand a peptic ulcer could be sufficiently managed by an operation for time if the disease by itself was a disease for time. We will have answers to most of these questions when we can overview 2–3 decades of SPV. Based on what we know today, SPV is superior to any other type of operation for duodenal ulcer.

Regarding gastric ulcer, the discussion remains open. There has been much evidence indicating that prepyloric (Johnson type III) ulceration, due to its similar pathogenesis, should be managed in the same way as duodenal ulcer. However, results reported by Amdrup, Becker and others have been disappointing. With its recurrence rate of 20%, SPV cannot be considered the procedure of choice in prepyloric gastric ulcer. Would an additional pyloroplasty give better results in this type of ulcer, pathogenetically connected with pyloric stenosis? This question has yet to be answered.

Equally disappointing are the results of SPV and ulcer excision in type I gastric ulcer. In addition to the difficulty of sparing the nerve of Latarjet in case of penetrating ulcer to the lesser omentum, SPV results in a high recurrence rate. More trials have to be done before a decision is possible as to whether or not there is any place at all for SPV in gastric ulcer surgery. At present, gastric resection is still the most reliable procedure.

In case of resection, a gastroduodenostomy (Billroth I) should be done, because of fewer side effects, preservation of the trophic effect of duodenal gastrin (Kelly) and a lower rate of gastric stump carcinoma. In young patients a reflux-preventing procedure as Roux gastroenterostomy or primary jejunal transposition should be considered. In any case, a simple gastrectomy of Billroth I type is still the safest procedure in gastric ulcer. One hundred years after Rydygier's first gastric resection in gastric ulcer [8], the Billroth I resection is still the procedure of choice in gastric ulcer. Whether or not a better method will be discovered in the future remains to be seen.

References

1. Kramer, N. (1882): Über Pylorusresektion. *Zentral Chir. 9*, 745.
2. Wölffler, A. (1881): Gastroenterostomie. *Zentral Chir. 8*, 705.
3. Pribram, B.O. (1923): Die Gastroenterostomie als Krankheit. *Klin. Wochenschr. 2*, 473–479.
4. Finsterer, H. (1918): Ausgedehnte Magenresektion bei Ulcus duodeni statt der einfachen Duodenalresektion bzw. Pylorusausschaltung. *Zentral Chir. 45*, 434.
5. Schreiber, H.W. (1972): Vagotomie ohne Drainage-Operation. *Langenbecks Arch. Chir. 332*, 205–211.
6. Schumpelick, V., Begemann, F. and Werner, B. (1979): *Die Refluxkrankheit des Magens*. Ferd. Enke Verlag, Stuttgart.
7. Deane, S.A., Youngs, D., Burdon, W. et al. (1980): Gastric microflora: effect of surgery and of cimetidine. (Abstracts). *Hepato-Gastroenterol. Suppl. 1980*, 256.
8. Rydygier, L. (1882): Die erste Magenresektion bei Magengeschwür. *Zentral Chir. 9*, 198.

Future approaches to the treatment of ulcer disease*

K.G. Wormsley**
Ninewells Hospital, Dundee, Scotland

In order to provide rational therapy for gastric and duodenal ulcers, we have to determine whether ulcers of the gastric or duodenal mucosa are merely ordinary wounds or whether the development and persistence of the ulcers depend upon a specific imbalance between local aggressive and defensive factors. In other words, do peptic ulcers have an underlying cause or causes similar to, for example, varicose ulcers (which show chronicity and phasic clinical activity like peptic ulcers)? If peptic ulcers are nonspecific wounds, in order to treat rationally, we should be studying the processes involved in wound healing and, if necessary, factors in the environment of the wound which delay healing. These environmental factors may, of course, be luminal or mucosal. However, factors which prevent healing of ulcer wounds are not necessarily aggressive in the sense that such factors result in ulceration of an intact mucosa while, conversely, defective healing attributable to mucosal abnormality does not necessarily have any bearing on defence against injury. In other words, the factors resulting in mucosal breakdown and ulceration need not be (and probably are not) the same as the factors responsible for the retarded healing of ulcers.

Quite apart from the therapeutic implications of the distinction between the aggressive and defensive factors involved in ulcerogenesis and the factors which prevent or promote wound healing, we have to realise that it may not be possible to detect, or measure, the latter factors when the mucosa is intact. Conversely, factors which we can identify as capable of causing or preventing mucosal injury may, or may not, have some effect on the healing of wounds (but, in any case, these aspects must be tested quite separately).

* Based on the round table discussion 'Future research directions in the medical therapy of ulcer disease'. Discussants were C. Johansson, W. Domschke, J. Hansky, S.J. Konturek, K.-Fr. Sewing and K.G. Wormsley (moderator).
** The author is in receipt of a Research grant from the Scottish Hospital Endowments Research Trust.

In ulcer disease, is there an excess of aggressive factors which must be reduced therapeutically (defining aggressive as factors which cause ulceration and/or prevent healing)? The traditional aggressive factors – which are considered to be present in abnormally great amounts especially in patients with duodenal ulcer – are luminal and comprise the acid and pepsin of gastric juice. That these intraluminal aggressive factors are involved in ulcer disease has been inferred from the therapeutic efficacy of drugs (and surgical procedures) which apparently achieve ulcer healing (and prevent relapse) by inhibiting the secretion of gastric juice or by neutralizing intraluminal acid [1]. However, while the inference regarding the basis of therapeutic efficacy may be correct, there are potential conceptual and operational problems. The latter aspect – the assumed identification of some ulcer-healing property – is what I would like to discuss in connection with urogastrone.

This peptide was shown to be virtually identical with epidermal growth factor (EGF/UG) [2]. EGF has been shown to increase the healing rate of experimental gastric ulcers [3, 4]. It was at first assumed that the ulcer-healing effects of EGF/UG were attributable to the powerful gastric inhibitory effects exerted by both peptides [5, 6] – and this may, of course, be true, but it may also not be so simple. EGF/UG is mitogenic and promotes the growth of epidermal, endodermal and some mesodermal cells [7], and promotes repair of epithelial wounds [8], properties which could, obviously, be involved in the ulcer-healing effects of the peptide. However, in addition to these 2 quite different actions, EGF/UG also increases the resistance of the gastric mucosal barrier to disruption by ethanol [9], perhaps in part because the peptide has also been shown to stimulate the biosynthesis of prostaglandins in some cells [10] and prostaglandins do, of course, exert cytoprotective effects [11]. A different aspect of the actions of EGF/UG, which may also be related to the barrier-strengthening effects of the peptide, is the stimulation of the production by fibroblasts and vascular endothelial cells of an extracellular glycoprotein (LETS protein) which increases cell adhesiveness [12]. We therefore have a choice of 3 different effects which might account for ulcer healing: gastric inhibition; growth and repair promoting; and mucosal barrier strengthening.

That, however, is not the end of our problems. It has recently been shown that EGF/UG inhibits the replication of some viruses [13]. There has also recently been renewed interest in a possible viral etiology of ulcer disease, in view of the close parallelisms between the clinical features of, for example, infection with herpes simplex virus and duodenal ulceration [14]. We cannot, therefore, exclude the possibility that EGF/UG acts as an anti-viral agent when healing ulcers.

It is clearly impossible at present to select from among the 4 or more possible modes of action that effect of EGF/UG which is responsible for healing ulcers. I suppose that further analysis of each of these roles is going to be worthwhile when we consider how to heal ulcers and keep them healed. What is certain is that continuing to focus our interest on one of these possibilities is not necessarily going to get us much further in the treatment of ulcers.

Perhaps ulcerogens of environmental origin are as important luminal aggressive factors as gastric juice. These ulcerogens include not only the anti-inflammatory drugs, but also ubiquitous industrial chemicals such as nitriles which could (for example as a consequence of sequestration in bile) attain especially high concentrations in the duodenum. Clearly, if luminal ulcerogens of a chemical nature were involved in ulcer disease, prophylactic avoidance would be the treatment of choice, although identification and production of antagonists might be necessary if the materials were industrially irreplaceable. Similarly, if dietary materials or chemicals were converted to ulcerogens as a result of endogenous metabolism (genetically restricted, perhaps, to ulcer patients), then that aspect might provide a focus for therapeutic intervention.

The fact that many drugs seem to heal ulcers without much apparent influence on the luminal content of gastric juice has again drawn attention to the role of potential systemic aggressive factors. Under this heading, we must consider psychic, infectious and chemical influences. The therapeutic implications of the renewed interest in the psychic aspects of ulcer disease have been emphasized by the efficacy of placebo in healing ulcers and, more important, by the recent use of psychotropic drugs such as trimipramine in the treatment of ulcers. Similarly, recent interest in the possibility that viral infections are involved in the production of ulcers has been reinforced by the finding that both EGF and derivatives of carbenoxolone have antiviral activity.

In addition to potential systemic influences, there may also exist local mucosal aggressive factors, with appropriate therapeutic implications. For example, if ulcerogenesis depends on vascular abnormalities, or immunological reactions, or imbalance of paracrine peptides, rational treatment may involve approaches quite different from those being considered at present.

It has often been proposed that ulcer disease represents some form of imbalance dependent on defective defensive mechanisms. Deficiencies in nonspecific (e.g. secretion of mucus) and specific (e.g. the secretion of bicarbonate) intraluminal defensive mechanisms have been sought and some therapeutic approaches (e.g. the use of carbenoxolone to stimulate mucus secretion; the use of bismuth compounds to coat the ulcers; and the use of secretin injections to stimulate bicarbonate secretion) have been directed to augmenting such supposed defensive mechanisms.

More important, it has been suggested that peptic ulceration depends in some way on defective or abnormal gastric or duodenal mucosa. In this connection, we know very little about normal defensive mechanisms, because we do not know against what the mucosa has to defend itself (except infection). That is to say, we do not know whether there are some potentially injurious factors (e.g., gastric juice) against which mucosal defence is continuously necessary or whether most aggressive factors are opportunistic (and obviously the therapeutic implications are different). Alternatively, do latent aggressive factors, which do not affect the normal mucosa, become aggressive under certain circumstances (such as mucosal injury)? Or are there defensive mechanisms which become operative only in the presence of a wounded mucosa (like all the wound-healing factors) because identification and strengthening of these factors, or replacement if deficient, may be what we ought to be seeking. While some information is available about the general aspects of replication of the surface cells of the gastric and duodenal mucosa, we know very little about the processes of wound repair in the upper alimentary tract and even less about potential abnormalities of these processes in defective mucosa. Not much attention has yet been paid to the potentially very important aspect of therapeutic promotion of wound healing (although, of course, agents such as EGF may act specifically in just that manner).

On the other hand, much importance and therapeutic attention has been paid to the phenomenon of cytoprotection, which comprises processes considered to be involved in the protection of the mucosa against injury by chemical and physical agents. It is not at all clear (to me) whether defective cytoprotection is relevant to human mucosal disease or ulceration and whether augmentation of cytoprotective processes improves, or results in, healing of ulcers.

Summarizing, the therapeutic implications of imbalance between aggressive and defensive factors depend on whether there is, normally, such interaction and whether imbalance results in the production of ulceration. It also has to be confirmed that such relationships and imbalances are operative under pathological conditions (i.e., in the presence of ulceration) since, alternatively, it seems possible that factors which are quite innocuous in the presence of normal alimentary mucosa may become aggressive towards ulcerated mucosa while defence may involve some entirely different protective reactions which are not evident under normal circumstances (with intact mucosa).

The rational basis of the treatment of peptic ulceration therefore depends on the satisfactory solution of unresolved problems rather than on intuitive extrapolation from (admittedly often effective) current forms of treatment.

References

1. Wormsley, K.G. (1979): *Duodenal ulcer*, Vol. 2. Eden Press, Montreal and Churchill Livingstone, Edinburgh.
2. Gregory, H. (1975): Isolation and structure of urogastrone and its relationships to epidermal growth factor. *Nature 257*, 325.
3. Koffman, C.G., Berry, J. and Elder, J.B. (1977): A comparison of cimetidine and epidermal growth factor in the healing of experimental gastric ulcer. *Br. J. Surg. 64*, 830.
4. Gregory, H., Bower, J.M. and Willshire, I.R. (1978): Urogastrone and epidermal growth factor. In: *Growth Factors*, Volume 48, Colloquim B3, p. 75. Eds: K.W. Kastrup and J.H. Nielsen. Pergamon Press, Oxford.
5. Bower, J.M., Camble, R., Gregory, H. et al. (1975): The inhibition of gastric acid secretion by epidermal growth factor. *Experientia 31*, 825.
6. Elder, J.B., Ganguli, P.C., Gillespie, I.E. et al. (1975): Effect of urogastrone on gastric secretion and plasma gastrin levels in normal subjects. *Gut 16*, 887.
7. Gospodarowicz, D., Greenburg, G., Bialecki, H. and Zetter, B.R. (1978): Factors involved in the modulation of cell proliferation in vivo and in vitro: The role of fibroblast and epidermal growth factors in the proliferative reponse of mammalian cells. *In Vitro 14*, 85.
8. Carpenter, G. (1978): The regulation of cell proliferation: Advances in the biology and mechanism of action of epidermal growth factor. *J. Invest. Dermatol. 71*, 283.
9. Pilot, M.A., Deregnaucourt, J. and Code, C.F. (1979): Epidermal growth factor increases resistance of the gastric mucosal barrier to ethanol in rats. *Gastroenterology 76*, 1217.
10. Levine, L. and Hassid, A. (1977): Epidermal growth factor stimulates prostaglandin biosynthesis by canine kidney (MDCK) cells. *Biochem. Biophys. Res. Commun. 76*, 1181.
11. Robert, A. (1979): Cytoprotection by prostaglandins. *Gastroenterology 77*, 761.
12. Chen, L.B., Gudor, R.C., Sun, T.T. et al. (1977): Control of a cell surface major glycoprotein by epidermal growth factor. *Science 195*, 776.
13. Knox, G.E., Reymolds, D.W., Cohen, S. and Alford, C.A. (1978): Alteration of the growth of cytomegalovirus and herpes simplex virus type I by epidermal growth factor, a contaminant of crude human chorionic gonadotropin preparation. *J. Clin. Invest. 61*, 1635.
14. Borg, I. and Andren, L. (1980): Herpes simplex virus as the possible cause of peptic ulcer. *Scand. J. Gastroenterol. 15*, (In press).

Closing remarks

M.I. Grossman
Veterans Administration Wadsworth Medical Center, Los Angeles, California, U.S.A.

These closing remarks are my opinions about topics covered which I feel need emphasis and about topics not covered which I think ought to be mentioned. The first section of the program dealt with epidemiology. Although some investigators have found that true incidence rates, the number of new cases per unit population per year, have shown no trend for change during recent years, in sharp contrast others in reports on hospitalizations, complications and deaths in Scotland, England, and the United States have shown sharp decreases in these secondary indices of ulcer disease during the past 2 decades.

It is obvious that we urgently need studies, done simultaneously on the same population, in which true incidence and secondary indices, such as hospitalizations, complications, and deaths, are both measured. Until that is done, we shall not know whether the apparent discrepancy between data is due to differences in the disease in different countries or to a true discordance between incidence rates, which are apparently staying constant, and secondary manifestations such as hospitalizations which may be changing because of changes in the severity of the disease or changes brought about by changes in management of the disease.

With regard to genetic factors, I think there will be an 'explosion' of continuing identification of additional physiological abnormalities which have a genetic basis. I mentioned hyperpepsinogenemia, rapid gastric emptying, and antral G-cell hyperfunction. Certainly many other physiological abnormalities are likely to be shown to have a genetic basis. Only a few family pedigrees are needed to provide convincing evidence that a given physiological abnormality and ulcer disease cosegregate and therefore are genetically linked. I wish it were possible to find an equally simple and effective means of identifying environmental factors because I feel sure that these are as important as genetic factors but are much more difficult to identify and to link unequivocally to ulcer disease.

For environmental factors, the usual procedure is to develop a strong hypothesis as to which factor or factors might be involved and then mount a large epidemiological study to test the hypothesis. Perhaps progress can be speeded by looking for interaction of genetic and environmental factors. It seems likely that persons with certain genetic traits will be found to be susceptible to certain environmental factors. There are of course many examples of this kind of genetic-environmental interactions in other diseases.

So far, only 2 environmental factors have been firmly established, namely, smoking cigarettes and prolonged use of acetylsalicylic acid. A recent study showed that persons taking 1 g of acetylsalicylic acid per day in an attempt to prevent recurrence of myocardial infarction had a 6-fold increase in incidence of hospital-diagnosed peptic ulcer [1].

In several recent studies, endoscopy was done on all patients receiving long-term treatment with ant-inflammatory drugs [2, 3]. There was a very high incidence of gastric lesions, including a surprisingly large number of gastric ulcers. An important question in this area is whether any of the many substitutes for acetylsalicylic acid that have been introduced in the last few years is less ulcerogenic than acetylsalicylic acid. Do they produce fewer true gastric ulcers? There is evidence that some of them produce less dyspepsia, occult bleeding, and the minor erosions seen over a short period of time. However, none of these new agents has been studied over long enough periods, 3–6 months, to determine whether the incidence of true gastric ulcer is lower than with acetylsalicylic acid.

I believe that the topic of mucosal defense will occupy our minds and efforts a great deal in the near future. We shall be looking for defects in mucosal defense in patients with peptic ulcer and we shall be testing agents which strengthen mucosal defense as treatments of ulcer disease. It has been known for a long time that in both gastric and duodenal ulcer the vast majority of patients have normal acid and pepsin secretions, so there is something wrong on the other side of the equation. Until recently, mucosal defense was an abstract concept. We had no methods for measuring it. Now methods are becoming available which may help us decipher the nature of the defect in mucosal defense. The greatest promise in this area lies with the prostaglandins because there can be no doubt that they play an extremely important role in protecting the mucosa.

There are 2 important questions about prostaglandins which require an answer. First, how do prostaglandins exert this protective action? What is the mechanism? There are several possible mechanisms. They are known to inhibit acid secretion, increase mucus and bicarbonate secretion, and increase blood flow. But which, if any, of those possibilities are the relevant ones? For example, we have recently developed a method for the direct measurement of the thickness of the gel layer of mucus on the surface of the gastric mucosa and have shown that prostaglandins can as much as triple the thickness of that layer. However, it remains to be determined whether that is the relevant action producing the protection afforded by the prostaglandins.

The second question concerns the therapeutic action of prostaglandins. Do they promote healing of ulcers by a mechanism other than inhibition of acid secretion? The work being done by Dr. Johansson, from Sweden, is of particular importance. As she reported at this meeting, she has already shown that oral prostaglandin E_2 (PGE_2) in a dose which has no antisecretory effect completely abolishes the increase in the occult bleeding that is produced by an anti-inflammatory drug. She is now using that same oral dose of PGE_2, a dose which does not inhibit gastric acid secretion, to test whether it has a therapeutic effect in duodenal ulcer. This is a particularly important study because it will establish whether prostaglandins are capable of producing a therapeutic effect in ulcer disease, apart from their ability to inhibit gastric acid secretion.

With regard to the regulation of gastric acid secretion, we have come a long way. Although there have been the usual kinds of bickering and slight differences of opinion among those of us who devote a great part of our lives to discussing such matters, there is also a great deal of commonality, understanding and agreement in this area. We agree that the parietal cell has separate receptors for histamine and cholinergic agents and probably also for gastrin. We agree that only histamine acts through adenosine $3',5'$-phosphate. Now that we have the ability to isolate the individual cell types, such as the acid-secreting cell, attention will turn to the neighboring cells, such as the histamine-producing cell and the somatostatin-producing cell, in order to determine their influence on the overall process. The advent of the H_2-blocking drugs has shown that histamine is of central importance in regulating acid secretion. The study of the isolated histamine cell will tell us how the synthesis, storage, and release of histamine is regulated. The old question of whether stimulants such as gastrin and cholinergic agents release histamine should soon be answered. These new methods now available, in which it is possible to dissect the mucosa, to disperse cells and to concentrate those that we want to study, will continue to be an extremely powerful tool for the study of many aspects of gastrointestinal physiology.

The section on experimental ulcer models reminded me that such models always have been and probably always will be of very limited value. There are a number of reasons for this statement: first, the heterogeneity of ulcer disease has been emphasized, so the thought of developing an ideal ulcer model is just as wrong as the thought of finding *the* cause of ulcer disease. There are many causes of ulcer disease, and therefore there would have to be many models to mimic the human disease − if that should be a desirable thing to do.

May I remind you that the greatest advance in the treatment of ulcer disease in recent years has been the development of the histamine H_2-antagonists. They were not discovered by the use of an ulcer model but by the development of an idea − the idea of the inhibition of the action of histamine on gastric acid secretion. Thus, although I feel that ulcer models have *a* place, it is a very limited place both in understanding the causative mechanisms of ulcer disease and in testing for new drugs.

With regard to the pathophysiology of ulcer disease, we are still learning more every day and discovering new abnormalities which have not previously been recognized. In future studies, the emphasis should be on demonstrating defects in mucosal resistance. I return again to the application of genetic methods to determine whether these new abnormalities which are constantly being discovered are of genetic origin or whether they have environmental causes and, if they have environmental causes, whether it is possible to determine what they are.

Diagnosis has not made great strides in comparison with other aspects of ulcer disease. Returning to some very old-fashioned principles might be useful. Dr. Peterson gave us an excellent talk about the symptoms of ulcer disease, but there has been no scientific study of the symptoms of ulcer disease, particularly as they relate to the clinical course and prognosis of the disease. If real progress is to be made, with regard to the questions about which drug is for which patient, and which patient is to be referred for surgery, real predictors must be found. Those predictors are just as likely to be identified by taking extremely careful histories as by doing any other type of fancy study.

Endoscopy has enabled us to do precise studies on healing of duodenal ulcer which could not have been accomplished without it. If we had a very simple diagnostic test, a noninvasive test that could be applied repeatedly, it would revolutionize the study of ulcer. Endoscopy is reliable but it is cumbersome. In the area of diagnosis, I think that endoscopy will become the primary method of diagnosis, as it already has in many places. It will happen last in the United States for the obvious reason that in that country the price of endoscopy is so much higher than radiology at present.

In medical treatment, as I have already indicated, the great advance has been the advent of the H_2-blockers which now dominate the field of medical treatment. More potent H_2-blockers will soon be in general use. We do not yet know whether they will be more effective in the sense of healing more ulcers or healing them sooner. I was surprised that Dr. Olbe did not mention one of the most promising developments in drug therapy, a drug which appears to inhibit acid secretion by a completely different mechanism. This mechanism is specific inhibition of the enzyme described by Dr. Sachs, the potassium-activated ATPase, which is the final step of acid secretion and apparently found only in the parietal cell and nowhere else in the body. If this drug is specific in its action, acting only on that process so that it will therefore inhibit all acid secretion and have no other action, and if it will do so effectively for long periods of time, it will indeed be an exciting discovery.

On the other side of the equation, there are drugs which increase the defensive properties of the mucosa. At the top of that list, as I have already mentioned, are the prostaglandins. There are others, too – bismuth has been mentioned in passing, but no more than that. Doing a simple tally, bismuth comes out as well as any drug that has been tested by good controlled clinical trials – and there have been many controlled clinical trials of it. In fact, bismuth even has a slight advantage over cimetidine in that in the trials on gastric ulcer, it is unequivocally effective whereas the situation with cimetidine is rather clouded. Because bismuth is an old drug, does not taste very nice, and there is no glamorous theory about how it might act, it tends to be discarded.

Carbenoxolone is in the same category as bismuth. It is not an important drug for use in clinical therapy because of its high toxicity, but nevertheless it is important because it has the capability of healing ulcers, although it is not understood exactly how it works. Finding out how carbenoxolone works would be important. Elucidation of the mechanism of action of therapeutic agents gives us fresh insights into normal and disturbed physiology.

Regarding surgical treatment, I wish to comment on 2 topics. The first is the occurrence of gastric cancer after surgery for peptic ulcer. In a recent study at the Memorial Sloan-Kettering Cancer Center in New York, persons who had surgical treatment of peptic ulcer had a 3-fold increase in risk of gastric cancer as compared with medically-treated peptic ulcer [4]. The risk of gastric cancer was just as high after surgery for duodenal ulcer as for gastric ulcer. The most surprising finding was that the risk was just as high in those with a drainage procedure as in those with partial gastrectomy. Since cancers tend to develop 15–20 years after ulcer surgery, the large crop of patients who were treated with a drainage procedure is just now ripening and we should be alert to this. Surveys should be done of patients who had drainage procedures for treatment of peptic ulcer 15 or more years ago to determine the incidence of asymptomatic cancer of the stomach.

The other remark I wish to make about surgical treatment concerns the so-called Visick grading. I have no objection to the principle of grading surgical outcomes. However, with the Visick grading, both a recurrence and what I call a 'gastric cripple' fall into the same grade, Visick IV. By 'gastric cripple' I mean a patient who would gladly give his operation back to the surgeon in exchange for his old ulcer − he believes that the cure is worse than the disease. If a recurrence is Visick IV, then a 'gastric cripple' should be much higher in number. Putting these 2 in the same Visick grading has caused considerable confusion. By Visick grading, proximal gastric vagotomy looks no better than truncal vagotomy with antrectomy or truncal vagotomy and drainage. However, when recurrences are put in a separate category, it is clear that proximal gastric vagotomy has a much lower incidence of 'gastric cripples' than other operations. Recurrence is usually responsive to treatment. We do not have effective treatments for 'gastric cripples'.

My final comment is in regard to the effect of treatment with H_2-blockers on the long-term outcome of the disease. These drugs speed healing in the short-term and decrease recurrences when taken for months or years. It is plausible to assume that a decrease in recurrences would be accompanied by a decrease in complications. But this is an assumption and like all assumptions must be put to the test. At present we do not know whether treatment with H_2-blockers or any of the other agents which have been shown to be effective in speeding healing decreases the number of hospitalizations, complications, operations, and deaths from ulcer disease. It is an important question and efforts to answer it should be made.

References

1. Aspirin Myocardial Infarction Study Research Group (1980): A randomized, controlled trial of aspirin in persons recovered from myocardial infarction. *J. Am. Med. Assoc. 243*, 661.
2. Silvoso, G.R., Ivey, K.J., Butt, J.H. et al. (1979): Incidence of gastric lesions in patients with rheumatic disease on chronic aspirin therapy. *Ann. Intern. Med. 91*, 517.
3. Caruso, I. and Bianchi Porro, G. (1980): Gastroscopic evaluation of anti-inflammatory agents. *Br. Med. J. 1*, 75.
4. Papachristou, D.N., Agnanti, N. and Fortner, J.G. (1980): Gastric carcinoma after treatment of ulcer. *Am. J. Surg. 139*, 193.

Genetic heterogeneity of ulcer disease: an overview

I.M. Samloff
Harbor General Hospital, UCLA Medical Center, Torrance, California, U.S.A.

The diagnostic category peptic ulcer can be defined by 3 characteristics: an anatomic defect (a hole in the mucosa of the stomach or duodenum), a physiologic characteristic (the presence of acid and pepsin in the gastric secretion) and a pathogenetic mechanism (too much acid-pepsin for the degree of mucosal resistance).

A major difficulty in defining the cause or causes of the mucosal defect is that only one of its determinants, acid-pepsin, can be measured. The other, mucosal resistance, cannot be measured, and the factors that contribute to its existence are not well defined. Consequently, any amount of acid-pepsin must be considered too much in a patient with a peptic ulcer.

Peptic ulcer patients have a wide range of values for acid-pepsin output, but most have values within the normal range. Most patients with values above normal have a duodenal ulcer, but only a minority of these have a known cause for their hypersecretion, such as hypergastrinaemia. At first, an elevated serum gastrin level with hypersecretory peptic ulcer disease was thought to be specific for a gastrin-secreting tumour (gastrinoma). With time, it was recognized that gastrinoma could be an isolated phenomenon or could be a component of the autosomal dominant syndrome, multiple endocrine adenomatosis, Type I. The latter is an example of a genetic form of peptic ulcer: the imbalance between acid-pepsin and mucosal resistance is caused by too much acid-pepsin, which is caused by an elevated serum gastrin level, which is caused by a gastrinoma, which is caused by a single gene defect. In this disorder, an elevated serum gastrin level is a subclinical marker of genetic predisposition to peptic ulcer. It is elevated in all clinically-affected family members (those with active ulcer disease) and also in some clinically-unaffected members [1]. The finding of hypergastrinaemia in unaffected members, who are clearly at high risk of developing an ulcer, may be an indication for preventative medical therapy [2].

Another rare autosomal dominant syndrome is duodenal ulcer in association with several neurological abnormalities [3]. The primary cause of the imbalance between peptic aggression and mucosal resistance is not known in this type of ulcer disease.

Two other diseases known to cause hypergastrinaemic peptic ulcer are antral G-cell hyperplasia and antral G-cell hyperfunction; some cases of the latter disease may also have a genetic basis [4].

Hypergastrinaemic peptic ulcer consists of a number of distinct diseases. A general characteristic of this subgroup of patients is massive hypersecretion, but this characteristic is not specific for hypergastrinaemia. Thus there must be other causes of hypersecretory peptic ulcer. The possibilities are numerous. One intriguing observation is that the serum IgG fraction from some of these patients is a potent stimulant of acid secretion [5]; thus, there may be an immunologic type of hypersecretory peptic ulcer.

Compared with controls, the average normogastrinaemic duodenal ulcer patient has a significantly higher rate of acid-pepsin secretion, larger parietal cell mass [6], greater responsiveness of the parietal cells to pentagastrin and gastrin [7, 8] and higher serum gastrin response to meals [9], and an impairment of the ability of intragastric acid and fat to inhibit gastrin release [10, 11]. The popular concept that duodenal ulcer is primarly due to excessive acid-pepsin, rather than to diminish mucosal resistance, is a generalization which is not applicable to all patients, however, as neither acid hypersecretion itself nor any one of the physiologic abnormalities, mentioned above, which might contribute to acid hypersecretion, is present in every patient with a duodenal ulcer. It is possible that 'ordinary' duodenal ulcer also consists of several distinct diseases. We have not, however, been able to distinguish between the different types until recently, due in part to the prevailing view that genetic predisposition to peptic ulcer is due to the additive effect of an indeterminate number of genes, each having a minor and unspecified effect (polygenic). It has been proposed that genetic heterogeneity is a better explanation for the genetics of peptic ulcer than polygenic inheritance [12]; that is, that peptic ulcer is composed of several diseases which are caused by the action and interaction of different but discrete genetic and environmental factors. Hypergastrinaemic peptic ulcer as a component of the autosomal dominant syndrome, multiple endocrine adenomatosis, Type I, as already noted, is an example of a type of ulcer attributable to a single gene defect; acetylsalicylic acid-associated gastric ulcer may be an example of a type of ulcer due to environmental agent. Although genetic-environmental interaction has not been excluded, the high incidence of asymptomatic gastric ulcer in rheumatic patients receiving chronic acetylsalicylic acid therapy [13] and the finding that some of these ulcers form in normal, rather than in gastritic, mucosa [14] suggest that acetylsalicylic acid-associated gastric ulcer may be aetiologically distinct from other types of gastric ulcer, with too little mucosal resistance implied as the pathogenetic mechanism.

The genetic uniqueness of individuals probably underlies differences in susceptibility and resistance to many common diseases. The evidence that duodenal ulcer and gastric ulcer have a genetic component and, at the same time, that they are genetically-distinct diseases has come from several types of genetic studies. These studies have shown that the incidence of duodenal ulcer, but not gastric ulcer, is increased in the first-degree relatives of patients with duodenal ulcer; that the incidence of gastric ulcer, but not duodenal ulcer, is increased in the relatives of gastric ulcer patients; that the ulcer site tends to be concordant in identical twin pairs; that the incidence of blood group A is increased in patients with simple gastric ulcer; and that the incidence of blood group O and ABH non-secretor status is increased in patients with duodenal ulcer. However, neither duodenal ulcer nor gastric ulcer can be attributed to a single gene defect, as neither aggregates in families according to a simple Mendelian pattern of inheritance. This does not exclude the possibility of Mendelian inheritance for the genetic predispositions (genotypes) to duodenal ulcer and gastric ulcer, nor does it exclude the possibility of more than one genotype for each type of ulcer.

The demonstration of Mendelian inheritance of a genetic predisposition requires a subclinical marker for that predisposition. As previously noted, elevated serum gastrin level is a subclinical marker of the genetic predisposition to peptic ulcer in families with the autosomal dominant syndrome, multiple endocrine adenomatosis, Type I. Similarly, erythrocyte glucose-6-phosphate dehydrogenase deficiency is a subclinical marker of the genetic predisposition to one type of haemolytic anaemia. It is inherited as an x-linked trait, but causes no symptoms until the individual is exposed to an environmental agent such as acetylsalicylic acid or primaquine.

Since subclinical markers are present in both clinically-affected and unaffected individuals, they can be used to delineate heterogeneity within an apparently homogeneous clinical disorder, to clarify the genetics of a particular disease, to identify the environmental factors that convert genetic predisposition to active disease and to investigate the mechanisms by which gene-environment interaction produces the disease.

It now appears that some abnormalities identified in cross-sectional studies of duodenal ulcer, none of which is present in all patients with duodenal ulcer, are subclinical markers of the genetic predisposition to different types of duodenal ulcer. The best example of this is serum pepsinogen I level: results of several studies confirm that, in some ulcer families, an elevated level is inherited as an autosomal dominant trait [15, 16]. Other traits with a familial basis are an increased rate of gastric emptying [17] and post-prandial hypergastrinaemia [4].

Blood group O and ABH non-secretor status have not proven to be useful subclinical markers of the genetic predisposition to duodenal ulcer, because of their common occurrence in the general population. Bloodgroup O genes may play a part in determining the severity of duodenal ulcer: blood group O patients have been found to have a higher rate of bleeding and perforation [18, 19]. ABH secretor genes determine the ability of individuals to secrete these antigens; since they are glycoprotein constituents of gastric mucus, their absence might alter the ability of mucus to protect the mucosa. However, some authors discount the idea that mucus has a role in mucosal resistance [20, 21]; this judgement may be premature, though, as it is likely that the initial battle between the forces of peptic aggression and mucosal resistance starts in the mucus layer. The surface epithelial cells secrete mucus and small amounts of bicarbonate. It has been suggested that, by providing a mixing barrier to H^+ and HCO_3^-, mucus establishes a pH gradient between the gastic lumen and the mucosal surface [22]. The thickness and the viscosity of the mucus layer would influence the effectiveness of this barrier. These factors are in turn influenced by pepsin, since native mucus is a substrate for pepsin and hydrolysed mucus is unable to form a gel [23]; whether the blood group antigens alter the susceptibility of mucus to digestion is not known, but merits investigation.

Other heterogeneities also require investigation, such as the heterogeneity of pepsinogen and its active enzymes, the pepsins. What we have been measuring for many years as gastric pepsin is the combined proteolytic activities of many pepsins having different pH optima and specific activities against protein substrates having no direct relevance to gastric mucus or the gastroduodenal mucosa. The structure and activity of hydrochloric acid is the same regardless of its origin; the pepsins, however, are proteins that differ structurally and functionally, both within and among species, and it is possible that certain molecular forms of pepsin are more 'ulcerogenic' than others.

Based on the importance of genetic factors and the accumulating evidence that chronic peptic ulcer disease in humans is a genetically heterogeneous disease, one can only agree with Jennewein and Hammer that no single ideal model of peptic ulcer is known [21], nor is such a model likely to be known. Animal models have contributed importantly to our understanding of the role of acid-pepsin in the pathogenesis of peptic ulcer, of the factors that regulate acid-pepsin secretion and contribute to mucosal resistance, and of agents that might facilitate ulcer healing. However, this information relates more to the general problem of acid-peptic diseases than to the specific problem of chronic peptic ulcer. Numerous questions remain. How many of the physiologic abnormalities in duodenal ulcer and gastric ulcer are genetic traits? What is their mode of inheritance? What combinations of abnormalities are there? Are certain psychological factors relevant to certain types of ulcer? What are the environmental agents which convert certain genetic predispositions to active disease? Are there differences in the natural history and response to therapy among the different ulcer genotypes? These important questions and many more can be dealt with only by integrating physiologic, psychologic, epidemiologic and genetic studies to delineate the diseases which together constitute the diagnostic category, peptic ulcer.

References

1. Lamers, C.B., Stadil, F. and Van Tongeren, J.H. (1978): Prevalence of endocrine abnormalities in patients with Zollinger-Ellison syndrome and their families. *Am. J. Med. 64*, 607.
2. McCarthy, D.M. (1978): Report of the United States experience with cimetidine in Zollinger-Ellison syndrome and other hypersecretory states. *Gastroenterology 74*, 453.
3. Neuhauser, G., Daly, R.F., Magnelli, N.C. et al. (1976): Essential tremor, nystagmus and duodenal ulceration. *Clin. Genet. 9*, 81.
4. Calam, J., Taylor, I.L., Dockray, G.J. et al. (1979): A subgroup of duodenal ulcer (DU) patients with familial G-cell hyperfunction and hyperpepsinogenaemia. *Gut 20*, A934.
5. Dubi, S., Gasztoryi, G. and Lenkey, B. (1980): Immunoglobulin-stimulated superacidity in duodenal ulcer. *Acta Med. Scient. Hung. 37*, 51.
6. Cox, A.J. (1952): Stomach size and its relation to chronic peptic ulcer. *Am. Med. Assoc. Arch. Pathol. 54*, 407.
7. Isenberg, J.I., Grossman, M.I., Maxwell, V. and Walsh, J.H. (1975): Increased sensitivity to stimulation of acid secretion by pentagastrin in duodenal ulcer. *J. Clin. Invest. 55*, 330.
8. Lam, S.K., Isenberg, J.I., Grossman, M.I. et al. (1980): Gastric acid secretion is abnormally sensitive to endogenous gastrin released after peptone meals in duodenal ulcer patients. *J. Clin. Invest. 65*, 555.
9. Trudeau, W.L. and McGuigan J.E. (1970): Serum gastrin levels in patients with peptic ulcer disease. *Gastroenterology 59*, 6.
10. Walsh, J.H., Richardson, C.T. and Fordtran, J.S. (1975): pH dependence of acid secretion and gastrin release in normal and ulcer subjects. *J. Clin. Invest. 55*, 462.
11. Gross, R.A., Isenberg, J.I., Hogan, D. and Samloff, I.M. (1978): The effect of fat on meal-stimulated duodenal acid load, duodenal pepsin load, and serum gastrin in duodenal ulcer and normal subjects. *Gastroenterology 75*, 357.
12. Rotter, J.I. and Rimoin, D.L. (1977): Peptic ulcer disease – a heterogeneous group of disorders? *Gastroenterology 73*, 604.

13. Silvoso, G.R., Ivey, K.J., Butt, J.H. et al. (1979): Incidence of gastric lesions in patients with rheumatic diseases on chronic aspirin therapy. *Ann. Intern. Med. 91*, 517.

14. McDonald, W.C. (1973): Correlation of gastric mucosal histology and aspirin intake in chronic gastric ulcer. *Gastroenterology 65*, 381.

15. Rotter, J.I., Sones, J.W., Samloff, I.M. et al. (1979): Duodenal ulcer disease associated with elevated serum pepsinogen I: An inherited autosomal dominant disorder. *N. Engl. J. Med. 300*, 63.

16. Rotter, J.I., Petersen, G.M., Samloff, I.M. et al. (1979): Genetic heterogeneity of hyperpepsinogenemic I and normopepsinogenemic I duodenal ulcer disease. *Ann. Intern. Med. 91*, 372.

17. Rotter, J.I., Rubin, R., Meyer, J.H. et al. (1979): Rapid gastric emptying – an inherited pathophysiologic defect in duodenal ulcer? *Gastroenterology 76*, 1229.

18. Langman, M.J.S. and Doll, R. (1965): ABO blood group and secretor status in relation to clinical characteristics of peptic ulcers. *Gut 6*, 270.

19. Evans, D.A.P., Horwich, L., McConnell, R.B. and Bullen, M.F. (1968): Influence of the ABO blood groups and secretor status on bleeding and perforation of duodenal ulcer. *Gut 9*, 319.

20. Cooke, A.R. (1980): Environmental aspects of ulcer disease. This publication, pp. 27–36.

21. Jennewein, H.M. and Hammer, R. (1980): Animal models of ulcer disease. This publication, pp. 37–48.

22. Heatley, N.G. (1959): Mucosubstance as a barrier to diffusion. *Gastroenterology 37*, 313.

23. Allen, A. and Garner, A. (1980): Mucous and bicarbonate secretion in the stomach and their possible role in mucosal protection. *Gut 21*, 249.

Editorial note

The Editors, Professors Holtermüller and Malagelada, would like to thank the following participants who took an active part in the discussions during the Symposium.

Arnold, R. - Göttingen, F.R.G.

Barth, H. - Constance, F.R.G.
Basso, N. - Rome, Italy
Becker, H.D. - Göttingen, F.R.G.
Bonfils, S. (Chairman) - Paris, France
Bonnevie, O. - Frederiksberg, Denmark
Brunner, H. - Vienna, Austria

Caspary, W. - Hanau, F.R.G.
Classen, M. - Frankfurt, F.R.G.
Clemencon, C. - Olten, Switzerland
Clowdus, B. - Göttingen, F.R.G.
Cooke, A.R. - Kansas City, KS, U.S.A.
Creutzfeldt, W. (Chairman) - Göttingen, F.R.G.

Demling, L. - Erlangen-Nürnberg, F.R.G.
Dölle, W. (Chairman) - Tübingen, F.R.G.
Domschke, W. - Erlangen, F.R.G.

Ewe, K. - Mainz, F.R.G.

Farthmann, E.H. - Homburg (Saar), F.R.G.
Festen, H. - Nijmegen, The Netherlands
Feurle, G. - Heidelberg, F.R.G.
Fritsch, W.P. - Düsseldorf, F.R.G.

Goebell, H. - Essen, F.R.G.
Grossman, M.I. (Chairman) - Los Angeles, CA, U.S.A.

Gugler, R. - Bonn, F.R.G.
Guth, P.H. - Los Angeles, CA, U.S.A.

Halter, F. - Bern, Switzerland
Hansky, J. - Melbourne, Australia
Heiden-Müller, - Ulm, F.R.G.
Herzog, P. - Mainz, F.R.G.
Hobsley, M. - London, U.K.
Holtermüller, K.-H. (Chairman) - Mainz, F.R.G.
Hotz, J.J. - Essen, F.R.G.

Isenberg, J.I. - San Diego, CA, U.S.A.

Jennewein, H.M. - Ingelheim, F.R.G.
Johansson, C. - Stockholm, Sweden
Johnston, D. - Leeds, U.K.

Kaess, H. - Munich, F.R.G.
Kelly, A. (Chairman) - Rochester, MN, U.S.A.
Konturek, S.J. - Krakow, Poland
Kronberg, O. - Odense, Denmark
Kümmerle, F. (Chairman) - Mainz, F.R.G.

Langman, M.J.S. - Nottingham, U.K.
Lewin, M.J.-M. - Paris, France
Lezochi, - Rome, Italy
Liavaag, I. - Oslo, Norway
Lieher, H. - Würzburg, F.R.G.
Lorenz, W. (Chairman) - Marburg, F.R.G.

Malagelada, J.-R. (Chairman)
Rochester, MN, U.S.A.
Massarrat, S. - Marburg, F.R.G.
Mazzacca, G. - Naples, Italy
Misiewicz, J.J. - London, U.K.
Miyake, T. - Kyoto, Japan

Navert, H. - Sherbrooke, Canada

Olbe, L. - Göteborg, Sweden

Peerenboom, H. - Düsseldorf, F.R.G.
Peskar, B.M. - Freiburg, F.R.G.
Petersen, H. - Trondheim, Norway
Peterson, W.L. - Dallas, TX, U.S.A.

Robert, A. - Kalamazoo, MI, U.S.A.
Rune, S.J. - Copenhagen, Denmark

Sachs, G. - Birmingham, AL, U.S.A.

Schiessel, R. - Vienna, Austria
Schmid, E. - Göppingen, F.R.G.
Schwedes, U. - Frankfurt, F.R.G.
Sewing, K.-F. - Tübingen, F.R.G.
Singer, M.V. - Essen, F.R.G.
Sonnenberg, A. - Düsseldorf, F.R.G.
Spencer, - London, U.K.
Strohmeyer, G. (Chairman) - Düsseldorf,
F.R.G.

Troidl, H. - Kiel, F.R.G.
Tytgat, G.N. - Amsterdam, The
Netherlands

Walan, A. - Linköping, Sweden
Waldron-Edward, D. - Quebec, Canada
Wastell, C. - London, U.K.
Weis, H.J. - Bamberg, F.R.G.
Wormsley, K.G. (Chairman) - Dundee,
Scotland

Acknowledgments

To Dr. Peter Herzog, Mainz, coeditor of the German edition of the book we are particularly indebted for his enthusiastic support in arranging the meeting and his help in the reviewing and editing process. An especial note of thanks to Mrs. Gisela Leineweber and Ms. Guardice Grube for their tireless secretarial help during the organisation of the symposium and the editing of the book.

K.-H. Holtermüller
J.-R. Malagelada

Subject index

Author index